The Neuropsychology of
Mental Illness

The Neuropsychology of Mental Illness

Edited by

Stephen J. Wood
Melbourne Neuropsychiatry Centre and ORYGEN Research Centre, Departments of Psychiatry and Psychology,
The University of Melbourne, Australia

Nicholas B. Allen
Melbourne Neuropsychiatry Centre and ORYGEN Research Centre, Departments of Psychiatry and Psychology,
The University of Melbourne, Australia

Christos Pantelis
Melbourne Neuropsychiatry Centre and ORYGEN Research Centre, Departments of Psychiatry and Psychology,
The University of Melbourne, Australia

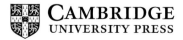

CAMBRIDGE
UNIVERSITY PRESS

CAMBRIDGE UNIVERSITY PRESS
Cambridge, New York, Melbourne, Madrid, Cape Town, Singapore,
São Paulo, Delhi

Cambridge University Press
The Edinburgh Building, Cambridge CB2 8RU, UK

Published in the United States of America by
Cambridge University Press, New York

www.cambridge.org
Information on this title: www.cambridge.org/9780521862899

First published 2009

Printed in the United Kingdom at the University Press, Cambridge

*A catalogue record for this publication is available from the British
Library*

Library of Congress Cataloging-in-Publication Data

The neuropsychology of mental illness / edited by Stephen J. Wood,
Nicholas B. Allen, Christos Pantelis.
     p. ; cm.
   Includes bibliographical references and index.
   ISBN 978-0-521-86289-9 (hardback)
1. Mental illness–Physiological aspects. 2. Mental illness–Psychological
aspects. 3. Neuropsychology. I. Wood, Stephen J. II. Allen, Nicholas B.
III. Pantelis, Christos.
   [DNLM: 1. Mental Disorders–physiopathology. 2. Mental
Disorders–psychology. 3. Neuropsychology. WM 140 N4957 2009]
   RC455.4.B5N477 2009
   616.89–dc22

                                                              2009024545

ISBN 978-0-521-86289-9 Hardback

To our wives for all their support
Amanda, Sabura and Kimberley

Contents

vii

Contents

The color plates are to be found between pages 388 and 389.

Foreword

It is just over 30 years since the publication of the influential article by psychiatrist George Engel (Engel, G. (1977). The need for a new medical model: a challenge for biomedicine. *Science*, **196**, 129–136). The paper was a significant attempt to bridge the gap between psychiatrists and other medical colleagues to enable "psychiatry to become better integrated with medical practice." The result was what has become known as the "biopsychosocial model," almost universally accepted as a way to treat human individuals simultaneously as biological organisms, as psychological beings with subjective feelings and also as members of diverse social groups. Despite this serious attempt to find a unitary home for the previously disassembled humans, the model paradoxically retained an even sharper separation between the biology, the psychology and the social issues of "mental" diseases. The idea that humans exist in two separate worlds, the "physical" and the "mental" still hovers over much of modern medicine and popular philosophy. The spectre of the proverbial Cartesian dualism of a *res extensa*, the world of matter, and the *res cogitans,* the world of the mind, still lives on.

This encyclopedic volume represents a significant contribution to the process of bridging this gap by bringing together workers in many diverse areas, all focusing on the disturbances of mental life, whether caused by genetic, biological or life experiences. The very title "neuropsychology," linking the "mental" to the "neuro," reflects a precise philosophical choice of accepting that the mental world is founded solidly on the neural circuits of the brain. With this aim the editors provide a remarkable resource of modern advances in the field. Yet, reading together the many in-depth chapters paradoxically reinforces the feeling that the desired unity is still somewhat out of reach. Nevertheless this volume will enable readers and the authors themselves to compare notes and decide whether to accelerate the process of unification under a broad neuroscientific perspective or to retain, or even to increase, the distances by insisting on the "independence" of their own field.

The primary importance of the feeling of unity of individuals is the recurrent motif of this comprehensive handbook. This unity is achieved by an ongoing interaction between individuals and the environment, as a whirling dance of the self with the rest of the world, which includes paradoxically the very self.

The simple conceptual framework of the experiential–existential loop that I discuss below may be helpful in providing the means to weave elements for such unity within the extensive collection of diverse articles. This framework is based on our evolutionary past, and is consistent with much of the available scientific literature.

The evolution of the brain probably started from a primordial set of functional loops made of (1) sensory neurons, which encode changes of various physical energies into neural signals, (2) integrating neurons and (3) motor neurons that transform neural activity into mechanical energy. Survival required this primordial sensorimotor loop to be dynamically adapted to the imperatives of detecting, evaluating and selecting amongst the actions to ensure food, water, shelter and defense, and reproduction. The already complex loop for immediate actions and reactions, limited nevertheless the primordial horizon of existence to the present. Evolution has been accompanied by the appearance of increasingly longer, superimposed neural loops that form our brain. With the increased complexity of such a hierarchical neural system, organisms like us, in addition to living in the present, acquired the ability to project their fictitious experiences both in the past, as memory and in the future, as expectations and imagination. Indirect experiences of the past and the future could be successfully integrated with the immediate experiences of the present. Horizons of existence beyond the present thereby become unlimited.

At every new level of superimposed neural loops, corresponding to broader horizons, adaptive processes are still required for detection, evaluation and decision for action. At the higher levels neural circuits for perception, emotions and decision-making become the corresponding loops for survival in the extended horizons.

Increased awareness of the environment, of one's body and of one's intentions via the internal "corollary discharges," evolved in parallel. Awareness of other similar beings also developed in parallel, with "mirror neuron systems" playing critical roles. Humans are the result of the evolutionary accretion of these superimposed loops adapted to extend "horizons" in time and space and yet also adapted to the present. The unified self is the result of a crafted construction that goes on throughout life.

The balance between "voluntary" top-down influences, interacting with internal standards based on prior experiences, and sensory-driven bottom-up influences reflect the need to apportion actions to the present or delaying many for the future. This perhaps is the origin of the sense of freedom.

The task to maintain an integrated unity in the face of many choices for action available within the extended horizon is an ongoing challenge for each person. It is not surprising that such a delicate dynamic balance to avoid any mismatch between what is experienced subjectively and what is "out there" is not always achieved. Indeed, new emerging levels that are usually acquired originally with awareness, become more automatic, moving below the horizon of consciousness and are thus not easily corrected. The gradual automatization of the lower loops probably generates the inner feeling that top-down "voluntary" influences are effortful, while bottom-up influences are effortless. Was this the origin of the clash between will and flesh? Between spirit and matter?

The increased dependence from frontal lobe circuits for delaying and inhibiting actions are revealed in the very syndromes of frontal disinhibition and various types of acquired sociopathy, perhaps evolutionary prices to pay for the flexibility of goal-directed behaviour in an ever-changing environment.

Many of the difficulties confronting neuropsychology in deciding what are the more fundamental levels of interplay of the organisms with the world can be brought back to the complexity of multiple superimposed loops. The concepts of bottom-up and top-down within these loops begin to make sense of otherwise incomprehensible observations in clinical and experimental neuropsychology.

For example, perception disorders, thought disorders and disorders of executive function may simply represent disturbances of the higher levels of the experiential–existential loop, which still requires detection, evaluation and action selection.

The terms appearing across this volume such as "underlie," "cause," "entail," "mechanisms," used to refer to the relationship between states of the brain and states of mind, reflect the philosophical uncertainties about the nature of such a relationship. Despite serious attempts of philosophers to live with the consequences of the Cartesian dualism, the mind irreducible to the biology of the brain, most contributors of this handbook provide convincing evidence that mental states are always accompanied by more or less subtle bodily states and vice versa. Hence, the sensible search for new markers, signs and symptoms of mental disorders.

What about principles of intervention for mental disorders? There is an apparent incompatibility between the choice of intervening either on the fundamental biological pathology of the brain or on the life experiences and human interactions that appear to have generated the disorders. This alternative has divided generations of professionals involved in mental and neurological disorders. Yet the framework of multiple levels of existential loops may help to overcome the apparent incompatibility of views. A pharmacological agent or a genetic disorder affecting some aspect of synaptic transmission are bound to have effects on the state of the entire system of superimposed loops. Similarly, words (psychological therapies) will modify the state of higher loops, and thus the synaptic transmission in these. This reciprocal interdependence of the biological on the psychological (and social) is the unavoidable consequence of the functional architecture of the hierarchical system of existential loops.

The brain, core of such loops, is a single biological organ evolved for the adaptation of bodily functions, social interactions and awareness of the world and the self (consciousness).

The editors should be commended for providing a path for the difficult, but not impossible, process of bringing human existence under a single perspective.

Marcello Costa, FAA
Professor of Neurophysiology

Marcello Costa, is a Fellow of the Australian Academy of Science (FAA) and Professor of Neurophysiology at Flinders University in Adelaide, South Australia. He was educated in Argentina and Italy where he obtained his medical degree before moving to Australia. He has been involved in research and teaching neuroscience for over 40 years. He was one of the founders of the Australian Neuroscience Society, becoming its President for a term in the 1990s. He has increasingly become interested in the broader issues of how to navigate across the many neural domains, while maintaining scientific rigor and without trivializing the problems inherent in such cross-disciplinary dialogue.

Preface

A neuropsychological approach to understanding various mental disorders has flourished over the last two decades, and particularly over the decade or so since the publication of a book on the neuropsychology of schizophrenia by one of us (Pantelis *et al.*, 1996). Since then, the field has evolved and matured tremendously, with an exponential rise in the number of publications in this area. While the largest body of work has been in schizophrenia, the methods and approaches of neuropsychology have begun to inform our understanding of all psychiatric disorders. Neuropsychology has been of particular importance in helping to unravel the mechanisms underlying brain function, and has helped us to understand the impact of treatments on various abilities and their relevance to functional outcome in psychiatric disorders. Indeed, our motivation to produce this book evolved from our growing interest in a neuropsychological approach *across* such disorders, and to inform the interface of neuropsychology with other neurobiological approaches, such as neuroimaging and genetics. We have brought together some of the world's leading experts in the field to discuss approaches, conditions and future directions.

The book is divided into a number of sections, including an introductory section that lays out the rationale for examining neuropsychological processes within clinical disorders. The study of these processes provides a complementary approach to diagnostically oriented approaches to neuropsychological dysfunction. Given that dysfunction in some processes is common across disorders, this approach has the potential to offer new insights into etiology and diagnosis. In the second section various experts summarize and critique the methodological approaches used in the study of neuropsychological processes within mental illness, and discuss future directions and innovations, including the use of sophisticated analysis methods to complement traditional approaches in order to address unique questions. Section 3 covers each of the major disorders, and is particularly interesting in providing a "state of the art" summary of neuropsychological findings for each condition. The final section considers whether the neuropsychology of consciousness is an appropriate integrative rubric under which to conceptualize these disorders, and represents a "trialogue" between neuroscientists, psychiatrists and philosophers. This section is unique in that the contributors of each chapter offer a commentary on the other chapters on this theme.

We hope that this book will be valuable to all who are interested in studying the healthy as well as the disordered brain, not only those from the fields of psychology, neuroscience, psychiatry and philosophy, but also all who have an interest in understanding how our brains work.

The editors thank all the authors who have contributed to this volume. Special thanks to Renée Testa for helping with proofing the various chapters, and to Barbara Stachlewski for her assistance in the final stages of the book.

Reference

Pantelis, C., Nelson, H. E. & Barnes, T. R. E. (1996). *Schizophrenia: A Neuropsychological Perspective.* London: John Wiley.

Contributors

Nicholas B. Allen
ORYGEN Youth Health Research Centre and
Department of Psychology
University of Melbourne
Parkville, VIC, Australia

Stephanie Assuras
Department of Psychology
Queens College and The Graduate Center
of the City University of New York
Flushing, NY, USA

Robert M. Bilder
Jane and Terry Semel Institute for Neuroscience
and Human Behavior, Lynda and Stewart
Resnick Neuropsychiatric Hospital
David Geffen School of Medicine at UCLA
Los Angeles, CA, USA

Joan C. Borod
Department of Psychology
Queens College and The Graduate Center of the City
University of New York
Flushing, NY, USA, & Department of Neurology
Mount Sinai School of Medicine
New York, NY, USA

John L. Bradshaw
School of Psychology Psychiatry and Psychological
Medicine
Monash University
Clayton, VIC
Australia

Warrick J. Brewer
ORYGEN Youth Health Research Centre
The University of Melbourne
Parkville, VIC
Australia

Ariel Brown
Clinical and Research Programs in Pediatric
Psychopharmacology and Adult ADHD
Massachusetts General Hospital
Boston, MA, USA

Nik Brown
Department of Computer Science
University of Calfornia at Los Angeles
Los Angeles, CA, USA

Tyrone Cannon
Jane and Terry Semel Institute for Neuroscience and
Human Behavior
Department of Psychology
David Geffen School of Medicine at UCLA
Los Angeles, CA, USA

Audrey Carstensen
Brain Research Institute
David Geffen School of Medicine at UCLA
Los Angeles, CA, USA

Cameron S. Carter
Departments of Psychiatry and Psychology
University of California, Davis
UC Davis Imaging Research Center
Sacramento, CA, USA

Luke Clark
Department of Experimental Psychology
University of Cambridge
Cambridge, UK

Phyllis Chua
School of Psychology, Psychiatry and Psychological
Medicine
Monash University
Clayton, VIC
Australia

Thilo Deckersbach
Department of Psychiatry
Massachusetts General Hospital/Harvard Medical
School
Charlestown, MA, USA

Richard A. Depue
Laboratory of Neurobiology of Personality
Department of Human Development
Cornell University
Ithaca, NY, USA

Tali Ditman
Department of Psychology,
Tufts University &
Department of Psychiatry
Massachusetts General Hospital
Boston, MA, USA

Aleksey Dumer
Department of Psychology
Queens College and The Graduate Center of the City
University of New York
Flushing, NY, USA

David E. Fleck
Department of Psychiatry
University of Cincinnati
Cincinnati, OH, USA

Lara Foland-Ross
Laboratory of Neuroimaging
Brain Research Institute
David Geffen School of Medicine at UCLA
Los Angeles, CA, USA

Judith M. Ford
Department of Psychiatry
University of California, San Francisco
San Francisco, CA, USA

Nelson Freimer
Center for Neurobehavioral Genetics
Jane and Terry Semel Institute for Neuroscience and
Human Behavior
David Geffen School of Medicine at UCLA
Los Angeles, CA, USA

Paolo Fusar-Poli
Neuroimaging Section
King's College London Institute of Psychiatry

De Crespigny Park
London, UK

Nathan A. Gates
Department of Psychology
Queens College and The Graduate Center of the City
University of New York
Flushing, NY, USA

Terry E. Goldberg
Psychiatry Research
Zucker Hillside Hospital
Glen Oaks, NY
Albert Einstein College of Medicine
New York City, NY, USA

George Graham
Department of Philosophy
Georgia State University
Atlanta, GA, USA

Igor Grant
Department of Psychiatry
University of California, San Diego
La Jolla, CA, USA

Melissa J. Green
School of Psychiatry
University of New South Wales & Black Dog Institute
Prince of Wales Hospital
Randwick, NSW
Australia

Michelle M. Halfacre
Department of Psychology
Queens College and The Graduate Center of the City
University of New York
Flushing, NY, USA

Wendy Heller
Psychology Department and Beckman Insititute for
Advance Science and Technology
University of Illinois at Urbana-Champaign
Champaign, IL, USA

John D. Herrington
University of Illinois at Urbana-Champaign
Urbana, IL, USA

Garry D. Honey
University of Cambridge
Department of Psychiatry

Brain Mapping Unit
Cambridge, UK

Jennifer E. Iudicello
Joint Doctoral Program in Clinical Psychology
San Diego State University
University of California, San Diego
San Diego, CA, USA

Henry J. Jackson
Department of Psychology
University of Melbourne
Parkville, VIC
Australia

J. David Jentsch
Department of Psychology
University of California, Los Angeles
Los Angeles, CA, USA

Donald Kalar
Department of Psychology
David Geffen School of Medicine at UCLA
Los Angeles, CA, USA

Paul Keedwell
Department of Psychological Medicine
Cardiff University Hospital
Cardiff, Wales, UK

Ester Klimkeit
Monash University Centre for Developmental
Psychiatry and Psychology
Monash Medical Centre
Clayton, VIC
Australia

Nancy S. Koven
Department of Psychology
Bates College
Lewiston, ME, USA

Donna A. Kreher
Department of Psychology
Tufts University
Medford, MA, USA

Gina R. Kuperberg
Department of Psychiatry, Mass. General Hospital
and Athinoula A. Martinos Center of Biomedical
Imaging, & Department of Psychology,

Tufts University
Boston, MA, USA

Edythe London
Jane and Terry Semel Institute for Neuroscience and
Human Behavior
Department of Pharmacology
David Geffen School of Medicine at UCLA
Los Angeles, CA, USA

Dan I. Lubman
ORYGEN Research Centre
The University of Melbourne
Parkville, VIC
Australia

Daniel H. Mathalon
Department of Psychiatry
University of California, San Francisco
San Francisco, CA, USA

Patrick D. McGorry
ORYGEN Research Centre
The University of Melbourne
Parkville, VIC
Australia

Philip McGuire
Neuroimaging Section
King's College London Institute of Psychiatry
De Crespigny Park
London, UK

George R. Mangun
Center for Mind and Brain
Departments of Psychology and Neurology
University of California, Davis
Davis, CA USA

Gregory A. Miller
University of Illinois at Urbana-Champaign
Urbana, IL, USA

Albert Newen
Department of Philosophy
University of Tuebingen
Germany

Jack B. Nitschke
Departments of Psychiatry and Psychology
University of Wisconsin at Madison
Madison, WI, USA

xvii

Jaak Panksepp
Department of VCAPP
College of Veterinary Medicine
Washington State University
Pullman, WA, USA

Christos Pantelis
Melbourne Neuropsychiatry Centre
The University of Melbourne & Melbourne Health
National Neuroscience Facility (NNF)
Carlton South, VIC
Australia

Mary Philips
Director of Functional Neuroimaging Program
Department of Clinical Psychiatry
Western Psychiatric Institute
University of Pittsburgh Medical Centre
Pittsburgh, PA, USA

Russell A. Poldrack
Departments of Psychology and Psychiatry &
Biobehavioral Sciences UCLA
Los Angeles, CA, USA

Scott L. Rauch
Psychiatry for Neuroscience Research
Massachusetts General Hospital/Harvard Medical School
Charlestown, MA, USA

Susan M. Ravizza
Department of Psychology
Michigan State University
East Lansing, MI, USA

Steven Paul Reise
Department of Psychology
Franz Hall, UCLA
Los Angeles, CA, USA

Nicole Rinehart
Center for Developmental Psychology and Psychiatry
School of Psychology Psychiatry and Psychological
Medicine
Monash University
Nottinghill, VIC
Australia

Angela Rizk-Jackson
Brain Research Institute
David Geffen School of Medicine at UCLA
Los Angeles, CA, USA

Trevor W. Robbins
Department of Experimental Psychology
University of Cambridge
Cambridge, UK

Tamara A. Russell
Macquarie Centre for Cognitive Science
Macquarie University
North Ryde, NSW
Australia

Fred W. Sabb
Jane and Terry Semel Institute for Neuroscience and
Human Behavior
Department of Psychology
David Geffen School of Medicine at UCLA
Los Angeles, CA, USA

Cary R. Savage
Hoglund Brain Imaging Center
Department of Psychiatry and Behavioral Sciences
Kansas University Medical Center
Kansas City, KS, USA

Kimberley R. Savage
Department of Psychology
Queens College and The Graduate Center of the City
University of New York
Flushing, NY, USA

J. Cobb Scott
Joint Doctoral Program in Clinical Psychology
San Diego State University
University of California, San Diego
San Diego, CA, USA

Marc L. Seal
Melbourne Neuropsychiatry Centre
The University of Melbourne & Melbourne Health
National Neuroscience Facility (NNF)
Carlton South, VIC, Australia

Larry J. Seidman
Harvard Medical School Departments of
Psychiatry at Beth Israel Deaconess Medical
Center and Massachusetts General Hospital
Boston, MA, USA

Paula K. Shear
Department of Psychology
University of Cincinnati
Cincinnati, OH, USA

Marisa M. Silveri
Cognitive Neuroimaging Laboratory
McLean Brain Imaging Center
Belmont, MA, USA

Nadia Solowij
School of Psychology
University of Wollongong
Wollongong, NSW, Australia and,
Schizophrenia Research Institute
Sydney, NSW, Australia

Laura Southgate
Section of Eating Disorders
Psychological Medicine
King's College London Institute of Psychiatry
De Crespigny Park
London, UK

G. Lynn Stephens
Department of Philosophy
University of Alabama at Birmingham
Birmingham, AL, US

D. Stott Parker
Department of Computer Science
University of Calfornia at Los Angeles
Los Angeles, CA, USA

Stephen M. Strakowski
Department of Psychiatry
Center for Imaging Research
University of Cincinnati College of Medicine
Cincinnati, OH, USA

Simon A. Surguladze
Division of Psychological Medicine & Psychiatry
King's College London Institute of Psychiatry
De Crespigny Park
London, UK

Kate Tchanturia
Section of Eating Disorders
Psychological Medicine
King's College London Institute of Psychiatry
London, UK

René Testa
Melbourne Neuropsychiatry Centre
University of Melbourne and Melbourne Health

National Neuroscience Facility
Carlton South, VIC
Australia, and
Monash University
School of Psychology, Psychiatry and
Psychological Medicine
Clayton, VIC, Australia
Sunshine Hospital
St Albans, VIC, Australia

Janet Treasure
Department of Academic Psychiatry
Guy's Hospital
King's College London Institute of Psychiatry
London, UK

Eve M. Valera
Clinical and Research Programs in Pediatric
Psychopharmacology and in Psychiatric
Neuroscience
Department of Psychiatry
Massachusetts General Hospital\Harvard Medical
School
Charlestown, MA, USA

Kai Vogeley
Department of Psychiatry
University of Cologne
Cologne, Germany

Anthony P. Weiss
Department of Psychiatry
Massachusetts General Hospital and Harvard Medical
School
Boston, MA, USA

Sarah Whittle
ORYGEN Research Centre & Melbourne
Neuropsychiatry Centre
The University of Melbourne
VIC, Australia

Stephen J. Wood
Melbourne Neuropsychiatry Centre
The University of Melbourne & Melbourne Health
National Neuroscience Facility (NNF)
Carlton South, VIC
Australia

xix

Steven Paul Woods
Department of Psychiatry
University of California, San Diego
La Jolla, CA, USA

Murat Yücel
ORYGEN Research Centre & Melbourne
Neuropsychiatry Centre

The University of Melbourne and Melbourne Health
Parkville, VIC
Australia

Deborah A. Yurgelun-Todd
Brain Institute
University of Utah
Salt Lake City, UT, USA

Neuropsychological processes

Why examine neuropsychological processes in mental illness?

In the first section of this volume we have included a series of chapters that examine the neuropsychological mechanisms that underlie a range of basic psychological processes with relevance to understanding mental illness. There are a number of reasons for beginning the volume in this way. First, many neuropsychological processes are more amenable to objective measurement than the core symptoms of mental disorder (which often rely on self report for their "gold-standard" measurement through diagnostic interviews – see Jackson and McGorry, Chapter 12, this volume). As such, neuropsychological evaluation of basic psychological functions may ultimately be used to aid diagnosis, especially in cases where self report is impaired.

Furthermore, although still far from complete, the brain bases for many neuropsychological functions have been established to some degree. In contrast, our understanding of the neural correlates of psychiatric symptoms is much more hazy. Studying neuropsychological processes may help our understanding of which brain regions are involved, and when they first show dysfunction. Consistent with this is the observation that although genetic risk factors for mental illness are well established (McGuffin *et al.*, 2002), many scientists conjecture that the relationship between genetic vulnerability and disease phenotypes will be clarified if intermediate phenotypes or endophenotypes are also included in models (Beauchaine *et al.*, 2008; Meyer-Lindberg & Weinberger, 2006). Because these intermediate markers fall along the causal chain between the distal genotype and disease they are likely to be more strongly associated with both the disease phenotype and the genotype than these latter variables will be with each other (Gottesman & Gould, 2003). As such, the examination of intermediate phenotypes and endophenotypes can be critical in both identifying the specific alleles associated with risk for psychopathology, and also in developing a mechanistic understanding of the particular neurobiological and behavioral expressions of the genotype that are proximally involved in the transition for risk to disorder. The neuropsychological processes examined here constitute an important set of such potential intermediate phenotypes (Abbott, 2008).

Furthermore, although the diagnostic system treats disorders as categorical entities, most disorders do not satisfy strict taxometric criteria for classes (Haslam, 2003). In other words, in many cases we are imposing a categorical distinction where none exists in nature. Associated with this issue are the facts that comorbidity between diagnoses is common (Jacobi *et al.*, 2004; Kessler *et al.*, 2005), and that similar symptoms are often observed across different disorders (Krueger, 1999). Examining basic neuropsychological process in mental disorder may therefore help to clarify the nature of the distinction between disordered and non-disordered states in a more principled way, and also may help to explain the patterns of comorbidity between diagnostic entities.

Finally, many analyses of the definition of mental disorder have emphasized that understanding the nature of disordered psychological and neuropsychological function is critical to the distinction between disordered and non-disordered states. For example Wakefield's "Harmful Dysfunction" analysis of mental disorder (Wakefield, 1999) proposes that mental disorder must have two properties. "Harmful" refers to the fact that the features of the disorder cause significant harm to a person under present cultural circumstances. This first criterion is therefore partially defined by the current social and cultural context. However, in order to qualify as a true mental disorder the condition must also result from the inability of some internal mental mechanism to perform its "natural function." In this context "natural function" is defined as the ability of that mechanism to perform the task for which the mechanism was "designed" by evolution. In other words, one strong implication of this analysis is that one must begin with an understanding of the natural (or evolutionarily designated) neuropsychological *functions* of the brain, before neuropsychological *dysfunction* (and therefore mental disorder itself), can be defined.

With these considerations in mind, we felt that it was appropriate to begin the volume by surveying the neuropsychology of a range of basic process that are implicated in mental disorder. The section begins with a chapter by Silveri and Yurgelun-Todd on the role of developmental processes. They conclude that neuropsychological evaluation of children and adolescents can reveal important changes in cognitive function that may relate to later onset of psychopathology, and note the important role that risk status and age must have in interpreting such evaluations. They note the importance of differentiating between the normal trajectory of cognitive development, delayed achievement of developmental milestones and cognitive deficits associated with risk for psychiatric illness.

This chapter is followed by contributions addressing sensory and perceptual processes (by Klimkeit and Bradshaw). They note that while anomalies of perceptual processes are good models that partly explain higher-level neuropsychiatric dysfunction, the link between perception and action will ultimately be critical to our understanding of the neuropsychological basis of psychiatric disorder. Accordingly, motor executive processes are reviewed by Rinehart, Chua and Bradshaw. The potential etiological relevance of neuromotor dysfunction has long been noted in a number of psychiatric disorders, especially autism and schizophrenia. However, developments in our understanding of the connectivity between the prefrontal cortex, basal ganglia and cerebellum has resulted in renewed interest in the application of neuromotor assessment in psychiatry. Rinehart and colleagues particularly note advances in our understanding of higher-order awareness and control of "action," mirror neurons, the concept of affordances, utilization behavior and extreme neurological motor conditions such as the anarchic hand, and explore what these findings may have to offer our understanding of mental illness.

Whittle, Yücel and Allen provide an overview of neurobiological models of emotion, with an emphasis on the specific neuropsychological systems involved in the perception of emotional stimuli, the experience of emotion, and its regulation. Herrington, Koven, Heller, Miller and Nitschke then examine the links between emotion, personality and psychopathology, with a specific emphasis on the role of asymmetry of brain function in these processes. They note the benefit of integrating multiple theoretical perspectives from personality psychology with theories regarding the frontal lateralization of emotion. They conclude that determining which psychological construct best explains lateralization in the frontal lobes may depend on which area of the frontal cortex is being examined. They suggest that hemodynamic imaging will be an invaluable tool for addressing these questions, and explore the appropriate data analytic techniques.

The role of language is explored by Kuperberg, Ditman, Kreher and Goldberg, and they show how paradigms at various levels of language including words, sentences, and discourse, can be used to study neuropsychiatric disorders. They provide a broad theoretical framework to help understand the relationships between these levels of dysfunction and to help guide future theoretically motivated studies of language, particularly in schizophrenia. Seal and Weiss examine associative memory and note several challenges exist for associative memory research in mental illness. One is to make more extensive use of memory research in the neuropsychology of non-psychotic disorder such as depression and obsessive-compulsive disorder. Increasing the sensitivity and specificity of associative memory tasks to both cognitive processes and brain regions is also an important challenge. They also note that exploring the molecular and genetic mechanisms that underlie memory dysfunction in mental illness is a critical priority for future research.

Attentional control and selection is addressed by Ravizza, Mangun and Carter. They note that the ability to control attention involves the interaction of specific cortical and subcortical neural networks influencing multiple stages of information processing. They conclude that to elucidate the neural mechanisms of attention, and its abnormalities in mental illness, it is essential to investigate and characterize attentional processes at a variety of levels of information processing. Likewise, Testa and Pantelis note that although the evidence of a fractionated executive system in mental illness is strong, the use of different executive tests to assess unique cognitive functions is an important challenge for future research in the area.

Clark and Robbins then explore the neuropsychology of decision-making, particularly implicating prefrontal cortical pathology in the decision-making deficits observed in mental illness. Once again, they note that developing assessment methods that isolate the various subcomponents of these neuropsychological functions is a significant challenge, albeit one upon which significant progress is being made. Finally, Russell and Green examine the neuropsychology of social cognition. Given the prominence of social dysfunction in those suffering from mental illness, understanding the neural networks subserving social cognition may prove to be particularly important for identifying the neuropathology of major psychiatric disorders, and is likely to be pertinent to the formulation of effective treatments for social cognitive disturbances in these individuals. They also address the critical question of domain specificity with respect to social cognitive processes and conclude that while neuropsychological studies suggest that social cognition cannot be fully accounted for by domain-general processes (such as attention, memory or executive function), this does not warrant an overarching conclusion that social cognition is completely independent of domain-specific processes.

In sum, this collection of chapters provides the reader with a series of up-to-date reviews of the neuropsychology of basic psychological functions as they pertain to mental illness. Critically, they also clearly lay out the future research agenda that must be addressed in order for examination of these processes to continue to advance our understanding of mental illness.

References

Abbott, A. (2008). The brains of the family. *Nature*, **454**, 154–157.

Beauchaine, T. P., Hinshaw, S. P. & Gatzke-Kopp, L. (2008). Genetic and environmental influences on behavior. In T. P. Beauchaine & S. P. Hinshaw (Eds.), *Child and Adolescent Psychopathology* (pp. 58–90). Hoboken, NJ: John Wiley & Sons.

Gottesman, I. I. & Gould, T. D. (2003). The endophenotype concept in psychiatry: etymology and strategic intentions. *American Journal of Psychiatry*, **160**, 636–645.

Haslam, N. (2003). Categorical versus dimensional models of mental disorder: the taxometric evidence. *Australian and New Zealand Journal of Psychiatry*, **37**(6), 696–704.

Jacobi, F., Wittchen, H. U., HöLting, C. *et al.* (2004). Prevalence, co-morbidity and correlates of mental disorders in the general population: results from the German Health Interview and Examination Survey (GHS). *Psychological Medicine*, **34**(4), 597–611.

Kessler, R. C., Berglund, P., Demler, O. *et al.* (2005). Lifetime prevalence and age-of-onset distributions of DSM–IV disorders in the National Comorbidity Survey Replication. *Archives of General Psychiatry*, **62**(6), 593.

Krueger, R. F. (1999). The structure of common mental disorders. *Archives of General Psychiatry*, **56**(10), 929–931.

McGuffin, P., Owen, M. J. & Gottesman, II. (2002). *Psychiatric Genetics and Genomics*. New York, NY: Oxford University Press.

Meyer-Lindenberg, A. & Weinberger, D. R. (2006). Intermediate phenotypes and genetic mechanisms of psychiatric disorders. *Nature Review Neuroscience*, **7**(10), 818–827.

Wakefield, J. C. (1999). Evolutionary versus prototype analyses of the concept of disorder. *Journal of Abnormal Psychology*, **108**(3), 374–399.

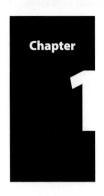

Developmental neuropsychology: normative trajectories and risk for psychiatric illness

Marisa M. Silveri and Deborah A. Yurgelun-Todd

Introduction

Examination of neuropsychological functioning, both in healthy populations and in individuals with brain injury, has provided important information with regard to lateralization of cognitive function, sex differences in neuropsychological performance, functional differences associated with disconnection syndromes, and cognitive capacity at various developmental stages. Studies of neuropsychological performance conducted at different maturational levels have helped identify abnormalities associated with childhood disorders, including chromosomal and genetic disorders, structural abnormalities, prematurity and low birth weight, infections, toxic damage, nutritional disorders, anoxic disorders, traumatic brain injury, focal neurological disorders, convulsive disorders, hemispherectomy and other effects of surgical manipulations (Spreen et al., 1995b). The utility of neuropsychological assessment in children and adolescents with neuropathologic conditions is not only to provide information regarding their progress in achieving normative developmental milestones but also to provide a framework for the identification of brain dysfunction and for the development of remediation strategies.

Significant development of the central and peripheral nervous systems occurs throughout early life, with major alterations being observed from infancy to adolescence (for review, see Huttenlocher, 1994). These rapidly evolving systems include the sensory systems (auditory, visual, chemical senses, somesthetic), motor systems (pyramidal and extrapyramidal) and integrative higher-order systems (association areas, reticular formation and brainstem chemical pathways, language areas) (Spreen et al., 1995a). Both structural and functional changes in these systems

permit the rapid improvements in cognitive abilities observed from infancy through late adolescence.

To date a large body of research has focused not only on structural brain development, but also on the maturation of individual neuropsychological domains and the process by which these domains become integrated during development (Webb et al., 2001). It is known that both genetic and experiential factors play a role in how brain networks develop (Nelson, 2000; Williamson et al., 2003). Furthermore, brain maturation and cognitive function have been shown to be sensitive to the timing of both toxic exposure and environmental experience (see Knudsen, 2004; Thompson & O'Quinn, 1979). This dynamic process of brain maturation therefore raises special challenges for the neuropsychological evaluation of children and adolescents.

Neuropsychological domains

Neuropsychological assessment is aimed at measuring cognitive-intellectual ability. Cognition is the process of knowing or thinking, and in childhood age-related changes in cognition occur, including quantitative increments in cognitive ability. Early researchers considered cognitive processing capacity as a unitary measure, however this approach proved limited, since deficits may be found in a specific cognitive area while performance in other cognitive functional areas remains essentially intact (Lezak, 1995). This led clinicians and researchers to focus on the assessment of separate functional domains. In general, these domains include attention, memory, executive function, language, visuospatial function, and processing speed, which are described in greater detail below.

The Neuropsychology of Mental Illness, ed. Stephen J. Wood, Nicholas B. Allen and Christos Pantelis. Published by Cambridge University Press. © Cambridge University Press 2009.

Attention

Attention encompasses a number of functions, including four different commonly reported components: divided attention, the ability to perform two tasks simultaneously; sustained attention, the ability to maintain attention over an extended time; selective attention, the ability to filter out irrelevant information to focus on the task attention; and attentional switching, the ability to switch between attention sets. Attentional capacity can vary significantly depending on mood state and level of arousal, as well as maturational level. The neural substrate for attention is thought to lie within a complex set of networks including the frontal cortex, the posterior parietal cortex and the reticular formation (Stuss & Benson, 1984).

Memory

Memory is an active process that records information from the past so that it may be used in the present. It involves a number of processes including encoding, storage and retrieval. Memory deficits are most often due to retrieval and encoding problems rather than limitations in storage capacity. Anatomical regions implicated in memory involve multiple bilateral brain regions, with the hippocampus and the frontal lobes being particularly important. Working memory involves short-term maintenance, sorting and manipulation of new and retrieved information; and is often considered a component of the attentional domain. Brain regions important for working memory include the prefrontal cortex and the inferior parietal lobule (Goethals et al., 2002), as well as the visual association area, the inferior temporal cortices and portions of the cerebellum (Berman et al., 1995).

Visuospatial function

Visuospatial function encompasses the ability to visualize objects in space. Tasks that measure visuospatial function include tests of mental rotation and spatial localization, both of which require intact parietal lobes, particularly in the right hemisphere (Benton, 1985; Heilman & Van Den Abell, 1980). The visual features of an object are processed via a pathway from the occipital to the temporal cortex, called the ventral stream, and the spatial locations are processed via a pathway from the occipital to the parietal cortex, called the dorsal stream (Ungerleider & Mishkin, 1982). Studies have shown that cerebral blood flow increases are significantly higher in the right parietal lobe during rotational tests, and that subjects with lesions in their right parietal lobe perform worse on mental rotation tasks than both normal controls and subjects with lesions in their left parietal lobe (Ditunno & Mann, 1990; Papanicolaou et al., 1987).

Language

Language processes can be divided into three categories, including expressive speech, object naming and language comprehension. Studies involving the electrical stimulation of the brain have implicated three main cortical areas of interest regarding language processes: the anterior language area (Broca's area), the posterior language area (Wernicke's area), and the supplementary language area (the supplementary motor area) (Penfield & Jasper, 1954; Penfield & Perot, 1963; Penfield & Roberts, 1959). Broca's area in the inferior frontal gyrus is largely responsible for language processing and speech production, and Wernicke's area in the superior temporal gyrus is important for speech comprehension (Lezak, 1995). These processes are lateralized to the left hemisphere in most individuals. The posterior-inferior temporal gyrus has been identified as the "naming center" of the brain, and is important for object naming (Penfield & Roberts, 1959).

Speed of processing

Speed of processing typically measures the required time to complete a specific cognitive task (Reitan & Wolfson, 1985; Smith, 1991). Multiple brain regions are involved in this function, although white matter integrity is thought to be particularly important, since the size of axons and the thickness of myelin are predictors of speed of processing (Gao et al., 1999). Changes in white matter that are associated with a reduction in processing speed may also affect performance in other cognitive domains, such as attention and working memory.

Executive function

Executive functions include a broad range of processes involved in implementing goal-oriented behavior. These processes include inhibitory function, mental flexibility and planning. These behaviors are dependent on multiple cortical networks including prefrontal areas and posterior association areas, particularly the dorsolateral prefrontal cortex. Spontaneous flexibility in particular is reliant on the frontal cortex, whereas reactive flexibility requires intact cortical-striatal interconnections (Eslinger & Grattan, 1993).

Age-related increases in cognitive capacity are thought to reflect brain maturational changes. During childhood and adolescence these neurobiological changes are paralleled by greater functional capacity, as well as more efficient synchronization of function between individual cognitive domains. Neuropsychological measures can provide estimates of overall intellectual ability and can assist in the identification of deficits within functional domains. It is this approach that has provided the greatest insights into the neuropsychological changes associated with psychiatric disorders.

Considerations in the assessment of children

It is important that appropriately designed neuropsychological tests are used to evaluate children. Often, adult tests are modified for use with younger populations; however, these may not provide an accurate functional assessment, because children and adolescents may not have fully developed the skills required. Further, tests designed to assess specific adult abilities may not accurately reflect the same cognitive features in children. Age-appropriate tests are clearly required to accurately assess the cognitive skills of children and adolescents, in order to consider the varying abilities associated with different developmental stages.

There are additional challenges involved in pediatric neuropsychological assessments, including the need to be aware of and account for several factors that can affect the test performance of children in different age groups. These include attentional capacity, including distractibility, as well as the level of social skill of the child. Issues related to mood, including stress and anxiety, are also important considerations when interpreting performance data, given the fear associated with separation from a parental figure, new locations and/or testing situations.

Developmental neuropsychology milestones

Cognition during infancy is largely observed as information processing. These maturing processes include the development of attention, learning and inhibitory function. Bornstein *et al.* (2006) conducted a large-

scale study to measure information processing, as indexed by habituation to novel stimuli, in children examined at 4, 6, 18, 24 and 49 months of age. Habituation efficiency observed at 4 months was shown to predict performance observed on the Denver Developmental Screening Test (6 months), the Mental Development Scale (18 months), the British English MacArthur Communicative Developmental Inventory (24 months) and the Wechsler Preschool and Primary Scale of Intelligence Revised (49 months). The authors concluded that subtle differences during the development of a cascade of age-appropriate achievements could influence later academic success.

Significant improvements in cognitive processing speed and intellectual functioning have been shown to continue into childhood and adolescence, with the most dramatic improvements occurring in the development of executive functions including abstract thought, organization, decision-making and planning, and response inhibition (Anderson, 2001; Klenberg *et al.*, 2001; Rosso *et al.*, 2004; Williams *et al.*, 1999). Recent neuroimaging studies have provided evidence for changes in brain structure and function being commensurate with improvements in cognitive abilities. For instance, rapid brain re-organization has been shown to include changes in white and gray matter, each of which undergo distinct developmental patterns, with white matter increasing (reflecting myelination) and gray matter decreasing (reflecting synaptic pruning). There is a growing body of evidence demonstrating significant relationships between brain structure and function with cognitive processing speed and performance (Casey *et al.*, 1997; Reiss *et al.*, 1996; Sowell *et al.*, 2001; Yurgelun-Todd *et al.*, 2002). Age-related improvements in higher-order cognitive domains, including executive functions, are thought to be related not only to a marked re-organization of the frontal lobe (Giedd *et al.*, 1999; Pfefferbaum *et al.*, 1994; Sowell *et al.*, 1999, 2001), but also to improved functional white matter connectivity within and between brain regions during adolescence (Giedd *et al.*, 1999; Pfefferbaum *et al.*, 1994).

In summary, rapid improvements in cognitive function are observed from infancy through adolescence, as well as into adulthood. Neuropsychological assessment of a variety of cognitive domains show distinct developmental patterns, with the development of information processing occurring very early in life and more complex, higher-order cognitive abilities, such as abstraction capacity and planning, that come online during adolescence and into adulthood. Thus, examination of normative developmental patterns of cognitive function, as well as delays or impairments in cognition, provide an informative framework for understanding and identifying individual profiles of cognitive performance deficits later in life. In addition, alterations in cognitive abilities observed in the first decades of life may reflect risk factors for the later onset of psychiatric illness.

Neuropsychological deficits: risk for psychiatric illness

As indicated earlier, studying neuropsychological performance in children serves as a valuable strategy for identifying potential risk factors associated with the development of psychiatric illness. Over the past 50 years, a number of studies have been conducted to examine neuropsychological performance in children, with the goal of identifying areas of cognitive function that might be associated with onset of psychiatric illness. In general, three types of research studies have been reported: (1) genetic high risk for psychiatric illness in children of one or both parents with a psychiatric disorder; (2) large-scale longitudinal examination of population birth cohorts; (3) short-term longitudinal examination of male conscripts; and (4) follow-back studies of pre-illness levels of cognitive functioning in adults inflicted with a psychiatric illness. Results from genetic high risk and population birth cohort and conscript studies will be briefly examined and discussed to highlight the approaches used in earlier investigations.

The majority of the genetic high-risk studies conducted during the last 50 years examined children of parents with schizophrenia (for review, see Niemi et al., 2003). Sixteen high-risk studies were conducted between 1952 and 1994, requiring that at least one parent (predominantly the mother) meet criteria for schizophrenia (Niemi et al., 2003). There have been a significant number of additional investigations conducted since 1994, which have examined children and adolescents who are the offspring of schizophrenic parents (e.g. see Byrne et al., 1999; Cornblatt et al., 1999; Cornblatt & Keilp, 1994; Davalos et al., 2004; Goldstein et al., 2000; Sorensen et al., 2006), although only one recent high-risk study examined cognitive performance in offspring of bipolar parents (McDonough-Ryan et al., 2002). The comparison

groups in these studies varied, but included cohorts of children of psychiatrically healthy parents, children of parents with depressive disorder, children of parents with a physical illness, and less frequently, children of parents with manic-depression illness, or bipolar disorder.

Several large-scale cohort studies also have been conducted. These studies have typically followed thousands of participants from childhood into adulthood. Individuals are examined on clinical and cognitive measures at specified intervals, with the objective of identifying variables that may predict later onset of psychosis. As with the high-risk studies, the majority of the cohort studies have been conducted to examine adult onset of schizophrenia (for review see Jones & Tarrant, 2000). These studies include, but are not limited to, the British 1946 birth cohort (Jones et al., 1994; Jones & Done, 1997), the British 1958 National Child Development Study (Done et al., 1994; Jones & Done, 1997), the North Finland 1966 birth cohort (Isohanni et al., 1997; Rantakallio, 1988), the 1949–1950 Swedish Conscript Study (David et al., 1997; Malmberg et al., 1998) and the Israeli Conscript Study (Davidson et al., 1999). While these studies have focused on identifying risk factors associated with schizophrenia, additional data have been reported for risk for affective and bipolar disorders (Done et al., 1994; Isohanni et al., 1997; Jones et al., 1994; Rantakallio, 1988; van Os et al., 1997).

It has been suggested that the paucity of developmental investigations focusing on risk factors for bipolar illness is due to difficulty with diagnostic classification and limited numbers of patients with first-onset bipolar disorder within samples ideal for cohort studies. Thus, most cohort studies utilize a general affective disorder category. Furthermore, it is possible that cognitive risk factors for some forms of bipolar illness, which may have an earlier age of onset than schizophrenia, are difficult to detect against a background of rapidly changing cognitive abilities observed during the first two decades of life. The results of genetic high risk and population cohort studies are discussed below, as they relate to the manifestation of schizophrenia, bipolar disorder and depression. Although not a topic reviewed in this chapter, a number of investigations have also found abnormalities in social and emotional functioning during childhood and adolescence to be associated with heightened risk for the development of schizophrenia (e.g. Done et al.,

1994) and affective disorders (Dworkin *et al.*, 1991, 1994; Gotlib *et al.*, 2005).

Schizophrenia

Risk for schizophrenia has been studied extensively in children of parents with schizophrenia, with such studies examining a wide range of clinical, experimental and cognitive measures.

Genetic high-risk studies have documented abnormalities in intelligence quotient (IQ), attention, executive functioning and verbal memory in high-risk children relative to psychiatrically healthy children or children at risk for affective disorder, although study findings have been inconsistent. For instance, a number of studies have documented lower intelligence quotient (IQ) in high-risk children relative to healthy comparison children (Byrne *et al.*, 1999; Goldstein *et al.*, 2000; Goodman, 1987; Neale *et al.*, 1984; Rieder *et al.*, 1977), while other studies have failed to find such differences (Klein & Salzman, 1984; Lifshitz *et al.*, 1985; Mednick & Schulsinger, 1968; Sameroff *et al.*, 1984; Sohlberg, 1985; Worland & Hesselbrock, 1980; Worland *et al.*, 1982, 1984). Impairments in attention observed in high-risk children relative to comparison children have been observed on some (Cornblatt *et al.*, 1999; Cornblatt & Keilp, 1994; Erlenmeyer-Kimling & Cornblatt, 1992; Erlenmeyer-Kimling *et al.*, 2000; Mirsky, 1988; Nuechterlein, 1984; Schreiber *et al.*, 1992; Weintraub, 1987) but not all neuropsychological measures of attention (Driscoll, 1984). Furthermore, there is evidence that high-risk children demonstrate abnormalities in other functional domains including working memory (Davalos *et al.*, 2004), executive functioning (Byrne *et al.*, 1999), math and spelling (Ayalon & Merom, 1985; Mirsky, 1988), verbal skills (Davalos *et al.*, 2004; Weintraub, 1987), verbal memory (Erlenmeyer-Kimling *et al.*, 2000) and perceptual motor speed (Mirsky, 1988; Sorensen *et al.*, 2006).

Cohort and conscript studies examining risk for the development of schizophrenia have likewise reported evidence for attenuated levels of IQ during development, which was associated with later development of schizophrenia (Cannon *et al.*, 2002; David *et al.*, 1997; Done *et al.*, 1994; Jones *et al.*, 1994; Jones & Done, 1997; Malmberg *et al.*, 1998). Deficits in verbal and non-verbal abilities, as well as mathematical skills and organizational abilities have also been reported in cohorts of children examined prior to

their later manifestation of schizophrenia (Cannon *et al.*, 2002; Davidson *et al.*, 1999; Jones *et al.*, 1994; Jones & Done, 1997).

Cohort studies, given their longitudinal nature, are particularly well suited to characterize developmental neuropsychology milestones and the role of such development on the risk for future psychopathology. For instance, subjects in the British 1946 birth cohort were examined prospectively at 11 time points prior to age 16 (Wadsworth, 1987). Thirty cases of schizophrenia were diagnosed from this birth cohort, with these subjects demonstrating later attainment of developmental milestones during the course of the study (Jones *et al.*, 1994; Jones & Done, 1997). Subjects from the British 1958 National Child Development Study were examined at birth, 7, 11, 16 and 23 years. Twenty-nine subjects from this cohort were later diagnosed with schizophrenia. Manifestation of schizophrenia was associated with pre-schizophrenic reductions in verbal and performance IQ, delayed advancement in mathematics and reading, and lower levels of general knowledge (Done *et al.*, 1994; Jones & Done, 1997). Children and adolescents were examined from ages 7–12 and again in mid-adulthood in the New York High-Risk Project. Verbal memory deficits, gross motor abnormalities and deficits in attention observed early in life predicted 83%, 75% and 58%, respectively, of adult cases of schizophrenia from this sample (Erlenmeyer-Kimling *et al.*, 2000).

Conscript studies may provide more limited information with regard to cognitive risk for psychiatric illness, as individuals who are conscripts are typically males aged 18 or older that are involuntarily enrolled in military service (i.e. "drafted"). Data from conscript studies have likewise found significant relationships between low IQ and manifestation of schizophrenia (David *et al.*, 1997; Davidson *et al.*, 1999; Malmberg *et al.*, 1998). Although these studies similarly offer a longitudinal perspective, changes observed during a younger course of cognitive development may be more informative. For instance, in the 1949–1950 Swedish Conscript Study, males were examined at age 18 and again up to 13 years after the initial assessment (David *et al.*, 1997; Malmberg *et al.*, 1998). In the Israeli Conscript Study, males were first examined at age 16 or 17 and then re-examined between 4 and 10 years after initial assessment (Davidson *et al.*, 1999). Cohort studies, given the younger age period and more repetitive assessments, may therefore be more sensitive in characterizing developmental abnormalities associated with risk for psychiatric illness. Nevertheless, findings from conscript studies suggest that estimates of less efficient intellectual functioning were associated with a broad category of psychotic disorders. It is important to note, however, that high-risk studies typically have documented more marked abnormalities across a greater number of cognitive domains (as opposed to IQ alone) than cohort and conscript studies, underscoring the influential roles of both genetics and environmental factors on manifestation of psychiatric illness.

In summary, high-risk, cohort and conscript studies of children have indicated that attenuated maturational increases in IQ as well as deficits in several cognitive domains may be associated with later development of the disorder. Diminished psychomotor function, delayed achievement of developmental milestones, and attention deficits are all cognitive domain abnormalities that have been associated with increased risk of developing schizophrenia.

Bipolar and depressive illness

The majority of studies of individuals at risk for bipolar disorder have been conducted during adulthood rather than during childhood or adolescence (Ferrier et al., 2004; Gourovitch et al., 1999; Keri et al., 2001; Zalla et al., 2004). Cognitive changes have not been consistently reported in adult high-risk populations (Kremen et al., 1998), as several adult studies have documented cognitive deficits in psychiatrically healthy relatives of people with schizophrenia but not in relatives of bipolar patients (Clark et al., 2005; Gilvarry et al., 2000; MacQueen et al., 2004; Schubert & McNeil, 2005). However, a number of studies examining neuropsychological functions in adult unaffected relatives of bipolar patients have reported poorer performances (Gourovitch et al., 1999; Sobczak et al., 2003; Zalla et al., 2004). These investigators suggest that deficits in verbal memory, attention and psychomotor function may be associated with risk for bipolar disorder. There is a paucity, however, of child and adolescent genetic high-risk (Decina et al., 1983; Kestenbaum, 1979; McDonough-Ryan et al., 2002; Worland & Hesselbrock, 1980) or cohort studies (Isohanni et al., 1997; Rantakallio, 1969), and there are no conscript studies that are aimed at examining developmental cognitive deficits associated with bipolar illness.

There is evidence for a relative impairment on measures of performance ability (PIQ) versus verbal abilities (VIQ) in high-risk children compared with psychiatrically healthy controls (Decina et al., 1983; Kestenbaum, 1979; McDonough-Ryan et al., 2002). However, not all high-risk studies have found this deficit; Worland & Hesselbrock (1980) reported that VIQ, PIQ and general IQ did not differ between the offspring of manic depressives and non-psychiatric control children. Interestingly, of the 6 offspring of parents with manic depression and the 17 offspring of parents with unipolar depression, the offspring of manic-depressive parents demonstrated lower VIQ than offspring of parents with unipolar depression. There was also evidence from a high-risk sample of delayed achievement of cognitive milestones in individuals from the North Finland 1966 birth cohort, however, no distinction was found between subjects who developed either schizophrenia or bipolar illness (Isohanni et al., 1997; Rantakallio, 1988). There have also been no significant differences in overall IQ found between children of bipolar parents and children of non-psychiatric parents (Grigoroiu-Serbanescu et al., 1989; Todd et al., 1994).

Surprisingly, there also are limited high-risk investigations that specifically focus on the role of neuropsychological deficits associated with major depressive disorder. Often, children of parents with depression are included as comparison subjects in studies examining children of parents with schizophrenia and bipolar disorder. To this end, the majority of studies that have included children with high-risk for depression have failed to find consistent cognitive impairments relative to healthy controls and offspring of parents with other psychopathologies. For instance, two studies failed to find differences in IQ between groups of children at risk for depression as compared with children of psychiatrically healthy parents (Pellegrini et al., 1986; Weissman et al., 1987). Furthermore, in the 1946 National Survey of Health and Development cohort study, although subtle decrements in educational test scores were associated with onset of affective disorder during adulthood, more pervasive cognitive abnormalities were only observed when the onset of affective disorder occurred during childhood (van Os et al., 1997). Similarly, only small differences on educational tests were found in prodromal children, whereas more marked deficits were observed in pre-schizophrenic children from the 1958 National Child Development Study (Done et al., 1994; Jones & Done, 1997).

In summary, there are relatively few developmental cognitive data that suggest risk for acquiring bipolar disorder. Reduced performance IQ compared with verbal IQ has been associated with increased risk for bipolar disorder, as well as delayed achievement of developmental milestones in children prior to the appearance of both schizophrenia and bipolar disorder. Evidence for cognitive impairments associated with risk for development of major depressive disorder tends to be more subtle, and appears limited to small differences on educational tests, as compared with the more pronounced deficits observed for verbal memory, attention, estimated intellectual capacity (IQ) and other complex cognitive deficits observed in children at risk for schizophrenia and bipolar illness.

Conclusion

Neuropsychological evaluation of children and adolescents can reveal important changes in cognitive function that may relate to later onset of psychopathology. There are several limitations that should be considered when identifying these deficits as potential risk factors for the later manifestation of psychiatric illness. First, data collected from children at high risk should be interpreted cautiously, as there can be increased incidence of prodromal symptoms and presence of other psychopathological traits that could contribute to the observed neuropsychological profile. In addition, children at high risk for psychosis may be exposed to a greater number of environmental stressors as a result of being reared in a household with one or two parents with a diagnosable psychiatric condition. Importantly, the age of assessment must be considered when examining the neuropsychological functioning of children, given that multiple and rapid changes in cognitive abilities are occurring during childhood and adolescence.

Cognitive impairments observed in both high-risk and cohort studies do not consistently predict psychiatric illness, as a large number of subjects who have measurable deficits during development (even in the high-risk group) do not go on to develop schizophrenia or other psychiatric illnesses. It is important to consider then, the presence of adaptive or compensatory strategies that may help overcome cognitive vulnerabilities associated with risk for psychiatric illness. In younger children, it may be particularly difficult to identify neuropsychological deficits when cognitive tasks are complex or effortful. For instance, test performance on measures of executive function and attentional capacity would be expected to differ between children and older adolescents, given the significant maturation of the frontal cortex during this age period. Therefore it is essential to differentiate between the normal trajectory of cognitive development, delayed achievement of developmental milestones and cognitive deficits associated with risk for psychiatric illness. In summary, the study of cognitive processes provides empirical research findings that complement diagnostic evaluation. Previous investigations have identified deficits in a number of functional domains including attention, verbal memory and estimated level of intellectual functioning that may predict the onset of psychiatric illness. Future studies should characterize the normative trajectory of neuropsychological function and the neurobiological correlates associated with compensatory mechanisms that would in turn improve early diagnosis and treatment approaches.

Acknowledgments

This work was supported by K01 AA014651 (MMS) and R01 MH069840 (DYT).

References

Anderson, V. (2001). Assessing executive functions in children: biological, psychological, and developmental considerations. *Pediatric Rehabilitation*, 4(3), 119–136.

Ayalon, M. & Merom, H. (1985). The teacher interview. *Schizophrenia Bulletin*, **11**(1), 117–120.

Benton, A. (1985). Some problems associated with neuropsychological assessment. *Bulletin on Clinical Neuroscience*, **50**, 11–15.

Berman, K. F., Ostrem, J. L., Randolph, C. *et al.* (1995). Physiological activation of a cortical network during performance of the Wisconsin Card Sorting Test: a positron emission tomography study. *Neuropsychologia*, 33(8), 1027–1046.

Bornstein, M. H., Hahn, C. S., Bell, C. *et al.* (2006). Stability in cognition across early childhood. A developmental cascade. *Psychological Science*, 17(2), 151–158.

Byrne, M., Hodges, A., Grant, E., Owens, D. C. & Johnstone, E. C. (1999). Neuropsychological assessment of young people at high genetic risk for developing schizophrenia compared with controls: preliminary findings of the Edinburgh High Risk Study (EHRS). *Psychological Medicine*, **29**(5), 1161–1173.

Cannon, M., Caspi, A., Moffitt, T. E. *et al.* (2002). Evidence for early-childhood, pan-developmental impairment specific to schizophreniform disorder: results from a longitudinal birth cohort. *Archives of General Psychiatry*, **59**(5), 449–456.

Casey, B. J., Trainor, R., Giedd, J. *et al.* (1997). The role of the anterior cingulate in automatic and controlled processes: a developmental neuroanatomical study. *Developmental Psychobiology*, **30**(1), 61–69.

Clark, L., Kempton, M. J., Scarna, A., Grasby, P. M. & Goodwin, G. M. (2005). Sustained attention-deficit confirmed in euthymic bipolar disorder but not in first-degree relatives of bipolar patients or euthymic unipolar depression. *Biological Psychiatry*, **57**(2), 183–187.

Cornblatt, B., Obuchowski, M., Roberts, S., Pollack, S. & Erlenmeyer-Kimling, L. (1999). Cognitive and behavioral precursors of schizophrenia. *Development and Psychopathology*, **11**(3), 487–508.

Cornblatt, B. A. & Keilp, J. G. (1994). Impaired attention, genetics, and the pathophysiology of schizophrenia. *Schizophrenia Bulletin*, **20**(1), 31–46.

Davalos, D. B., Compagnon, N., Heinlein, S. & Ross, R. G. (2004). Neuropsychological deficits in children associated with increased familial risk for schizophrenia. *Schizophrenia Research*, **67**(2–3), 123–130.

David, A. S., Malmberg, A., Brandt, L., Allebeck, P. & Lewis, G. (1997). IQ and risk for schizophrenia: a population-based cohort study. *Psychological Medicine*, **27**(6), 1311–1323.

Davidson, M., Reichenberg, A., Rabinowitz, J., Weiser, M., Kaplan, Z. & Mark, M. (1999). Behavioral and intellectual markers for schizophrenia in apparently healthy male adolescents. *American Journal of Psychiatry*, **156**(9), 1328–1335.

Decina, P., Kestenbaum, C. J., Farber, S. *et al.* (1983). Clinical and psychological assessment of children of bipolar probands. *American Journal of Psychiatry*, **140**(5), 548–553.

Ditunno, P. L. & Mann, V. A. (1990). Right hemisphere specialization for mental rotation in normals and brain damaged subjects. *Cortex*, **26**(2), 177–188.

Done, D. J., Crow, T. J., Johnstone, E. C. & Sacker, A. (1994). Childhood antecedents of schizophrenia and affective illness: social adjustment at ages 7 and 11. *British Medical Journal* **309**(6956), 699–703.

Driscoll, R. (1984). Intentional and incidental learning in children vulnerable to psychopathology. In N. F. Anthony, E. J. Anthony, L. C. Wynne & J. E. Rolf (Eds.), *Children at Risk for Schizophrenia: A Longitudinal Perspective* (pp. 320–326). New York, NY: Cambridge University Press.

Dworkin, R. H., Bernstein, G., Kaplansky, L. M. *et al.* (1991). Social competence and positive and negative symptoms: a longitudinal study of children and adolescents at risk for schizophrenia and affective disorder. *American Journal of Psychiatry*, **148**(9), 1182–1188.

Dworkin, R. H., Lewis, J. A., Cornblatt, B. A. & Erlenmeyer-Kimling, L. (1994). Social competence deficits in adolescents at risk for schizophrenia. *Journal of Nervous and Mental Diseases*, **182**(2), 103–108.

Erlenmeyer-Kimling, L. & Cornblatt, B. A. (1992). A summary of attentional findings in the New York High-Risk Project. *Journal of Psychiatric Research*, **26**(4), 405–426.

Erlenmeyer-Kimling, L., Rock, D., Roberts, S. A. (2000). Attention, memory, and motor skills as childhood predictors of schizophrenia-related psychoses: the New York High-Risk Project. *American Journal of Psychiatry*, **157**(9), 1416–1422.

Eslinger, P. J. & Grattan, L. M. (1993). Frontal lobe and frontal-striatal substrates for different forms of human cognitive flexibility. *Neuropsychologia*, **31**(1), 17–28.

Ferrier, I. N., Chowdhury, R., Thompson, J. M., Watson, S. & Young, A. H. (2004). Neurocognitive function in unaffected first-degree relatives of patients with bipolar disorder: a preliminary report. *Bipolar Disorder*, **6**(4), 319–322.

Gao, W. Q., Shinsky, N., Ingle, G. *et al.* (1999). IGF-I deficient mice show reduced peripheral nerve conduction velocities and decreased axonal diameters and respond to exogenous IGF-I treatment. *Journal of Neurobiology*, **39**(1), 142–152.

Giedd, J. N., Blumenthal, J., Jeffries, N. O. *et al.* (1999). Brain development during childhood and adolescence: a longitudinal MRI study. *Nature Neuroscience*, **2**(10), 861–863.

Gilvarry, C., Takei, N., Russell, A. *et al.* (2000). Premorbid IQ in patients with functional psychosis and their first-degree relatives. *Schizophrenia Research*, **41**(3), 417–429.

Goethals, I., Audenaert, K., Jacobs, F. *et al.* (2002). Toward clinical application of neuropsychological activation probes with SPECT: a spatial working memory task. *Journal of Nuclear Medicine*, **43**(11), 1426–1431.

Goldstein, J. M., Seidman, L. J., Buka, S. L. *et al.* (2000). Impact of genetic vulnerability and hypoxia on overall intelligence by age 7 in offspring at high risk for schizophrenia compared with affective psychoses. *Schizophrenia Bulletin*, **26**(2), 323–334.

Goodman, S. H. (1987). Emory University Project on Children of Disturbed Parents. *Schizophrenia Bulletin*, **13**(3), 411–423.

Gotlib, I. H., Traill, S. K., Montoya, R. L., Joormann, J. & Chang, K. (2005). Attention and memory biases in the offspring of parents with bipolar disorder: indications

11

from a pilot study. *Journal of Child Psychology and Psychiatry*, **46**(1), 84–93.

Gourovitch, M. L., Torrey, E. F., Gold, J. M. *et al.* (1999). Neuropsychological performance of monozygotic twins discordant for bipolar disorder. *Biological Psychiatry*, **45**(5), 639–646.

Grigoroiu-Serbanescu, M., Christodorescu, D., Jipescu, I. *et al.* (1989). Psychopathology in children aged 10–17 of bipolar parents: psychopathology rate and correlates of the severity of the psychopathology. *Journal of Affective Disorders*, **16**(2–3), 167–179.

Heilman, K. M. & Van Den Abell, T. (1980). Right hemisphere dominance for attention: the mechanism underlying hemispheric asymmetries of inattention (neglect). *Neurology*, **30**(3), 327–330.

Huttenlocher, P. R. (1994). Synaptogenesis in human cerebral cortex. In G. Dawson & K. W. Fischer (Eds.), *Human Behavior and the Developing Brain* (pp. 137–152). New York, NY: Guilford Press.

Isohanni, M., Makikyro, T., Moring, J. *et al.* (1997). A comparison of clinical and research DSM-III-R diagnoses of schizophrenia in a Finnish national birth cohort. Clinical and research diagnoses of schizophrenia. *Society of Psychiatry and Psychiatric Epidemiology*, **32**(5), 303–308.

Jones, P., Rodgers, B., Murray, R. & Marmot, M. (1994). Child development risk factors for adult schizophrenia in the British 1946 birth cohort. *Lancet*, **344**(8934), 1398–1402.

Jones, P. B. & Done, D. J. (1997). From birth to onset: a developmental perspective of schizophrenia in two national birth cohorts. In M. S. Keshavan & R. M. Murray (Eds.), *Neurodevelopment and Adult Psychopathology* (pp. 119–136). New York, NY: Cambridge University Press.

Jones, P. B. & Tarrant, C. J. (2000). Developmental precursors and biological markers for schizophrenia and affective disorders: specificity and public health implications. *European Archives in Psychiatry and Clinical Neuroscience*, **250**(6), 286–291.

Keri, S., Kelemen, O., Benedek, G. & Janka, Z. (2001). Different trait markers for schizophrenia and bipolar disorder: a neurocognitive approach. *Psychological Medicine*, **31**(5), 915–922.

Kestenbaum, C. J. (1979). Children at risk for manic-depressive illness: possible predictors. *American Journal of Psychiatry*, **136**(9), 1206–1208.

Klein, R. H. & Salzman, L. F. (1984). Response-contingent learning in children at-risk. In N. F. Watt, E. J. Anthony, L. C. Wynne & J. E. Rolf (Eds.), *Children at Risk for Schizophrenia: A Longitudinal Perspective* (pp. 371–375). New York, NY: Cambridge University Press.

Klenberg, L., Korkman, M. & Lahti-Nuuttila, P. (2001). Differential development of attention and executive functions in 3- to 12-year-old Finnish children. *Development and Neuropsychology*, **20**(1), 407–428.

Knudsen, E. I. (2004). Sensitive periods in the development of the brain and behavior. *Journal of Cognitive Neuroscience*, **16**(8), 1412–1425.

Kremen, W. S., Faraone, S. V., Seidman, L. J., Pepple, J. R. & Tsuang, M. T. (1998). Neuropsychological risk indicators for schizophrenia: a preliminary study of female relatives of schizophrenic and bipolar probands. *Psychiatry Research*, **79**(3), 227–240.

Lezak, M. D. (1995). *Neuropsychological Assessment* (3rd edn.). New York, NY: Oxford University Press.

Lifshitz, M., Kugelmass, S. & Karov, M. (1985). Perceptual-motor and memory performance of high-risk children. *Schizophrenia Bulletin*, **11**(1), 74–84.

MacQueen, G. M., Grof, P., Alda, M., Marriott, M., Young, L. T. & Duffy, A. (2004). A pilot study of visual backward masking performance among affected versus unaffected offspring of parents with bipolar disorder. *Bipolar Disorder*, **6**(5), 374–378.

Malmberg, A., Lewis, G., David, A. & Allebeck, P. (1998). Premorbid adjustment and personality in people with schizophrenia. *British Journal of Psychiatry*, **172**, 308–313.

McDonough-Ryan, P., DelBello, M., Shear, P. K. *et al.* (2002). Academic and cognitive abilities in children of parents with bipolar disorder: a test of the nonverbal learning disability model. *Journal of Clinical and Experimental Neuropsychology*, **24**(3), 280–285.

Mednick, S. A. & Schulsinger, F. (1968). Some premorbid characteristics related to breakdown in children with schizophrenic mothers. In D. Rosenthal & S. S. Kety (Eds.), *Transmission of Schizophrenia* (pp. 267–292). Oxford, UK: Pergamon Press.

Mirsky, A. F. (1988). The Israeli high-risk study. In *Relatives at Risk for Mental Disorders* (Dunner, D. L. & Gershon, E. S., eds). New York, NY: Raven Press.

Neale, J. M., Winters, K. C. & Weintraub, S. (1984). Information processing deficits in children at high-risk for schizophrenia. In *Children at Risk for Schizophrenia: A Longitudinal Perspective* (Watt, N. F., Anthony, E. J., Wynne, L. C. & Rolf, J. E., eds), pp. 264–277. New York, NY: Cambridge University Press.

Nelson, C. A. (2000). Neural plasticity and human development: the role of early experience in sculpting memory systems. *Developmental Science*, **3**, 115–130.

Niemi, L. T., Suvisaari, J. M., Tuulio-Henriksson, A. & Lonnqvist, J. K. (2003). Childhood developmental abnormalities in schizophrenia: evidence from high-risk studies. *Schizophrenia Research*, **60**(2–3), 239–258.

Nuechterlein, K. (1984). Sustained attention among children vulnerable to adult schizophrenia and among hyperactive children. In N. F. Watt, E. J. Anthony, L. C. Wynne & J. E. Rolf (Eds.), *Children at Risk for Schizophrenia: A Longitudinal Perspective* (pp. 304–312). New York, NY: Cambridge University Press.

Papanicolaou, A. C., Deutsch, G., Bourbon, W. T. *et al.* (1987). Convergent evoked potential and cerebral blood flow evidence of task-specific hemispheric differences. *Electroencephalography and Clinical Neurophysiology*, **66**(6), 515–520.

Pellegrini, D., Kosisky, S., Nackman, D. *et al.* (1986). Personal and social resources in children of patients with bipolar affective disorder and children of normal control subjects. *American Journal of Psychiatry*, **143**(7), 856–861.

Penfield, W. & Jasper, H. (1954). *Epilepsy and the Functional Anatomy of the Human Brain*. Boston, MA: Little Brown.

Penfield, W. & Perot, P. (1963). The brain's record of auditory and visual experience. A final summary and discussion. *Brain*, **86**, 595–696.

Penfield, W. & Roberts, L. (1959). *Speech and Brain Mechanisms*. New York, NY: Oxford University Press.

Pfefferbaum, A., Mathalon, D. H., Sullivan, E. V. *et al.* (1994). A quantitative magnetic resonance imaging study of changes in brain morphology from infancy to late adulthood. *Archives of Neurology*, **51**(9), 874–887.

Rantakallio, P. (1969). Groups at risk in low birth weight infants and perinatal mortality. *Acta Paediatrica Scandinavica*, **193**(Suppl.), 1.

Rantakallio, P. (1988). The longitudinal study of the northern Finland birth cohort of 1966. *Paediatric and Perinatal Epidemiology*, **2**(1), 59–88.

Reiss, A. L., Abrams, M. T., Singer, H. S., Ross, J. L. & Denckla, M. B. (1996). Brain development, gender and IQ in children. A volumetric imaging study. *Brain*, **119** (Pt 5), 1763–1774.

Reitan, R. M. & Wolfson, D. (1985). *The Halstead-Reitan Neuropsychological Test Battery*. Tucson, AZ: Neuropsychology Press.

Rieder, R. O., Broman, S. H. & Rosenthal, D. (1977). The offspring of schizophrenics. II. Perinatal factors and IQ. *Archives of General Psychiatry*, **34**(7), 789–799.

Rosso, I. M., Young, A. D., Femia, L. A. & Yurgelun-Todd, D. A. (2004). Cognitive and emotional components of frontal lobe functioning in childhood and adolescence. *Annals of the New York Academy of Science*, **1021**, 355–362.

Sameroff, A., Barocas, R. & Seifer, R. (1984). The early development of children born to mentally ill women. In N. F. Watt, E. J. Anthony, L. C. Wynne & J. E. Rolf (Eds.), *Children at Risk for Schizophrenia: A Longitudinal Perspective* (pp. 482–513). New York, NY: Cambridge University Press.

Schreiber, H., Stolz-Born, G., Heinrich, H., Kornhuber, H. H. & Born, J. (1992). Attention, cognition, and motor perseveration in adolescents at genetic risk for schizophrenia and control subjects. *Psychiatry Research*, **44**(2), 125–140.

Schubert, E. W. & McNeil, T. F. (2005). Neuropsychological impairment and its neurological correlates in adult offspring with heightened risk for schizophrenia and affective psychosis. *American Journal of Psychiatry*, **162**(4), 758–766.

Smith, A. (1991). *Symbol Digit Modalities Test*. Los Angeles, CA: Western Psychological Services.

Sobczak, S., Honig, A., Schmitt, J. A. & Riedel, W. J. (2003). Pronounced cognitive deficits following an intravenous L-tryptophan challenge in first-degree relatives of bipolar patients compared to healthy controls. *Neuropsychopharmacology*, **28**(4), 711–719.

Sohlberg, S. C. (1985). Personality and neuropsychological performance of high-risk children. *Schizophrenia Bulletin*, **11**(1), 48–60.

Sorensen, H. J., Mortensen, E. L., Parnas, J. & Mednick, S. A. (2006). Premorbid neurocognitive functioning in schizophrenia spectrum disorder. *Schizophrenia Bulletin*, **32**(3), 578–583.

Sowell, E. R., Delis, D., Stiles, J. & Jernigan, T. L. (2001). Improved memory functioning and frontal lobe maturation between childhood and adolescence: a structural MRI study. *Journal of the International Neuropsychology Society*, 7(3), 312–322.

Sowell, E. R., Thompson, P. M., Holmes, C. J., Jernigan, T. L. & Toga, A. W. (1999). In vivo evidence for post-adolescent brain maturation in frontal and striatal regions. *Nature Neuroscience*, **2**(10), 859–861.

Spreen, O., Risser, A. H. & Edgell, D. (eds) (1995a). Development of functional systems. In *Developmental Neuropsychology*, pp. 37–56. Oxford, UK: Oxford University Press.

Spreen, O., Risser, A. H. & Edgell, D. (1995b). *Developmental Neuropsychology*. Oxford, UK: Oxford University Press.

Stuss, D. T. & Benson, D. F. (1984). Neuropsychological studies of the frontal lobes. *Psychology Bulletin*, **95**(1), 3–28.

Thompson, O'Quinn (1979). *Developmental Disabilities: Etiologies, Manifestations, Diagnoses, and Treatments*. New York, NY: Oxford University Press.

Todd, R. D., Reich, W. & Reich, T. (1994). Prevalence of affective disorder in the child and adolescent offspring of a single kindred: a pilot study. *Journal of the American Academy of Child and Adolescent Psychiatry*, **33**(2), 198–207.

Ungerleider, L. G. & Mishkin, M. (1982). Two cortical visual systems. In D. J. Ingle, M. A. Goodale & R. J. W. Mansfield (Eds.), *Analysis of Visual Behavior*. Cambridge, MA: MIT Press.

van Os, J., Jones, P., Lewis, G., Wadsworth, M. & Murray, R. (1997). Developmental precursors of affective illness in a general population birth cohort. *Archives of General Psychiatry*, **54**(7), 625–631.

Wadsworth, M. E. (1987). Follow-up of the first national birth cohort: findings from the Medical Research Council National Survey of Health and Development. *Paediatric and Perinatal Epidemiology*, **1**(1), 95–117.

Webb, S. J., Monk, C. S. & Nelson, C. A. (2001). Mechanisms of postnatal neurobiological development: implications for human development. *Developmental Neuropsychology*, **19**(2), 147–171.

Weintraub, S. (1987). Risk factors in schizophrenia: the Stony Brook High-Risk Project. *Schizophrenia Bulletin*, **13**(3), 439–450.

Weissman, M. M., Wickramaratne, P., Warner, V. *et al.* (1987). Assessing psychiatric disorders in children. Discrepancies between mothers' and children's reports. *Archives of General Psychiatry*, **44**(8), 747–753.

Williams, B. R., Ponesse, J. S., Schachar, R. J., Logan, G. D. & Tannock, R. (1999). Development of inhibitory control

across the life span. *Developmental Psychology*, **35**(1), 205–213.

Williamson, D. E., Coleman, K., Bacanu, S. A. *et al.* (2003). Heritability of fearful-anxious endophenotypes in infant rhesus macaques: a preliminary report. *Biological Psychiatry*, **53**(4), 284–291.

Worland, J. & Hesselbrock, V. (1980). The intelligence of children and their parents with schizophrenia and affective illness. *Journal of Child Psychology and Psychiatry*, **21**(3), 191–201.

Worland, J., Janes, C. L., Anthony, E. J., McGinnis, M. & Cass, L. (1984). St. Louis Risk Research Project: comprehensive progress report of experimental studies. In N. F. Watt, E. J. Anthony, L. C. Wynne & J. E. Rolf (Eds.), *Children At Risk for Schizophrenia: A Longitudinal Perspective* (pp. 105–147). New York, NY: Cambridge University Press.

Worland, J., Weeks, D. G., Weiner, S. M. & Schechtman, J. (1982). Longitudinal, prospective evaluations of intelligence in children at risk. *Schizophrenia Bulletin*, **8**(1), 135–141.

Yurgelun-Todd, D. A., Killgore, W. D. & Young, A. D. (2002). Sex differences in cerebral tissue volume and cognitive performance during adolescence. *Psychology Report*, **91**(3), 743–757.

Zalla, T., Joyce, C., Szoke, A., Schurhoff, F. *et al.* (2004). Executive dysfunctions as potential markers of familial vulnerability to bipolar disorder and schizophrenia. *Psychiatry Research*, **121**(3), 207–217.

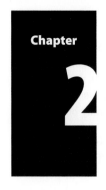

Processes and mechanisms in neuropsychiatry: sensory-perceptual

Ester Klimkeit and John L. Bradshaw

Despite there being only few simple and purely sensory (or even perceptual) disturbances per se in psychiatric disorders, sensory-perceptual abnormalities may help us better understand their neurobiological underpinnings. Sensory-perceptual distortions are also observed in neurological conditions such as neglect, neuropsychiatric conditions such as disorders of misidentification (e.g. Frégoli syndrome), and in non-neurological, non-psychiatric populations including phantom limb phenomenon and synesthesia. The two different medical fields, psychiatry and neurology, often adopt different explanations for these sensory disturbances, where the psychiatrist will often assume the absence of organic causes, whilst the neurologist will take the opposite view. This occurs even though both fields may merely be encountering different aspects of disorders of the same brain systems. For example, the neurological basis of prosopagnosia likely mirrors the underlying processes (or deficits) in the psychiatric disorders of Capgras and Frégoli syndromes, while the complex visual hallucinations observed in the ictal phenomena of temporal lobe epilepsy and the thought disturbance of schizophrenia may be comparable and therefore amenable to similar treatment (Starr & Sporty, 1994). In this chapter we will bridge the traditional divide between psychiatry and neurology, and outline our understanding of some selected instances of anomalous sensory processes in these often difficult-to-differentiate neuropsychiatric conditions.

Synesthesia

Synesthesia offers insight into anomalous perceptual processes, which are not dysfunctional or detrimental to daily living. This condition commonly involves an intra-modal form of synesthesia, in which a stimulus evokes an additional, unusual response within the same modality. For instance, an individual "sees" vivid colours when looking at certain digits, letters or words; these synesthetic colors may appear "out in space" or merely in their "mind's eye." However, in some rare individuals, stimulation in one sensory modality results in a vivid involuntary sensory experience in another (Rich, 2004; Rich & Mattingley, 2002), where, for example, some synesthetes will "see" colors when they hear particular sounds, whereas others have specific taste sensations when they read certain words. These experiences are unusual, as whilst it is common for a perfume or a tune to suddenly and powerfully evoke vivid associations or images, usually we do not literally "see red" when hearing a gratuitous insult, or "feel blue" when things go badly wrong.

The relationship for an individual between the stimulus and synesthetic experience is highly consistent over time, and has usually been present since early childhood; affected individuals are usually surprised to learn that others do not share these experiences. While the prevalence of synesthesia has been estimated variously as between 1 in 2000 and 1 in 25 000, our own Australian data (Rich et al., 2005) provide estimates of around 1 in 1150 for females and 1 in 7150 for males, with a strong familial component.

Synesthetes cannot generally suppress their experiences voluntarily, and conscious identification of a letter or digit seems necessary to elicit a synesthetic color (Mattingley et al., 2001). In respect of this lack of voluntary control and the necessity of awareness of the inducing stimulus, synesthesia may provide a model for some forms of induced hallucinatory states in psychopathology. Two broad and different explanations for synesthesia have been proposed: synesthesia is mediated by either normal neural and cognitive architecture or by special neuroanatomical and/or neurophysiological mechanisms that are only present in synesthetes (Rich & Mattingley, 2002). Rich *et al.* (2005) found that in a subset of 150 lexical-color synesthetes, for whom letters, digits and words induce color experiences, there was a striking consistency in the colors induced by certain letters and digits. Thus "R" frequently elicited red; "Y," yellow; and "D," brown. Given that a similar, but less consistent, association was identified in a non-synesthetic control group, it suggests that early learning experiences may be involved in determining these sensory perceptual experiences that are common to all individuals. These learning experiences, particularly for synesthetes, may determine particular patterns of lexical-color associations that could generalize to other words or information sequences (e.g. days of the week, number and letter sequences).

If anomalous neural architecture occurs in synesthesia, it may take the form of additional synaptic connections between brain regions responsible for processing auditory and color perception, or may even stem from inadequate neural pruning (apoptosis). A small PET study of response to auditory words has shown that color-word synesthetes, like non-synesthetes, show activation of areas concerned with language and visual feature integration including the perisylvian regions, as well as the posterior temporal cortex and parieto-occipital junction (Paulesu *et al.*, 1995).

Synesthesia provides an opportunity for investigating variable interconnections between different sensory systems, and the most significant advances towards a biological and cognitive model of synesthesia will probably emerge through future functional imaging and transcranial magnetic stimulation studies.

Phantom limbs

Up to 98% of amputees may report phantom limbs following limb loss or deafferentation (Giummarra *et al.*, 2007); often the experience is of phantom pain, though each amputee experiences a unique combination of spontaneous and evoked phantom sensations. While phantom phenomena do not represent a psychopathological condition per se, the condition may provide a good model with which more complex hallucinatory experiences can be compared. Phantom sensations may occur for a number of reasons, including physical loss of a limb, deafferentation, sensory root loss or spinal injury. In the case of an amputee, even though he or she knows that the limb is missing, the phantom experience may be so powerful and compelling that he or she may be tempted to use, rely or even stand on the missing limb. Parietal damage can induce experiences of supernumerary limbs, such as a ghost arm or a third arm perceived to emerge from the chest. More unusual phantom phenomena have been reported following removal of a breast, penis, eye, bladder or rectum. Such phantom sensations may be painful or characterized by functional sensations, e.g. of urination or erection after penis removal. Phantom limbs occur less commonly in instances of congenital limb deficiency (aplasia) or early limb loss (in 20%; Melzack *et al.*, 1997). While phantom limbs are typically experienced soon after limb loss, they may develop many years later; they may be transient, fade gradually or persist permanently.

In instances where the phantom is perceived as fixed, it may be possible to reinstate voluntary phantom movement by providing false and illusory visual feedback (via mirrors) of a moving limb corresponding in shape, size and spatial position to the phantom (Frith *et al.*, 2000). The reafference theory (see the following chapter) offers one explanation as to why this may occur. It proposes that the mirror-derived visual feedback allows the reafference predictors to be updated; consequently the efference copies produced in parallel with the motor commands bring about changes in the predicted position of the missing limb that correspond to what the patient observes in the mirror. Thus the individual, while neurologically intact and retaining full insight into the situation, experiences powerful illusory perceptions.

Older theories propose that phantom sensations result from impulses generated in the stump; however this explanation was inadequate, as it did not explain aplasic phantom limbs. More recently, disturbances have been invoked in the body schema (an internal, dynamic representation of the body's spatial properties), or in the body's structural description (a topological map of body part locations). Re-organization of the somatosensory homunculus occurs after amputation and is strongly correlated with phantom limb pain (Knecht *et al.*, 1998). Internal representations of the body appear to be stored in the parietal cortex where there is multimodal convergence of visual, vestibular, proprioceptive and efference copy inputs (Ventre-Dominey *et al.*, 2003). The neuromatrix concept (Melzack, 1990) extends these ideas, as an innate, genetically determined representation of the body in the parietal lobe that is continuously modified by sensorimotor and emotional experience throughout the lifespan. Phantom limb perception is seen to derive from excessive neuromatrix activity, despite an absence of somatosensory input following amputation. This consequently leads to a wide range of sensations from excruciating pain to orgasm. The neuromatrix concept can also accommodate the rarer phantom experiences, usually also free of pain, with congenital limb loss or aplasia. It is also compatible with the high incidence of referred sensations from the mouth/face region to the phantom hand/arm (Ramachandran & Blakeslee, 1998), given the strong functional connectivity between the adjacent cortical representations of the hand and face regions.

Phantom phenomena are regarded as a more complex perceptual disturbance than synesthesia, and may also throw light upon body integrity identity disorder. The latter is characterized by a desire, often beginning in childhood or adolescence, to amputate a healthy limb (First, 2005). Most cases desire amputation (apotemnophilia) of a lower limb to "restore my true identity or optimal shape." When sexual arousal is associated with the condition, some individuals report being attracted to other amputees (acrotomophilia). It is possible that, during an emotional state, patterns of neural activity from sensory input from the genitals and lower limbs (that are represented closely adjacent in the cortical homunculus) reinforce a desire to amputate the lower limbs (Kell *et al.*, 2005).

Phantom limb phenomena also have links with conditions such as synesthesia and unilateral neglect (discussed later in this chapter), and also with the concept of mirror neurons. Mirror neurons, discussed in detail in the following chapter, refer to neurons observed to "fire" during the observation of actions performed by others. These are active during action preparation and in initiation and communication, and may also play a role in the phantom phenomenon. The activity of mirror neurons may indeed reinforce the internal representation of a limb within the body schema, even when the limb has failed to develop (Brugger *et al.*, 2000). A link with synesthesia comes from the report that visual perception of touch elicited conscious tactile experiences in a female synesthete (Blakemore *et al.*, 2005). This "mirrored-touch" synesthetic experience was assessed by fMRI. Results indicated higher somatosensory cortex and left premotor cortex activation in the synesthete, and activation in the anterior insula cortex not seen in controls, during the observation of touch. The authors interpreted these findings as evidence for an overactive mirror system for touch. A link between phantom limb and unilateral neglect phenomena is suggested by the report that vestibular caloric stimulation (which laterally biases attention) provoked temporary perception of a normal phantom limb in a substantial group of amputees who previously did not experience phantoms (André *et al.*, 2001). In others who currently experienced deformed or painful phantom limbs, caloric stimulation led to temporary replacement of the abnormal phantom with a non-painful normal phantom. This evidence suggests that vestibular bias can trigger reconstruction of the global body schema.

"Missing" and supernumerary limbs

After peripheral deafferentation, a patient may develop a "phantom" even though the deafferented limb is still there. A phantom may be contained within the space occupied by the real limb, or separated from it in space and be regarded as supernumerary (Kew *et al.*, 1997). In other cases, patients do not develop phantoms, but become unaware of the limb unless it is continually present in vision; otherwise it seemingly fades from consciousness, presumably due to the absence of sensory information or feedback from the limb. Hemianesthesia after right inferior parietal damage can result in similar problems (see Frith *et al.*, 2000, for a review). Patients can only initiate simple movements in the absence of continuing visual feedback, to provide information about limb position prior to, during and after movement.

McGonigle *et al.* (2002) report the case of a stroke patient (right frontomesial lesion) who sporadically experienced a supernumerary "ghost" left arm, which occupied the position the real left arm had occupied around a minute earlier. Frith *et al.* (2000) review other instances of apparent supernumerary limbs, noting that the estimated position of a limb involves the integration of information from motor commands (in moving a limb to new target positions) and sensory feedback (relating to old and new positions attained). Failure to integrate these two sources of information (e.g. because of defective sensory feedback) could lead to the experience of a supernumerary limb. Conversely, additional failure to receive signals indicating absence of intended movement in an already paralyzed limb may lead to the false belief that the limb can be, and indeed has successfully been, moved. Even normal healthy individuals may falsely believe that they have moved a limb when they have not (Ramachandran & Blakeslee, 1998). Imaging studies would be helpful in understanding how these phenomena occur.

Unilateral (hemispatial) neglect

Right parietal or parieto-frontal damage may result in the patient's apparent unawareness or inability to acknowledge the existence of objects or events in contralateral (i.e. left) hemispace. Right neglect after left hemisphere damage is much less common, which may be a result of spatial, attentional and emotional processes (including those relating even to language) being commonly represented on the right. This raises the possibility of whether unilateral (hemispatial) neglect is a disorder of spatial perception or attention (indeed, it is often referred to as hemi-inattention).

Parton et al. (2004) and Bradshaw & Mattingley (1995) have both reported that patients typically attend to items towards the same (ipsilesional) side as their brain damage. Patients with neglect may habitually collide with "unnoticed" and often large obstacles on their left, or even be unaware of people in extrapersonal (left) space; however, there are cases that require careful clinical testing before it becomes apparent. Individuals may not acknowledge or, in severe cases, actively disown their own contralateral body parts. In such cases, if attention can somehow be drawn towards their neglected side, the patient may "confabulate" and ascribe it as belonging to someone else. Some patients may also fail to use their contralesional limbs even if they have little or no weakness (commonly known as "motor neglect"). Other patients can also deny that they have any perceptual or motor control difficulties (anosognosia), if any are actually present.

Neglect, as a function of either individual differences or of task requirements, may extend to the left side of any object, irrespective of its location within peripersonal space (object-based neglect); alternatively, it may be linked specifically to the left side of

space (scene-based neglect). It may also be limited to near (peripersonal) space, or to far (extracorporeal) space. Neglect may be transiently corrected, alleviated or compensated for by a variety of vestibular maneuvers. These may include caloric irrigation of the auditory meatus on one side (cold water to the contralateral or warm to the ipsilateral ear), or rapid rotation on, for example, an office chair, so as to effect apparent attentional redirection (see Buxbaum, 2006 for a review).

Unattended material, of which the patient is apparently unaware, may still bias how the individual is perceiving or interpreting material that he/she are aware of, or attending to. Therefore, it is apparent that the material in the neglected side is still available for sophisticated preattentive or implicit processing, even though it is below the threshold for conscious awareness – a phenomenon reminiscent of blindsight in the cortically blind (Weiskrantz, 1986). Neglect is also not necessarily limited to the visual modality, as tactile and auditory neglect are not uncommon.

Clearly the neglect syndrome is a heterogeneous condition, resulting from various combinations of component cognitive deficits involving injury to several regions, circuits or systems, including the inferior parietal, inferior frontal, striatal or even medial temporal regions. One phenomenon, "extinction," is still debated as to whether it is a mild form of neglect, or a syndrome in its own right. Extinction occurs when a patient's visual fields are intact, but he or she fails to report a contralesional stimulus when it is presented simultaneously with an ipsilesional stimulus; this can sometimes occur in a different sensory modality. Just as many regions of the brain participate at different levels and to different extents in different aspects of attentional processes, so too in neuropsychiatric disturbances of attention we encounter different degrees of perseveration and loss of range of component functions, often with fluctuating levels of insight, depending upon vestibular factors (affecting orientation), neurotransmitter status (arousal levels) and site and extent of pathology.

Asomatognosia and pathological embodiment

Patients with asomatognosia typically describe parts of their body as missing from corporeal awareness. Despite the disturbance being usually attributed to right parietal damage, the patient generally has pre-servation of insight, in contrast to neglect or extinc-tion syndromes (Arzy *et al.*, 2006). Asomatognosia may be modified by touching or looking at the body part, suggesting multisensory (parietal) mechanisms in awareness and embodiment of body parts. Arzy *et al.* (2006) present a case study of a patient who reported that parts of her left arm had disappeared, enabling her to see the table on which her arm was resting, as if the latter was transparent.

Hallucinations and delusions

Hallucinations involve perception without an external stimulus (Sims, 2003) and are common to both orga-nic and psychiatric disorders. Verbal hallucinations in psychotic disorders and in temporal and parietal lobe epilepsy have been linked to activity in cortical areas that are normally concerned with the perception of external speech (Behrendt & Young, 2004). Report-edly, speaking or reading aloud is effective in allevia-ting hallucinations, suggesting that it is possible that hallucinations may involve generation of inner speech and rely on similar neural substrates as speech (Seal *et al.*, 2004). Delusions, that is, false beliefs held with extraordinary conviction (Sims, 2003), are also common to psychiatric and organic conditions and are considered in greater detail below, in the context of passivity delusions and delusional misidentification disorders.

Delusions of control in psychosis

Patients with schizophrenia often exhibit a failure of reality monitoring, claiming that their actions, emo-tions and thoughts are under external "alien" control, rather than under their own volitional control – even though what they actually end up doing may still be more or less appropriate (Bradshaw, 2001). This dif-ficulty in determining the agency of purposive actions is known as passivity delusions (Sims, 2003). These abnormal experiences may arise through a lack of awareness of one's actual intentions or thought pro-cesses, which are misattributed to outside sources. As with alien limb phenomena and unilateral neglect, parietal and cingulate cortices are likely involved (Maruff *et al.*, 2005; Spence *et al.*, 1997). Whether it is a matter of subvocal speech, as in hallucinations, or possibly of thought processes, as in delusions, or of actions demanded by the current situation, the

patients may be unable to recognize them as their own (Frith, 1992); it is as if there is a failure of the ability to self-monitor and of the feedforward (re-afference or corollary discharge) system that normally comes into play whenever we undertake voluntary actions. Such a goal-seeking and recursively error-correcting comparator system enables us to match forward projections (neural copies) of likely experi-ences of each upcoming response with the actual consequences and feedback of that action. The system has to distinguish sensations caused directly by the body's own movement, from those arriving extrane-ously from the environment. Our ability to do this and to predict the consequences of our actions may explain why we cannot successfully tickle ourselves, unless we create a simulacrum of alien control by introducing a short time lag into a device that enables us to deliver delayed tickling stimuli to ourselves. Interestingly, in addition to possible disorders of self-attribution, patients with schizophrenia *can* experience self-tickling (Wolpert *et al.*, 1998).

Frith *et al.* (2000) propose a close variant of the above formulation, suggesting that experience of alien control arises from a lack of awareness of predicted limb positions; thus patients are unaware of the exact specification of the movement. They are aware of their goal, of the intention to move, and of the move-ment having occurred, but not of having *initiated* the movement. "It is as if the movement, although intended, has been initiated by some external force" (Frith *et al.*, 2000, p. 1784). They note, too, that patients have difficulty remembering the precise details of actions made in the absence of feedback. They also have difficulty distinguishing between cor-rect visual feedback about the position of their hand, and false feedback when the image of the hand they see (via a system of mirrors and screens, see above) is in fact that of another person making the same move-ment. Maruff *et al.* (2005) found that compared with other patients with schizophrenia, those with passivity delusions showed reductions in gray matter volume in the left prefrontal and the right parietal region, including parts of the primary somatosensory cor-tex. Such observations are compatible with Frith's hypothesis that passivity phenomena arise from dys-function in the prefrontal association cortex where intentions to act are generated, and in the parietal association cortex where the sensory consequences of motor actions are modeled.

Delusional misidentification syndromes

Most patients suffering delusional misidentification syndromes are diagnosed with schizophrenia or mania. Misidentification syndromes are also associated with high rates of organic etiology e.g. Alzheimer's disease, dementia and head trauma (Edelstyn & Oyebode, 1999). Capgras syndrome is the most frequently reported, characterized by the belief that a person, usually someone well known to the patient, has been replaced by an almost identical impostor (Edelstyn & Oyebode, 1999). Thus a woman may believe that her spouse and children have been replaced by doubles, typically with evil intent. Small differences in appearance or behaviour are often reported by patients to distinguish between the person and the imagined impostor. Delusions can also involve inanimate objects and animals. For example, Edelstyn et al. (1996) reported a case where a patient believed that family members were stealing his personal belongings and replacing them with identical but inferior doubles.

Frégoli syndrome, named after an Italian actor and mimic who had great skill in changing his appearance, is characterized by the patient's belief that a familiar person is able to take on different physical forms and adopt another's appearance (Förstl et al., 1991). It is as if biographical information for a certain person is automatically accessed and applied, regardless of whom is present (Bradshaw & Mattingley, 1995). In the syndrome of intermetamorphosis a person is believed to have been changed into someone else entirely with altered identity and physical appearance (Edelstyn & Oyebode, 1999). In the syndrome of subjective doubles, another person is believed to have taken on the physical characteristics and identity of oneself (Bradshaw & Mattingley, 1995). The belief that a physical location has been duplicated is referred to as reduplicative paramnesia (Förstl et al., 1991). In this condition, a patient may insist that the hospital he or she is in has been duplicated and relocated from one site to another, so that the two hospitals coexist in different places at the same time (Anderson, 1988). Misidentification of place is the misidentification syndrome most frequently associated with neurological disease (Förstl et al., 1991).

The face misidentification phenomena in misidentification disorders have led to comparisons with prosopagnosia, an organic condition in which recognition of familiar faces is impaired. Misidentification of strangers in Frégoli and intermetamorphosis suggests impairment in visual processing. Frégoli patients may perform more poorly on face recognition relative to word recognition tasks, and show impaired ability to detect subtle visual differences in animal stimuli (Edelstyn et al., 1996). In light of these deficits in processing non-facial stimuli, and the fact that inanimate objects are often implicated in misidentification syndromes, the authors argued that explanations of misidentification disorders should not be confined to models of face processing, but should be extended to models of visual recognition in general. However, Rojo et al. (1991) reported Capgras syndrome in a blind person, suggesting that it cannot be purely visual.

A quarter of a century ago, Ungerleider & Mishkin (1982) proposed the concept of two parallel, though interconnected, visual systems within the primate brain: a largely automatic and unconscious "dorsal" system in the posterior parietal cortex which sets the spatial context within which objects, events and actions take place; and a "ventral" (inferior occipito-temporal) pathway responsible at a more conscious level for object recognition. Quite separately, different classes of retinal ganglion cell have been identified which project to separate target layers in the lateral geniculate nucleus: the parvocellular (P) and magnocellular (M) streams (Desimone & Ungerleider, 1989). Differing (amongst other features) in their respective capacities to respond preferentially to higher or lower spatial frequencies, projections from the M stream are abundantly represented in the parietal cortex, and those from the P stream tend to terminate in the inferotemporal cortex.

More recently, the idea of two semi-independent but complementary visual systems has been further developed (Goodale & Milner, 2004, p. 97); the ventral stream is seen as delivering a rich, detailed and largely conscious representation of object identities within the world scene, while the dorsal stream delivers fast, accurate, automatic and largely unconscious information about objects in the required egocentric coordinates for action. This differentiation of visual processing was demonstrated in a case study by Goodale & Milner (2004) who describe a patient unable to consciously and deliberately copy a slant shown as a target display with a hand-held card, but nevertheless retained the ability to adopt the requisite slanted posture so as to "post" the card in a tilted slot. Ellis & Young (1990) also suggested that Capgras syndrome and prosopagnosia reflect differential impairment in ventral and dorsal visual pathways. The ventral pathway, responsible for conscious face recognition, connects with the visual cortex, and may be impaired in prosopagnosia. Similarly, the dorsal pathway, responsible for giving the face its emotional significance, connects the visual system with limbic structures; it may be impaired in Capgras syndrome, resulting in a distorted sense of familiarity. The cognitive dissonance resulting from normal face recognition (intact ventral stream) coupled with the absence of the feeling of familiarity (impaired dorsal stream) is proposed as the basis of this misidentification disorder. Evidence of absence of familiarity in Capgras patients comes from an experiment which recorded skin conductance responses during the showing of a series of familiar and unfamiliar faces. Unlike controls, who showed greater skin conductance to familiar than unfamiliar faces, Capgras patients failed to discriminate between such faces in terms of the degree of their autonomic arousal (Ellis *et al.*, 1997).

Autoscopia, out-of-body and near-death experiences

Individuals with near-death experiences typically report dissociative symptoms like depersonalization, increased alertness and often give various descriptions of mystic consciousness (Sims, 2003). They often describe out-of-body experiences and the impression of seeing their own body (autoscopy) from their out-of-body perspective. Autoscopy occurs in individuals with various psychiatric and organic conditions such as emotional disturbance, delirium, epilepsy, drug addiction and alcoholism (Hamilton, 1985). The German folklore, that you will die if you see your double ("Doppelgänger"), may relate to the fact that autoscopy is often associated with cerebrovascular disorders or severe infectious diseases affecting the parietal lobe (Hamilton, 1985). Out-of-body experiences differ from autoscopic hallucinations, in that in the latter a double of oneself is seen without the sensation of having left one's body. Blanke & Arzy (2005) define an out-of-body experience as an experience of "disembodiment (location of the self outside one's body), the impression of seeing the world from a distant and elevated visuo spatial perspective (extracorporeal egocentric perspective), and the impression of seeing one's own body (or autoscopy) from this elevated perspective" (p. 11). These episodes are often

associated with vestibular sensations of elevation and floating and 180 degree inversion of one's body.

Brugger *et al.* (2006) distinguish between autoscopic hallucinations (visual perception of an exact mirror image of oneself, whole or part) and heautoscopy (confrontation with one's double, which may or may not mirror one's appearance). Heautoscopic echopraxia (imitation of bodily movements by the double) gives rise to the illusion that it is the Doppelgänger that contains the real mind, and may be accompanied by feelings of depersonalization, alienation from one's own body and dizziness. The authors review cases of polyopic heautoscopy, with multiple copies of the body and self, suggestive of multiple mappings of the body. They emphasize the specific importance of lesions at the temporo-occipitoparietal junction.

Depersonalization symptoms are not only found in near-death experiences or heautoscopic echopraxia, but also in a variety of psychiatric disorders. Depersonalization symptoms in psychiatric patients with depersonalization disorder positively correlate with increased parietal activity (Simeon *et al.*, 2000). Similarly, dissociative responses in patients with posttraumatic stress disorder associate with greater activation in the parietal lobe, occipital lobe and middle temporal gyri, as well as increased activation in the inferior frontal gyrus, medial prefrontal cortex, medial frontal gyrus and anterior cingulate gyrus (Lanius *et al.*, 2002). Out-of-body experiences and autoscopic hallucinations have been reported in various neurological conditions, such as epilepsy and migraine, and psychiatric conditions such as schizophrenia, depression, anxiety and dissociative disorders (Blanke *et al.*, 2004).

Out-of-body experiences may occur in 10% of the normal population (Blanke & Arzy, 2005). Parietal, temporal and occipital lobe involvement has again been implicated (Zamboni *et al.*, 2005). Blanke *et al.* (2002) reported a case where an out-of-body experience and visual body part illusions resulted after stimulation at the right temporoparietal junction. Blanke *et al.* (2004) postulate that an out-of-body experience follows failure to integrate sensory information regarding the body (proprioceptive, tactile and visual information) coupled with vestibular dysfunction, leading to disintegration between personal (vestibular) space and extrapersonal (visual) space. Dysfunction in the temporoparietal junction, which contains the vestibular cortex and is also implicated in neglect, is proposed. Brain damage to this area has been associated with vestibular sensations and feelings of agency (Blanke & Arzy, 2005).

Conclusion

It is not coincidental that the parietal lobe, an area of sensory convergence, plays a major role in most of the conditions we have reviewed. While we discuss possible sensory-perceptual underpinnings of abnormal sensory processes, we note that Roediger (1990) emphasized that there might be two potential processes whereby an organism might perceive external objects or events: a data-driven bottom-up hierarchical process of gradual and successive combination of lower-level analyses and outputs and also, in contrast, an "intelligent," concept-driven, top-down process that is almost akin to inspired guessing and which operates from an acquired knowledge of stored statistical properties and predictive probabilities.

The motor theory of speech perception (Liberman *et al.*, 1967), for example, embodies these principles. Speech perception involves the motor system in a process of auditory-to-articulatory mapping so as to access a phonetic code with motor properties (Wilson *et al.*, 2004). Similarly, in conversation, we tend to hear just what we have come to expect from the statistical nature (probabilities) of the phonological or semantic context. Indeed the errors ("confusions") made by listeners to "noisy" (i.e. unclear) speech tend to reflect the contextually likely upcoming articulatory *gestures* of the speaker (as if the listener is trying in real time to guess-ahead the next utterance from the speaker's vocal apparatus), rather than the resultant acoustic consequences (phonemes). The idea that perception is somehow linked, conceptually and pragmatically, to potential action is discussed in detail in the following chapter.

While anomalies of fundamental perceptual processing are good models, and partly explanatory of higher-level neuropsychiatric dysfunction, perception drives potential action, and anomalies at both levels must play equal roles in understanding the syndromes of neuropsychiatry.

References

André, J. M., Martinet, N., Paysant, J., Beis, J. M. & Le Chapelain, L. (2001). Temporary phantom limbs evoked by vestibular caloric stimulation in amputees. *Neuropsychiatry Neuropsychology and Behavioral Neurology*, 14(3), 190–196.

Anderson, D. N. (1988). The delusion of inanimate doubles: implications for understanding the Capgras phenomenon. *British Journal of Psychiatry*, **153**, 694–699.

Arzy, S., Overney, L. S., Landis, T. & Blanke, O. (2006). Neural mechanisms of embodiment: asomatognosia due to premotor damage. *Archives of Neurology*, **63**, 1022–1025.

Behrendt, R. P. & Young, C. (2004). Hallucinations in schizophrenia, sensory impairment, and brain disease: a unifying model. *Behavioral and Brain Sciences*, **27**, 771–830.

Blakemore, S. J., Bristow, D., Bird, G., Frith, C. & Ward, J. (2005). Somatosensory activations during the observation of touch and a case of vision-touch synaesthesia. *Brain*, **128**(Pt 7), 1571–1583.

Blanke, O. & Arzy, S. (2005). The out-of-body experience: disturbed self-processing at the temporo-parietal junction. *Neuroscientist*, **11**(1), 16–24.

Blanke, O., Landis, T., Spinelli, L. & Seeck, M. (2004). Out-of-body experience and autoscopy of neurological origin. *Brain*, **127**, 243–258.

Blanke, O., Ortigue, S., Landis, T. & Seeck, M. (2002). Stimulating illusory own-body perceptions. *Nature*, **419**, 269–270.

Bradshaw, J. L. (2001). *Developmental Disorders of the Frontostriatal System: Neuropsychological Neuropsychiatric and Evolutionary Perspectives*. Hove, UK: Psychology Press.

Bradshaw, J. L. & Mattingley, J. B. (1995). *Clinical Neuropsychology: Behavioral and Brain Science*. San Diego, CA: Academic Press.

Brugger, P., Blanke, O., Regard, M., Bradford, D. T. & Landis, T. (2006). Polyopic heautoscopy: case report and review of the literature. *Cortex*, **42**(5), 661–784.

Brugger, P., Kollias, S. S., Muri, R. M., Crelier, G. & Hepp-Reymond, M. (2000). Beyond remembering; Phantom sensations of congenitally absent limbs. *Proceedings of the National Academy of Sciences USA*, **97**(11), 6167–6172.

Buxbaum, L. J. (2006). On the right (and left) track: twenty years of progress in studying hemispatial neglect. *Cognitive Neuropsychology*, **23**(1), 184–201.

Desimone, R. & Ungerleider, L. G. (1989). Neural mechanisms of visual processing in monkeys. In F. Boller & J. Grafman (Eds.), *Handbook of Neuropsychology* (Vol. 2, pp. 267–299). Amsterdam: Elsevier.

Edelstyn, N. M. J. & Oyebode, A. F. (1999). A review of the phenomenology and cognitive neuropsychological origins of the Capgras syndrome. *International Journal of Geriatric Psychiatry*, **14**, 48–59.

Edelstyn, N. M. J., Riddoch, M. J., Oyebode, F., Humphreys, G. W. & Forde, E. (1996). Visual processing in patients with Frégoli syndrome. *Cognitive Neuropsychiatry*, **1**(2), 103–124.

Ellis, H. D. & Young, A. W. (1990). Accounting for delusional misidentifications. *British Journal of Psychiatry*, **157**, 239–248.

Ellis, H. D., Young, A. W., Quayle, A. H. & de Pauw, K. W. (1997). Reduced autonomic responses to faces in Capgras delusion. *Proceedings of the Royal Society of London B*, **264**(1384), 1085–1092.

First, M. B. (2005). Desire for amputation of a limb: paraphilia, psychosis or a new type of identity disorder. *Psychological Medicine*, **35**, 919–928.

Förstl, H., Almeida, O. P., Owen, A. M., Burns, A. & Howard, R. (1991). Psychiatric, neurological and medical aspects of misidentification syndromes: a review of 260 cases. *Psychological Medicine*, **21**, 905–910.

Frith, C. D. (1992). *The Cognitive Neuropsychology of Schizophrenia*. Hove, UK: Lawrence Erlbaum Associates.

Frith, C. D., Blakemore, S. J. & Wolpert, D. M. (2000). Abnormalities in the awareness and control of action. *Philosophical Transactions of the Royal Society of London B Biological Sciences*, **355**(1404), 1771–1788.

Goodale, M. & Milner, D. (2004). *Sight Unseen: An Exploration of Conscious and Unconscious Vision*. Oxford, UK: Oxford University Press.

Giummarra, M., Gibson, S., Georgiou-Karistianis, N. & Bradshaw, J. (2007). Central mechanisms in phantom limb perception: the past, present and future. *Brain Research Reviews*, **54**(1), 219–232.

Hamilton, M. (1985). *Fish's Clinical Psychopathology* (2nd edn.). Bristol, UK: John Wright and Sons.

Kell, C., von Kriegstein, K., Rosler, A., Kleinschmidt, A. & Laufs, H. (2005). The sensory cortical representation of the human penis: revisiting somatotopy in the male homunculus. *Journal of Neuroscience*, **25**(25), 5984–5987.

Kew, J. J., Halligan, P. W., Marshall, J. C., *et al.* (1997). Abnormal access of axial vibrotactile input to deafferentated somatosensory cortex in human upper limb amputees. *Journal of Neurophysiology*, **77**, 2735–2764.

Knecht, S., Henninngsen, H., Hohling, C. *et al.* (1998). Plasticity of plasticity? Changes in the pattern of perceptual correlates of reorganization after amputation. *Brain*, **121**, 717–724.

Lanius, R. A., Williamson, P. C., Boksman, K. *et al.* (2002). Brain activation during script-driven imagery induced dissociative responses in PTSD: a functional magnetic resonance imaging investigation. *Biological Psychiatry*, **52**, 305–311.

Liberman, A. M., Cooper, F. S., Shankweiler, D. P. & Studdert-Kennedy, M. (1967). Perception of the speech code. *Psychological Review*, **74**(6), 431–461.

Maruff, P., Wood, S. J., Velakoulis, D. *et al.* (2005). Reduced volume of parietal and frontal association areas in patients with schizophrenia characterised by passivity delusions. *Psychological Medicine*, **35**, 783–789.

Mattingley, J. B., Rich, A. N., Yelland, G. & Bradshaw, J. L. (2001). Unconscious priming eliminates automatic binding of colour and alphanumeric form in synaesthesia. *Nature*, **410**(6828), 580–582.

McGonigle, D. J., Hanninen, R., Salenius, S. *et al.* (2002). Whose arm is it anyway? An fMRI case study of supernumerary phantom limb. *Brain: a Journal of Neurology*, **125**(6), 1265–1274.

Melzack, R. (1990). Phantom limbs and the concept of a neuromatrix. *Trends in Neurosciences*, **13**(3), 88–92.

Melzack, R., Isreal, R., Lacroix, R. & Schultz, G. (1997). Phantom limbs in people with congenital limb deficiency or amputation in early childhood. *Brain*, **120**, 1603–1620.

Parton, A., Malhotra, P. & Husain, M. (2004). Hemispatial neglect. *Journal of Neurology Neurosurgery and Psychiatry*, **75**(1), 13–21.

Paulesu, E., Harrison, J., Baron-Cohen, S. *et al.* (1995). The physiology of coloured hearing: a PET activation study of colour-word synaesthesia. *Brain*, **118**, 661–676.

Ramachandran, V. S. & Blakeslee, S. (1998). *Phantoms in the Brain*. New York, NY: William Morrow.

Rich, A. N. (2004). *An Investigation of the Cognitive and Neural Mechanisms Underlying Lexical-Colour Synaesthesia*. PhD thesis. University of Melbourne, Melbourne.

Rich, A. N. & Mattingley, J. B. (2002). Anomalous perception in synaesthesia: a cognitive neuroscience perspective. *Nature Reviews Neuroscience*, **3**(1), 43–52.

Rich, A. N., Bradshaw, J. L. & Mattingley, J. B. (2005). A systematic, large-scale study of synaesthesia: implications for the role of early experience in lexical-colour associations. *Cognition*, **98**(1), 53–84.

Roediger, H. L. (1990). Memory metaphors in cognitive psychology. *Memory and Cognition*, **8**, 231–246.

Rojo, V. I., Caballero, L., Iruela, L. M. & Baca, E. (1991). Capgras syndrome in a blind patient. *American Journal of Psychiatry*, **148**, 1272.

Seal, M. L., Aleman, A. & McGuire, P. K. (2004). Compelling imagery, unanticipated speech and deceptive memory: neurocognitive models of auditory verbal hallucinations in schizophrenia. *Cognitive Neuropsychiatry*, **9**(1/2), 43–72.

23

Simeon, D., Guralnik, O., Hazlett, E. A. *et al.* (2000). Feeling unreal: A PET study of depersonalisation disorder. *American Journal of Psychiatry*, **157**, 1782–1788.

Sims, A. (2003). *Symptoms in the Mind: An Introduction to Descriptive Psychopathology* (3rd edn.). London: Saunders.

Spence, S. A., Brooks, D. J., Hirsch, S. R. *et al.* (1997). A PET study of voluntary movement in schizophrenic patients experiencing passivity phenomena (delusions of alien control). *Brain*, **120**, 1997–2011.

Starr, A. & Sporty, L. D. (1994). Similar disorders viewed with different perspectives. A challenge for neurology and psychiatry. *Archives of Neurology*, **51**(10), 977–980.

Ungerleider, L. G. & Mishkin, M. (1982). Two cortical visual systems. In D. Ingle, M. A. Goodale & R. J. W. Mansfield (Eds.), *Analysis of Visual Behavior* (pp. 549–586). Cambridge, MA: MIT Press.

Ventre-Dominey, J., Nighoghossian, N. & Denise, P. (2003). Evidence for interacting cortical control of vestibular function and spatial representation in man. *Neuropsychologia*, **41**, 1884–1898.

Weiskrantz, L. (1986). *Blindsight: A Case Study and Implications*. New York, NY: Oxford University Press.

Wilson, S. M., Saygin, A. P., Sereno, M. I. & Iacoboni, M. (2004). Listening to speech activates motor areas involved in speech production. *Nature Neuroscience*, 7(7), 701–702.

Wolpert, D. M., Miall, R. C. & Kawato, M. (1998). Internal models in the cerebellum. *Trends in Cognitive Sciences*, **2**, 338–347.

Zamboni, G., Budriesi, C. & Nichell, P. (2005). "Seeing oneself": a case of autoscopy. *Neurocase*, **11**, 212–215.

Chapter 3

Processes and mechanisms in neuropsychiatry: motor-executive processes

Nicole Rinehart, Phyllis Chua and John L. Bradshaw

Introduction

"The irritating historical division between neurology and psychiatry is at its most arbitrary in the field of movement disorders" (Lennox & Lennox, 2002, p. 28).

The introduction and differentiation of "extrapyramidal motor disorders" from "pyramidal disorders," by Wilson in 1912, heralded a major paradigm shift (Rogers, 1992). Wilson conceptualized disorders that had traditionally been regarded as "psychiatric" or "functional," such as Parkinson's disease, as extrapyramidal. In addition, he also described a group of patients with motor symptoms, the majority of whom also experienced psychiatric symptoms with diagnoses of hysteria or schizophrenia. Although neurology and psychiatry have continued to develop along separate lines, disorders such as Parkinson's disease, Huntington's disease and Gilles de la Tourette syndrome (GTS), which straddle the neurology and psychiatry boundary, highlight the importance of understanding both motor and psychological processes in these and other conditions. This may offer insight into the neural correlates and clinical management of these disorders.

This chapter will discuss the relevance of the neuromotor circuitry and recent theoretical advances in motor theories that relate to the underlying neuropathophysiology of these disorders.

Neuromotor circuitry

The basal ganglia and cerebellum are key neural structures in the brain's motor circuitry. The basal ganglia are comprised of the caudate, putamen, globus pallidus and substantia nigra. The caudate and putamen form the striatum, and the putamen and globus pallidus are referred to as the lentiform nucleus. Generally speaking the striatum is the input layer of the basal ganglia and lentiform nucleus the output layer. Basal ganglia efferents are inhibitory to the thalamus. The cerebellar hemispheres are functionally analogous input layers of the cerebellum; however, unlike the striatum which receives afferents directly from the cortices, the cerebellum receives cortical input via pontine nuclei that then project via mossy fibers to the cortex of the cerebellum. The three deep cerebellar structures, the fastigial, dentate and interposed nuclei, have excitatory projections to the thalamus and can be conceived in simple terms as the output layer.

The basal ganglia and cerebellum both project via the thalamus to widespread areas of the cortex, influencing motor and cognitive functioning. Disorders such as Parkinson's disease and Huntington's diseases, with discrete and well-defined neuropathology, have served as a model for basal ganglia dysfunction. Similarly, diseases such as Friedreich's ataxia with known cerebellar pathology serve as models for cerebellar influence on the cortex. While the basal ganglia play a central role in the initiation and mediation of movements, the cerebellum is more involved in controlling and tempering end-stage movement (Bradshaw & Mattingley, 1995); for example, cerebellar lesions result in movements which are inaccurate, rough and variable (Robinson & Fuchs, 2001). Although traditionally the roles of these structures were conceived as purely motor, there is converging evidence indicating damage to basal ganglia and cerebellum can have deleterious consequences for cognitive functioning (Glickstein, 2006).

The Neuropsychology of Mental Illness, ed. Stephen J. Wood, Nicholas B. Allen and Christos Pantelis. Published by Cambridge University Press. © Cambridge University Press 2009.

Conceptual advances in motor theory: affordances and mirror neurons, motor control models

The general clumsiness (e.g. "dropping things") so often described in psychiatric disorders may eventually be more carefully re-defined and understood in the context of *"affordances."* Similarly, problems with motor imitation skills may lead to motor learning difficulties to be interpretable via the concept of *"mirror neurons."* Motor control models such as feed forward, motor overflow and the role of top-down influences, as well as attention, may contribute to our understanding of the more complex motor phenomena.

Affordances

The concept of two complementary visual systems (Ungerleider & Mishkin, 1982), a dorsal system located in the posterior parietal cortex and a ventral system located in the inferior occipito-temporal cortex responsible for unconscious and conscious object identification respectively, underlies the notion of affordance. When picking up a cup, we typically do so via the handle, not the body of the receptacle; many such objects elicit "use-appropriate" hand postures, reflecting the accessing of stored ("dorsal stream") information about object identity and potential utility. Indeed, the central nervous system as a whole has necessarily evolved in the service of potential action. Such "preparation for action," largely the province of the dorsal stream, highlights an important new theoretical concept of *affordance*, which is a central component of ecological psychology (Gibson, 1979). Affordances, generally, are properties of the environment taken relative to an observer's standpoint. Thus representations for action that are elicited by an object's visual affordance serve to potentiate motor components (a specific hand position or posture to adopt), so that a response and action is initiated. Intraparietal regions may extract such affordance information for the premotor cortex in due course to initiate and execute appropriate action (Taira *et al.*, 1990). How we represent the sensory or perceptual world arises partly from affordances using a repertoire of stored actions; actions that are developed on the basis of interactions between the visual attributes of an object and the conscious, deliberate and contextually relevant goal of the observer. An object's

possibilities for action, namely its affordances, are built directly into its perceptual representation. Therefore, perceptual and motor processes are inextricably linked, i.e. perception as potential or implicit action, and action in a perceptually relevant context. Indeed, according to this view, objects may potentiate a range of actions associated with them, irrespective of the intentions of the viewer.

When such potentiation overrides intentionality, we may see *utilization behavior*; this can occur when distractedly picking up and toying with an object, or when prefrontal damage and inhibitory dysfunction are present. Following bilateral medial frontal lobe damage the patient may display a compulsive, inappropriate urge to use objects in sight. Such utilization behavior is thought to manifest from a supervisory-system deficit (Della Sala, 2005; Frith *et al.*, 2000). The patient may offer confabulatory explanations for such behavior, given that they often seem unaware of the inappropriateness of the behavior. This situation of course contrasts with our own realization when abstractedly and absent-mindedly, for example, taking off all our clothes when we only intended to change our socks.

An extreme example of such behavior is the *anarchic hand* phenomenon. While patients after parietal damage with optic ataxia (Balint's syndrome, see Perenin & Vighetto, 1988) or certain forms of apraxia have great difficulty picking up, grasping or manipulating objects which they can see quite clearly, patients showing the anarchic hand sign may complain that a hand makes apparently purposeful, complex, smooth and well-formed movements of its own accord, and quite contrary to the patient's own intention or will (Della Sala, 2005). The patients are aware of their limb's bizarre and potentially hazardous behavior, but cannot inhibit it. They often refer to the feeling that one of their hands behaves as if it had a will of its own, but never deny that this capricious hand is part of their own body – as can happen with severe unilateral neglect (Parton *et al.*, 2004). Thus self-ownership of actions is apparently separable from awareness of actions; affected patients are aware of their anarchic hand, which they know is part of their own anatomy and not a robotic counterfeit, yet they disown its actions. Affected patients typically have medial frontal lobe damage, in the vicinity of the supplementary motor area (SMA), on the side contralateral to the wayward hand. The SMA is known (Cunnington *et al.*, 1996) to be responsible for converting self-generated (as opposed to externally initiated) intentions into self-initiated action sequences or motor subroutines related to internal drives. Environmentally relevant movement sequences can, instead, be initiated by the alternative, lateral, premotor system. This system, remaining intact in the patient with an anarchic hand, will now take over and drive the patient's hand, to their consternation, according to triggering events or objects encountered in the external environment. Note that the term "alien hand," often used as a synonym for the anarchic hand (Marchetti & Della Sala, 1998), means a range of different things to different authors, and perhaps is best seen as uncooperative behavior or posturing by a hand which especially is felt to be somehow foreign to or "estranged" from its owner (hemisomatognosia), and may or may not require alternative (to SMA involvement) or additional callosal damage (Bundick & Spinella, 2000; Chan & Liu, 1999).

Mirror neurons

This essential and inextricably linked interrelatedness of perception and action is also played out in the recent discovery and account of mirror neurons (Arbib, 2005; Rizzolatti & Craighero, 2004). *Canonical neurons*, abundant in the rear section of the monkey's arcuate sulcus (part of area F5), may fire whenever a particular object is seen, as a function of its shape, size and spatial orientation. They may also fire when an animal is presented with a graspable object, irrespective of whether this is followed up by an actual grasping response (cf. the concept of affordances, above), or alternatively when a specific response or response sequence is initiated. They do not fire, however, when the individual merely observes actions performed by another. Conversely, *mirror neurons*, first identified in the convexity of area F5 of the primate frontal cortex, and now thought to be widely distributed in the brain, are active both when the monkey performs certain actions, *and when they observe actions performed* by another monkey or person. In this way, unlike canonical neurons, mirror neurons do *not* respond when objects alone are presented (Rizzolatti & Craighero, 2004). Mirror neurons represent a mechanism for object-directed action capable of coupling the observation of another's actions and their execution, as if they were performing the actions observed themselves.

Consequently, we must now add a third term to the relation between *perception* and *action*;

simulation. Understanding others' beliefs, intentions and actions is an important social ability – "theory of mind" – possibly deficient in certain developmental disorders of the fronto-striatal system such as autism (Happe, 1999) and schizophrenia (Brune, 2005). While a mere visual representation, without involvement of the motor system, can describe the superficial, visible aspects of another agent's movement, it fails to provide information critical for understanding "action semantics" (Nelissen *et al.*, 2005). That is, what the action concerns, its goal and context. Likewise action information, without knowledge concerning object identity, again can only tell half the story. We need to combine information about object identity with semantic information about the action. This may be the role of mirror neurons, in matching observed actions with their corresponding internal motor representations. Nelissen *et al.* (2005) report that the monkey's frontal lobe hosts multiple representations of others' actions. Representations located caudally in F5 seem to be context-dependent, activated only when the agent is seen, while representations in rostral F5 and prefrontally code the action. In humans area 44, a probable homolog of monkey F5, plays a fundamental role in speech; the motor theory of speech perception (Liberman *et al.*, 1967) posits an active, if tacit, recreation of the speaker's articulatory intentions. Parenthetically, it is also noteworthy that the canonical neurons of monkey F5 receive input from the anterior parietal sulcus in the form of neural codes for *affordances* e.g. grasping (Taira *et al.*, 1990).

While the classical studies of the mirror system indicate that some of the same motor regions are activated both when performing and when observing a movement, there is also evidence that such motor activity may even occur *prior* to observing another's action. Thus the mere knowledge of the likelihood of another's upcoming movement may be sufficient to excite the observer's mirror-motor system (Kilner *et al.*, 2004). This would enable (as in the motor theory of speech perception) one to anticipate rather than to merely react to another's actions.

Neurons responding to the observation of actions done by others are not present only in area F5. Movements effective in eliciting neural responses in the cortex of the superior temporal sulcus include walking, turning the head, bending the torso, and goal-directed hand and arm movements (Rizzolatti & Craighero, 2004). However, the mirror system may not necessarily be restricted to motor functions.

Blakemore *et al.* (2005) report a new form of synesthesia, where visual perception of touch elicited conscious tactile experiences in the observer. This may have occurred because the mirror system for touch (parietal and premotor cortices and superior temporal sulcus) proved overactive (as shown by fMRI) and above the normal threshold for conscious tactile perception. Pain, too, when observed in others, may excite the observer's mirror system and lead to painful sensations (Avenanti *et al.*, 2005; Bradshaw & Mattingley, 1995). As Singer & Frith (2005) note, we all have a remarkable and largely involuntary capacity to share the experience of others; for example, yawns are infectious, and we wince when we see another person trap her fingers in a door.

Two main hypotheses have been advanced on the underlying function of mirror neurons; they might mediate imitation or more likely are the basis of action understanding (Rizzolatti & Craighero, 2004). Each time an individual sees an action performed by another, neurons representing that action are activated in the observer's premotor cortex. This automatically induced motor representation of the observed action corresponds to the representation that is spontaneously executed during self-generated action. Thus, a role of the mirror system can be regarded as the transformation of visual information into knowledge, and actions performed by another become messages that are understood without any cognitive mediation. On the basis of this, the mirror-neuron system provides a potential mechanism from which language may have evolved, probably via an oral-manual stage. The mirror neuron hypotheses have been used to explain the diverse motor, social and communicative impairments which characterize pervasive developmental disorders (see Williams *et al.*, 2001), and may be invoked to account for neuromotor impairments which we see across the psychiatry spectrum.

Motor control models

Feed forward models

Prior knowledge can also enable us to predict the sensory changes resulting from movements. The "forward model" proposes that prior knowledge based on intended actions can modify perception. The "forward dynamic model" allows the prediction of the trajectory of the limb movement in space and time, whilst the "forward output model" predicts the

tactile and kinesthetic sensations resulting from the movement (Frith, 2005). Environmentally appropriate responding towards a goal demands production and control of sequences of requisite muscle contractions, in the context of initial sensory input and feedback that is consequent upon action. Note must also be made of the current configurations of joint angles and limb postures prior to implementation of the motor commands (Frith *et al.*, 2000). Just prior to movement initiation, a predictor, receiving an efference copy from the initiating motor system, estimates the movements' likely sensory consequences (reafference). In this way compensation can be made for the sensory effects of movement and, secondly, in the event of response error, corrections can be initiated.

Several studies have shown that forward modelling is abnormal in patients with schizophrenia when they have to consciously attend to their actions; however no abnormalities in implicit, automatic use of forward modelling such as anticipatory adjustments of grip force when picking up objects were noted in such patients. Different areas may be involved: the frontal cortex for initiating actions, the sensory areas to process the consequences of actions, and the anterior cingulate cortex to detect discrepancies. Disconnections between these brain areas may explain the different symptoms reported in schizophrenia (Frith, 2005), and disconnections between the frontal and parietal regions may account for the misperception of limb positions in delusions of control. The absence of delusional explanations in neurological patients with lesions in these brain regions, e.g. anarchic hand after parietal lobe lesions, is noteworthy. Additional concepts such as "intentional binding" which draws together cause and effect in perceived time may bridge such gaps. Intentional binding occurs when, for example, we put together cause (e.g. we push a button or watch someone else push a button) and effect (e.g. the resulting sound). There may be exaggerated intentional binding in patients with schizophrenia, perhaps explaining incorrect attribution of agency in those with delusions of control or persecution.

Motor control and attention

While we can attend to and be aware of our intended movements and perform movement sequences in imagination; *fast, overlearnt and automatic responding is typically best achieved below the level of conscious awareness.* We may only be aware of our movements when they deviate from what we intend or expect to occur.

It may be that young people with motor coordination problems who have difficulty with automatic responding (e.g. catching a ball) are processing at a more conscious level that results in a slowed, awkward motor response falling short of the target behavior. Operating at a more conscious level in this way would perhaps place greater demands on the attentional and executive control centers of the brain (i.e. the prefrontal and cortico-thalamo-cortical circuitry), which are typically impaired in neurodevelopmental disorders.

This fits with the phenomenon of *kinesia paradoxa*, where "the individual who typically experiences severe difficulties with the most simple of movements" (e.g. running) "may suddenly perform complex, skilled movements" (e.g. running and trying to get a ball) (Leary & Hill, 1996, p. 41). For example, individuals with Asperger's disorder have been described as showing considerable dexterity in drawing, model building, or playing a computer game (particularly if the topic is one of special interest, and therefore benefits from the child's directed attention) (Leary & Hill, 1996). Yet, they show abnormalities in everyday, simple motor tasks such as walking or catching a ball, often appearing uncoordinated and clumsy. It may be that individuals with autism or Asperger's disorder exhibit more skillful movement on these (seemingly) more difficult tasks because attention becomes more focused, either because they become obsessed with a particular motor task (e.g. computer games) or more complex tasks have more cues embedded (e.g. verbal instructions, visual cues) to focus the individual's attention, which enables motor functioning to become automated.

These observations suggest that prefrontal input (mediating focused attention) to the cerebellum and possibly basal ganglia are able to play an important modulatory role in motor behavior. In addition the thalamus, an area that is neuroanatomically anomalous in autism (Tsatsanis *et al.*, 2003), has major connections to both the cerebellum and basal ganglia fronto-striatal circuitry; it has also been implicated in such paradoxical motor improvements when compromised and may play a mediating role in such "kinesia paradoxa" (Mennemeier *et al.*, 1996).

Our understanding of how attentional focus interacts with motor functioning is at the heart of understanding how movement abnormalities may translate to functional impairment in a psychiatric context. Unlike the movement disorder of more classic neurological disorders such as Parkinson's disease, movement disorders that appear in a developmental psychiatric context, with multiple circuitry involvement (e.g. involving the thalamus, basal ganglia, cerebellum, fronto-striatal region) are less likely to be "fixed" (e.g. shuffling, uncoordinated gait) or "consistent" (e.g. continually postured arms), and may be more contextually dependent.

Motor overflow

Motor overflow refers to the involuntary movement which can sometimes accompany voluntary movement. Three forms of motor overflow have been described: (1) associated movement when involuntary movement occurs in non-homologous muscles in either the ipsilateral or contralateral limbs; (2) contralateral mirror movement when directly observable involuntary movements occur in homologous muscles contralateral to the voluntary movements; and (3) contralateral motor irradiation when involuntary movements detected on electromyogram occur in homologous muscles contralateral to the voluntary movements (Hoy *et al.*, 2004). Most theories on the etiology of motor overflow such as transcallosal facilitation and ipsilateral activation theory have focused on potential cortical origins, although the possibility of subcortical contribution remains. Motor overflow has been described in several populations including normal adults under effortful conditions, children under the age of ten, and the elderly, and is pronounced in Huntington's disease, Parkinson's disease, obsessive-compulsive disorder and schizophrenia. In Huntington's disease, abnormal intracortical inhibition and resultant disinhibition of ipsilateral descending fibers have been postulated to be responsible for the motor overflow (Hoy *et al.*, 2004). In contrast, there is evidence of corpus callosum abnormalities in patients with schizophrenia, which can result in greater transcallosal facilitation (Hoy *et al.*, 2004).

Neuromotor dysfunction and mental disorders
Disorders usually first diagnosed in infancy, childhood or adolescence

Neuromotor soft signs identified in early childhood (e.g. 6–10 years of age) are now increasingly recognized as an early marker of various developmental problems and later-onset psychiatric disorders (Bergman *et al.*, 1997). As movement is affected by the aberrant neurodevelopmental processes which appear to be associated with, and in some cases define, many early-onset psychiatric disorders, neuromotor assessment tasks have much to offer in the way of improving diagnostic definition and conceptualizations of comorbidity. Neuromotor assessment tools may also act as important neurobiological probes to brain dysfunction in disorders where imaging has so far been unable to make strong inroads into neuropathological processes. Thus, while neuromotor assessment may, on the surface, seem more at home with the study of "frank" movement disorders, such as Parkinson's and Huntington's disease, it is perhaps the neurodevelopmental psychiatric disorders associated with much less obvious structural and discernable functional brain abnormality, which may stand to benefit the most from such investigations.

The majority of childhood psychiatric disorders involve motor disturbance to a greater (e.g. autism) or lesser degree (e.g. learning disabilities). The inclusion of a seemingly "neurological" condition such as Developmental coordination disorder (DCD) in the *Diagnostic and Statistical Manual of Mental Disorders* (DSM – IV-TR; American Psychiatric Association, 2000), underscores Lennox & Lennox's (2002) point about the "irritating historical division between neurology and psychiatry . . ." (p. 28). Developmental coordination disorder involves a range of possible disruptions to motor development and activities including delays in meeting motor milestones (e.g. sitting, crawling and walking), general clumsiness (e.g. "dropping things"), subaverage performance in sports and/or poor handwriting. It is interesting to note that disorders such as autism and Asperger's disorder, both associated with movement disorders, cannot be comorbidly diagnosed with DCD. Attention-deficit hyperactivity disorder (ADHD), on the other hand, a disorder which also involves marked motor coordination impairment (Barkley, 1997), can be comorbid with DCD, but not with autism and Asperger's disorder. The issue of comorbidity has been described as an "important if vexatious issue in psychopathology" (Bradshaw, 2001, p. 259). It may be that movement coordination problems are a risk factor for a multitude of psychiatric disorders which involve "extrapyramidal" structures such as the basal ganglia and cerebellum. These structures form cortico-thalamo-cortical re-entrant loops and play a key role in selecting, inhibiting, releasing, filtering, modulating and automatizing cognitive-motor function (Bradshaw, 2001). There is a potential relationship between concomitant comorbid conditions and greater involvement of the cortico-thalamo-cortical circuitry (Bradshaw, 2001). It is not uncommon to find that an individual with autism or Asperger's disorder may show clinically significant signs of motor coordination disorder, ADHD, depression and anxiety (Tonge *et al.*, 1999).

In relation to pervasive developmental disorders, in particular autism and Asperger's disorder, there has been much speculation about several issues including: the validity of separate diagnostic labeling, issues of diagnostic comorbidity, the role of movement abnormality in the clinical expression of the disorders, and the role of the basal ganglia and cerebellum. As a result these disorders are perhaps the best "model" to exemplify how neuromotor investigation has advanced, and may further advance, clinical child psychiatry and psychology.

Case focus: autism and Asperger's disorder. An example of how neuromotor investigation has the potential to offer new insights into etiology and diagnosis

The clinical focus in disorders such as autism and Asperger's disorder has traditionally been directed to the more salient social and communicative impairments. Research criteria in DSM–IV-TR separates children with autism and Asperger's disorder based on language and intellectual functioning criteria. There is a tendency for individuals diagnosed with Asperger's disorder to continue to be conceptualized as having a "milder" variant of autism, with the terms Asperger's disorder (AD) and high-functioning autism (HFA) often used interchangeably.

Instrumented gait analysis may play an important adjunctive role in the assessment and differential diagnosis of psychiatric disorders. In the context of autism and AD this approach has revealed distinct patterns of *cerebellar gait variability* which are a distinguishing feature of autism (cf: non-clinical populations) in children from 4–6 years of age (usual age of diagnosis) through to adolescence (Rinehart *et al.*, 2006c, 2006d). Moreover, there is some evidence that atypical movement disturbances impacting on crawling may be observable in autism as young as infancy, and appear before the diagnostically relevant social-communicative signs (Teitelbaum *et al.*, 1998). Similar retrospective findings have been reported in the schizophrenia literature (Schiffman *et al.*, 2004). The observation that autism is associated with greater "cerebellar" gait variability than AD (the latter is perhaps more a basal ganglia fronto-striatal gait disorder) is consistent with the general body of research which has particularly focused on cerebellar deficits in autism (Courchesne, 1999). This is also consistent with upper-body kinematic analysis which reveals that individuals with autism, but not Asperger's disorder, show cerebellar-like deficits in accurately modulating later stages of movement in order to efficiently "home-in" on targets (Rinehart *et al.*, 2006a).

DSM-IV-TR only hints that motor functioning is differentially affected by these disorders; for example, "motor clumsiness and awkwardness" (p. 81) is described as a feature of Asperger's disorder, and "abnormalities of posture" (for example, walking on tiptoe, odd hand movements and body postures) (p. 71) as a feature of autistic disorder. Neuromotor investigations, however, may more accurately dissociate between these disorders. For example, in contrast to the DSM-IV-TR description above, blindly rated video observational analysis by gait experts has revealed that *both* autism *and* AD may be associated with motor clumsiness; however, AD may be dissociated from autism more on the basis of abnormalities in terms of head and trunk posture (Rinehart *et al.*, 2006b). These observable upper-body postural abnormalities fit well with Damasio & Maurer's (1978) "Parkinsonian" view of autism, given the putative role of the basal ganglia in regulating postural alignment and axial motor control (Morris & Iansek, 1996).

A key feature of basal ganglia dysfunction is that it leads to a failure to maintain preparedness for movement ("motor set"), and is thought to result clinically in a mismatch between desired and actual movement (Morris & Iansek, 1996). Anecdotally, individuals with HFA (and AD) report difficulty in playing sport because there is a mismatch between wanting to "catch a ball" and actually catching the ball, noting that they tend to "duck" from the ball or move away at the last minute. Analysis of movement-related-potential activity (MRPs) over the supplementary motor area (a region which receives main input

from basal ganglia via the thalamus, and outputs to the primary motor cortex and back to the basal ganglia) reveals a reduced early component of the MRP similar to that observed in patients with Parkinson's disease (Cunnington *et al.*, 1995); this is consistent with the suggestion that autism may be associated with difficulties in maintaining adequate "motor set." The finding of normal post-movement MRP activity, which contrasts with Parkinson's disease (Cunnington *et al.*, 1995), suggests the presence of an intact "motor cue" for efficient running of well-learned motor sequences, and is consistent with clinical observation that individuals with autism do not have difficulty with well-learned movement sequences.

Disorders usually first diagnosed in late adolescence and adulthood

The role of neuromotor investigation is well established in psychiatric research of adult mental disorders. A detailed criticism of these findings in specific disorders will be covered in later chapters. Neuromotor dysfunction in adult mental disorders ranges from soft signs to more defined phenomena. In 1874, Kahlbaum described catatonia as an "insanity of tension" (Pfuhlmann & Stöber, 2001) referring to the abnormal mental and motor manifestations which he considered as a distinct clinical entity. Contemporary psychiatric classification systems such as ICD–10 and DSM–IV consider catatonia as a subtype of schizophrenia, despite the occurrence of catatonic features in affective and medical conditions.

The interrelated nature of motor and psychiatric phenomena is revealed in the observations of abnormal activity ranging from seemingly aimless pacing, restlessness or over- or under-activity, to more seemingly purposeful behaviors such as compulsive touching, self-mutilation and aggressive behaviors in patients with severe psychiatric disorders preceding the introduction of neuroleptics in 1954 (Rogers, 1992). The side-effects associated with the introduction of neuroleptics to treat psychosis, i.e. dystonia, akinesia and tardive dyskinesia, as well as antiparkinsonian medications to treat Parkinson's disease, i.e. psychoses, visual hallucinations and acute brain syndrome, only serve to emphasize the integral role of the basal ganglia and associated circuits in both groups of disorder. Oculomotor disturbances in these disorders suggest involvement of the dopaminergic system and frontal lobe.

A case exemplar of neuromotor and psychiatric abnormality is Gilles de la Tourette's syndrome (GTS), which is characterized by multiple vocal and motor tics and accompanied by many comorbid behavioral and cognitive problems such as obsessive-compulsive disorder, ADHD, learning difficulties, depression and anxiety (Bradshaw, 2001). The tics are preceded by an increasing sensation of tension relieved upon their release, which is often forceful and potentially self-injurious. Tics may be briefly suppressed or incorporated into a seemingly purposeful movement. Although not common, GTS is often associated with repetitive or obscene gestures or speech such as echopraxia, echolalia, palilalia, copropraxia and coprolalia. Not surprisingly, a disinhibitory response to the Simon task in the incongruent condition has been observed in GTS (Bradshaw, 2001). Deficits in visuomotor integration tasks such as Rey Osterrieth Complex Figure copying have been consistently reported (Bradshaw, 2001). It is unclear whether deficits on motor tasks, such as Purdue Pegboard or finger tapping, are secondary to this visuomotor integration deficit. Eye movement abnormalities have also been found. The occurrence of tics in other pathological conditions affecting this region such as carbon monoxide poisoning, encephalitis lethargica (Stern, 2000) and volumetric changes in the basal ganglia support a basal ganglia dysfunction theory. All evidence indicates failure of the striatopallidal gating of motor, cognitive and limbic pathways resulting in the inability to suppress impulsivity. A more complex model involving aberrant activity in the sensorimotor, executive, language and paralimbic circuits has been suggested by PET studies (Stern, 2000).

Obsessive-compulsive disorder (OCD) is often seen as the cognitive counterpart of GTS, although there are important differences such as the ideational component and the overfocusing of attention in OCD. The main symptoms of OCD are recurrent, intrusive thoughts, impulses or images (obsessions) often accompanied by ritualistic behaviors (compulsions) that cannot be resisted without increasing anxiety. Recent research has hinted at subtle differences in OCD populations depending on the presence of tics or soft neurological signs. Tic-related OCD has an earlier onset in childhood, is commoner in boys and responds less well to selective serotonin inhibitors alone (Bradshaw, 2001). The content of the OCD symptoms varies depending on the presence or absence of tics, with contamination themes and rituals being more common in non tic-related OCD, and the need to touch or rub, blinking or staring rituals, the need for symmetry, and intrusive aggressive images being more common in OCD with comorbid tics. Kinematic analysis of handwriting to assess subtle motor dysfunction found differences between responders and non-responders to combined sertraline and behavior therapy (Mergl, 2005).

The high prevalence of depression in motor disorders such as Parkinson's disease, Huntington's disease and Wilson's disease, as well as the recognition of the psychomotor symptoms of depression, have led to increased interest in using these specific basal ganglia diseases as models to study depression (Sobin, 1998). Some researchers continue to argue that the incidence of depression in these motor disorders is a psychological reaction to a chronic illness, whilst others view the depression and the motor manifestations equally as manifestations of underlying brain abnormalities. The observation that depression can precede the onset of motor symptoms of Huntington's disease by many years, and can occur in those who may not be aware of their being at risk for the disorder, provides support for the latter (Peyser & Folstein, 1990). The view that depression is reactive to stress and has no underlying cerebral pathology should therefore be rejected.

The psychomotor symptoms observed in major depression including slowed movement, shuffling gait, stooped posture, soft and monotonous speech, facial immobility and purposeless movements of the limbs and trunk, closely mimic the symptoms of Parkinson's disease. Psychomotor retardation has been correlated with reduced blood flow in the left dorsolateral prefrontal cortex (DLPFC) and left angular gyrus (Bench, 1993). Similar neuroimaging findings in patients with diminished speech in aphasia and chronic schizophrenia implicate the role of the left DLPFC in volitional and intentional activities, and in interconnecting with the anterior cingulate. The angular gyrus plays an important role in visuospatial orientation and attention. In contrast, marked motor agitation has been associated with increased blood flow in the inferior parietal lobe and the cingulate cortex, which plays a role in drive and affect and connects with the higher association cortex (Bench, 1993). Neuropsychological deficits of executive dysfunction in major depression provide further support for involvement of the frontostriatal circuit in some subtypes of major depression (Bradshaw, 2001). Similar neuroimaging and neurocognitive findings in schizophrenia (described in Chapter 26) also implicate frontostriatal circuit abnormalities (Pantelis *et al.* 1992, 1997).

The significance of other motor abnormalities co-existing with other psychiatric phenomena is less well-defined. Neurological soft signs characterized by abnormalities in motor, sensory and integrative functions have been used as probes for non-specific central nervous system defects. Neurological soft signs in schizophrenia have been linked with genetic and environmental factors, such as intrauterine and perinatal trauma, and are hypothesized as non-specific markers of vulnerability to psychoses. A better understanding of the presence of neurological soft signs in other mental disorders as diverse as antisocial personality disorder (Lindberg *et al.*, 2004) and post-traumatic stress disorder (Gurvits *et al.*, 1997) may elucidate the underlying pathology of these disorders that have traditionally been regarded as falling more into the psychiatric realm.

Neuromotor assessment and research

Formal neurological examination including gait analysis and assessment for extrapyramidal symptoms as markers of basal ganglia involvement, e.g. muscular rigidity, bradykinesia, resting tremor and flexion posture, is an important part of neuropsychiatric assessment. Instruments such as the Geriatric Movement Disorders Assessment that include ratings on the Simpson Extrapyramidal Side Effect Scale (Simpson & Angus, 1970), the Abnormal Involuntary Movement Scale and the Neurological Evaluation Scale and Unified Huntington's Disease Rating Scale, can all provide quantitative measures for use in research. A variety of tools such as ambulatory activity monitors with solid state memory, along with kinematic analysis of handwriting using digitizing graphic tablets (Mergl, 2005), the Purdue Pegboard, and other reaction-timed and motor-coordination tasks can enhance and quantify clinically observable and more subtle motor behaviors.

While in the past instrumented neurological examination (e.g. gait analysis) and EEG have been described as "non-contributory" (p. 64) in a developmental psychiatric assessment context (Graham *et al.*, 2001), it might be that the future coupling of EEG and movement tasks, together with systematic gait analysis using clinical technologies that are commercially available, may greatly improve our definition of early-onset psychiatric disorders.

Other relatively new technologies such as transcranial magnetic stimulation (TMS) also open up new possibilities for investigating psychiatric disorders. Transcranial magnetic stimulation is a non-invasive means of stimulating nerve cells (in excitatory or inhibitory fashion) in superficial areas of the brain, providing a powerful method for the study of motor cortical function. Transcranial magnetic stimulation applied to the motor cortex of human subjects has been extensively used to investigate normal motor cortical physiology and disease states (Fitzgerald *et al.*, 2002). Transcranial magnetic stimulation methods have a significant advantage over other methods of assessment of motor function as they are completely independent of motivation, attention and other elements of higher cognitive function (Fitzgerald *et al.*, 2002). Possible comorbid impairments must be taken into account when we are assessing neuromotor functioning in a psychiatric context.

Eye movements "whose premotor structures and descending commands are the best understood of any motor system" may also play a role in expanding our clinical and neurobiological understanding of psychiatric disorders (Robinson & Fuchs, 2001). The most important advantage of applying this approach to these complex cognitive–motor disorders is that the ocular motor system, truly a window directly in to the brain, has a reduced number of degrees of freedom of movement and little in the way of plastic or inertial forces. Therefore, output closely mirrors the command signals and the cognitive influences on them.

While conventional clinical diagnosis of early-onset psychiatric disorders may take place informally (e.g. observation of skills during play, drawing), and sometimes with the use of standardized tests of motor ability such as the Bruininks–Osertesky test (Bruininks, 1978) and the Movement Assessment Battery for Children (Henderson & Sugden, 1992), future diagnosis of these disorders may include instrumented gait analysis, motor cortical EEG analysis, TMS, and ocular motor assessment; all of which will shed greater light on the neurobiological underpinnings of these disorders and thereby have *early* intervention and management implications.

Summary

The etiological relevance of neuromotor dysfunction has now been established as a key focus of clinical research for a number of psychiatric disorders such as autism and schizophrenia. Renewed interest in the application of neuromotor assessment in the psychiatric arena occurs in parallel to critical developments in our understanding of the neural connectivity of the prefrontal cortex, basal ganglia and cerebellum (Hoshi *et al.*, 2005). Conceptual advances have been made in our understanding of higher-order awareness and control of "action," mirror neurons, the concept of affordances, utilization behavior, and extreme neurological motor conditions such as the anarchic hand, all of which may form part of the larger landscape for understanding the complex cognitive–motor processing dysfunctions that occurs in people with mental illness.

References

American Psychiatric Association (2000). *Diagnostic and Statistical Manual of Mental Disorders, Fourth Edition – Text Revision*. Washington, DC: American Psychiatric Association Press.

Arbib, M. A. (2005). From monkey-like action recognition to human language: an evolutionary framework for neurolinguistics. *Behavioral and Brain Sciences*, **28**(2), 105–124.

Avenanti, A., Bueti, D., Galati, G. & Aglioti, S. M. (2005). Transcranial magnetic stimulation highlights the sensorimotor side of empathy for pain. *Nature Neuroscience*, **8**(7), 955–960.

Barkley, R. A. (1997). Behavioral inhibition, sustained attention, and executive functions: constructing a unifying theory of ADHD. *Psychological Bulletin*, **121**(1), 65–94.

Bench, C. J. (1993). Regional cerebral blood flow in depression measured by positron emission tomography: the relationship with clinical dimensions. *Psychological Medicine*, **23**, 579–590.

Bergman, A. J., Wolfson, M. A. & Walker, E. E. (1997). Neuromotor functioning and behaviour problems in children at risk for psychopathology. *Journal of Abnormal Child Psychology*, **25**(3), 229–237.

Blakemore, S. J., Bristow, D., Bird, G., Frith, C. & Ward, J. (2005). Somatosensory activations during the observation of touch and a case of vision-touch synaesthesia. *Brain*, **128**(7), 1571–1583.

Bradshaw, J. L. (2001). *Developmental Disorders of the Frontostriatal System: Neuropsychological, Neuropsychiatric and Evolutionary Perspectives*. Hove, UK: Psychology Press.

Bradshaw, J. L. & Mattingley, J. B. (1995). *Clinical Neuropsychology: Behavioral and Brain Science*. San Diego, CA: Academic Press.

Bruininks, R. H. (1978). *Bruininks–Oseretsky Test of Motor Proficiency*. Circle Pines, MN: American Guidance Service.

Brune, M. (2005). Theory of mind in schizophrenia: a review of the literature. *Schizophrenia Bulletin*, **31**(1), 21–42.

Bundick, T., Jr. & Spinella, M. (2000). Subjective experience, involuntary movement, and posterior alien hand syndrome. *Journal of Neurology, Neurosurgery and Psychiatry*, **68**(1), 83–85.

Chan, J.-L. & Liu, A. B. (1999). Anatomical correlates of alien hand syndromes. *Neuropsychiatry Neuropsychology and Behavioral Neurology*, **12**(3), 149–155.

Courchesne, E. (1999). An MRI study of autism: the cerebellum revisited. *Neurology*, **52**(5), 1106–1107.

Cunnington, R., Bradshaw, J. L. & Iansek, R. (1996). The role of the supplementary motor area in the control of voluntary movement. *Human Movement Science*, **15**, 627–647.

Cunnington, R., Iansek, R., Bradshaw, J. L. & Phillips, J. G. (1995). Movement-related potentials in Parkinson's disease: presence and predictability of temporal and spatial cues. *Brain*, **118**, 935–950.

Damasio, A. R. & Maurer, R. G. (1978). A neurological model for childhood autism. *Archives of Neurology*, **35**, 777–786.

Della Sala, S. (2005). The anarchic hand. *The Psychologist*, **18**(10), 606–609.

Fitzgerald, P. B., Brown, T. L. & Daskalakis, Z. J. (2002). The application of transcranial magnetic stimulation in psychiatry and neurosciences research. *Acta Psychiatrica Scandinavica*, **105**, 324–340.

Frith, C. (2005). The neural basis of hallucinations and delusions. *C.R. Biologies*, **328**, 169–175.

Frith, C. D., Blakemore, S. J. & Wolpert, D. M. (2000). Abnormalities in the awareness and control of action. *Philosophical Transactions of the Royal Society of London B Biological Sciences*, **355**(1404), 1771–1788.

Gibson, J. J. (1979). *The Ecological Approach to Visual Perception*. London: Erlbaum.

Glickstein, M. (2006). Thinking about the cerebellum. *Brain*, **129**, 288–292.

Graham, P., Turk, J. & Verhulst, F. (2001). *Child Psychiatry: A Developmental Approach*. Oxford: Oxford University Press.

Gurvits, T. S., Glibertson, M. W., Lasko, N. B., Orr, S. P. & Pitman, R. K. (1997). Neurological status of combat veterans and adult survivors of sexual abuse PTSD. *Annals of the New York Academy of Science*, **21**, 468–471.

Happe, F. (1999). Autism: cognitive deficit or cognitive style. *Trends in Cognitive Sciences*, **3**, 216–222.

Henderson, S. E. & Sugden, D. A. (1992). *Movement Assessment Battery for Children*. Sidcup, Kent: The Psychological Corporation Ltd.

Hoshi, E., Tremblay, L., Feger, J., Carras, P. L., & Strick, P. L. (2005). The cerebellum communicates with the basal ganglia. *Nature Neuroscience*, **11**, 1491–1493.

Hoy, K. E., Fitzgerald, P. B., Bradshaw, J. L., Armatas, C. A. & Georgiou-Karistianis, N. (2004). Investigating the cortical origins of motor overflow. *Brain Research Reviews*, **46**, 315–327.

Kilner, J. M., Vargas, C., Duval, S., Blakemore, S. J. & Sirigu, A. (2004). Motor activation prior to observation of a predicted movement. *Nature Neuroscience*, 7(12), 1299–1301.

Leary, M. R. & Hill, D. A. (1996). Moving on: autism and movement disturbance. *Mental Retardation*, **34**(1), 39–53.

Lennox, B. R. & Lennox, G. G. (2002). Mind and movement: the neuropsychiatry of movement disorders. *Journal of Neurology, Neurosurgery, and Psychiatry*, **72**(Suppl. 1), 28–31.

Liberman, A. M., Cooper, F. S., Shankweiler, D. P. & Studdert-Kennedy, M. (1967). Perception of the speech code. *Psychological Review*, **74**(6), 431–461.

Lindberg, N., Tani, P., Stenberg, J.-H. *et al.* (2004). Neurological soft signs in homicidal men with antisocial personality disorder. *European Psychiatry*, **19**, 433–437.

Marchetti, C. & Della Sala, S. (1998). Disentangling the alien and anarchic hand. *Cognitive Neuropsychiatry*, **3**, 191–207.

Mennemeier, M., Crosson, B., Williamson, D. J. *et al.* (1996). Tapping, talking and the thalamus: possible influence of the intralaminar nuclei on basal ganglia function. *Neuropsychologia*, **35**(2), 183–193.

Mergl, R. (2005). Can a subgroup of OCD patients with motor abnormalities and poor therapeutic response be identified? *Psychopharmacology*, **179**, 826–837.

Morris, M. E. & Iansek, R. (1996). Characteristics of motor disturbance in Parkinson's disease and strategies for movement rehabilitation. *Human Movement Science*, **15**, 649–669.

Nelissen, K., Luppino, G., Vanduffel, W., Rizzolatti, G. & Orban, G. A. (2005). Observing others: multiple action representation in the frontal lobe. *Science*, **310**(5746), 332–336.

Pantelis, C., Barnes, T. R. E. & Nelson, H. E. (1992). Is the concept of frontal-subcortical dementia relevant to schizophrenia? *British Journal of Psychiatry*, **160**, 442–460.

Pantelis, C., Barnes, T. R. E., Nelson, H. E. *et al.* (1997). Frontal-striatal cognitive deficits in patients with chronic schizophrenia. *Brain*, **120**, 1823–1843.

Parton, A., Malhotra, P. & Husain, M. (2004). Hemispatial neglect. *Journal of Neurology, Neurosurgery and Psychiatry*, **75**(1), 13–21.

Perenin, M. T. & Vighetto, A. (1988). Optic ataxia: a specific disruption in visuomotor mechanisms. I. Different aspects of the deficit in reaching for objects. *Brain*, **111**(3), 643–674.

Peyser, C. E. & Folstein, S. E. (1990). Huntington's disease as a model for mood disorders. Clues from neuropathology and neurochemistry. *Molecular and Chemical Neuropathology*, **122**, 99–119.

Pfuhlmann, B. & Stöber, G. (2001). The different conceptions of catatonia: historical overview and critical discussion. *European Archives of Psychiatry and Clinical Neurosciences*, **251**(Suppl.1), 1/4–1/7.

Rinehart, N. J., Bellgrove, M. A., Bradshaw, J. L., Brereton, A. V. & Tonge, B. J. (2006a). An examination of movement kinematics in young people with high-functioning autism and Asperger's disorder: further evidence for a motor planning deficit. *Journal of Autism and Developmental Disorders*, **36**, 757–767.

Rinehart, N. J., Tonge, B., Bradshaw, J. L. *et al.* (2006b). Movement-related potentials in high-functioning autism and Asperger's disorder. *Developmental Medicine and Child Neurology*, **48**, 272–277.

Rinehart, N. J., Tonge, B., Iansek, R. *et al.* (2006c). Gait function in newly diagnosed children with autism: cerebellar and basal ganglia related motor disorder. *Developmental Medicine and Child Neurology*, **48**, 819–824.

Rinehart, N. J., Tonge, B. J., Bradshaw, J. L., *et al.* (2006d). Gait function in high-functioning autism and Asperger's disorder: evidence for basal-ganglia and cerebellar involvement. *European Child and Adolescent Psychiatry*, **15**, 256–264.

Rizzolatti, G. & Craighero, L. (2004). The mirror-neuron system. *Annual Reviews of Neuroscience*, **27**, 169–192.

Robinson, F. R. & Fuchs, A. F. (2001). The role of the cerebellum in voluntary eye movements. *Annual Review of Neuroscience*, **24**, 981–1004.

Rogers, D. (1992). Motor disorder in psychiatry. In *Towards a Neurological Psychiatry*. Chichester, UK: John Wiley and Sons.

Schiffman, J., Walker, E., Ekstrom, M. *et al.* (2004). Childhood videotaped social and neuromotor precursors of schizophrenia: a prospective investigation. *American Journal of Psychiatry*, **161**, 2021–2027.

Simpson, G. M. & Angus, J. W. S. (1970). A rating scale for extrapyramidal side effects. *Acta Psychiatrica Scandinavica*, **Suppl.**, 11–19.

Singer, T. & Frith, C. (2005). The painful side of empathy. *Nature Neuroscience*, **8**(7), 845–846.

Sobin, C. (1998). The motor agitation and retardation scale: a scale for the assessment of motor abnormalities in depressed patients. *Journal of Neuropsychiatry*, **10**, 85–92.

Stern, E. (2000). A functional neuroanatomy of tics in Tourette syndrome. *Archives of General Psychiatry*, **57**, 741–748.

Taira, M., Mine, S., Georgopoulos, A. P. & Murata, A. S. H. (1990). Parietal cortex neurons of the monkey related to the visual guidance of hand movement. *Experimental Brain Research*, **83**, 29–36.

Teitelbaum, P., Teitelbaum, O., Nye, J. Fryman, J. & Maurer, R. G. (1998). Movement analysis in infancy may be useful for early diagnosis of autism. *Proceedings of the National Academy of Sciences: Psychology*, **95**, 13982–13987.

Tonge, B., Brereton, A., Gray, K. M. & Einfield, S. L. (1999). Behavioural and emotional disturbance in high functioning autism and Asperger's disorder. *Autism*, 3(2), 117–130.

Tsatsanis, K. D., Rourke, B. P., Klin, A., *et al.* (2003). Reduced thalamic volume in high-functioning individuals with autism. *Biological Psychiatry*, **53**, 121–129.

Ungerleider, L. G. & Mishkin, M. (1982). Two cortical visual systems. In D. J. Ingle, M. H. Goodale & J. W. Mansfield (Eds.), *Analysis of Visual Behavior* (pp. 549–586). Cambridge, MA: MIT Press.

Williams, J. H. G., Whiten, A., Suddendorf, D. I. & Perrett, D. I. (2001). Imitation, mirror neurons and autism. *Neuroscience and Biobehavioral Reviews*, **25**, 287–295.

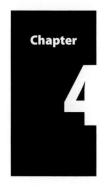

The neurobiology of the emotion response: perception, experience and regulation

Sarah Whittle, Murat Yücel and Nicholas B. Allen

Introduction

Emotion is a complex phenomenon that influences, and is influenced by, every aspect of human experience. It is unconditionally tied to our perceptions and interpretation of stimuli; the content of our memories and the means by which they are encoded and retrieved; our attentional capacity and other executive functioning; and our motivations to think and act in specific ways. Given such widespread significance, it is not surprising that there have been centuries of research dedicated to understanding the neural bases of emotion.

Understanding how emotion is represented in the brain has nevertheless proved to be a difficult task; primarily due to its complexity, and the difficulty in operationalizing and measuring this construct. Emotion has been described as a set of physiological, phenomenological and facial expression changes evoked in relation to appraisals of situations (Beer & Lombardo, 2007). Accordingly, a large amount of research has been dedicated to understanding the neural processes associated with the perception of emotional stimuli, and the production of physiological arousal and subjective feeling states (Adolphs & Damasio, 2000). Much of this research has treated these processes as a single entity; however, recent evidence suggests that they may be governed by neurally distinct mechanisms. Further, emotion regulation is also an important component of the emotion response. Emotion regulation refers to control processes aimed at manipulating when, where, how and which emotions are experienced and expressed (Ochsner & Gross, 2005). This aspect of emotional functioning has traditionally been overlooked, which is largely attributable to the fact that most of the early emotion research was conducted with animals, which

likely lack a number of the higher-order neural functions required for this task. Only relatively recently has the recognition of these diverse aspects of emotion been translated into human neuropsychological research. Particularly, research utilizing sophisticated neuroimaging techniques has begun to shed light on the complex spatial and temporal neural architecture of the emotion response.

This chapter aims to present an integrated overview of the neural bases of three major components of the emotion response: (1) emotion perception (i.e. the identification and appraisal of emotional stimuli); (2) emotion experience (i.e. the production of a specific affective state in response to a stimulus, including physiological arousal, conscious feeling and emotional behavior); and (3) the regulation of the affective state and emotional behavior, which may occur consciously or unconsciously. For each component, relevant evidence from human neuroimaging research (and also from lesion studies, where appropriate) is presented. These methodologies offer greater spatial resolution than previous methodologies for examining brain–behavior relationships, and hence have provided the means for more fine-grained investigation of the neural correlates of the components of the emotion response. Following this, there will be a discussion of how the identified brain regions might work together in neural circuits that underlie the unfolding emotion response. The chapter will conclude with a brief discussion of how deficits in the brain circuitry underlying the emotion response may contribute to the etiology of a number of psychiatric disorders.

Emotion perception

The initial identification and appraisal of an affective stimulus is the first process comprising the emotion

---

The Neuropsychology of Mental Illness, ed. Stephen J. Wood, Nicholas B. Allen and Christos Pantelis. Published by Cambridge University Press. © Cambridge University Press 2009.

response. An affective stimulus may be a stimulus with inherent affective properties such as an emotionally expressive face or sound, or a neutral stimulus that has been conditioned to elicit an affective response. The amygdala and insula are two key structures that have been implicated in emotion perception.

The amygdala

The amygdala is an ovoid gray matter structure situated bilaterally on the superomedial wall of the temporal lobes. Research suggests this structure is involved in the modulation of vigilance to emotionally salient stimuli, and in the initial and largely subconscious assignment of affective significance to sensory events (LeDoux, 1993; Ochsner & Schacter, 2000). Widespread cortical and subcortical connections subserve the transfer of information processed in the amygdala for subsequent emotional learning and behavior. The amygdala has been primarily implicated in the processing of negative affective stimuli, particularly fearful or threatening in nature. Lesions of the amygdala have resulted in impairments in the response to fear stimuli in both visual (Young et al., 1995) and auditory (Scott et al., 1997) domains. Functional imaging (i.e. functional magnetic resonance imaging [fMRI] or positron emission tomography [PET]) studies have documented increased amygdala activation during exposure to fearful and other unpleasant stimuli (Schwartz et al., 2003; Zald, 2003). Trait measures of behavioral inhibition or anxiety (where there is chronic sensitivity to threat) have been correlated with amygdala activity during exposure to a range of affective stimuli (Etkin et al., 2004; Reuter et al., 2004; Schienle et al., 2005).

Whilst there is a wealth of evidence for the involvement of the amygdala in the perception of aversive stimuli, functional imaging studies have also reported amygdala activity with exposure to pleasurable stimuli, indicating a complex role for the amygdala in affective processing. Amygdala activation has been reported during exposure to positive photographs (Hamann et al., 2002), positive emotional words (Hamann & Mao, 2002), erotic stimuli (Ferretti et al., 2005) and pleasant tastes (Small et al., 2003). It has been suggested that the amygdala's apparent role in processing both negative and positive affective stimuli may stem from its broader role in the processing of any stimuli that are of biological relevance, and also novel, ambiguous or highly arousing (Whalen,

1998; Zald, 2003). The apparent negative bias in the literature (i.e. majority of studies showing amygdala associations with negative stimuli) may arise from the fact that aversive stimuli are usually arousing to a greater degree than pleasant stimuli.

Recent research suggests that an individual's characteristic style of perceiving and responding to affective stimuli may affect the degree of attentional processing afforded to specific affective stimuli by the amygdala. Canli (2004) reported a series of fMRI studies whereby individual differences in trait extraversion and neuroticism predicted differential amygdala responses to affective stimuli. In one study increased amygdala activation to pleasant pictures was correlated with self-reported extraversion, whilst increased activation to negative stimuli was correlated with neuroticism. Such findings highlight a complex role for the amygdala in affective processing, and suggest that an important direction for future investigation of the neural bases of emotion will be to incorporate measures of trait-level individual difference factors.

The insula

The insula cortex, a part of the extended limbic system, lies bilaterally at the deepest point of the lateral sulcus, which separates the temporal lobe from the inferior parietal cortex. The anterior insula cortex in particular has been implicated in emotion perception, with evidence that it may convey representations of affective sensory information to the amygdala, with which it has dense bilateral connections (Augustine, 1996). The insula cortex has been implicated in the recognition and processing of disgusting stimuli, with patients with insula lesions exhibiting deficits in the recognition of facial and vocal expressions of disgust (Calder et al., 2000). Functional MRI studies have reported insula activation with the perception of facial expressions of disgust (Phillips et al., 1997) and during unpleasant taste perception (Small et al., 1999). Although insula activation has been frequently associated with disgust, there is increasing evidence of a broader role for this brain structure in emotion processing (Schienle et al., 2002). Insula activation has been implicated in the processing of fear stimuli (Buchel et al., 1998), pain perception (Gelnar et al., 1999), and the making of judgments about facial expressions of a number of emotions including disgust and happiness (Gorno-Tempini et al., 2001).

Emotion production, experience and emotion-dependent learning and decision-making

Once a stimulus has been perceived as affectively salient, a myriad of responses may be triggered, including autonomic and somatic symptoms, subjective feeling, facial and other bodily expressions, and associated behavior. Paradigms employed to examine these responses include conditioning and mood induction via extended exposure to affective stimuli or autobiographical recall. Success of the paradigm is typically assessed retrospectively via self-report. Trait mood measures (i.e. chronic emotional experience) may also be correlated with brain structure or function. Incentive motivation and reward or punishment-related decision-making paradigms can also be integrated into a review of emotional experience, as these processes involve desire, attainment or avoidance of a particular favorable or unfavorable affective state. Both the amygdala and the insula have been implicated in the experiential (in addition to the perceptual) components of the emotional response. The rostral and ventral anterior cingulate cortex (ACC), medial orbitofrontal cortex and ventral striatum (VS) also appear to be uniquely involved in emotion production and experience.

The amygdala

In addition to its role in the initial identification of affective stimuli, the amygdala has been suggested to be important for learning about the affective consequences of stimuli, which is an important process for guiding future affect-related decision-making and behavior. Again, the majority of evidence suggests a primary involvement in aversive learning (Adolphs & Damasio, 2000; Davidson & Irwin, 1999; Davidson et al., 2000a; Ochsner & Schacter, 2000). Fear conditioning has been reported to be reduced in patients with amygdala lesions (Bechara et al., 1995), and has been associated with amygdala activation in healthy individuals (Buchel et al., 1999). Amygdala activation has further been reported in response to both the induction and maintenance of both positive and negative emotional states (Davidson et al., 1999; Schaefer et al., 2002). The size of the amygdala has been correlated with self-reported dysthymia in patient populations (Tebartz van Elst et al., 1999), whilst amygdala activation has been reported during anticipation of pleasant taste (O'Doherty, 2004) and monetary reward (Knutson et al., 2001). Drugs of abuse possess extremely high appetitive motivational value in drug-dependent individuals, and in such individuals, increased activation of the amygdala has been reported with craving (i.e. desire to use) and anticipation of drug administration (Bonson et al., 2002; Lingford-Hughes et al., 2003).

The insula

The insula cortex has also been implicated in the generation of affective states in response to emotional stimuli. For example, imaging studies have reported insula activation during induced sadness and anticipatory anxiety, during recall of internally generated emotion (Reiman et al., 1997) and during the experience of guilt (Shin et al., 2000), highlighting the involvement of the insula in the generation of particularly aversive affective experience. The importance of trait differences in emotional functioning has been suggested by findings that individuals that rate highly on measures of trait anxiety show particularly high insula activity during the anticipation of emotionally negative stimuli (Simmons et al., 2006).

Furthermore, associations between insula activation and autonomic arousal (e.g. heart rate and heart-rate variability), and visceral changes associated with facial emotion processing have been reported (Critchley et al., 2005). It has been suggested that the insula cortex provides the neural substrate that links emotional distress, anticipatory processing and autonomic arousal (Simmons et al., 2006).

Ventral/rostral anterior cingulate cortex

The anterior cingulate cortex (ACC) is situated bilaterally on the medial walls of the frontal lobes. It is a functionally heterogeneous region, involved in a vast array of cognitive, emotional, motor, nociceptive and visuospatial functions (Bush et al., 2000). There is strong evidence that the region of the ACC lying ventral and rostral to the corpus callosum is preferentially related to affective processes (Bush et al., 2000, 2002), with the ventral region particularly implicated in the production of somatic and autonomic emotional responses via efferent connections to autonomic, endocrine and visceral effectors (Nauta, 1971). Early animal studies report that electrical stimulation of the ventral ACC results in increased heart rate, blood pressure and respiration, as well as increased distress vocalizations and emotional facial expression (see Allman *et al.*, 2001). Lesions to this area also cause a variety of changes in emotional behavior, ranging from apathy to anxiety (Angelini *et al.*, 1981; Levin & Duchowny, 1991). A number of functional imaging studies have reported increased activity in the ventral/rostral ACC with the induction of various emotions. For example, induced sadness in healthy individuals has been reported to result in increased activity in the ventral/rostral ACC (Liotti *et al.*, 2000), and higher resting activity in the ventral/rostral ACC has been observed in individuals with higher self-reported trait negative affectivity as measured by the Positive and Negative Affect Schedule (PANAS; Zald *et al.*, 2002).

The ventral and rostral ACC have also been implicated in reward processing and motivated behavior. The ventral ACC appears to be involved in the experience of emotional states resulting from rewarding outcomes, whilst the rostral ACC appears to be involved in the mediation of the representation of reward values, and stimulating motivated behavior. Increased activity in these regions has been reported during reward-based decision-making in gambling tasks (Bush *et al.*, 2002; Rogers *et al.*, 2004; Williams *et al.*, 2004); with craving, desire and positive mood in cocaine addicts during drug administration (Breiter *et al.*, 1997; Volkow *et al.*, 2005); and during sexual arousal in healthy men (Rauch *et al.*, 1999).

Increased rostral ACC activity has also been reported in the context of social affective functioning, with activations reported to correlate with feelings of social exclusion (Somerville *et al.*, 2006), with maternal distress during exposure to sounds of infant cries (Lorberbaum *et al.*, 2002), but also with feelings of romantic and maternal love during exposure to visual stimuli of loved ones (Bartels & Zeki, 2004).

Medial orbitofrontal cortex

The orbitofrontal cortex (OFC) occupies the ventral surface of the frontal lobes of the cortex. The OFC has been ascribed a prime role in multi-modal stimulus-reinforcement associative learning, which is the type of learning that is often involved in emotion. It has been suggested that different subregions of the OFC subserve different aspects of this function (Kringelbach & Rolls, 2004). The functional importance of a medial-lateral parcellation of the OFC has been

emphasized, with the medial OFC related to the monitoring, learning and memory of the reward value of stimuli, and the lateral OFC related to the evaluation of punishers, which when detected may lead to a change in ongoing behavior (Elliott *et al.*, 2000; Öngür *et al.*, 2003). A posterior-anterior distinction of function has also been suggested, with more complex or abstract reinforcers (such as monetary gain and loss) represented more anteriorly and less complex reinforcers (such as taste) more posteriorly (Kringelbach & Rolls, 2004).

The medial OFC (which often includes parts of rostral and ventral ACC, and may be termed ventromedial PFC) has particularly been implicated in the production of reward-related emotional states and behaviors. Activation of the medial OFC has been reported during the monitoring of rewarding stimuli during gambling tasks (Rogers *et al.*, 2004), and with increased desire and craving in cocaine addicts during drug administration (Volkow *et al.*, 2005). Kringelbach (2005) suggests that the medial OFC is important for the subjective experience of positive affect associated with rewarding stimuli, and cites studies that have demonstrated a correlation between medial OFC activation with the subjective pleasantness of tastes and odors, as well as the feeling of rush associated with administration of stimulant drugs in drug-naïve subjects. Increased activation of the medial OFC has also been reported in mothers whilst viewing pictures of their infants, with the increases proportional to the degree of increase in felt positive affect (Nitschke *et al.*, 2004). Further, increased activation in this region has been associated with emotional expression. For example, a PET study reported increased medial OFC activity to increase with smiling and laughter during exposure to visual comics (Iwase *et al.*, 2002).

Ventral striatum

The ventral striatum (VS) is the most inferomedial part of the striatal (or subcortical) part of the brain, which primarily comprises the nucleus accumbens. The VS is a core region of the brain reward system and associated dopaminergic innervations from the ventral tegmental area (Schultz, 2000). There is evidence that the VS plays a key role in encoding the motivational salience of stimuli and encouraging appetitive or reward-dependent behaviors (Berridge & Robinson, 2003). Although much of this evidence comes from animal studies showing an involvement of the VS in the modulation of both unconditioned and learned rewarding behaviors (Berridge, 2003; Cardinal *et al.*, 2002), there is also some supportive human evidence. For example, increased activity in this region has been reported with subjective measures of craving in cocaine users following cocaine infusion (Breiter *et al.*, 1997). Dopamine release in the VS has been associated with naturally rewarding experiences such as food, sex (Giuliano & Allard, 2001) and the use of certain drugs (Heinz *et al.*, 2004). It has been suggested that in substance abuse, dopaminergic dysfunction in the ventral striatum may bias the brain reward system toward excessive attribution of incentive salience to substance-associated stimuli.

It has been suggested that the VS is necessarily involved in positive feeling states associated with the anticipation and attainment of rewarding stimuli (Berridge & Robinson, 2003). Supporting this, activity in the VS has been reported during picture-induced positive affect (Sutton, 1997), exposure to positive auditory stimuli (Blood & Zatorre, 2001; Hamann & Mao, 2002) and during sexual arousal in men (Rauch *et al.*, 1999). Self-reported happiness with the anticipation of increasing monetary reward has also been shown to correlate with activity in this region (Knutson *et al.*, 2001).

Emotion regulation

An individual's ability to regulate their emotion governs the duration, intensity and type of emotion experienced, with important implications for mental health. An increasing amount of theory and research into emotion regulation has suggested the existence of a variety of regulation processes, which may occur at either the conscious or unconscious level, and may develop or be emphasized at different stages of life (Gross, 1998; Rothbart & Derryberry, 1981). The existing neuroimaging literature has highlighted an important distinction between unconscious (or automatic) control processes and conscious (or cognitive/effortful) control processes. Automatic control processes have been investigated primarily by extinction paradigms, which involve the cessation of a conditioned affective response via repeated pairing of a conditioned stimulus with a neutral outcome. Automatic regulation has also been inferred from findings of increased brain activity correlated with decreased

physiological responding to emotional stimuli. Two main cognitive emotion-regulation strategies have been identified in the literature: reappraisal and suppression. *Reappraisal* involves the cognitive transformation of emotional experience; for example, reframing an aversive event in neutral or positive terms. *Suppression* involves the inhibition of reactions to emotional stimuli; that is, changing one's affective state once an emotion has been triggered by an affective stimulus (e.g. thinking of a pleasant scenario when in an aversive mood). Although these two types of emotion-regulation strategies may differ in their effectiveness (John & Gross, 2004), both have implicated similar brain regions. Both automatic and cognitive regulation processes are considered below, with a relatively more detailed discussion presented for the roles of the hippocampus, lateral OFC, dorsolateral prefrontal cortex (DLPFC) and dorsal ACC in cognitive emotion regulation.

Automatic regulatory processes

In addition to a role in experiential aspects of emotion, the medial OFC appears to have a role in the regulation of emotional behavior occurring at an unconscious or automatic level. It has been suggested that this may occur as a result of direct and indirect connections with subcortical structures involved in eliciting emotion-related autonomic responses, including the amygdala and ventral striatum (Kim & Jung, 2006). There is evidence from both human and animal studies that the medial OFC is involved in the extinction of conditioned fear. Enhanced activation in the medial OFC has been reported with the extinction of olfactory fear conditioning (Gottfried & Dolan, 2004). Further, fear association has been found to remain post extinction, suggesting that the involvement of this region in extinction represented the regulation (or inhibition) of fear expression. Also, recall of fear extinction learned the previous day has been correlated with medial OFC fMRI activity (Phelps *et al.*, 2004) and cortical thickness in this area (Milad *et al.*, 2005).

Cognitive regulatory processes
Dorsal anterior cingulate cortex and dorsolateral prefrontal cortex

There is evidence that the dorsal region of the ACC is preferentially involved in cognitive and executive processes. The dorsal ACC has been implicated in a range of such processes including attention, error monitoring and inhibitory control (Bush *et al.*, 2002). Strong reciprocal connections to the lateral prefrontal cortex and supplementary and premotor areas are suggested to be important for the integration of information processed in the dorsal ACC with higher cognitive processes (such as working memory) and the translation of cognitive processes into physical action (Vogt *et al.*, 1995). The DLPFC in particular has been theorized to work closely with the dorsal ACC in a network subserving cognitive control; while the dorsal ACC is involved in evaluative processes indicating when control needs to be engaged, the DLPFC is responsible for the strategic implementation of control over one's thoughts and actions in line with specific goals or task-oriented behaviors (Botvinick *et al.*, 2001; MacDonald *et al.*, 2000).

There is evidence that the dorsal ACC and DLPFC are involved in such control functions specifically related to affective behavior. Both reappraisal and suppression emotion-regulation paradigms have been found to elicit activation in the dorsal ACC and DLPFC (Levesque *et al.*, 2003, 2004; Ochsner *et al.*, 2004; Ohira *et al.*, 2006; Phan *et al.*, 2005).

Lateral orbitofrontal cortex

It has been suggested that the primary role of the lateral OFC is to respond to signals of punishment by regulating behavior and emotion to maximize adaptive outcomes (Elliott *et al.*, 2000). The lateral OFC has been implicated in the inhibition of aggressive and other socially inappropriate behaviors and emotions. Damage to this area results in increased general irritability, inappropriate overt emotional displays (Barrash *et al.*, 2000) and anger and hostility (Berlin *et al.*, 2004). Lateral OFC activation has been reported during the viewing of angry faces (Blair *et al.*, 1999) and induction of anger via autobiographical recall (Dougherty *et al.*, 1999). In these studies it is suggested that the observed activation may represent attempts to inhibit reactions to, or feelings of anger. Lateral OFC activation, in addition to the dorsal ACC and DLPFC (to which the lateral OFC is highly interconnected), is also often reported with conscious efforts to regulate emotional response by suppression or reappraisal strategies (Levesque *et al.*, 2003; Ochsner *et al.*, 2004). Activity in this region has also been associated with suppression of the influence of negative emotional stimuli on subsequent behavior (Beer *et al.*, 2006).

Hippocampus

The hippocampus has a long-established role in spatial processing and certain forms of memory. It has become increasingly apparent however that the hippocampus plays a more general role in information processing and behavioral regulation, and that these various functions may be distributed throughout the hippocampus. It has been recently proposed that there are two main subregions of the hippocampus: a dorsal region that has a preferential role in spatial learning and memory, and a ventral region that has a preferential role in the regulation of anxiety-related behaviors (Bannerman *et al.*, 2004; Gray, 1982; Gray & McNaughton, 2000). It has been suggested that when there is conflict between the tendency to approach cues associated with reward and the tendency to avoid cues associated with negative affect, the hippocampus outputs a signal that increases the weight or valence of affectively negative information, therefore decreasing the tendency to approach a goal. Pathological anxiety is thought to result from hippocampal dysfunction (hyperactivity), whereby there is a greatly increased perception of threat in situations involving conflicting stimuli, and an increase in the suppression of approach-related actions and cognitions. Most of the research driving this model has been with rodents, however, there is a wealth of supportive human research showing relationships between measures of hippocampal function and structure and anxiety-related phenomena (Barros-Loscertales *et al.*, 2006; Rauch *et al.*, 2003; Rusch *et al.*, 2001).

Neural systems for emotion

Thus far, evidence has been presented for the contribution of a number of cortical, limbic and subcortical brain regions in three major components of emotion: the perception/identification of emotional stimuli, the production and experience of the affective state, and the regulation of this state. A few specific cortical regions have been shown to be important for more than one of these cognitive processes. The amygdala and insula have been implicated in the identification of the emotional significance of an environmental stimulus, as well as the production of the affective state and emotional behavior. Although it is difficult to design paradigms to examine the neural correlates of these components separately (e.g. passive viewing of emotional stimuli indexes emotion perception but will also likely trigger a felt and expressed affective state), findings do indicate that there are some brain structures likely to be involved in a single component. For example, the ventral ACC appears to be preferentially involved in the production of autonomic responses accompanying the experience of emotion (Blumberg *et al.*, 2000). Although not given substantial focus in this chapter, there does appear to be some neural specificity for different types of emotions. For example, the ventral ACC has been predominantly implicated in sadness, whilst the ventral striatum appears to be particularly involved in pleasant emotion and reward-related behaviors. Hemispheric laterality may be an important factor influencing the type and valence of emotional response; this issue is covered in greater detail in Chapter 16.

A point of discussion critical to a comprehensive understanding of the neural bases of emotion concerns neural circuits or systems. Animal and post-mortem research has provided much knowledge about anatomical connections in the brain. More recently, with the rapid advancement in brain-imaging technologies, functional and structural brain connectivity can be studied in vivo. Together, this research is strongly suggestive of the aforementioned regions working together in neural systems underlying the unfolding emotional response; from the perception of emotional stimuli, to the production, experience and regulation of the emotional state and behavior. Consistent with what is known about cortical architecture, a number of such neural models have recently been proposed (Mayberg, 2003; Phillips *et al.*, 2003a). These models are consistent in emphasizing the contribution of two reciprocally connected brain systems underlying emotion. A "ventral" system, including the amygdala, insula, ventral striatum, and ventromedial PFC (including ventral/rostral regions of the ACC and medial OFC), appears to be important for the identification of the emotional significance of affective stimuli, the production of affective states, and the automatic regulation of autonomic responses to affective stimuli. A "dorsal" system, including the hippocampus, dorsal ACC and lateral areas of the dorsal PFC and OFC, exerts a predominant role in higher-order executive processes such as attention, error monitoring, response selection, working memory, and planning, and appears to be

important for the effortful rather than automatic regulation of affective states.

A relationship between these two systems is suggested by evidence that components of each often exhibit concerted activity in functional imaging studies of cognitive and affective processing. For example, during the down-regulation of emotion via reappraisal, but also with other paradigms whereby effortful cognitive processing is required, increased activity in dorsal ACC, DLPFC and lateral OFC, in concert with decreases in amygdala and/or ventromedial PFC activity, have been observed (Hariri *et al.*, 2003; Ochsner *et al.*, 2004). Conversely, during mood induction, a reciprocal pattern of activity in dorsal regions and ventral ACC has been reported; specifically, negative mood has been associated with decreases in dorsal ACC and DLPFC and increases in ventral ACC activity (Mayberg *et al.*, 1999).

It must be noted that this idea of two interconnected systems underlying emotion is certain to be oversimplified. These systems are likely to be made up of subsystems, and include a number of other cortical and subcortical structures not mentioned in the current discussion (see Tekin & Cummings, 2002). However, the proposed model is a useful framework for thinking about the neural basis of emotion, and provides a testable basis for future research.

Implications for psychopathology

Specific abnormalities in the functioning of the dorsal and/or ventral emotion systems, or the connections between these systems, may be associated with abnormalities in emotional behavior or regulation, and result in the generation of symptomatology characteristic of a range of psychiatric disorders. Although a thorough discussion of the links between affective neuroscience and psychopathology is beyond the scope of this chapter, and indeed has been attempted elsewhere (e.g. Phillips *et al.*, 2003b), we can provide a general heuristic that can be used to organize the potential associations between the structures and systems reviewed in the chapter and some of the basic dimensions of psychiatric symptomatology. For example, Krueger (1999) examined the underlying structure of symptoms of common mental disorders in a large community sample. He found that two broad factors accounted for most of the variance; internalizing and externalizing. Within the internalizing factor there were two distinguishable subfactors that included symptoms of fear versus anxious misery. Such empirically driven models of the structure of symptoms are a good starting place to explore the potential association between the neurobiological systems that underlie affective functioning and symptoms of psychopathology.

Dysfunction of the dorsal system and its regulatory connections with the ventral system (particularly those regions implicated in negative affect such as the amygdala and insula) may result in uncontrolled functioning of ventral structures. This may trigger exaggerated affective and autonomic responses and behavior that are driven by somewhat primitive or instinctive reactions to affective stimuli. This type of dysfunction may underlie symptoms characteristic of fear disorders such as attentional biases toward negative emotional stimuli and the experience of excess levels of negative emotions, as well as deficits in various executive skills (Davidson *et al.*, 2002). Hyperfunction of certain dorsal system structures (particularly the hippocampus) may also result in mood and anxiety-related symptomatology (cf. anxious misery; Krueger, 1999) in the case where there is excessive inhibition of ventral regions (such as the ventral striatum and medial OFC) involved in reward-based motivation and approach behaviors (Gray & McNaughton, 2000). Dysfunction of dorsal structures such as the lateral OFC might also explain symptomatology characteristic of certain externalizing disorders, such as abnormally increased levels of anger, aggression, or tendencies to approach rewards in a socially inappropriate manner (Davidson *et al.*, 2000b). Additionally, hypofunction of the ventral system might underlie externalizing symptomatology, whereby individuals may engage in risky or socially inappropriate behaviors as a compensatory mechanism for low baseline-levels of affect, particularly low fearfulness and sensitivity to punishment (Chambers & Potenza, 2003). These conjectures regarding the links between the neural systems of emotion and mental illness are merely illustrative, but do show how examining the neuropsychology of basic affective processes may motivate innovative conceptualizations of etiology, nomenclature and potentially even treatment. However, a significant research effort will be required before such promises are realized.

There is much existing evidence for both structural and functional abnormalities in a number of the above-mentioned structures in a variety of psychopathologies, as well as emerging evidence that

dysfunction of the connections between dorsal and ventral system structures might be key to many of these disorders (Mayberg *et al.*, 1999; Phillips *et al.*, 2003b). As such, further research aiming to investigate the functioning of the identified neural structures and systems underlying the emotion response will likely be a fruitful approach to a more informative characterization of psychopathology, and a greater understanding of etiological mechanisms and eventually treatment planning.

References

Adolphs, R. & Damasio, A. R. (2000). Neurobiology of emotion at a systems level. In J. C. Borod (Ed.), *The Neuropsychology of Emotion* (pp. 194–213). New York, NY: Oxford University Press.

Allman, J. M., Hakeem, A., Erwin, J. M., Nimchinski, E. & Hof, P. (2001). The anterior cingulate cortex: the evolution of an interface between emotion and cognition. *Annals of the New York Academy of Sciences*, **935**, 107–117.

Angelini, L., Mazzucchi, A., Picciotto, F., Nardocci, N. & Broggi, G. (1981). Focal lesion of the right cingulum: a case report in a child. *Journal of Neurology Neurosurgery and Psychiatry*, **44**(4), 355–357.

Augustine, J. R. (1996). Circuitry and functional aspects of the insular lobe in primates including humans. *Brain Research Reviews*, **22**, 229–244.

Bannerman, D. M., Rawlins, J. N. P., McHugh, S. B. *et al.* (2004). Regional dissociations within the hippocampus – memory and anxiety. *Neuroscience and Biobehavioral Reviews*, **28**, 273–283.

Barrash, J., Tranel, D. & Anderson, S. W. (2000). Acquired personality disturbances associated with bilateral damage to the ventromedial prefrontal region. *Developmental Neuropsychology*, **18**(3), 355–381.

Barros-Loscertales, A., Meseguer, V., Sanjuan, A. *et al.* (2006). Behavioral inhibition system activity is associated with increased amygdala and hippocampal gray matter volume: a voxel-based morphometry study. *Neuroimage*, **33**(3), 1011–1015.

Bartels, A. & Zeki, S. (2004). The neural correlates of maternal and romantic love. *Neuroimage*, **21**(3), 1155–1166.

Bechara, A., Tranel, D., Damasio, H., Adolphs, R., Rockland, C. & Damasio, A. (1995). Double dissociation of conditioning and declarative knowledge relative to the amygdala and hippocampus in humans. *Science*, **269**(5227), 1115–1118.

Beer, J. S. & Lombardo, M. V. (2007). Insights into emotion regulation from neuropsychology. In J. J. Gross (Ed.),

Handbook of Emotion Regulation (pp. 69–86). New York, NY: Guilford Publications.

Beer, J. S., Knight, R. T. & D'Esposito, M. (2006). Controlling the integration of emotion and cognition – the role of frontal cortex in distinguishing helpful from hurtful emotional information. *Psychological Science*, **17**(5), 448–453.

Berlin, H. A., Rolls, E. T. & Kischka, U. (2004). Impulsivity, time perception, emotion and reinforcement sensitivity in patients with orbitofrontal cortex lesions. *Brain*, **127**(5), 1108–1126.

Berridge, K. C. (2003). Pleasures of the brain. *Brain and Cognition*, **52**, 106–128.

Berridge, K. C. & Robinson, T. E. (2003). Parsing reward. *Trends in Neurosciences*, **26**(9), 507–513.

Blair, R. J. R., Morris, J. S., Frith, C. D., Perrett, D. I. & Dolan, R. J. (1999). Dissociable neural responses to facial expressions of sadness and anger. *Brain*, **122**, 883–893.

Blood, A. J. & Zatorre, R. J. (2001). Intensely pleasurable responses to music correlate with activity in brain regions implicated in reward and emotion. *Proceedings of the National Academy of Sciences*, **98**(20), 11818–11823.

Blumberg, H. P., Stern, E., Martinez, D. *et al.* (2000). Increased anterior cingulate and caudate activity in bipolar mania. *Biological Psychiatry*, **48**, 1045–1052.

Bonson, K. R., Grant, S. J. & Contoreggi, C. S. (2002). Neural systems and cue-induced cocaine craving. *Neuropsychopharmacology*, **263**, 376–386.

Botvinick, M. M., Braver, T. S., Barch, D. M., Carter, C. S. & Cohen, J. D. (2001). Conflict monitoring and cognitive control. *Psychological Review*, **108**(3), 624–652.

Breiter, H. C., Gollub, R. L., Weisskoff, R. M. *et al.* (1997). Acute effects of cocaine on human brain activity and emotion. *Neuron*, **19**(3), 591–611.

Buchel, C., Dolan, R. J., Armony, J. L. & Friston, K. J. (1999). Amygdala-hippocampal involvement in human aversive trace conditioning revealed through event-related functional magnetic resonance imaging. *Journal of Neuroscience*, **19**(24), 10869–10876.

Buchel, C., Morris, J., Dolan, R. J. & Friston, K. J. (1998). Brain systems mediating aversive conditioning: an event-related fmri study. *Neuron*, **20**, 947–957.

Bush, G., Luu, P. & Posner, M. I. (2000). Cognitive and emotional influences in anterior cingulate cortex. *Trends in Cognitive Sciences*, **4**(6), 215–222.

Bush, G., Vogt, B. A., Holmes, J. *et al.* (2002). Dorsal anterior cingulate cortex: a role in reward-based decision making. *Proceedings of the National Academy of Sciences*, **99**(1), 523–528.

Calder, A. J., Keane, J., Manes, F., Antoun, N. & Young, A. W. (2000). Impaired recognition and experience of disgust following brain injury. *Nature Neuroscience*, **3**, 1077–1078.

Canli, T. (2004). Functional brain mapping of extraversion and neuroticism: learning from individual differences in emotion processing. *Journal of Personality*, **72**(6), 1105–1132.

Cardinal, R. N., Parkinson, J. A., Hall, J. & Everitt, B. J. (2002). Emotion and motivation: the role of the amygdala, ventral striatum, and prefrontal cortex. *Neuroscience and Biobehavioral Reviews*, **26**, 321–352.

Chambers, R. A. & Potenza, M. N. (2003). Neurodevelopment, impulsivity, and adolescent gambling. *Journal of Gambling Studies*, **19**(1), 53–84.

Critchley, H. D., Rotshtein, P., Nagai, Y. *et al.* (2005). Activity in the human brain predicting differential heart rate responses to emotional facial expressions. *Neuroimage*, **24**, 751–762.

Davidson, R. J. & Irwin, W. (1999). The functional neuroanatomy of emotion and affective style. *Trends in Cognitive Sciences*, **3**(1), 11–21.

Davidson, R. J., Abercrombie, H., Nitschke, J. B. & Putnam, K. (1999). Regional brain function, emotion and disorders of emotion. *Current Opinion in Neurobiology*, **9**, 228–234.

Davidson, R. J., Jackson, D. C. & Kalin, N. H. (2000a). Emotion, plasticity, context, and regulation: perspectives from affective neuroscience. *Psychological Bulletin*, **126** (6), 890–909.

Davidson, R. J., Pizzagalli, D., Nitschke, J. B. & Putnam, K. (2002). Depression: perspectives from affective neuroscience. *Annual Review of Psychology*, **53**, 545–574.

Davidson, R. J., Putnam, K. M. & Larson, C. L. (2000b). Dysfunction in the neural circuitry of emotion regulation: a possible prelude to violence. *Science*, **289** (5479), 591–594.

Dougherty, D. D., Shin, L. M., Alpert, N. M. *et al.* (1999). Anger in healthy men: a PET study using script-driven imagery. *Biological Psychiatry*, **46**(4), 466–472.

Elliott, R., Dolan, R. J. & Frith, C. D. (2000). Dissociable functions in the medial and lateral orbitofrontal cortex: evidence from human neuroimaging studies. *Cerebral Cortex*, **10**, 308–317.

Etkin, A., Klemenhagen, K. C., Dudman, J. T. *et al.* (2004). Individual differences in trait anxiety predict the response of the basolateral amygdala to unconsciously processed fearful faces. *Neuron*, **44**(6), 1043–1055.

Ferretti, A., Caulo, M., Del Gratta, C. *et al.* (2005). Dynamics of male sexual arousal: distinct components of brain activation revealed by fMRI. *Neuroimage*, **26**(4), 1086–1096.

Gelnar, P. A., Krauss, B. R., Sheehe, P. R., Szeverenyi, N. M. & Apkarian, A. V. (1999). A comparative fMRI study of cortical representations for thermal painful, vibrotactile, and motor performance tasks. *Neuroimage*, **10**(4), 460–482.

Giuliano, F. & Allard, J. (2001). Dopamine and sexual function. *International Journal of Impotence Research*, 3(Suppl.), S18–S28.

Gorno-Tempini, M. L., Pradelli, S., Serafini, M. *et al.* (2001). Explicit and incidental facial expression processing: an fMRI study. *Neuroimage*, **14**(2), 465–473.

Gottfried, J. A. & Dolan, R. J. (2004). Human orbitofrontal cortex mediates extinction learning while accessing conditioned representations of value. *Nature Neuroscience*, **7**(10), 1144–1152.

Gray, J. A. (1982). *The Neuropsychology of Anxiety*. Oxford: Oxford University Press.

Gray, J. A. & McNaughton, N. (2000). *The Neuropsychology of Anxiety* (2nd edn.). Oxford: Oxford University Press.

Gross, J. J. (1998). The emerging field of emotion regulation: an integrative review. *Review of General Psychology*, **2**(3), 271–299.

Hamann, S. B. & Mao, H. (2002). Positive and negative emotional verbal stimuli elicit activity in the left amygdala. *Neuroreport*, **13**(1), 15–19.

Hamann, S. B., Ely, T. D., Hoffman, J. M. & Kilts, C. D. (2002). Ecstasy and agony: activation of the human amygdala in positive and negative emotion. *Psychological Science*, **13**(2), 135–141.

Hariri, A. R., Mattay, V. S., Tessitore, A., Fera, F. & Weinberger, D. R. (2003). Neocortical modulation of the amygdala response to fearful stimuli. *Biological Psychiatry*, **53**(6), 494–501.

Heinz, A., Siessmeier, T., Wrase, J. *et al.* (2004). Correlation between dopamine d2 receptors in the ventral striatum and central processing of alcohol cues and craving. *American Journal of Psychiatry*, **161**(10), 1783–1789.

Iwase, M., Ouchi, Y., Okada, H. *et al.* (2002). Neural substrates of human facial expression of pleasant emotion induced by comic films: A PET study. *Neuroimage*, **17**(2), 758–768.

John, O. P. & Gross, J. J. (2004). Healthy and unhealthy emotion regulation: personality processes, individual differences, and life span development. *Journal of Personality*, **72**(6), 1301–1333.

Kim, J. J. & Jung, M. W. (2006). Neural circuits and mechanisms involved in pavlovian fear conditioning: a critical review. *Neuroscience and Biobehavioral Reviews*, **30**(2), 188–202.

Knutson, B., Adams, C. M., Fong, G. W. & Hommer, D. (2001). Anticipation of increasing monetary reward selectively recruits nucleus accumbens. *Journal of Neuroscience*, **21**(16), RC159.

Kringelbach, M. L. (2005). The human orbitofrontal cortex: linking reward to hedonic experience. *Nature Reviews Neuroscience*, **6**(9), 691–702.

Kringelbach, M. L. & Rolls, E. T. (2004). The functional neuroanatomy of the human orbitofrontal cortex: evidence from neuroimaging and neurophysiology. *Progress in Neurobiology*, **72**, 341–372.

Krueger, R. F. (1999). The structure of common mental disorders. *Archives of General Psychiatry*, **56**, 921–926.

LeDoux, J. E. (1993). Emotional networks in the brain. In M. Lewis & J. M. Haviland (Eds.), *Handbook of Emotions* (pp. 109–118). New York, NY: Guilford Press.

Levesque, J., Eugene, F., Joanette, Y. *et al.* (2003). Neural circuitry underlying voluntary suppression of sadness. *Biological Psychiatry*, **53**(6), 502–510.

Levesque, J., Joanette, Y., Mensour, B. *et al.* (2004). Neural basis of emotional self-regulation in childhood. *Neuroscience*, **129**(2), 361–369.

Levin, B. & Duchowny, M. (1991). Childhood obsessive-compulsive disorder and cingulate epilepsy. *Biological Psychiatry*, **30**(10), 1049–1055.

Lingford-Hughes, A. R., Davies, S. J. C., McIver, S. *et al.* (2003). Addiction. *British Medical Bulletin*, **65**, 209–222.

Liotti, M., Mayberg, H. S., Brannan, S. L. *et al.* (2000). Differential limbic-cortical correlates of sadness and anxiety in healthy subjects: implications for affective disorders. *Biological Psychiatry*, **48**, 30–32.

Lorberbaum, J. P., Newman, J. D., Horwitz, A. R. *et al.* (2002). A potential role for thalamocingulate circuitry in human maternal behavior. *Biological Psychiatry*, **51**(6), 431–445.

MacDonald, A. W., Cohen, J. D., Stenger, V. A. & Carter, C. S. (2000). Dissociating the role of the dorsolateral prefrontal and anterior cingulate cortex in cognitive control. *Science*, **288**(5472), 1835–1838.

Mayberg, H. S. (2003). Modulating dysfunctional limbic-cortical circuits in depression: towards development of brain-based algorithms for diagnosis and optimised treatment. *British Medical Bulletin*, **65**, 193–207.

Mayberg, H. S., Liotti, M., Brannan, S. K. *et al.* (1999). Reciprocal limbic-cortical function and negative mood: converging PET findings in depression and normal sadness. *American Journal of Psychiatry*, **156**(5), 675–682.

Milad, M. R., Quinn, B. T., Pitman, R. K. *et al.* (2005). Thickness of ventromedial prefrontal cortex in humans is correlated with extinction memory. *Proceedings of the National Academy of Sciences*, **102**(30), 10706–10711.

Nauta, W. J. H. (1971). The problem of the frontal lobe: a reinterpretation. *Journal of Psychiatric Research*, **8**, 167–187.

Nitschke, J. B., Nelson, E. E., Rusch, B. D. *et al.* (2004). Orbitofrontal cortex tracks positive mood in mothers viewing pictures of their newborn infants. *Neuroimage*, **21**(2), 583–592.

O'Doherty, J. P. (2004). Reward representations and reward-related learning in the human brain: insights from neuroimaging. *Current Opinion in Neurobiology*, **14**(6), 769–776.

Ochsner, K. N. & Gross, J. J. (2005). The cognitive control of emotion. *Trends in Cognitive Sciences*, **9**(5), 242–249.

Ochsner, K. N. & Schacter, D. L. (2000). A social cognitive neuroscience approach to emotion and memory. In J. C. Borod (Ed.), *The Neuropsychology of Emotion* (pp. 163–193). New York, NY: Oxford University Press.

Ochsner, K. N., Ray, R. D., Cooper, J. C. *et al.* (2004). For better or for worse: neural systems supporting the cognitive down- and up-regulation of negative emotion. *Neuroimage*, **23**(2), 483–499.

Ohira, H., Nomura, M., Ichikawa, N. *et al.* (2006). Association of neural and physiological responses during voluntary emotion suppression. *Neuroimage*, **29**(3), 721–733.

Öngür, D., Ferry, A. T. & Price, J. L. (2003). Architectonic subdivision of the human orbital and medial prefrontal cortex. *Journal of Comparative Neurology*, **460**, 425–449.

Phan, K. L., Fitzgerald, D. A., Nathan, P. J. *et al.* (2005). Neural substrates for voluntary suppression of negative affect: a functional magnetic resonance imaging study. *Biological Psychiatry*, **57**(3), 210–219.

Phelps, E. A., Delgado, M. R., Nearing, K. I. & LeDoux, J. E. (2004). Extinction learning in humans: role of the amygdala and VMPFC. *Neuron*, **43**(6), 897–905.

Phillips, M. L., Drevets, W. C., Rauch, S. L. & Lane, R. D. (2003a). Neurobiology of emotion perception i: the neural basis of normal emotion perception. *Biological Psychiatry*, **53**(5), 504–514.

Phillips, M. L., Drevets, W. C., Rauch, S. L. & Lane, R. D. (2003b). The neurobiology of emotion perception ii: implications for major psychiatric disorders. *Biological Psychiatry*, **53**(5), 515–528.

Phillips, M. L., Young, A. W., Senior, C. *et al.* (1997). A specific neural substrate for perceiving facial expressions of disgust. *Nature*, **389**(6650), 495–498.

Rauch, S. L., Shin, L. M., Dougherty, D. D. *et al.* (1999). Neural activation during sexual and competitive arousal in healthy men. *Psychiatry Research*, **91**(1), 1–10.

Rauch, S. L., Shin, L. M. & Wright, C. I. (2003). Neuroimaging studies of amygdala function in anxiety

disorders. *Annals of the New York Academy of Sciences*, **985**, 389–410.

Reiman, E., Lane, R., Ahern, G. *et al.* (1997). Neuroanatomical correlates of externally and internally generated human emotion. *American Journal of Psychiatry*, **154**(7), 918–925.

Reuter, M., Stark, R., Hennig, J. *et al.* (2004). Personality and emotion: test of Gray's personality theory by means of an fMRI study. *Behavioral Neuroscience*, **118**(3), 462–469.

Rogers, R. D., Ramnani, N., Mackay, C. *et al.* (2004). Distinct portions of anterior cingulate cortex and medial prefrontal cortex are activated by reward processing in separable phases of decision-making cognition. *Biological Psychiatry*, **55**(6), 594–602.

Rothbart, M. K. & Derryberry, D. (1981). Development of individual differences in temperament. In M. E. Lamb & A. L. Brown (Eds.), *Advances in Developmental Psychology* (Vol. 1, pp. 37–86). Hillsdale, NJ: Lawrence Erlbaum Associates.

Rusch, B. D., Abercrombie, H. C., Oakes, T. R., Schaefer, S. M. & Davidson, R. J. (2001). Hippocampal morphometry in depressed patients and control subjects: relations to anxiety symptoms. *Biological Psychiatry*, **50**(12), 960–964.

Schaefer, S. M., Jackson, D. C., Davidson, R. J. *et al.* (2002). Modulation of amygdalar activity by the conscious regulation of negative emotion. *Journal of Cognitive Neuroscience*, **14**(6), 913–921.

Schienle, A., Schafer, A., Stark, R., Walter, B. & Vaitl, D. (2005). Relationship between disgust sensitivity, trait anxiety and brain activity during disgust induction. *Neuropsychobiology*, **51**(2), 86–92.

Schienle, A. C., Stark, R., Walter, B. *et al.* (2002). The insula is not specifically involved in disgust processing: an fMRI study. *Neuroreport*, **13**(16), 2023–2026.

Schultz, W. (2000). Multiple reward systems in the brain. *Nature Reviews Neuroscience*, **1**, 199–207.

Schwartz, C. E., Wright, C. I., Shin, L. M. *et al.* (2003). Differential amygdalar response to novel versus newly familiar neutral faces: a functional MRI probe developed for studying inhibited temperament. *Biological Psychiatry*, **53**, 854–862.

Scott, S. K., Young, A. W., Calder, A. J. *et al.* (1997). Impaired auditory recognition of fear and anger following bilateral amygdala lesions. *Nature*, **385**(6613), 254–257.

Shin, L. M., Dougherty, D. D., Orr, S. P. *et al.* (2000). Activation of anterior paralimbic structures during guilt-related script-driven imagery. *Biological Psychiatry*, **48**(1), 43–50.

Simmons, A., Strigo, I., Matthews, S. C., Paulus, M. P. & Stein, M. B. (2006). Anticipation of aversive visual stimuli is associated with increased insula activation in anxiety-prone subjects. *Biological Psychiatry*, **60**(4), 402–409.

Small, D. M., Gregory, M. D., Mak, Y. E. *et al.* (2003). Dissociation of neural representation of intensity and affective valuation in human gustation. *Neuron*, **39**(4), 701–711.

Small, D. M., Zald, D. H., Jones-Gotman, M. *et al.* (1999). Human cortical gustatory areas: a review of functional neuroimaging data. *Neuroreport*, **10**(1), 7–13.

Somerville, L. H., Heatherton, T. F. & Kelley, W. M. (2006). Anterior cingulate cortex responds differentially to expectancy violation and social rejection. *Nature Neuroscience*, **9**(8), 1007–1008.

Sutton, S. K. (1997). Asymmetry in prefrontal glucose metabolism during appetitive and aversive emotional states: An FDG-PET study. *Psychophysiology*, **34**, S89.

Tebartz van Elst, L., Woermann, F. G., Lemieux, L. & Trimble, M. R. (1999). Amygdala enlargement in dysthymia – a volumetric study of patients with temporal lobe epilepsy. *Biological Psychiatry*, **46**, 1614–1623.

Tekin, S. & Cummings, J. L. (2002). Frontal-subcortical neuronal circuits and clinical neuropsychiatry: an update. *Journal of Psychosomatic Research*, **53**, 647–654.

Vogt, B. A., Nimchinsky, E. A., Vogt, L. J. & Hof, P. R. (1995). Human cingulate cortex – surface-features, flat maps, and cytoarchitecture. *Journal of Comparative Neurology*, **359**(3), 490–506.

Volkow, N. D., Wang, G. J., Ma, Y. M. *et al.* (2005). Activation of orbital and medial prefrontal cortex by methylphenidate in cocaine-addicted subjects but not in controls: relevance to addiction. *Journal of Neuroscience*, **25**(15), 3932–3939.

Whalen, P. J. (1998). Fear, vigilance, and ambiguity: initial neuroimaging studies of the human amygdala. *Current Directions in Psychological Science*, **7**(6), 177–188.

Williams, Z. M., Bush, G., Rauch, S. L., Cosgrove, G. R. & Eskandar, E. N. (2004). Human anterior cingulate neurons and the integration of monetary reward with motor responses. *Nature Neuroscience*, **7**(12), 1370–1375.

Young, A. W., Aggleton, J. P., Hellawell, D. J. *et al.* (1995). Face processing impairments after amygdalotomy. *Brain*, **118**(1), 15–24.

Zald, D. H. (2003). The human amygdala and the emotional evaluation of sensory stimuli. *Brain Research Reviews*, **41**(1), 88–123.

Zald, D. H., Mattson, D. L. & Pardo, J. V. (2002). Brain activity in ventromedial prefrontal cortex correlates with individual differences in negative affect. *Proceedings of the National Academy of Sciences USA*, **99**(4), 2450–2454.

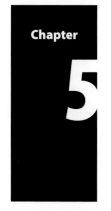

Frontal asymmetry in emotion, personality and psychopathology: methodological issues in electrocortical and hemodynamic neuroimaging

John D. Herrington, Nancy S. Koven, Wendy Heller, Gregory A. Miller and Jack B. Nitschke

Introduction

It is well established that depression and anxiety are associated with abnormal patterns of asymmetric brain activity, particularly in frontal regions (Heller *et al.*, 1998). Data in support of this finding have highlighted the relative roles of left and right frontal regions in positive and negative emotions, respectively (Davidson & Irwin, 1999). In recent years it has become increasingly clear that asymmetric brain function can be understood not only in terms of theories of emotion, but also in terms of specific personality constructs. Despite decades of EEG research identifying frontal asymmetries in emotion and personality, these findings have been largely unreplicated by hemodynamic studies (e.g. functional MRI and PET). This chapter will briefly review evidence regarding the contribution of frontal brain asymmetries to understanding components of emotion, motivation and personality. The review will be followed by a more detailed consideration of how frontal brain asymmetries can and should be measured using hemodynamic imaging. Examples of recent studies from our laboratories that illustrate some of the methodologies discussed will also be presented (Herrington *et al.*, 2005; Herrington *et al.*, under review; Nitschke *et al.*, 2006).

Emotion and frontal brain asymmetries

Evidence in favor of frontal brain asymmetries for emotion, personality and psychopathology comes from numerous methodologies. Clinical case studies have shown that damage to the right hemisphere is

associated with euphoric mood states, whereas damage to the left hemisphere results in dysphoric mood states (Borod, 1992; Gainotti, 1972). These findings parallel some studies of patients undergoing intracarotid sodium amytal testing, where one hemisphere of the brain is temporarily deactivated (Alema *et al.*, 1961; Lee *et al.*, 1987; but see Stabell *et al.*, 2004). Eye movement, electroconvulsive therapy (ECT) and epilepsy studies have shown a similar pattern (Bear & Fedio, 1977; Decina *et al.*, 1985; Flor-Henry, 1979; Myslobodsky & Horesh, 1978). Finally, over the past two decades, numerous EEG studies have documented both state and trait changes in affect related to lateralized activity in frontal regions (Coan & Allen, 2004; Davidson *et al.*, 2002).

Findings regarding the role of the frontal cortex in emotion and personality have been informed by specific models of the structure of emotion. Factor-analytic and multidimensional scaling approaches have shown that basic emotions (e.g. happiness, fear, etc.) can be represented by a two-dimensional structure with axes representing valence (pleasant vs unpleasant) and arousal (Russell, 1980). This structure is the basis for the circumplex model of emotion, which has been applied to the interpretation of brain activity (Heller *et al.*, 1997, 1998; Nitschke *et al.*, 1999). We and others have suggested that the pleasant/unpleasant axis (valence) can be used to describe patterns of relative activity in the frontal cortex among non-clinical samples, and that abnormalities in these patterns are related to personality (Schmitke & Heller, 2004) and psychopathology, particularly depression and anxiety

Note: Portions of this chapter were previously published in *The Biology of Personality and Individual Differences* edited by Turhan Canli, and are reprinted here with permission from Guilford Press (pending).

disorders (for review, see Coan & Allen, 2004; Heller *et al.*, 1998).

The study of frontal lateralization of function has advanced the understanding of various forms of psychopathology, particularly mood and anxiety disorders. For example, Heller and colleagues (Heller *et al.*, 1995, 1997; Keller *et al.*, 2000; Nitschke *et al.*, 1999) have argued that it is important to interpret frontal asymmetries for emotion and psychopathology in the context of the common co-occurrence of depression and anxiety. Their work is informed by an influential model positing that mood and anxiety disorders share a general distress factor referred to as negative affect (Clark & Watson, 1991). Like the circumplex model, negative affect is a concept derived from factor analytic studies of emotion. In fact, positive and negative affect are terms for the axes formed after implementing a factor rotation on the circumplex model (Watson & Tellegen, 1985). The two dimensions of Watson and Tellegen's rotated circumplex model differ interpretively from the original in that they subsume arousal, and place pleasant and unpleasant emotions on separate dimensions (rather than on a single valence dimension). Hence, the rotated model better characterizes variance when positive and negative affect function in parallel, operating simultaneously but independently. Given that depression and anxiety are commonly viewed as sharing high negative affect but not low positive affect (characteristic of depression alone), the rotated circumplex model is an appealing framework from which to examine these two conditions (Clark & Watson, 1991).

Because elevated negative affect is related to frontal asymmetry in favor of the right hemisphere, depression and anxiety would both be expected to show right-lateralized patterns of frontal activity (Davidson, 2004). This common pattern would appear to suggest that measures of frontal lateralization cannot be used to distinguish depression and anxiety. However, some research suggests that frontal lateralization may be related to other dimensions of emotion along which depression and anxiety do differ. In particular, several studies have shown that a specific dimension of anxiety called anxious apprehension (e.g. worry) is related to increased left hemisphere activity, possibly resulting in a pattern of frontal asymmetry distinct from depression (Heller *et al.*, 1997, 1998; Nitschke *et al.*, 1999). The robustness and reliability of this finding remain unclear, as comorbidity is seldom controlled in studies of depression and anxiety. An additional possibility is that both negative affect and anxious apprehension dimensions capture unique variance in frontal lateralization. Depression and anxiety may therefore share brain asymmetries in some regions of frontal cortex but not others. Appropriate electromagnetic or hemodynamic imaging studies using well-characterized clinical samples will be essential to answering these questions.

Personality and frontal brain asymmetries

In recent years it has become increasingly apparent that frontal brain asymmetries can also be understood in terms of specific personality dimensions. Numerous studies have posited that frontal lateralization associated with emotion reflects approach and avoidance motivation; with left activity more associated with approach motivation, and right activity reflecting avoidance motivation (Davidson, 1992, 1998). Because most positive emotions are associated with approach motivation and negative emotions with avoidance motivation, the valence and motivation perspectives are highly overlapping. Anger, however, typically involves both unpleasant valence and approach motivation. Based on findings examining anger, a series of studies have argued that the valence/arousal dimensions may not account for the frontal asymmetry data as well as a motivational dimension dichotomized as approach/withdrawal (Harmon-Jones, 2004). Recent work by Wacker *et al.* (2003), however, has emphasized that affective states can be characterized by both valence and motivational direction (e.g. anger is unpleasant, but could be accompanied by approach motivation or withdrawal motivation, depending on the circumstances). Furthermore, recent evidence suggests that the left-lateralized activity associated with anger is attributable to a dimension of anger that is associated with anxious apprehension, rather than approach motivation (Stewart *et al.*, 2008). Regardless, evidence that valence may be an important source of variance in the degree to which different brain regions are involved in cognition (Herrington *et al.*, 2005; Perlstein *et al.*, 2002) indicates that it remains an important variable in investigations of emotion/cognition interactions.

A central goal of personality psychology has been to identify the basic structures of personality, and the valence and motivation models are just two of several approaches that have been used to classify personality

Who's Who in America - 2011

Special Listee Prices:

	PAYMENT ENCLOSED	BILL ME
CLASSIC EDITION	Save over 65%!	Save over 60%!
	$789.00	$789.00
	$247.00	$280.00
DELUXE EDITION	PAYMENT ENCLOSED	BILL ME
	Save over 65%!	Save over 60%!
	$830.00	$830.00
	$277.00	$297.00

WA65C Classic Edition reference market price $789. WA65DLX Deluxe Edition reference market price $830.
Scheduled publication date: October 2010.

WA65N

☐ *Personalize your book* (optional)

Print Listee's name here: _____

[grid of boxes for characters]

All engraving will appear in upper and lower case - up to 28 characters. Allow boxes for punctuation and spaces between names/initials. Please use English letters only. Returns on personalized books will only be accepted for defects or errors in production.

*Please remit payment in U.S. dollars. For residents of NJ, NY & PA, include sales tax on total cost of order. IL include tax on book cost only. Orders will be charged applicable sales tax unless properly accompanied by a Tax-Exemption Certificate or resale. Canadian customers please include 6% for Goods and Services Tax except residents of NB, NL, and NS who must include 14%. When purchased for business or professional reference use, this book may be a tax-deductible expense. For information on wire transfer payments, call customer service at 1-800-473-7020. Please allow 8-12 weeks for shipping outside the U.S. **All returns must be submitted within 30 days.**

Payment Options:

Price: $ _____

Add shipping/handling: **U.S.: $34.95; Outside U.S.: $65.00** + $ _____

*Applicable Sales tax + $ _____

TOTAL = $ _____

☐ Check or money order enclosed. (Please make checks payable to Marquis Who's Who)

☐ Please charge my: ☐ MasterCard ☐ VISA ☐ American Express

Card #: _____

Expiration Date: _____ Security Code: _____

Cardholder's Name: _____

Shipping Information: Item cannot be shipped to a P.O. Box

☐ Business Address ☐ Residential Address

Name: _____

Business: _____

Address: _____

City: _____ State/Province: _____

Country: _____ ZIP: _____

Phone: _____

Email: _____ ☐ Personal ☐ Bus.

Signature: _____ Date: _____

Order not valid without signature

Who'sWho in America® · 2011

For over a century, **Who's Who in America** has remained the authoritative biographical resource chronicling the achievements of America's most notable men and women from every field of endeavor. With this special discount, only available to listees, the 2011 (65th) Edition will be a welcome addition to your home or office library, serving as a permanent record of your accomplishments.

Special Offer: Personalize your copy FREE of Charge!

Who's Who in America listees can have their names imprinted on the cover in elegant gold lettering—at no additional cost! First, choose from the Classic Edition or the distinguished Leather-Bound Deluxe Edition, then check the appropriate box if you would like your copy of the 2011 Edition imprinted with your name. For more information, or to place your order by phone, call toll-free **1-800-473-7020.** (Outside the U.S. and Canada, call 1-908-673-1000)

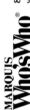

MARQUIS
Who'sWho®   890 Mountain Avenue • New Providence, NJ 07974 USA
www.marquiswhoswho.com • 1-800-473-7020

dimensions. These also include trait adjective systems (e.g. yielding descriptors such as extraversion, introversion). Although debate continues regarding the nature of proposed dimensions (e.g. nomenclature, number and orthogonality), these systems share the same core tenet that personality, at a basic level, consists of stable, heritable, biologically instantiated sensitivities to positive and negative stimuli (Elliot & Thrash, 2002). How one responds emotionally to positive and negative stimuli, how one regulates this response, and how the regulated response is characterized across experiential, language, behavioral, physiological and interpersonal domains are all questions that extend from this premise. Scholars have identified conceptual overlap between neuroticism–extraversion and negative temperament–positive temperament (Carver et al., 2000), behavioral inhibition–behavioral activation and negative temperament–positive temperament (Watson, 2000), and neuroticism–extraversion and behavioral inhibition–behavioral activation (Carver et al., 2000). Further empirical work, through factor-analytic and correlational studies, has identified relationships between extraversion and positive temperament and neuroticism and negative temperament (Clark & Watson, 1999); negative temperament and behavioral inhibition, as well as positive temperament and behavioral activation (Carver & White, 1994); extraversion and behavioral activation (Gomez et al., 2000); and neuroticism and behavioral inhibition (Diaz & Pickering, 1993).

Elliot & Thrash (2002) proposed that variance shared among these constructs be interpreted as approach and avoidance temperaments. "Approach temperament" subsumes the personality qualities associated with extraversion, the affective style associated with positive temperament, and the behavior patterns associated with the behavioral activation system (BAS). In contrast, "avoidance temperament" subsumes personality qualities associated with neuroticism, the affective style associated with negative temperament, and behavior patterns associated with the behavioral inhibition system (BIS) (Elliot & Thrash, 2002). This theoretical heuristic has been supported empirically through factor-analytic studies showing that measures of extraversion, neuroticism, positive temperament, negative temperament, BAS and BIS yield a two-factor structure (approach temperament and avoidance temperament) that is unaffected by response bias (Elliot & Thrash, 2002).

Recent support for the intersection of personality, psychopathology and emotional dimensions comes from work in our laboratory examining the relationship of approach and avoidance temperament, as defined by Elliot & Thrash (2002), to performance on neuropsychological tests sensitive to lateralized brain activity (Koven, 2003). In this study, relationships between approach and avoidance temperament, patterns of anterior brain asymmetry, situational strategies to regulate negative emotion (suppression and reappraisal), and the outcomes of these strategies on emotion processes were examined. Emotional responses to a situational stressor were measured via self-report, facial affect coding and salivary cortisol. Individuals characterized by approach temperament used reappraisal more advantageously than they did suppression. Reappraisal instructions were effective in reducing the degree of emotional responding in the self-report, behavioral and physiological domains. Individuals characterized by avoidance temperament, in contrast, were more adept at using suppression to achieve the same results. The suppression technique facilitated approximately the same magnitude of emotion regulation for avoidance-biased individuals as the reappraisal technique did for approach-biased individuals. However, suppression was slightly less effective for avoidance temperament participants than reappraisal was for approach temperament participants in down-regulating cortisol reactivity.

Of greatest relevance to this chapter, approach-biased participants outperformed avoidance-biased individuals on neuropsychological tests that required specialized cognitive functions of the left prefrontal cortex; whereas, avoidance-temperament participants excelled on neuropsychological tests involving specialized cognitive functions of the right prefrontal cortex (see Figure 5.1). These data complement findings from other studies that have used neuropsychological techniques in non-clinical samples to map relationships between patterns of anterior brain asymmetry and personality-, mood- and coping-related variables such as euphoric/dysphoric affect (Bartolic et al., 1999; Gray, 2001; Greene & Noice, 1988; Isen & Daubman, 1984; Isen et al., 1987), hostility (Williamson & Harrison, 2003), anxiety (Everhart & Harrison, 2002), verbal/non-verbal cognitive style (Elfgren & Risberg, 1998; Gevins & Smith, 2000), extraversion/introversion (Henderson, 1992), self-control (O'Connell et al., 1987), flexibility/rigidity (Regard, 1983), engagement/disengagement (Fogel,

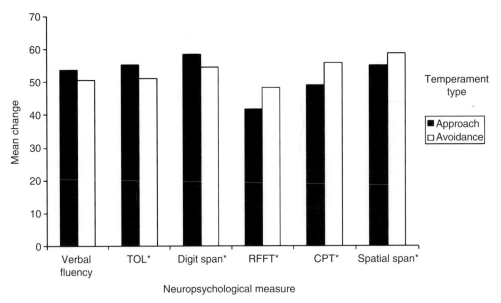

Figure 5.1. Mean change in neuropsychological test performance for approach- and avoidance-biased participants. The x-axis represents groups of individuals classified as having either an approach or avoidance temperament, according to a two-factor solution from a principal components analysis using subscales of the NEO Five Factor Inventory (Costa & McCrae, 1992), General Temperament Survey (Watson & Clark, 1993), and the Behavioral Inhibition System and Behavioral Activation System scales (Carver & White, 1994). The x-axis also represents neuropsychological tests related to left (Verbal Fluency Test: Gladsjo *et al.*, 1999; Tower of London (TOL): Culbertson & Zillmer, 2001; Digit Span subtest of the Wechsler Memory Scale, Third Edition: Wechsler, 1997) and right (Ruff Figural Fluency Test (RFFT): Ruff, 1996; Conners' Continuous Performance Test (CPT), Second Edition: Conners, 2000; Spatial Span subtest of the Wechsler Memory Scale, Third Edition: Wechsler, 1997) frontal hemisphere functions. The y-axis shows mean scores in *T*-score units. * indicates that mean difference between temperament types for the specified neuropsychological test is significant at $P < 0.05$. Figure based on Koven (2003).

2000) and self-enhancement coping style (Tomarken & Davidson, 1994). These studies provide strong evidence for hemisphericity of temperament variables. Specifically, that approach temperament which reflects behavioral approach, extraversion and positive temperament, is associated with greater left-trait anterior brain activity, whilst in contrast, avoidance temperament that encompasses behavioral inhibition, introversion and negative temperament, is associated with greater right-trait anterior brain activity. Moreover, these neuropsychological findings provide additional support for earlier studies suggesting that the two-dimensional models of extraversion/neuroticism, positive/negative temperament, and behavioral inhibition/activation are different conceptualizations of the same psychobiological substrates that contribute to personality, affective and motivation traits.

The considerable conceptual overlap between extraversion and neuroticism, approach and avoidance motivation, pleasant and negative emotion, and positive and negative affect suggests that extraversion and neuroticism should be associated with lateralized brain function (Koven, 2003). Although results in the literature have been mixed in this regard, Schmidtke & Heller (2004) reported that increased neuroticism was associated with decreased alpha activity (indicating elevated brain activity) recorded over the right hemisphere. However, this lateralization was localized to posterior and not anterior regions. Although the lack of frontal findings failed to provide evidence for anterior asymmetries, the posterior findings were consistent with the hypothesis that neuroticism would be positively correlated with arousal, as indexed by activity in right posterior cortex. Other studies have provided support for asymmetries in the predicted direction in anterior regions (Canli *et al.*, 1998).

In summary, a substantial amount of evidence indicates that lateralized activity in the frontal cortex is associated with specific dimensions of emotion and motivation; particularly positive emotion/approach motivation in favor of left frontal cortex, and negative emotion/avoidance motivation in favor of right frontal cortex. Data in support of this pattern comes from numerous methodologies, including brain-injury studies, intracarotid sodium amytal testing, EEG and others (Borod, 1992; Davidson, 2004;

Heller *et al.*, 1997, 1998; Lee *et al.*, 1987; Nitschke *et al.*, 1999). This lateralization appears to have both state and trait components, responding to experimentally induced changes in mood and characterizing the emotional experience of individuals with depression and anxiety (Coan & Allen, 2003). Studies examining frontal lateralization have traversed a variety of theoretical perspectives in psychology, including emotion, psychopathology and personality. The prominence of frontal brain lateralization research in human neuroscience attests to its potential importance for parsing complex, overlapping constructs such as depression and anxiety, or motivation and personality.

Frontal asymmetry, electrophysiology and hemodynamics

Numerous EEG studies have found lateralized frontal activity in emotion and personality, but studies using hemodynamic imaging generally have not (Coan & Allen, 2004; Wager *et al.*, 2003). We argue that this replication failure may stem from the widespread use of data-analytic strategies that are inappropriate for identifying asymmetric brain activity. This section will review neurophysiological techniques for examining lateralized brain activity, with particular emphasis on techniques used in hemodynamic imaging studies.

EEG and the study of frontal asymmetries

Coan & Allen (2004) estimated that over 70 published EEG studies have examined frontal asymmetries in emotion. As EEG methods have advanced, so has knowledge of the dynamics of these asymmetries. For example, analyses of spectral activity across frontal electrode sites have shown that important differences in left and right frontal activity in depression and anxiety are relative rather than absolute (Bell *et al.*, 1998; Bruder *et al.*, 1997; Gotlib *et al.*, 1998). Although data from EEG studies using few electrodes have generally supported the finding that individuals with depression and anxiety show relatively less left frontal activity, the limited spatial resolution of this methodology constrains the ability to localize this activity within the frontal cortex. Recent years have seen dramatic improvements in the spatial resolution of EEG, due primarily to increased electrode densities, more common availability of structural MRIs, and improved source localization techniques. However, many previous studies of brain

asymmetry have not capitalized on these advances. Very few of these EEG studies have reliably identified electrical signals from deep frontal regions (e.g. orbital and medial frontal cortex), as the observed scalp distribution of signals from these regions is often difficult to disambiguate from signals closer to the scalp (Davidson, 2004). The incorporation of structural and functional MRI information can greatly improve our ability to localize EEG signal in deep structures, but to date few studies of depression and anxiety have capitalized on this combined approach.

Positron emission tomography and fMRI have been used extensively in recent years to localize specific regions related to emotion, depression and anxiety (for reviews see Wager *et al.*, 2003, and Murphy *et al.*, 2003). Studies using these techniques can provide somewhat better localization information than EEG, particularly for deep structures. It is thus striking that virtually no PET or fMRI studies have robustly replicated the EEG asymmetry findings (Wager *et al.*, 2003). As discussed in the recent literature, this represents a significant problem, calling into question either the asymmetry itself or the methods used to measure it (Canli, 1999; Davidson, 1998, 2002; Davidson & Irwin, 1999; Herrington *et al.*, 2005; Nitschke *et al.*, 2006).

In their recent meta-analysis, Wager *et al.* (2003) concluded that there was only "limited support for valence-specific lateralization of emotional activity in frontal cortex" (p. 513) in the hemodynamic literature. When analyzing studies designed to assess brain activity during approach/withdrawal and positive/negative affective states, they found only a trend toward increased activity in left versus right frontal cortex for approach versus withdrawal, and no effect of hemisphere for positive compared with negative stimuli or states. However, an examination of their methods calls this null finding into question. Of critical importance is that most of the studies used in their meta-analysis did not actually directly test laterality effects. In an effort to compensate for this critical shortcoming, Wager *et al.* (2003) used a form of conjunction analysis in order to infer laterality effects in the studies they examined.[1] As explained below, conjunction analyses are frequently insensitive to laterality effects in PET and fMRI. Thus, reliance on this approach limits the conclusions that can be drawn. This criticism also applies to a meta-analysis by Murphy *et al.* (2003), who also examined PET and fMRI studies to test the anterior asymmetry hypothesis in non-clinical populations. They concluded that theories of anterior asymmetries "may be too coarse, in terms of both their neural underpinnings and the aspect of emotion under consideration" (p. 227). However, in the absence of hemodynamic imaging studies using robust asymmetry analyses, the conclusions of these meta-analyses cannot be accepted with confidence.

Because of the failure of hemodynamic methods to replicate EEG, it remains to be seen which (if any) specific areas of prefrontal cortex are driving the EEG laterality effects. Some researchers have argued that dorsolateral prefrontal cortex (DLPFC) is the key region relating frontal EEG lateralization to emotional valence and motivation (Davidson, 2004; Herrington et al., 2005; Nitschke et al., 2006). However, it is quite possible that, due to the relative ease with which EEG can detect signals from regions near the scalp surface, electrical activity from DLPFC may overshadow important lateralized activity in deeper structures. For example, in addition to DLPFC, ventromedial prefrontal cortex (VMPFC) and regions of anterior cingulate cortex play important roles in emotion (Damasio, 1994; Davidson et al., 2000; Drevets et al., 1997; Davidson & Irwin, 1999; Milad & Quirk, 2002). Although relatively few studies to date have postulated functional asymmetries in these regions, few direct tests of asymmetries have been applied to them.

Because of the relative consistency of EEG techniques and findings in this area over the past two decades, it can be argued that limitations in hemodynamic imaging paradigms, techniques and analyses are central to the failure of hemodynamic imaging to replicate EEG findings regarding frontal lateralization. The following sections examine theoretical and methodological areas where hemodynamic imaging studies may be falling short.

Hemodynamic imaging and the manipulation of emotion

Findings regarding frontal asymmetries in emotion turn crucially on what component of the emotion construct is under investigation. The distinction between recognition and experience of different emotions is particularly important, as self-reported emotional experience is more frequently related to patterns of frontal lateralization than is recognition performance (Canli, 1999; Heller, 1990; Davidson, 1992; Ekman et al.,

1990; Starkstein & Robinson, 1988). Studies examining self-reported emotional experience typically rely either on experimental mood manipulations or comparisons between groups of individuals exhibiting abnormal, stable patterns of emotional function (e.g. depression or anxiety). Canli (1999) noted that many hemodynamic imaging studies of emotion have focused only on the perception of affective stimuli rather than on other aspects of emotion processing, such as emotional experience. It is unclear whether hemodynamic studies have employed paradigms that examine changes in emotional experience to a lesser extent than have EEG studies. If so, robust laterality findings would be expected to occur less frequently in hemodynamic imaging studies.

Another critical issue is the extent to which specific psychophysiological measures alter moods. Although few, if any, data exist comparing individuals' emotional reactions to hemodynamic versus electrophysiological procedures, there is reason to suspect that the former may in fact be significantly more anxiety-inducing in ways that could artifactually foster different results for the two types of measures – both PET and MRI involve placement in tightly enclosed spaces, PET involves an intravenous injection and MRI involves very loud noise. It is unclear what effect these procedural factors have on experiments concerning the neurobiology of emotion and personality. It is possible that a procedurally induced baseline increase in negative affect may attenuate the relative effect of an experimental mood manipulation or group comparison. Ultimately, this attenuation may play some part in the failure of hemodynamic imaging studies of emotion to replicate the EEG frontal asymmetry findings.

Hemodynamic measures of brain asymmetry

Positron emission tomography and fMRI techniques for measuring brain asymmetry generally employ a few basic approaches, such as size/mass difference analyses, conjunction analyses, factorial designs and connectivity analyses (Friston, 2003). Almost no studies directly compared relative strengths and weaknesses of these four approaches. The following section briefly examines the utility of these approaches in revealing lateralized brain activity. An examination of 52 hemodynamic imaging studies of frontal asymmetries in emotion indicates that only a very small number used analyses that were sufficiently sensitive to hemispheric asymmetries.

Size/mass difference analysis

Some studies (Canli *et al.*, 1998) have examined laterality by counting the number of voxels within an active cluster, and comparing that with the number of voxels in an active cluster in the same region of the contralateral hemisphere. It would be important in a study using this method to specify the criteria used to select a contralateral cluster – e.g. what sort of search field is allowed to consider a contralateral cluster truly homologous. This issue is both difficult and non-trivial, given that in many respects the brain is not truly symmetric structurally or functionally. For example, the volume that is contralateral according to 3D coordinates may fall in a neighboring gyrus, such as a different portion of a somatotopic map, etc. As a consequence, it is difficult to assess the validity or generalizability of this approach in testing asymmetries. Furthermore, this technique is vulnerable to a more significant problem – it may take only cluster size into account and not cluster intensity. Some studies attempt to overcome this limitation by deriving some type of index that reflects both the size and intensity of a cluster (such as "cluster mass") or simultaneously using size and intensity thresholds (Maddock *et al.*, 2003). A third limitation of this strategy is that it ignores voxels that are just below the specified significance threshold. As a result, it is possible that a putative cluster in one hemisphere has a substantial amount of subthreshold activity, yet an observed voxel significance count of zero. Lastly, hemispheric asymmetries may be present in areas where activity in neither hemisphere reaches the a priori statistical threshold for inclusion in a cluster. A size/mass difference analysis would overlook such regions; even if a region fails to meet a statistical threshold in each hemisphere, they may still differ from one another were the test done. Overall, this technique can lead to unacceptably high false-positive or false-negative laterality findings.

Conjunction analysis

A so-called conjunction analysis involves a binary comparison of significant activity in two regions, conditions or groups (Friston, 2003). If a particular region is considered active based on a specific significance threshold, activity in that region can be considered asymmetric if the analogous region in the contralateral hemisphere does not exceed that same threshold. As discussed by Davidson & Irwin (1999)

and Friston (2003), this approach is problematic, as it does not directly test the *size* of the difference between a given region and its contralateral homologue. Failure to conduct a direct comparison violates basic tenets of conventional ANOVA. This approach drastically increases the vulnerability to both false-positives and false-negatives.

Factorial designs

A direct comparison of asymmetric activity can be obtained using a factorial design, where hemisphere is included as one of the factors (Davidson & Irwin, 1999; Friston, 2003). Very few hemodynamic studies examining the contribution of frontal regions to emotion have implemented this analytic strategy, and it is remarkably rare in hemodynamic studies in the cognitive neuroscience literature more generally. Although Friston (2003) outlined how it can be implemented in the program Statistical Parametric Mapping (SPM, one of the most widely used neuro-imaging statistical packages, http://www.fil.ion.ucl.ac.uk/spm), it is not directly integrated into the analysis component of the program or in most other commonly used programs. This is surprising, as the inclusion of hemisphere as a factor in an ANOVA design is consistent with basic statistical approaches across numerous disciplines, and is analytically trivial relative to the computations carried out by most hemodynamic imaging analysis packages.

Connectivity analyses

Connectivity analysis is another approach to examining hemispheric asymmetries (Friston, 2003). This approach examines coactivation patterns in two or more brain regions. It can be implemented in many ways, most simply with correlational designs using voxels or clusters of voxels as inputs over time, conditions or subjects. For example, Irwin *et al.* (2004) examined fronto-limbic correlations in depressed and non-depressed samples. A group-wise comparison of correlations between frontal and amygdalar regions using Fisher's R-to-Z test showed a significant group difference.

Structural equation modeling, independent components analysis and dynamic causal modeling are techniques for testing specific relationships among brain regions (Friston *et al.*, 1997). These techniques are presently rare in hemodynamic imaging studies, as they are computationally intensive and unfamiliar to most researchers, but they are receiving increasing attention.

Connectivity analyses can be used to address questions regarding brain asymmetries by examining the relationship between homologous (or non-homologous) regions in contralateral hemispheres. For example, a significant correlation between a frontal region in both hemispheres during an emotional task can indicate coordinated, bilateral activity. Correlations between paired regions can be calculated separately by subject group and then statistically compared to examine group differences in lateralized activity. Dynamic causal modeling and structural equation modeling can further the understanding of this sort of bilateral activity by testing whether activity in a subregion of one hemisphere is mediated or moderated by activity in a contralateral region (Friston, 2003). These and other techniques warrant considerably wider use in the systematic evaluation of brain asymmetries.

Methodological complexities in asymmetry analyses

Although some of the statistical techniques discussed above are relatively trivial to implement, additional methodological complexities exist that may be responsible for their underutilization. There is a great deal of confusion in fMRI research regarding exactly what, where and how much brain data should be submitted to statistical analyses. Functional MRI studies collect voxels of data that generally range in size from 1–10 mm per dimension, and then align and scale them to a standard anatomical template so that ideally each voxel for each participant will be coregistered. Commonly, statistics are then carried out independently for each voxel. However, variations in participants' brain anatomy and imperfections in standardization procedures essentially preclude each recorded voxel aligning with an identical part of the brain across an entire sample or vis-à-vis a standard brain template. This problem is particularly relevant to analyses carried out between homologous voxels in different hemispheres, as the two hemispheres often differ morphologically in ways that are not readily accounted for using typical fMRI alignment procedures.

A number of strategies can be employed to address this problem. Most fMRI studies do not draw conclusions based on the findings of individual voxels. Low-pass spatial filters are typically applied, blurring the signal from individual voxels across their neighbors. This has the effect of decreasing spatial resolution (mm scale) while expanding signal across larger areas that can be more reliably identified (many mm or cm).

However, because many areas of the brain lack obvious morphological landmarks that are discernable from fMRI images, even these larger areas may be difficult to define stereotactically. This problem is generally handled by creating some other type of boundary criterion to define signal from a number of voxels grouped together – either a predefined shape (e.g. a sphere encompassing all voxels within a specified radius) or a set of contiguous voxels that individually meet some statistical threshold. It is often unclear which of these approaches will most effectively minimize localization error on a given dataset. Few studies have systematically compared them, and none has done so within the context of measuring brain asymmetries.

Examples of lateralized activity measured by fMRI

Recently, some studies have emerged that implement direct tests of brain asymmetry using hemodynamic imaging techniques (Herrington *et al.*, 2005; Herrington *et al.*, under review; Nitschke *et al.*, 2006). Three of these will be examined here, with emphasis placed on their contributions to the neuroscience of emotion, as well as their approaches to measuring brain asymmetries.

Herrington *et al.* (2005) examined brain asymmetries associated with emotion using fMRI in an unselected sample of participants. The experimental paradigm was a variant on the color–word Stroop task using pleasant, neutral and unpleasant words as stimuli. In this emotional Stroop task participants name the color ink in which a series of emotional and neutral words are written while ignoring the meaning of the word. Changes in response time for emotionally valenced words are regarded as evidence of an effect of emotional information on cognition. This experiment set out to examine prefrontal cortical asymmetries for positive emotion using a factorial design.

Analyses explored a variety of techniques for isolating bilateral regions in DLPFC. The most effective technique combined low-pass spatial filtering with the selection of a set of contiguous voxels in left DLPFC that was statistically significant on a per-voxel basis when comparing data from the pleasant and unpleasant word conditions. Data from this cluster, as well as the homologous region in the right hemisphere were extracted and included as levels of an ANOVA factor. Functional image processing and analyses were implemented using FEAT (FMRI Expert Analysis Tool, FMRIB's Software Library, http://www.fmrib. ox.ac.uk/analysis/research/feat/) and SPSS. Each fMRI time series was motion-corrected, high-pass filtered (to remove drift in signal intensity), intensity normalized, and spatially smoothed using a 3D Gaussian kernel (FWHM = 7 mm) prior to analysis.

Statistical maps were generated for each participant's time-series data by applying a regression analysis to each intracerebral voxel (Woolrich *et al.*, 2001). The fitted model was designed to predict observed brain activity from explanatory variables representing pleasant and unpleasant trial blocks separately, convolved with a gamma variate function to model the hemodynamic response (Aguirre *et al.*, 1998; Miezin *et al.*, 2000). Each explanatory variable in these analyses yielded a voxel-by-voxel map of parameter estimates (β) representing the correlation between the explanatory variable (e.g. pleasant and unpleasant word conditions) and the observed data. These maps were then converted to t statistic maps by dividing each β by its standard error. Finally, each voxel in the t statistic maps was converted into a z statistic by comparing each t value to a Gaussianized t distribution that follows a z distribution.

For analyses across participants, z-maps representing the difference between pleasant and unpleasant word conditions for each participant were registered into a common stereotactic space (Talairach & Tornoux, 1988) using automated linear registration software (FMRIB's Linear Image Registration Tool, FMRIB's Software Library). Statistical analyses were carried out with MEDx v3.4 via paired t-tests comparing each participant's Z map to zero (zero indicating no valence effect for that voxel). For ease of interpretation, the resulting t-values for each voxel were then converted into z statistics following a Gaussianized t distribution (as above for individual participant's z-maps). This analysis was intended to identify specific regions for subsequent region of interest (ROI) analyses. The probability of obtaining false positives was minimized by assigning a relatively liberal statistical threshold concurrently with requiring a large cluster size. Thus, voxels were considered to show a significant valence effect if the z-score greater than 2.3 or less than -2.3 ($P < 0.01$, two-tailed, uncorrected) and comprised at least 20 contiguous voxels (Compton *et al.*, 2003; Forman *et al.*, 1995).

This analysis revealed a significant cluster of greater activity for pleasant words in left DLPFC (see Figure 5.2). The center of mass for this cluster

Left and right ROIs in DLPFC

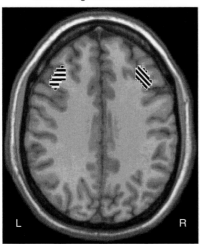

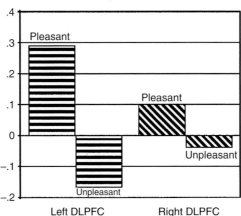

Average ROI *z*-scores for pleasant and unpleasant conditions

Figure 5.2. Differences in brain activity during presentation of pleasant versus unpleasant words. Left panel: Regions of interest (ROIs) used to quantify activity in left and right dorsolateral prefrontal cortex (DLPFC) on an axial image in radiological orientation (right hemisphere displayed on left) at a *z* coordinate of 34 mm. Right panel: Mean *z*-scores for pleasant and unpleasant word conditions in right and left DLPFC. *Z*-scores representing the relationship between brain activity and pleasant or unpleasant word conditions were averaged for all voxels inside the DLPFC ROIs. Figure and caption taken from Herrington *et al.* (2005).

was located at $x = -32$, $y = 24$ and $z = 42$ in Talairach & Tournoux (1988) coordinate space. The cluster was located in inferior and medial frontal gyri, with small intrusions into superior frontal and precentral gyri (between z coordinates of 20 and 62). In order to test the hypothesis regarding the conjoint effects of emotion, laterality and executive function, an ANOVA was implemented to examine activity within this DLPFC cluster and its homolog in the right hemisphere. Average z-scores were calculated for this cluster within each participant's z-maps representing significant activity during pleasant and unpleasant conditions. A repeated-measures ANOVA was carried out on these ROI scores to examine main effects and interactions for word valence (pleasant or unpleasant) and hemisphere. In line with the voxel-wise t-tests in the left hemisphere, the ANOVA revealed a main effect for valence, $F(1, 19) = 5.216$, $P = 0.034$, with more bilateral DLPFC activity for pleasant than for unpleasant words. Importantly, the valence effect varied by hemisphere, $F(1, 19) = 6.712$, $P = 0.018$, indicating more left than right DLPFC activity for pleasant than for unpleasant words. There was no main effect of hemisphere, $F(1, 19) = 0.017$, ns.

As predicted, the results revealed an asymmetric activation in favor of the left-hemisphere dorsolateral prefrontal cortex (DLPFC) for pleasant relative to unpleasant stimuli. This study is thus among the first to effectively use fMRI to complement EEG findings of asymmetric brain activity for emotion and to localize these findings within a specific frontal region.

Another important component of the study concerned the use of multiple techniques for isolating homologous regions. Although the paper focused on an area of DLPFC shown to be statistically significant on a per-voxel basis, other techniques were initially used as well, including extracting spherically shaped regions of data centered on the area of highest statistical significance within left DLPFC. These techniques yielded comparable results, converging on a significant interaction between pleasant versus unpleasant word conditions and left versus right DLPFC.

In summary, the results of Herrington *et al.* (2005) suggest that the consistency between EEG and fMRI studies of emotion and laterality will improve, to the extent that analysis methods in the two domains are similar. Including hemisphere as a factor in one's ANOVA is *de rigeur* in the EEG literature but is remarkably rare in the fMRI literature.

This problem is readily addressed with an ANOVA design that reflects hypotheses about hemispheric differences.

Although the approach in the Herrington *et al.* (2005) study of isolating activity in one hemisphere and examining its exact contralateral homolog proved sensitive to hemispheric asymmetries, this approach may overlook asymmetries in regions that are not exact mirror images of one another across hemispheres. Nitschke *et al.* (2006) demonstrated one solution to this problem. Their study focused on the role of emotion circuitry in anticipating aversive events. The paradigm used in their study involved the presentation of negative, high-arousal stimuli and neutral, low-arousal stimuli. A cue immediately preceding the stimulus indicated to participants whether a negative or neutral stimulus was about to be presented. Using an event-related design with variable intertrial intervals, the authors were able to examine brain activity during the anticipation, as well as perception of negative stimuli. The central finding of their study was that the anticipation of an aversive event engaged many of the same brain regions as the actual experience of the event – namely, amygdala, anterior insula, anterior cingulate cortex, dorsolateral prefrontal cortex and orbitofrontal cortex.

As with the Herrington *et al.* (2005) study, Nitschke *et al.* (2006) tested hypotheses about frontal asymmetries in emotion processes using a two-way ANOVA with stimulus valence (negative or neutral) and hemisphere as repeated measures. A comparison of activity between the negative and neutral trials revealed two significant clusters of activity in right DLPFC (see Figure 5.3). Instead of using these clusters to delineate a contralateral region for asymmetry analyses (as in Herrington *et al.*, 2005), they first dilated these clusters by 250%. The two-way ANOVA within these dilated clusters yielded significant condition by hemisphere interactions in the predicted direction (greater activity in right DLPFC compared with left, for negative compared with neutral trials), $F(1, 20) = 18.12$, $P < 0.001$, and $F(1, 20) = 17.87$, $P < 0.001$, respectively. Furthermore, the increase in right DLPFC activity during the anticipation of negative versus neutral stimuli was significantly predicted by levels of state and trait negative affect in the sample, $r = 0.71$, $P < 0.001$, and $r = 0.67$, $P < 0.001$ respectively, as measured by the Positive and Negative Affect Scale (PANAS; Watson & Clark, 1991). The same pattern of results was observed when dilations

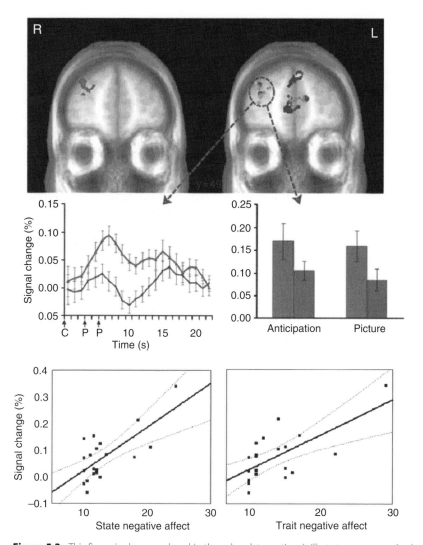

Figure 5.3. This figure is also reproduced in the color plate section. It illustrates greater activation for aversive than neutral trials across anticipation and picture periods in right dorsolateral prefrontal cortex (DLPFC) (Nitschke *et al.*, 2006). The brain image in the top left panel displays the results of a conjunction analysis, which identifies areas that activate more for aversive than neutral trials during both the anticipation period and the picture period when analyzed separately. For the top right brain image, colored areas showed a Valence main effect for the voxel-wise Period × Valence ANOVA ($P < 0.05$, corrected). Blue areas also showed greater activation for aversive than neutral trials during the anticipation period but not the picture period (aversive–neutral contrasts as indicated by corresponding voxel-wise *t* tests, $P < 0.05$, corrected). In contrast, purple areas also showed greater activation for aversive than neutral trials during the picture period but not the anticipation period (aversive–neutral contrasts, as noted above). Yellow areas showed greater activation for aversive than neutral trials for the Valence effect and for the aversive–neutral contrast for each period, whereas green areas for the Valence main effect did not meet the $P < 0.05$ (corrected) threshold for either contrast. The middle left panel shows time series plots of the circled clusters illustrating average percentage signal change across all time points of the aversive (red) and neutral (blue) trials. The onset of the 1-s picture presentation (P) occurred 3 s after warning cue (W) onset on half of the trials and 5 s after cue onset on the other half. In the middle right panel, bar graphs of the circled clusters illustrate average percentage signal change for the anticipation period and picture period separately. Error bars for time series plots and bar graphs are for confidence intervals (Cumming & Finch, 2005) around the mean after adjusting for between-subject variance (Loftus & Masson, 1994). The bottom panel shows scatter plots illustrating the positive relationship between negative affect and right DLPFC activation during the anticipation of aversive pictures.

Plots illustrate the relationship of greater activation for aversive than neutral trials during the anticipation period in the right dorsolateral prefrontal area depicted in the top panel to increases in state negative affect (left bottom panel; $r = 0.71$, $P < 0.001$) and trait negative affect (right bottom panel; $r = 0.67$, $P < 0.001$), as measured by the Positive and Negative Affect Schedule (PANAS; Watson *et al.*, 1988). R = right. L = left.

smaller than 250% were used and when no dilation was used, similar to the strategy employed by Herrington *et al.* (2005). Like Herrington *et al.* (2005), Nitschke *et al.* (2006) successfully replicated EEG findings of asymmetric frontal activity as a function of emotional valence. In addition, the findings of Nitschke and colleagues underscored the importance of examining how this asymmetry is modulated by individual difference variables (in their case, state and trait negative affect).

Individual differences were central to another study by Herrington (in preparation). Participants were selected by screening large groups of undergraduates and inviting selected subsets to participate in laboratory research. These subsets were chosen based on dimensions of depression and anxiety that have been shown to distinguish between these highly comorbid conditions (Nitschke *et al.*, 1999): the Anhedonic Depression and Anxious Arousal scales of the Mood and Anxiety Symptom Questionnaire (MASQ; Watson *et al.*, 1995a, 1995b) and the Penn State Worry Questionnaire (PSWQ; Meyer *et al.*, 1990; Molina & Borkovec, 1994). This study also used the emotional Stroop including blocks of pleasant, unpleasant or neutral trials. The primary hypothesis of this study was that both depression and anxiety would be associated with similar, abnormal patterns of frontal asymmetry within DLPFC.

Both Herrington *et al.* (2005) and Nitschke *et al.* (2006) examined asymmetries by averaging activity differences across voxels within regions of interest and submitting these averages to statistical analyses. Herrington *et al.* (under review) demonstrated another approach: instead of averaging across clusters of activity, they tested hemisphere effects separately for each voxel and its contralateral homolog. This approach has been proposed by Friston (2003), but to our knowledge has never been used in studies of hemispheric asymmetry in emotion (Matlab and C++ software had to be written expressly for this design, as none of the standard hemodynamic image analysis packages include it).

Statistical analyses followed a two-stage approach. At the first stage, parameter estimates were calculated representing the effect of pleasant and unpleasant words. The second stage focused on analyses across groups, conditions and hemispheres. A three-way mixed model ANOVA was implemented that estimated the fixed effects of group (Anxious Arousal, Anhedonic Depression and Control), brain activity as a function of emotional valence (pleasant versus unpleasant words) and hemisphere. Although not of interest by itself, the full ANOVA model included the random effect of participants within group in order to calculate appropriate mixed model error terms for each main effect and interaction of interest (see Kirk, 1994). Family-wise error was controlled by using Monte Carlo simulations to determine the probability of observing clusters of activity at a per-voxel threshold of $P < 0.01$.

Two areas of DLPFC were shown to be active in this study when implementing separate planned comparisons for Depression and Anxious Arousal groups versus Control, $F(1, 27) = 14.8$, $P = 0.001$ and $F(1, 30) = 8.5$, $P = 0.007$, respectively (see Figures 5.4 and 5.5). Responses to the pleasant word condition are particularly informative. The Control group activated DLPFC bilaterally for pleasant words, whereas the Depression group activated primarily the left DLPFC. These data suggest that depression may be characterized by an inability to bring DLPFC online bilaterally when presented with positive information. This is consistent with decades of literature showing abnormal responsiveness to pleasant affect (i.e. anhedonia) among individuals with depression (Klein, 1974; Rush & Weissenburger, 1994; Willner, 1993).

In contrast, when compared with the Anxious Arousal group, the Control group showed a lateralized pattern of activity for the pleasant word condition. This difference may reflect the fact that anxiety, unlike depression, is generally not associated with a lack of responsivity to positive stimuli per se (i.e. anhedonia; Watson *et al.*, 1995a). It is possible that the Depression versus Control contrast highlighted a region of DLPFC that is particularly responsive to pleasant stimuli among non-depressed individuals, manifesting as bilateral rather than unilateral activity. As the Anxious Arousal group did not differ from the Control group in self-reported Anhedonic depression, the location of the cluster in that contrast may have been driven less by activity during the pleasant word condition than was the case for the Depression versus Control contrast.

These findings are consistent with decades of EEG research on abnormal frontal asymmetries in depression and anxiety. However, they also raise new possibilities regarding where these asymmetries may be localized. In particular, the depression and anxiety groups both showed three-way interactions in the predicted direction, but in adjacent regions of

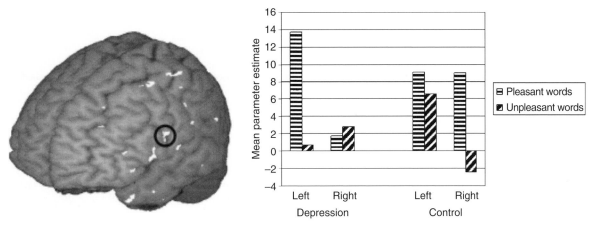

Figure 5.4. Significant three-way interaction between group (Depression versus Control), valence and hemisphere within the dorsolateral prefrontal cortex (DLPFC). The black circle in the left panel outlines the cluster, centered at ±50, 18, 20 in the coordinate space of Talairach & Tournoux (1988). The right panel displays histograms for parameter estimates at each factor level. The three-way interaction of average parameter estimates within this cluster is significant at $P < 0.001$ (corrected).

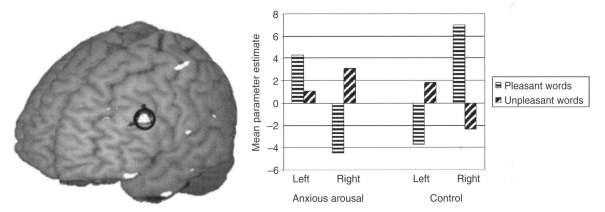

Figure 5.5. Significant three-way interaction between group (Anxious arousal versus Control), valence and hemisphere within the dorsolateral prefrontal cortex (DLPFC). The black circle in the left panel outlines the cluster, centered at ±-47, 24, 30 in the coordinate space of Talairach & Tournoux (1988). The right panel displays histograms for parameter estimates at each factor level. The three-way interaction of average parameter estimates within this cluster is significant at $P < 0.007$ (corrected).

DLPFC. Given the differences between the two clusters in average parameter estimates for the pleasant word condition, it is possible that specific areas of DLPFC are more responsive to positive emotion than other areas. Very few studies have examined functional heterogeneity within DLPFC, and no studies to date have done so with respect to emotion processes. Additional research is therefore critical to understanding whether the differential locations of these clusters maps reflect different components of depression and anxiety.

Conclusion

Recent research examining frontal brain function has demonstrated the benefit of integrating multiple theoretical perspectives from personality psychology with decades-old theories regarding the frontal lateralization of emotion (Elliot & Thrash, 2002; Schmidtke & Heller, 2004; Wacker et al., 2003). As pointed out by Wacker et al. (2003), the valence perspective on frontal asymmetry has persisted for about 20 years with very little direct examination of whether related constructs such as motivation or behavioral activation/inhibition may in fact capture the lateralization as well or better. Considerably more research is needed before findings regarding frontal asymmetry converge on one or more dimensions or resolve disagreements in favor of one dichotomy over another; for example, Wacker *et al.* (2003) and Elliot & Thrash (2002) reached somewhat different conclusions regarding whether one or many dimensions may be related to frontal lateralization. Whereas Wacker *et al.* found motivation (approach/avoidance temperament) to subsume numerous other constructions (extraversion and neuroticism, emotional valence, and behavioral activation and inhibition), Elliot & Thrash (2002) argued that the behavioral activation/inhibition best accounted for frontal lateralization and that valence and motivation models did not.

Which psychological construct best explains frontal lateralization may ultimately be dependent on which area of the frontal cortex is being examined. Few researchers have tried to reconcile models of specific frontal regions related to emotion with patterns of EEG frontal lateralization. Perspectives on the roles of frontal subregions in emotion generally focus on DLPFC, VMPFC and regions of anterior cingulate cortex (Davidson & Irwin, 1999). Although it has been suggested that the DLPFC in particular accounts for patterns of frontal EEG asymmetry (Davidson, 2004; Herrington *et al.*, 2005), VMPFC and anterior cingulate may also show lateralized activity patterns. For example, lateralized activity in VMPFC may be more related to approach/avoidance motivation or BIS/BAS than to valence, as VMPFC has been shown to play a role in the anticipation of rewards and punishments (Bechara *et al.*, 1994). Hemodynamic imaging could be an invaluable tool for addressing this and many other questions, if appropriate data-analytic techniques are used.

Acknowledgments

This work was supported by NIDA R21-DA14111, NIMH R01-MH61358, NIMH R01-MH74847, NIMH K08-MH63984, NIMH T32-MH19554, NIMH T32-MH14257, NIMH T32-MH18931, NICCHD P30-HD03352 to the Waisman Center, Carle Clinic, the Beckman Institute, and the HealthEmotions Research Institute. The authors thank Aprajita Mohanty, Joscelyn Fisher, Jennifer Stewart, Marie Banich, Andrew Webb, Joseph Barkmeier, Sid Sarinopoulos, Hillary Schaefer, Richie Davidson and Tracey Wszalek for their contributions to this research.

Endnote

1. This description of Wager *et al.*'s (2003) analysis holds if one defines conjunction analysis as including the binary examination of multiple regions within the same group or condition. Wager *et al.* (2003) conducted their meta-analysis by tallying the presence or absence of bilateral activity findings across emotion studies and statistically testing for the likelihood of obtaining these tallies. They went beyond typical conjunction analyses by directly testing the probabilities of finding multiple studies that had lateralized findings in a particular direction. But the underlying principle they used was conjunction – examining the co-occurrence, or lack thereof, of homologous activity across hemispheres.

References

Aguirre, G. K., Zarahn, E. & D'Esposito, M. (1998). The variability of human BOLD hemodynamic response. *Neuroimage*, **8**, 360–369.

Alema, G. Rosadini, G. & Rossi, G. F. (1961). Psychic reactions associated with intracarotid amytal injections and relation to brain damage. *Excerpta Medica*, **37**, 154–155.

Bartolic, E. I., Basso, M. R., Schefft, B. K., Glauser, T. & Titanic-Schefft, M. (1999). Effects of experimentally-induced emotional states on frontal lobe cognitive task performance. *Neuropsychologia*, **37**, 677–683.

Bear, D. M. & Fedio, P. (1977). Quantitative analysis of interictal behavior in temporal lobe epilepsy. *Archives of Neurology*, **34**, 454–467.

Bechara, A., Damasio, A., Damasio, H. & Anderson, S. (1994). Insensitivity to future consequences following damage to human prefrontal cortex. *Cognition*, **50**(1–3), 5–15.

Bell, I. R., Schwartz, G. E., Hardin, E. E., Baldwin, C. M. & Kline, J. P. (1998). Differential resting quantitative electroencephalographic alpha patterns in women with environmental chemical intolerance, depressives, and normals. *Biological Psychiatry*, **43**, 376–388.

Borod, J. C. (1992). Interhemispheric and intrahemispheric control of emotion: a focus on unilateral brain damage. *Journal of Consulting and Clinical Psychology*, **60**(3), 339–348.

Bruder, G. E., Stewart, J. W., Mercier, M. A. *et al.* (1997). Outcome of cognitive-behavioral therapy for depression: relation to hemispheric dominance for verbal processing. *Journal of Abnormal Psychology*, **106**, 138–144.

Canli, T. (1999). Hemispheric asymmetry in the experience of emotion: a perspective from functional imaging. *The Neuroscientist*, **5**(4), 201–207.

Canli, T., Desmond, J. E., Zhao, Z., Glover, G. & Gabrieli, J. D. E. (1998). Hemispheric asymmetry for emotional stimuli detected with fMRI. *Neuroreport*, **9**(14), 3233–3239.

Carver, C. S. & White, T. (1994). Behavioral inhibition, behavioral activation, and affective responses to impending reward and punishment: the BIS/BAS scales. *Journal of Personality and Social Psychology*, **67**, 319–333.

Carver, C. S. Sutton, S. & Scheier, M. F. (2000). Action, emotion, and personality: emerging conceptual integration. *Personality and Social Psychology Bulletin*, **26**, 741–751.

Clark, L. A. & Watson, D. (1991). Tripartite model of anxiety and depression: psychometric evidence and taxonomic implications. *Journal of Abnormal Psychology*, **100**, 316–336.

Clark, L. A. & Watson, D. (1999). Temperament: a new paradigm for trait psychology. In L. Pervin & O. John (Eds.), *Handbook of Personality: Theory and Research* (2nd edn), (pp. 399–423). New York, NY: Guilford Press.

Coan, J. A. & Allen, J. J. (2003). The state and trait nature of frontal EEG asymmetry in emotion. In K. Hugdahl & R. J. Davidson (Eds.), *The Asymmetrical Brain* (pp. 565–615). Cambridge, MA: MIT Press.

Coan, J. A. & Allen, J. J. (2004). Frontal EEG asymmetry as a moderator and mediator of emotion. *Biological Psychology*, **67**, 7–50.

Compton, R. J., Banich, M. T., Mohanty, A. *et al.* (2003). Paying attention to emotion: an fMRI investigation of cognitive and emotional stroop tasks. *Cognitive, Affective and Behavioral Neuroscience*, **3**(2), 81–98.

Conners, C. K. (2000). *Conners' Continuous Performance Test II: Computer Technical Guide and Software Manual.* [Computer software]. North Tonawanda, NY: Multi-Health Systems.

Costa, P., & McCrae, R. (1992). *Revised NEO Personality Inventory (NEO-PI-R) and Five Factor Inventory (NEO-FFI) Professional Manual.* Odessa, Fl.: Psychological Assessment Resources.

Culbertson, W. C., & Zillmer, E. A. (2001). *Tower of London – Drexel University (TOLDX).* North Tonawanda, NY: Multi-Health Systems.

Cumming, G. & Finch, S. (2005). Inference by eye: Confidence intervals and how to read pictures of data. *American Psychologist* **60**, 170–180.

Damasio, A. (1994). *Descarte's Error: Emotion, Reason and the Human Brain.* New York, NY: Avon Books.

Davidson, R. J. (1992). Emotion and affective style: hemispheric substrates. *Psychological Science*, **3**, 39–43.

Davidson, R. J. (1998). Anterior electrophysiological asymmetries, emotion, and depression: conceptual and methodological conundrums. *Psychophysiology*, **35**, 607–614.

Davidson, R. J. (2002). Anxiety and affective style: role of prefrontal cortex and amygdala. *Biological Psychiatry*, **51**, 68–80.

Davidson, R. J. (2004). What does the prefrontal cortex "do" in affect: perspectives on frontal EEG asymmetry research. *Biological Psychology*, **67**, 219–233.

Davidson, R. J. & Irwin, W. (1999). The functional neuroanatomy of emotion and affective style. *Trends in Cognitive Sciences*, **3**, 11–21.

Davidson, R. J., Pizzagalli, D., Nitschke, J. B. & Putnam, K. (2002). Depression: perspectives from affective neuroscience. *Annual Review of Psychology*, **53**(1), 545–574.

Davidson, R. J., Putnam, K. M. & Larson, C. L. (2000). Dysfunction in the neural circuitry of emotion regulation – a possible prelude to violence. *Science*, **289**, 519–594.

Decina, P., Sackeim, H. A., Prohovnik, I., Portnoy, S. & Malitz, S. (1985). Case report of lateralized affective states immediately after ECT. *American Journal of Psychiatry*, **142**, 129–131.

Diaz, A. & Pickering, A. (1993). The relationship between Gray's and Eysenck's personality spaces. *Personality and Individual Differences*, **15**, 297–305.

Drevets, W. C., Price, J. L., Simpson, J. R. *et al.* (1997). Subgenual prefrontal cortex abnormalities in mood disorders. *Nature*, **386**, 824–827.

Ekman, P., Davidson, R. J. & Friesen, W. V. (1990). Duchenne's smile: emotional expression and brain physiology, II. *Journal of Personality and Social Psychology*, **58**, 342–353.

Elfgren, C. I. & Risberg, J. (1998). Lateralized frontal blood flow increases during fluency tasks: influences of cognitive strategy. *Neuropsychologia*, **36**, 505–512.

Elliot, A. J., & Thrash, T. M. (2002). Approach-avoidance motivation in personality: approach and avoidance temperaments and goals. *Journal of Personality and Social Psychology*, **82**, 804–818.

Everhart, D. E. & Harrison, D. W. (2002). Heart rate and fluency performance among high- and low-anxious men following autonomic stress. *International Journal of Neuroscience*, **112**, 1149–1171.

Flor-Henry, P. (1979). On certain aspects of the localization of the cerebral systems regulating and determining emotion. *Biological Psychiatry*, **14**, 677–698.

Fogel, T. G. (2000). Patterns of perceptual asymmetries in the perception of chimeric faces: influences of depression, anxiety, and approach and withdrawal styles of coping. *Dissertation Abstracts International: Section B: The Sciences and Engineering*, **60**, 5223.

Forman, S. D., Cohen, J. D., Fitzgerald, M. *et al.* (1995). Improved assessment of significant activation in functional magnetic resonance imaging. *Magnetic Resonance in Medicine*, 33(5), 636–647.

Friston, K. J. (2003). Characterizing functional asymmetries with brain mapping. In K. Hugdahl & R. J. Davidson (Eds.), *The Asymmetrical Brain* (pp. 162–196). Cambridge, MA: MIT Press.

Friston, K. J., Buechel, C., Fink, G. R. *et al.* (1997). Psychophysiological and modulatory interactions in neuroimaging. *Neuroimage*, 6, 218–229.

Gainotti, G. (1972). Emotional behavior and hemispheric side of the lesion. *Cortex*, 8, 41–55.

Gevins, A. & Smith, M. E. (2000). Neuropsychological measures of working memory and individual differences in cognitive ability and cognitive style. *Cerebral Cortex*, 10, 829–839.

Gladsjo, J. A., Miller, S. W. & Heaton, R. K. (1999). *Norms for Letter and Category Fluency: Demographic Corrections for Age, Education, and Ethnicity*. Odessa, FL: Psychological Assessment Resources.

Gomez, R., Cooper, A. & Gomez, A. (2000). Susceptibility to positive and negative mood states: test of Eysenck's, Gray's, and Newman's theories. *Personality and Individual Differences*, 29, 351–365.

Gotlib, I., Ranganath, C. & Rosenfeld, P. (1998). Frontal EEG alpha asymmetry, depression, and cognitive functioning. *Cognition and Emotion*, 12, 449–478.

Gray, J. R. (2001). Emotional modulation of cognitive control: approach-withdrawal states double-dissociate spatial from verbal two-back task performance. *Journal of Experimental Psychology: General*, 130, 436–452.

Greene, T. R. & Noice, H. (1988). Influence of positive affect upon creative thinking and problem solving in children. *Psychological Reports*, 63, 895–898.

Harmon-Jones, E. (2004). Contributions from research on anger and cognitive dissonance to understanding the motivational functions of asymmetrical frontal brain activity. *Biological Psychology*, 67, 51–76.

Heller, W. (1990). The neurospychology of emotion: developmental patterns and implications for psychopathology. In N. L. Stein, B. Leventhal & T. Trabasso (Eds.), *Psychological and Biological Approaches to Emotion*. Hillsdale, NJ: Lawrence Erlbaum Associates.

Heller, W., Etienne, M. A. & Miller, G. A. (1995). Patterns of perceptual asymmetry in depression and anxiety: implications for neuropsychological models of emotion and psychopathology. *Journal of Abnormal Psychology*, 104, 327–333.

Heller, W., Nitschke, J. B., Etienne, M. A. & Miller, G. A. (1997). Patterns of regional brain activity differentiate types of anxiety. *Journal of Abnormal Psychology*, 106, 376–385.

Heller, W., Nitschke, J. B. & Miller, G. A. (1998). Lateralization in emotion and emotional disorders. *Current Directions in Psychological Science*, 7, 26–32.

Henderson, J. R. (1992). Introverts' and extroverts/ performance on the Wechsler Memory Scale – Revised. *Dissertation Abstracts International*, 53, 1064.

Herrington, J. D., Mohanty, A., Koven, N. S. *et al.* (2005). Emotion-modulated performance and activity in left dorsolateral prefrontal cortex. *Emotion*, 5, 200–207.

Herrington, J. D., Heller, W., Mohanty, A. *et al.* (under review). *Localization of asymmetric brain function in emotion and depression.*

Irwin, W., Anderle, M. J., Abercrombie, H. C. *et al.* (2004). Amygdalar interhemispheric functional connectivity differs between the non-depressed and depressed human brain. *Neuroimage*, 21, 674–686.

Isen, A. M. & Daubman, K. A. (1984). The influence of affect on categorization. *Journal of Personality and Social Psychology*, 46, 1206–1217.

Isen, A. M., Daubman, K. A. & Nowicki, G. P. (1987). Positive affect facilitates creative problem solving. *Journal of Personality and Social Psychology*, 52, 1122–1131.

Keller, J., Nitschke, J. B., Bhargava, T. *et al.* (2000). Neuropsychological differentiation of depression and anxiety. *Journal of Abnormal Psychology*, 109(1), 3–10.

Kirk, R. (1994). *Experimental Design: Procedures for the Behavioral Sciences*. Pacific Grove, CA: Brooks/Cole Publishing.

Klein, D. (1974). Endogenomorphic depression. *Archives of General Psychiatry*, 31, 447–451.

Koven, N. S. (2003). *An individual differences approach to emotion regulation using a neuropsychological model of approach and avoidance temperament*. Unpublished doctoral dissertation, University of Illinois at Urbana-Champaign, Illinois.

Lee, G. P., Loring, D. W., Meador, K. J. & Flanagan, H. F. (1987). Emotional reactions and behavioral complications following intracarotid sodium amytal injection. *Journal of Clinical and Experimental Neuropsychology*, 37, 565–610.

Loftus, G. R. & Masson, M. E. (1994). Using confidence intervals in within-subjects designs. *Psychonomic Bulletin & Review* 1, 476–490.

Maddock, R. J., Buonocore, M. H., Kile, S. J. & Garrett, A. S. (2003). Brain regions showing increased activation by threat-related words in panic disorder. *Neuroreport*, 14(3), 325–328.

Miezin, F. M., Maccotta, L., Ollinger, J. M., Petersen, S. E. & Buckner, R. L. (2000). Characterizing the hemodynamic response: effects of presentation rate, sampling procedure, and the possibility of ordering brain activity based on relative thinking. *Neuroimage*, **11**, 735–739.

Milad, M. R. & Quirk, G. J. (2002). Neurons in medial prefrontal cortex signal memory for fear extinction. *Nature*, **420**, 70–74.

Meyer, T. J., Miller, M. L., Metzger, R. L. & Borkovec, T. D. (1990). Development and validation of the Penn State Worry Questionnaire. *Behavior Research and Therapy*, **28**, 487–495.

Molina, S. & Borkovec, T. D. (1994). The Penn State Worry Questionnaire: psychometric properties and associated characteristics. In G. C. L. Davey & F. Tallis (Eds.), *Worrying: Perspectives on Theory, Assessment and Treatment* (pp. 265–283). Chichester: John Wiley & Sons.

Murphy, F. C., Nimmo-Smith, I. & Lawrence, A. D. (2003). Functional neuroanatomy of emotions: a meta-analysis. *Cognitive, Affective, and Behavioral Neuroscience*, **3**(3), 207–233.

Myslobodsky, M. S. & Horesh, N. (1978). Bilateral electrodermal activity in depressive patients. *Biological Psychology*, **6**(2), 111–120.

Nitschke, J. B., Heller, W., Palmieri, P. A. & Miller, G. A. (1999). Contrasting patterns of brain activity in anxious apprehension and anxious arousal. *Psychophysiology*, **36**, 628–637.

Nitschke, J. B., Sarinopoulos, I., Mackiewicz, K. L., Schaefer, H. S. & Davidson, R. J. (2006). Functional neuroanatomy of aversion and its anticipation. *Neuroimage*, **29**, 106–116.

O'Connell, T. R., Tucker, D. M. & Scott, T. B. (1987). Self-report of neuropsychological dimensions of self-control. In A. Glass (Ed.), *Individual Differences in Hemispheric Specialization* (pp. 267–282). *NATO ASI Series A: Life Sciences*, 130.

Perlstein, W. M., Elbert, T. & Stenger, V. A. (2002). Dissociation in human prefrontal cortex of affective influences on working memory-related activity. *Proceedings of the National Academy of Science USA*, **99**(3), 1736–1741.

Regard, M. (1983). Cognitive rigidity and flexibility: a neuropsychological study. *Dissertation Abstracts International*, **43**, 2714.

Ruff, R. M. (1996). *Ruff Figural Fluency Test*. Odessa, FL: Psychological Assessment Resources.

Rush, A. & Weissenburger, J. (1994). Melancholic symptoms features and DSM–IV. *American Journal of Psychiatry*, **151**, 489–498.

Schmidtke, J. I. & Heller, W. (2004). Personality, affect and EEG: predicting patterns of regional brain activity

related to extraversion and neuroticism. *Personality and Individual Differences*, **36**, 717–732.

Stabell, K. E., Andresen, S., Bakke, S. J. *et al.* (2004). Emotional responses during unilateral amobarbital anesthesia: differential hemispheric contributions? *Acta Neurologica Scandinavica*, **110**, 313–321.

Starkstein, S. E. & Robinson, R. G. (1988). Lateralized emotional responses following stroke. In M. Kinsbourne (Ed.), *Cerebral Hemisphere Function in Depression*. Washington, DC: American Psychiatric Press.

Stewart, J. L., Levin-Stilton, R., Sass, S. M., Heller, W. & Miller, G. A. (2008). Anger style, psychopathology, and regional brain activity. *Emotion*, **8**(5), 701–713.

Talairach, J. & Tornoux, P. (1988). *Co-planar Stereotactic Atlas of the Human Brain*. Stuttgart: Thieme.

Tomarken, A. J. & Davidson, R. J. (1994). Frontal brain activation in repressors and nonrepressors. *Journal of Abnormal Psychology*, **103**(2), 339–349.

Wacker, J., Heldmann, M. & Stemmler, G. (2003). Separating emotion and motivational direction in fear and anger: effects on frontal asymmetry. *Emotion*, **3**(2), 167–193.

Wager, T. D., Phan, K. L., Liberzon, I. & Taylor, S. F. (2003). Valence, gender, and lateralization of functional brain anatomy in emotion: a meta-analysis of findings from neuroimaging. *Neuroimage*, **19**(3), 513–531.

Watson, D. (2000). *Mood and Temperament*. New York, NY: Guilford Press.

Watson, D. & Clark, L. (1991). *The PANAS-X: Manual for the Positive and Negative Affect Schedule – Expanded Form*. University of Iowa.

Watson, D., & Clark, L. A. (1993). Behavioral disinhibition versus constraint: A dispositional perspective. In D. Wegener & J. Pennebaker (Eds.), *Handbook of Mental Control*, (pp. 506–527). New York: Prentice Hall.

Watson, D., Clark, L. A., & Tellegen, A. (1988). Development and validation of brief measures of positive and negative affect: the PANAS scales. *Journal of Personality and Social Psychology*, **54**(6), 1063–70.

Watson, D., Clark, L. A., Weber, K. *et al.* (1995a). Testing a tripartite model: II. Exploring the symptom structure of anxiety and depression in student, adult, and patient samples. *Journal of Abnormal Psychology*, **104**, 15–25.

Watson, D. & Tellegen, A. (1985). Toward a consensual structure of mood. *Psychological Bulletin*, **98**(2), 219–235.

Watson, D., Weber, K., Assenheimer, J. S. *et al.* (1995b). Testing a tripartite model: I. Evaluating the convergent and discriminant validity of anxiety and depression symptom scales. *Journal of Abnormal Psychology*, **104**, 3–14.

Wechsler, D. (1997). *Wechsler Memory Scale – Third Edition: Administration and Scoring Manual.* San Antonio, TX: The Psychological Corporation.

Williamson, J. B. & Harrison, D. W. (2003). Functional cerebral asymmetry in hostility: a dual task approach with fluency and cardiovascular regulation. *Brain and Cognition*, **52**, 167–174.

Willner, P. (1993). Anhedonia. In C. G. Costello (Ed.), *Symptoms of Depression* (Wiley Series on Personality Processes) (pp. 63–84). Oxford: John Wiley & Sons.

Woolrich, M. W., Ripley, B. D., Brady, M. & Smith, S. M. (2001). Temporal autocorrelation in univariate linear modeling of fMRI data. *Neuroimage*, **14**, 1370–1386.

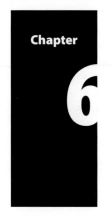

Chapter

6

Behavioral and electrophysiological approaches to understanding language dysfunction in neuropsychiatric disorders: insights from the study of schizophrenia

Gina R. Kuperberg, Tali Ditman, Donna A. Kreher and Terry E. Goldberg

Introduction

Language disturbances are characteristic of several neuropsychiatric disorders including schizophrenia, mania, Alzheimer's disease (and other dementias) and developmental disorders such as the autistic spectrum disorders. Yet it is only over the last 25 years that researchers have begun to study the language system in neuropsychiatric disorders from cognitive, psycholinguistic and neurophysiological perspectives. This chapter aims to review a selection of such studies to illustrate this progress, focusing primarily on schizophrenia. We begin with a summary of how clinical language disturbances in adult psychiatric disorders have traditionally been viewed. We then review selected studies at three basic levels of the language code – words (focusing on conceptual relationships within semantic memory), sentences (focusing on how words are combined to build up linguistic context and propositional meaning), and discourse (focusing on the generation of coherence links across more than one sentence). We then examine the relationship between abnormalities at each of these levels of language with cognitive dysfunction in more general domains, such as attention and working memory.

The functional neuroimaging literature examining the neuroanatomical basis of language abnormalities in neuropsychiatric disorders has generally lagged behind the cognitive behavioral and electrophysiological literatures (but see Kuperberg, 2009, for an overview of potential links between cognitive, electrophysiological and fMRI studies of language in schizophrenia). Although the focus of this chapter is on studies using behavioral and electrophysiological methods,

we conclude by discussing how a deeper understanding of the cognitive basis of language abnormalities might inform the design and interpretation of neuroanatomical and neuropharmacological studies, and how such a multifaceted approach might give new information about the underlying neuropathology of schizophrenia and other neuropsychiatric disorders.

Clinical language disturbances in psychosis: thought disorder and beyond

Clinically, the most obvious manifestation of language disturbances in adult psychiatric disorders is the disorganized unintelligible speech produced by patients during psychosis. This has traditionally been termed "thought disorder," reflecting the original perspective of psychopathologists who considered it an underlying disorder of thinking rather than a primary disturbance of language (Bleuler, 1911/1950; Kraepelin, 1971). Today, however, the term "thought disorder" is used purely descriptively without any assumptions about the complex relationship between thought and language (DSM–IV; American Psychiatric Association, 1990). Thought disorder occurs in mania as well as schizophrenia, but its most detailed characterization has been in schizophrenia. Building upon the detailed phenomenological descriptions of Schneider (1930) and others, clinical assessments of thought disorder such as the Thought, Language and Communication (TLC) scale (Andreasen, 1979a, 1979b), emphasize the "form" rather than the content

The Neuropsychology of Mental Illness, ed. Stephen J. Wood, Nicholas B. Allen and Christos Pantelis. Published by Cambridge University Press. © Cambridge University Press 2009.

of thought/speech, i.e. the way words and sentences are strung together. They include phenomena ranging from tangentiality (the shift in speech from one topic to another without obvious links between them), through neologisms (the use of non-words), as well as poverty of speech. Studies in the late 1970s and early 1980s established that some of these phenomena (including tangentiality, derailment, and incoherent speech) tended to occur more often in patients with positive than negative symptoms (Andreasen, 1979a, 1979b; Harvey et al., 1984; Oltmanns et al., 1985). These phenomena constitute "positive thought disorder." In contrast, phenomena such as "poverty of speech" co-occurred primarily with negative symptoms and were termed "negative thought disorder." Subsequent factor-analytic studies showed that positive thought disorder occurred more frequently with disorganized, non-goal directed behavior as opposed to hallucinations and delusions (Liddle, 1987, 1992; Andreasen et al., 1995). In DSM–IV (1990) positive thought disorder and disorganized behavior are now grouped together as constituting the "disorganization" subsyndrome of schizophrenia.

Original attempts to explain the various phenomena constituting positive thought disorder proposed concepts such as "loosening of association" (Bleuler, 1911/1950), "overinclusive thinking" (a tendency of patients to use concepts beyond their usual boundaries; Cameron, 1939, 1964), and concrete thinking (an inability to think abstractly; Goldstein, 1944). Some of these concepts, particularly Bleuler's "loosening of associations," were intended not only to describe the origins of positive thought disorder (disorganized speech output) itself, but to help explain the underlying cognitive basis of schizophrenia as a whole. In keeping with this idea, although many of the studies reviewed in the current chapter were originally inspired by the disorganized language output produced by some patients, it has become increasingly apparent that language abnormalities in schizophrenia are not confined to patients with positive thought disorder (although they are often more prominent in such patients), or to the language production system. Patients, with and without clinical evidence of thought disorder, can show clear abnormalities in language comprehension. Clinically, these abnormalities are usually subtler than the abnormalities evident in thought-disordered speech, but their study can yield valuable insights into fast, online word-by-word

processing mechanisms that may also be impaired during speech production. Moreover, the study of such mechanisms may also give insights into other symptoms of schizophrenia.

These observations, together with the identification of language disturbances in children at risk for schizophrenia (Cannon et al., 2002; Fuller et al., 2002; Ott et al., 2001), as well as in patients in their first episode of psychosis (Fuller et al., 2002; Hoff et al. 1999), suggest that a systematic study of the language system may give new insights into the neuropathogenesis of schizophrenia as a whole.

Single words and concepts: semantic memory structure and function

Most studies at the level of single words in neuropsychiatric disorders have examined how words are stored and accessed within semantic memory – an approach inspired by the observation that the speech of some psychotic patients is characterized by strings of word associations (Chaika, 1974). This section reviews studies adopting this perspective: we consider studies that have examined how patients with schizophrenia identify and name concepts, as well as investigations that have used both explicit and implicit measures to explore how such concepts are linked together through perceptual attributes, hierarchical relationships and semantic associations.

Semantic identification and naming

The identification and distinction of objects in the visual world is dependent on a hierarchical ventral visual pathway (Ungerleider & Haxby, 1994) that runs from primary visual cortex (V1) to extrastriate visual areas (V2 and V4) to the inferotemporal cortex, and is a major source of input to the prefrontal cortex. Some of the observed impairments in conceptual classification and identification in schizophrenia, discussed below, may arise because of deficits in visual perception rather than in cognitive semantic function. Although it has often been assumed that the ventral visual pathway is intact in schizophrenia, there has been surprisingly little research to back up this assumption. In one of the few paradigms to explicitly examine basic object identification in schizophrenia, Elvevaag et al. (2002b) asked patients to watch pictures of objects (e.g. a pear) morph into other objects (e.g. a lightbulb) and to indicate the frame in the morphing sequence at which the first object was no longer identifiable. Performances of patients and controls were nearly identical, suggesting that basic object perception was intact.

In humans, basic object identification is linked to the language system through our ability to name objects. Naming involves the activation and retrieval of lexical representations of both meaning and phonological form. Anomia, a word-finding impairment, is characteristic of several types of aphasic syndromes as well as other neurological disorders characterized by a loss of lexico-semantic knowledge such as Alzheimer's disease. Given the hypothesis that schizophrenia is associated with abnormalities in semantic processing, it has been of particular interest to determine how well patients with schizophrenia perform on naming tasks. Early studies suggested that patients with schizophrenia performed worse than controls on simple naming tasks (Faber & Reichstein, 1981), and in some cases as poorly as patients with fluent aphasia (Landre *et al.*, 1992) or Alzheimer's disease (Davidson *et al.*, 1996). Unlike Alzheimer's patients, however, schizophrenia patients improved their performance when given appropriate semantic cues (Laws *et al.*, 1998; Maas & Katz, 1992; McKenna *et al.*, 1994), suggesting that any deficit lay in the access and use of lexical knowledge rather than the loss of this knowledge. A more recent study of object naming by Denke & Goldberg (unpublished data) demonstrated that schizophrenia patients performed as well as healthy controls and significantly better than patients with mild Alzheimer's disease; there was no association between naming deficits and severity of positive thought disorder within the schizophrenia group – a finding that is consistent with previous observations (Aloia *et al.*, 1998; Goldberg *et al.*, 2000).

Explicit knowledge and use of semantic category

Concepts are not represented in isolation of one another, but are thought to be organized hierarchically according to domains and categories of knowledge within semantic memory. It is therefore important to examine whether schizophrenia patients' disordered use of concepts results from their abnormal organization within semantic memory. This issue has been investigated using both semantic production and categorization tasks.

Explicit production: semantic fluency

In semantic fluency tasks, participants are required to generate as many exemplars as possible from a given category (e.g. animals) in a defined time period (often one minute), with the assumption that abnormalities in the number and types of items produced will reveal abnormalities in the storage and retrieval of categorical semantic information. Patients with schizophrenia show mild-to-moderate difficulties on this test, producing fewer items per category than control participants. This impairment appears to be at least somewhat specific to producing semantic categorical information; several studies have demonstrated that patients are relatively less impaired on letter fluency tasks in which the requirement is to produce words beginning with a particular letter (Feinstein *et al.*, 1998; Goldberg *et al.*, 1998; Gourovitch *et al.*, 1996). A recent meta-analysis of studies directly comparing category and letter fluency, and controlling for factors like motivation, cooperation, symptomatology and IQ, confirmed a selective deficit on category fluency (Bokat & Goldberg, 2003). Kremen *et al.* (2003) came to a similar conclusion based upon a large well-controlled study that compared the performance of schizophrenia patients, bipolar patients and healthy controls.

The relationship between categorical fluency and thought disorder in schizophrenia is still unclear, however. While Aloia *et al.* (1996) found that the difference score between letter and semantic fluency performance accounted for a significant portion of thought disorder variability, later studies have not replicated this finding (Bokat & Goldberg, 2003).

Several approaches have been developed to examine the pattern of responses produced on semantic categorical fluency tasks. Allen & Frith (1983) and Allen *et al.* (1993) developed a methodology in which semantic fluency tests were repeatedly administered and the number of novel exemplars generated in each session tallied. They demonstrated that, given enough time, patients do eventually produce the same total number of category exemplars as controls. Elvevaag *et al.* (2002a) replicated this finding and went on to demonstrate that patients showed no category-specific deficits. These findings were interpreted as suggesting that there is no overall loss of semantic knowledge in schizophrenia patients: the impairment is in retrieving this knowledge in response to specific task demands.

Others have used multidimensional scaling, pathfinder and clustering techniques to examine relationships between words within superordinate categories in more depth (Allen & Frith, 1983; Aloia *et al.*, 1996; Paulsen *et al.*, 1996). These studies have suggested that patients are less likely than controls to group superordinate exemplars into related clusters and are more likely to produce bizarre associations. In addition, patients are slower than controls to produce items within a semantic cluster and to produce items that transition from one semantic cluster to the next. Taken together, these findings suggest that either the underlying organization of items stored within semantic memory is abnormal or that the process of retrieval is more disorganized in patients than in controls.

Explicit processing: knowledge of semantic category and semantic attributes

Although potentially useful, semantic fluency tasks are relatively uncontrolled, in that each individual generates different word lists and it is often difficult to derive objective quantitative measures of performance. To probe semantic memory structure in a more controlled fashion, several studies have examined participants' explicit semantic categorization judgments on controlled sets of stimuli.

The most basic type of categorization paradigm is to simply ask participants to decide whether or not an exemplar comes from a specified superordinate semantic category. There is some evidence that schizophrenia patients are slower and less accurate than controls in classifying common prototypes versus marginal exemplars. In two early studies, patients, relative to healthy controls, were slower to make a decision about whether a sparrow is a bird (a prototype) relative to whether a penguin is a bird (a marginal exemplar) (Chen *et al.*, 1994; Clare *et al.*, 1993; Gurd *et al.*, 1997). However, later studies did not replicate this finding (Elvevaag *et al.*, 2002b; McKenna *et al.*, 1994).

A second way of probing semantic knowledge is to ask participants to compare objects according to a particular perceptual semantic attribute, e.g. size. Cohen *et al.* (2005) capitalized on the so-called "distance effects" in size among real-world objects; this pertains to the longer reaction time (RT) to make size similarity judgments about two words or pictures that represent real-world objects of the same size versus different sizes. Despite having slower overall RTs, patients demonstrated a principled distance effect that did not differ from that of healthy controls.

A third method of probing categorical knowledge is to ask participants to classify words or objects using unspecified categories or dimensions. In the "triadic comparisons" test, participants view groups of three words and are asked to select the two words that are most similar. Each word triplet is a permutation derived from an overall word list in which words vary on two continuous dimensions: (1) living and non-living and (2) "associated with humans" and "not associated with humans." This information is not conveyed to the participants. Participants' responses are analyzed using multidimensional scaling methods to generate graphic maps of the structure of their semantic memories. Tallent *et al.* (2001) used this task with schizophrenia patients and demonstrated less-disorganized maps in patients than healthy controls. Interestingly, the degree of disorganization within these maps predicted severity of thought disorder over time. Moreover, in an unpublished study, Denke & Goldberg showed that these disorganized maps were specific to thought-disordered (TD) patients; they were not found in non-TD patients, patients with Alzheimer's disease or in healthy children.

Impairments in patients' use of categorical knowledge are also evident in declarative memory paradigms. When healthy controls learn a list of words, their recall is better if the list can be organized into semantic categories than if it consists of a sequence of unrelated words. This is thought to reflect the tendency to organize words in semantic memory during encoding (Craik & Lockhart, 1971; Kintsch, 1968). There is now fairly compelling evidence that patients with schizophrenia fail to spontaneously use such semantic categorization strategies during encoding. Several studies have reported that patients often produce largely unorganized word lists at recall (e.g. Iddon *et al.*, 1998; Koh *et al.*, 1973). Interestingly, most of these studies (Iddon *et al.*, 1998; Koh & Kayton, 1974), although not all (Gold *et al.*, 1992), have reported that if material is pre-organized, or if patients are given enough time to organize material during encoding, they do have the capacity to use semantic information to improve recall. Once again these results suggest that there is no overall loss of semantic knowledge in schizophrenia.

There has not been nearly as much study of semantic memory in bipolar disorder as in schizophrenia. However, recent studies suggest some impairments; Deckersbach *et al.* (2004, 2005) reported that bipolar patients can exhibit poorer organization during encoding than healthy controls, while other studies suggest that, despite using normal semantic clustering strategies during encoding, patients fail to make use of such strategies during recall (Bearden *et al.*, 2006a, 2006b).

Implicit knowledge of semantic and associative relationships

Another way of probing the structure and use of semantic memory is to manipulate semantic relationships between words but conceal the purpose of the study altogether from participants by asking participants to perform an orthogonal task. This yields implicit measures, which not only give information about the nature of categorical relationships between words within semantic memory, but also provide information about associative relationships between words that may not necessarily have semantic features in common. For example, "surgeon" and "scalpel" are associatively related but they are not categorically related and do not share semantic features.

Implicit production: word association tasks and the Latent Semantic Analysis

The classic method of probing implicit associative knowledge has been to use word association tasks in which participants are given a word and then asked to generate the first word (or series of words) that come to mind. Word association studies have a long history in psychiatry. Early experiments carried out by Bleuler, C. G. Jung and Kraepelin demonstrated that schizophrenia patients produced more idiosyncratic associations than normal controls (Jung, 1981). These findings were confirmed by some later studies (reviewed by Spitzer *et al.*, 1992). However, as discussed above with respect to semantic fluency, because word associations differ from individual to individual, it is often difficult to objectively measure the output produced.

Elvevaag *et al.* (2007) have recently addressed this issue by measuring the semantic coherence of words produced on association tasks using a Latent Semantic Analysis (LSA). The LSA derives a measure of coherence not simply on the basis of co-occurrence frequency, but also through examining the similarity of contexts in which words occur in a large text corpus (Landauer *et al.*, 1998). Elvevaag *et al.*'s

findings using this measure confirmed that schizophrenia patients' word associations were less semantically cohesive than those of healthy controls. Moreover, the associations produced by TD patients were less cohesive than those produced by non-TD patients.

Implicit processing: semantic priming

An even more objective method of implicitly assessing semantic memory structure and function is through the use of the semantic priming paradigm using an implicit task, such as lexical decision (LD: deciding whether a target word is a real word or a non-word) or word pronunciation (simply naming the target word). The semantic priming effect describes the faster response to target words (e.g. stripes) that are preceded by semantically related words (e.g. tiger), relative to semantically unrelated words (e.g. table) (Meyer & Schvaneveldt, 1971; Neely, 1991). This behavioral priming effect also has a neurophysiological correlate: the attenuation of the N400 event-related potential (ERP) – a negative-going waveform evoked *c.* 400 ms after the onset of a word – to primed versus unprimed targets (Bentin *et al.*, 1985; Rugg, 1985). This attenuation of the N400 amplitude is known as the N400 effect.

There have been numerous studies of semantic priming in schizophrenia over the past two decades and the literature is often contradictory: studies have reported normal priming, increased priming and decreased priming in patients relative to controls. Nonetheless, some consistencies do emerge, particularly when findings are examined in relation to types of experimental conditions (automatic versus controlled) used in each study. Below is a brief review of behavioral and ERP semantic priming studies in schizophrenia (for a more detailed review of the behavioral literature up to 2002, see Minzenberg *et al.*, 2002; for a recent meta-analysis of the behavioral literature, see Pomarol-Clotet *et al.*, 2008, and for a review of the ERP semantic priming literature, see Kuperberg, Kreher & Ditman, in press).

Automatic semantic priming in schizophrenia

Experimental conditions that bias towards automatic semantic priming are those in which the interval between the presentation of the prime and target (the stimulus onset asynchrony, SOA) is short (usually less than *c.* 400 ms), and in which the proportion of related words in the stimulus set (the relatedness proportion, RP) is small (usually less than 33%) (Neely, 1977). The mechanism most often invoked to explain the semantic priming effect under these conditions is the spread of activation within semantic memory (Anderson, 1983; Collins & Loftus, 1975), whereby the presentation of the first word (or prime) activates its internal representation, leading to an implicit, automatic spread of activation to nearby and related representations. If a second word, the target, corresponding to one of these partially pre-activated or primed representations is then presented, the individual's response to that target will be facilitated.

One theory proposed to account for the "loosening of associations" seen in thought disorder (TD) is that the spread of activation within semantic memory is abnormally heightened, leading to speech that is difficult to follow because it is dominated by such associations. Evidence for this theory is provided by findings that schizophrenia patients exhibit increased semantic priming under more automatic processing conditions. Manschreck et al. (1988) were the first to demonstrate increased semantic priming in TD patients relative to non-TD patients, psychiatric controls and healthy controls (using a LD task). Subsequent studies have confirmed "hyper-priming" in TD patients across a variety of SOAs (Spitzer et al., 1994), during word pronunciation tasks (Moritz et al., 2001a; Moritz et al., 2002) and even when participants viewed triplets, rather than pairs of words (Chenery et al., 2004). Others have reported increased cross-modal (across auditory and visual modalities) semantic priming (Surguladze et al., 2002), as well as increased priming, particularly to high-frequency words (Rossell & David, 2006) in patients with schizophrenia.

Other researchers, however, have failed to show increases in direct priming in schizophrenia under automatic conditions: equal priming in patients and controls has been demonstrated using LD (Barch et al., 1996; Blum & Freides, 1995), double LD (Besche-Richard et al., 2005; Chapin et al., 1989), and word pronunciation (Ober et al., 1995; Vinogradov et al., 1992) tasks. And a few behavioral studies (Henik et al., 1992; Ober et al., 1997; Vinogradov et al., 1992) and two ERP studies (Condray et al., 2003; Mathalon et al., 2002) have reported reduced direct semantic priming using LD tasks in schizophrenia using short SOAs.

All of the studies reviewed above used directly related word pairs (e.g. tiger-stripes). However, since closely associated words are presumably automatically activated by both schizophrenia patients and controls, the use of indirectly related word pairs during semantic priming paradigms may be a more stringent test for a heightened activation (or reduced inhibition) (Spitzer, 1993). In indirect semantic priming paradigms, the prime and target are related only through an unseen mediating word (e.g. "lion-stripes" via "tiger") (Balota & Lorch, 1986; Chwilla & Kolk, 2002; Kiefer et al., 1998; Kreher et al., 2006; McNamara & Altarriba, 1988; Weisbrod et al., 1999). Unlike direct priming, indirect semantic priming cannot be accounted for by alternative models of automatic semantic priming, and is best explained by spreading activation theory (Kreher et al., 2006; McNamara & Altarriba, 1988; Neely, 1991). The unseen mediating word is thought to be activated by the prime, and this spread of activation activates the target.

Spitzer et al. (1993) were the first to report increased indirect priming using a LD task under automatic conditions in TD patients, relative to both healthy individuals and non-TD patients (see also Moritz et al., 2001b). This finding has been replicated both using lateralized presentation (Weisbrod et al., 1998) and using a word pronunciation task (Moritz et al., 2002).

In an ERP study by Mathalon et al. (2002), patients showed a smaller amplitude of the N400 than controls to target words that were moderately (but not closely) related to their picture primes. This was interpreted as reflecting increased activation to these targets in schizophrenia patients. Of note, however, these word-pairs were not indirectly related, as they belonged to the same superordinate categories (e.g. camel – fox). In a more recent ERP study, Kreher et al. (2008) used a short SOA and an implicit task (semantic monitoring just on filler trials) to demonstrate increased spreading activation in TD schizophrenia patients. In the early part of the N400 time window (300–400 ms after target word onset), TD patients showed increased indirect semantic priming relative to non-TD patients and healthy controls, while the degree of direct semantic priming was increased in only the most severely thought-disordered patients. By 400–500 ms after target word onset, both direct and indirect semantic priming were generally equivalent across the three groups. These findings suggest that under automatic conditions, activation across the semantic network spreads further, within a shorter period of time, in specific association with positive thought disorder in schizophrenia.

However, experimental task also appears to play a role in whether hyper- or hypoactivation will be observed in schizophrenia patients relative to controls, even under "automatic" conditions. Kreher et al. (2009) used an explicit relatedness ratings task with the same group of patients and matched controls, who were presented with the same directly related, indirectly related and unrelated word pairs using the same SOA, and found that schizophrenia patients, as a whole, showed *reduced* direct and indirect N400 priming effects compared with healthy controls. Similarly, Kiang et al. (2008) reported reduced N400 effects to both directly and indirectly related targets in schizophrenia patients, compared with controls, using a LD task with a short SOA.

In sum, studies examining semantic priming under automatic conditions have generally revealed normal direct priming in schizophrenia patients as a whole, suggesting that implicit associative activity within the semantic network is normal in such patients. However, there is some evidence that TD patients show increased direct priming, and even more consistent evidence that TD patients show increased indirect priming under these automatic conditions. This suggests that, in patients with severe thought disorder, automatic activation may spread further (and possibly faster) across the semantic network. This may be due to hyperactivity and/or a failure of inhibition. Additionally, requiring a decision to each target word, through relatedness judgments or lexical decision can lead to a reduction in semantic priming in schizophrenia patients even when a short SOA and indirectly related word pairs are used. This is likely to occur because of the engagement of controlled semantic mechanisms which, as discussed below, are impaired in patients.

Controlled semantic priming in schizophrenia

Controlled priming mechanisms involve the generation of predictions or expectations (Becker, 1980), as well as attempts to match the semantic relationship between prime and target (Neely et al., 1989). They have most often been studied under experimental conditions using a long SOA and a high RP.

With the exception of Spitzer et al. (1993, 1994) who reported increased semantic priming in patients relative to controls, most studies carried out under such controlled conditions have demonstrated reduced

priming in schizophrenia. Using a pronunciation task, Aloia et al. (1998) found that TD patients exhibited less priming to both highly associated and moderately associated targets than non-TD patients, and less priming to the highly associated targets than healthy controls. Reduced priming in TD patients at longer SOAs has also been demonstrated using a LD task (Besche et al., 1997; Passerieux et al., 1997) and a variant of the double LD task with a low RP (Besche-Richard et al., 2005). Studies using multiple SOAs have found either reduced (Barch et al., 1996; Chenery et al., 2004) or normal (Henik et al., 1995) priming effects in patients relative to controls at long SOAs.

ERP studies have also reported reduced priming under controlled conditions in patients relative to controls (although see Koyama et al., 1991, 1994). For example, Grillon et al. (1991) reported two distinct subgroups of schizophrenic patients: one in which there was a reduced N400 effect, and one in which the N400 effect did not differ from that of controls, and Bobes et al. (1996) found that schizophrenia patients showed a smaller N400 effect than controls in a picture priming paradigm. There have also been reports of a reduced N400 effect using LD tasks by Kostova et al. (2003, 2005), particularly in TD patients. Others have reported reduced N400 effects both in medicated patients (Condray et al., 1999) and unmedicated patients (Condray et al., 1999; Hokama et al., 2003) at longer SOAs. Using a LD task, Kiang et al. (2008) reported reduced N400 effects in schizophrenia patients to both directly and indirectly related words at a long SOA; the reduction in semantic priming was correlated with delusions and hallucinations, but not with thought disorder. Another consistent finding under controlled processing conditions is that the peak latency of the N400 is delayed (Bobes et al., 1996; Condray et al., 1999; Grillon et al., 1991; Hokama et al., 2003; Koyama et al., 1991).

In sum, behavioral and ERP studies of controlled semantic priming suggest that priming is reduced in patients with schizophrenia relative to controls. This has generally been attributed to impaired controlled mechanisms of accessing information within semantic memory.

Single words and concepts: summary and discussion

The findings reviewed here suggest that semantic memory structure and function in schizophrenia requires further clarification. There are clearly aspects of semantic memory that are intact: patients perform just as well as healthy controls on simple object perception and some aspects of semantic categorization. Semantic fluency is impaired but, when given enough time, patients produce as many exemplars as controls. Moreover, under automatic experimental conditions patients generally show the same degree of semantic priming as healthy controls, and indeed, patients with thought disorder can show even greater priming effects than controls, suggesting that there may be some automatic hyperactivity within the network in these patients.

This set of findings is important because it sets schizophrenia apart from disorders such as Alzheimer's disease. There does not appear to be an overall loss of knowledge in schizophrenia: the main semantic problem appears to be one of access and/or retrieval, i.e. of using semantic knowledge effectively. This manifests in both explicit and implicit measures. On explicit semantic fluency, word association and categorization tasks, the pattern of responses in patients reveals an abnormality in the organization of semantic memory. Behavioral and ERP studies of implicit semantic memory function examining the semantic priming effect under controlled experimental conditions, suggest that patients fail to employ strategic semantic mechanisms to prime targets, leading to reduced priming.

Sentences, ambiguity and figurative language

As discussed above, thought-disordered speech can be dominated by associations between individual words. Importantly, such associations can result in a failure to build coherence within and across sentences. Consider the following sample of speech produced by a patient with schizophrenia, quoted by Maher (1983): "If you think you are being wise to send me a bill for money I have already paid, I am in nowise going to do so unless I get the whys and wherefores from you to me. But where the fours have been, then fives will be, and other numbers and calculations and accounts to your no-account ..." In this speech sample, the associations between the individual words are clear; what is unclear is the overall message the patient wishes to convey.

In this section we review studies examining how patients process and make use of contextual information within written and spoken language, at the level of sentences. We focus again on schizophrenia, as most of the work has been carried out in this area. We consider studies that have examined the predictability of the speech produced by schizophrenia patients, as well as studies exploring patients' abilities to predict words within text and to detect and integrate semantic anomalies in sentences. In addition, we review studies exploring the syntactic structure of patients' speech and examining how patients combine syntactic structure with the meaning of individual words during comprehension. Finally, we discuss studies that have explored patients' ability to select the most appropriate meanings of ambiguous words in context, and studies of non-literal language.

Semantic predictability and congruity

The traditional way of measuring language predictability is through the use of the Cloze technique, which requires healthy participants to produce the missing words in text (Taylor, 1953). If they tend to produce the same word, then this indicates that the text was highly predictable. An early schizophrenia study confirmed the clinical impression that patients' speech output was unpredictable (Salzinger et al., 1964). Moreover, when participants were provided with more context, it was harder to predict patients' speech (Salzinger et al., 1970, 1979). Later studies, however, suggested that unpredictable speech was only produced by patients with thought disorder (Hart & Payne, 1973; Manschreck et al., 1979). Impairments in the ability to make predictions about upcoming words in normal speech or text have also been identified in schizophrenia (Blaney, 1974; Honigfeld, 1963). This has been demonstrated using reverse Cloze procedures in which patients are asked to predict upcoming words in speech transcripts of healthy adults. Unlike healthy controls, the performance of acute schizophrenia patients deteriorates when more context is provided (de Silva & Hemsley, 1977).

Another method used to examine how patients use context within sentences is to introduce words that violate semantic contextual constraints. Some studies suggest that chronic schizophrenia patients can accurately judge the appropriateness of semantically anomalous sentences (Miller & Phelan, 1980); however, acutely psychotic patients (Anand et al., 1994) and TD patients (Kuperberg et al., 1998) appear to be relatively impaired. Furthermore, this relative insensitivity to semantic anomalies appears to be related to the state (i.e. impairment related to symptom exacerbation) rather than the trait (i.e. impairment independent of symptom exacerbation) of thought disorder (Kuperberg *et al.*, 2000).

Measurement of ongoing brain activity using ERPs can also offer insight into the effects of semantic anomalies. Event-related potential studies of sentence processing, like those of single words, have focused on the N400 waveform. In sentences, the N400 is evoked by words that are semantically incongruous or unexpected with their preceding context (Kutas & Hillyard, 1980, 1984) and is thought to reflect the difficulty of semantically integrating words into their preceding context (Holcomb, 1993). Although most studies have reported that the size of the N400 effect is normal in schizophrenia (Andrews *et al.*, 1993; Kuperberg *et al.*, 2006d; Nestor *et al.*, 1997; Niznikiewicz *et al.*, 1997; Ruchsow *et al.*, 2003), there have been some investigations demonstrating that it can be abnormally reduced (Adams *et al.*, 1993; Mitchell *et al.*, 1991; Ohta *et al.*, 1999; Sitnikova *et al.*, 2002). A reduced N400 effect is most evident when the anomalous words fall at the sentence-final position, which is when there are relatively high processing demands (see below for further discussion).

A number of investigators have also identified more negative N400 amplitudes to congruous words (Mitchell *et al.*, 1991; Nestor *et al.*, 1997; Niznikiewicz *et al.*, 1997; Ohta *et al.*, 1999), and incongruous words (Nestor *et al.*, 1997; Niznikiewicz *et al.*, 1997) in patients relative to controls. These data may reflect increased difficulty in semantically integrating words, regardless of whether the context is congruous or incongruous. Other studies, however, have failed to find such differences (Kuperberg *et al.*, 2006d; Ruchsow *et al.*, 2003). Finally, some studies report that the peak of the N400 is delayed, suggesting that integrative semantic processing occurs later in patients than controls (Mitchell *et al.*, 1991; Nestor *et al.*, 1997; Niznikiewicz *et al.*, 1997; Ohta *et al.*, 1999).

Syntax and the semantic-syntactic interface

Syntactic processing has often been considered relatively unimpaired in patients with schizophrenia. The evidence supporting this assumption comes from three early studies using the "click" paradigm in which a short burst of noise (the click) is delivered in the middle of a spoken clause (Fodor & Bever,

1965; Garrett *et al.*, 1966). In these studies, patients and controls perceived the click as occurring at or near a clause boundary, suggesting that patients were using normal syntactic constraints to guide perception (Carpenter, 1976; Grove & Andreasen, 1985; Rochester *et al.*, 1973), and that at least some implicit aspects of syntactic structural processing remained intact. This type of paradigm, however, does not index how well patients can combine syntactic structure with semantic information to assign thematic roles and build up overall meaning.

Thematic roles are the semantic roles that are occupied by each constituent of a sentence around a given action; these are generalizable across a variety of sentence meanings. For example, the Agent of a sentence is the performer of the main action and the Theme is the entity that undergoes the action. While thematic roles are assigned by the syntax, they are considered semantic in nature as they determine "who does what to whom" in a sentence. During normal language production and comprehension, syntax and semantics are combined, word by word, to assign thematic roles (although it is debated whether this combination occurs in a single stage of processing in a parallel constraint-based model (e.g. MacDonald *et al.*, 1994), or at a second stage of processing in a serial model (e.g. Frazier & Rayner, 1982)). In patients with schizophrenia, there is growing evidence for abnormalities in this combination of semantic and syntactic information.

One situation in which there is an increased demand for syntactic structure to be combined with the meaning of individual words is during the production or processing of syntactically complex sentences. In simple "canonical" sentences, the semantic order of constituents of English sentences (e.g. Agent–Action–Theme) corresponds to the syntactic order of constituents (e.g. Subject–Verb–Object). This is not necessarily true of more complex, non-canonical sentences where there is an increased demand on the production and processing systems to use syntactic rules to assign thematic roles. There is fairly compelling evidence that patients with schizophrenia are relatively impaired in processing syntactic complexity during both speech production and language comprehension.

The speech produced by schizophrenia patients is less complex than that of matched controls (Morice & Ingram, 1982; Thomas *et al.*, 1990). Reduced syntactic complexity is associated with negative symptoms and seems to be relatively unresponsive to treatment (Thomas *et al.*, 1990). Although some researchers have postulated that it may represent a premorbid marker of schizophrenia (Thomas *et al.*, 1990), a study examining the writing samples of children who later developed schizophrenia, compared with matched controls, did not find differences in syntactic complexity (Done *et al.*, 1998).

Complementing these findings in language production, studies of language comprehension have revealed impairments in patients' abilities to comprehend grammatically complex sentences. Condray *et al.* (1996, 2002) compared patients' accuracy on comprehension questions tapping into the assignments of thematic roles (e.g. "Who did what to whom?") and compared more complex, object-relative sentences (e.g. The senator that the reporter attacked admitted the error) to less complex, subject-relative sentences (e.g. The accountant that sued the lawyer read the paper). These sentences were presented at normal (i.e. conversational) and accelerated rates. Initial results (Condray *et al.*, 1996) demonstrated that accuracy in both schizophrenia patients and healthy adult controls was negatively impacted by both fast presentation rates and grammatical complexity. These results were replicated and extended by Bagner *et al.* (2003) using a larger sample size. A later study by Condray *et al.* (2002) indicated that, although both patients and controls were more accurate in answering questions about information in the main clause compared to embedded clause, the drop in accuracy between main and embedded clause questions was greater in patients than in controls.

A second situation in which there are increased demands for syntactic structure to be combined with the meaning of individual words is when potentially plausible thematic-semantic relationships contradict the implausible syntactic assignment of thematic roles. For example, in the sentence, "Every morning for breakfast the eggs would eat...", there is a potentially plausible thematic-semantic relationship between "eggs" and "eat" (eggs can be eaten) but the actual interpretation dictated by the syntax is impossible. Kuperberg *et al.* (2006c) recently showed that, when asked to judge the acceptability of such sentences, patients with schizophrenia were less sensitive to these types of anomalies than healthy controls: relative to controls, they showed smaller reaction time differences between these sentences and both non-violated sentences, e.g. "Every morning for

breakfast the boys would eat..." and sentences that were only incongruous with real-world knowledge, e.g. "Every morning for breakfast the boys would plant...."

Further evidence that patients show impairments in combining semantic and syntactic information comes from ERP studies. First, as mentioned above, in most of the ERP studies documenting an abnormally reduced N400 effect to semantic anomalies (versus non-violated words) within sentences, the anomalies occurred on the sentence-final word (Adams *et al.*, 1993; Mitchell *et al.*, 1991; Ohta *et al.*, 1999; Sitnikova *et al.*, 2002). The demands of integrating semantic with syntactic information are particularly great at the sentence-final position, when there is often an attempt to evaluate and "wrap-up" the meaning of the sentence as a whole (Friedman *et al.*, 1975).

Second, there have also been several reports of a reduced Late Positivity (or P600) following the N400 during sentence processing in schizophrenia (Adams *et al.*, 1993; Andrews *et al.*, 1993; Mitchell *et al.*, 1991; Nestor *et al.*, 1997). Although the theoretical relevance of the P600 has been debated (see Coulson *et al.*, 1998; Kuperberg, 2007; Osterhout & Hagoort, 1999), there is evidence that it reflects the increased demands of integrating semantic and syntactic information under certain circumstances. For example, when there is a potentially plausible semantic-thematic relationship ("eggs"–"eat"), but the actual interpretation dictated by the syntax is impossible ("At breakfast the eggs would eat...") (Kuperberg *et al.*, 2003c, 2006a, 2007), it is harder to integrate semantic and syntactic information to come up with this interpretation and a P600 effect is evoked.

A recent study by Kuperberg *et al.* (2006d) demonstrated that, unlike healthy controls, schizophrenia patients failed to evoke a Late Positive effect to these types of anomalies. Yet, in this study the same patients produced a normal N400 effect to violations of real-world knowledge, suggesting that they had no problem in accessing and combining the meanings of individual words based on real-world knowledge alone.

One important question is whether patients' poor performance when required to combine semantic and syntactic information is due to their impaired working memories (Lee & Park, 2005). The relationship between working memory function and syntactic-semantic combinatory processes has been extensively discussed in normal language processing (Caplan & Waters, 1999; Fedorenko *et al.*, 2006), and there is increasing evidence that the language processing system is influenced by top-down executive function and is therefore more dynamic than has been previously assumed (Kuperberg, 2007). There is some evidence that impairments on some of the measures discussed here are correlated with more general cognitive impairments (this is discussed later in this chapter). However, the precise nature and mechanisms of such links remain to be explored.

Lexical ambiguity

Being able to effectively build up and use context by combining semantic with syntactic information is particularly important for interpreting words that are lexically ambiguous. Context plays a critical role in constraining and selecting the most appropriate meaning of such words. One well-studied source of lexical ambiguity comes from homonyms – words that sound (homophones) and/or look (homographs) the same but have different conceptual representations. For example, in order to interpret the word "pen" in the sentence, "When the farmer bought a herd of cattle, he needed a new pen," one must use the preceding context to inhibit the inappropriate dominant meaning (a writing instrument) and to select the contextually appropriate subordinate meaning (a place where animals live).

In an early study, Chapman *et al.* (1964) asked healthy adults and schizophrenia patients to indicate the meaning (by selecting a response from several choices) of sentences containing homonyms, similar to the sentence above. Patients were more likely than healthy adults to misinterpret homonyms in terms of their dominant meanings, suggesting that they failed to use context to inhibit the prepotent response and to select the most appropriate meaning (see also Benjamin & Watt, 1969). In a more recent study, Bazin *et al.* (2000) examined the use of context to disambiguate homographs. Participants read sentences containing homographs that were preceded by contexts that biased towards the subordinate meaning of the homograph. In addition, they viewed sentence fragments without a biasing context. Resolution of the homograph was measured by whether participants completed sentence fragments according to the dominant or subordinate meaning. When no context was given, both patients and controls showed a similar

pattern of results: both groups used the dominant interpretation. Interestingly, when a biasing context preceded the homograph, TD patients relative to healthy controls and non-TD patients, failed to make use of this information and completed the sentences according to the contextually inappropriate dominant meaning of the homograph.

Titone *et al.* (2000) also examined the processing of homonyms using a cross-modal priming paradigm and a LD task. Participants listened to prime stimuli consisting of homonyms embedded in contexts that either moderately or strongly biased towards their subordinate meanings. Targets were related to either the dominant or subordinate meaning of the homonym. Priming of targets related to the dominant meanings of the homonyms indicated an ability to inhibit a prepotent response, as such targets were never contextually appropriate. Priming of targets related to the subordinate meanings of the homonyms indicated an ability to build-up and use context. Healthy adults only showed priming of words related to the subordinate meanings of the homographs, regardless of the strength of the context biasing, suggesting that they were able to inhibit the prepotent response as well as build-up and use context appropriately. Patients also showed priming of words related to the subordinate meaning of the homographs under both contextual biasing conditions. However, with a moderately biasing context, the dominant meaning was also activated, suggesting an inability to inhibit this meaning. When the context strongly biased towards the subordinate meaning of the homograph, patients were able to inhibit the dominant meaning. Thus, in patients, a strong global context was necessary to inhibit local, lexico-semantic associations.

Finally, there have been a few recent studies using ERPs to study how homographs are processed as language is built-up online. Using sentences that did not include any disambiguating context prior to the homonym (e.g. "The toast was sincere"), Salisbury and colleagues demonstrated that patients with schizophrenia were more likely to misinterpret homographs when the correct interpretation of a sentence required the subordinate meaning. This was reflected by larger N400 amplitude to sentence-final words that were consistent with a subordinate interpretation (Salisbury *et al.*, 2000; Salisbury *et al.*, 2002). Taking this a step further, Sitnikova *et al.* (2002) constructed sentences that included a disambiguating context prior to the homograph. Specifically, the first clause of each sentence biased towards either the dominant meaning (e.g. "Diving was forbidden from the bridge...") or the subordinate meaning (e.g. "The guests played bridge...") of a homograph, followed by a second clause that contained a critical word that was always semantically associated with the dominant meaning of the homonym (e.g. "...because the river had rocks in it"). As expected, healthy adults produced an N400 effect to contextually inappropriate words (e.g. to "river" when the initial context was "The guests played bridge"). Schizophrenia patients, however, showed an attenuated N400 effect, suggesting that they failed to use context to inhibit the dominant meaning of the homograph ("bridge") that primed "river". Critically, the same patients in the same study showed a normal N400 effect to unambiguously contextually incongruous words that, in half the sentences, were introduced towards the end of the second clause (e.g. "cracks" in "...because the river had cracks in it."). Taken together, these findings suggest that patients were able to use some aspects of context (perhaps the lexico-semantic relationships between individual words), but that they had specific difficulty in using global context to inhibit contextually inappropriate, dominant meanings of homographs.

Figurative language

Figurative language is often, by its very nature, ambiguous. Proverbs, metaphors and many idioms have both literal as well as figurative interpretations, posing a particular challenge to the comprehension system to select their most appropriate meaning. Healthy adults very quickly and easily understand the meanings of familiar idioms (e.g. Titone & Connine, 1994). Similarly, most healthy adults are able to interpret metaphor, although there is some debate over whether both the literal and figurative meanings or only the figurative meanings remain active during online processing (e.g. Kintsch, 2000).

Patients with schizophrenia have particular difficulties in understanding figurative language. Indeed, proverb interpretation is commonly used clinically to assess language and thought disturbances in schizophrenia (it constitutes one item on the PANSS; Kay et al., 1987). Misinterpretations usually take the form of an over-reliance on the literal meaning, sometimes triggering semantic associations. For example, when

asked to interpret the proverb, "Gold goes in at any gate except heaven's," one patient responded, "There's jewelry, there's platinum. They use it on your teeth for filling. There's gold in churches. There's gold in the mosque areas; like Lincoln's tomb" (example taken from Harrow & Quinlan, 1985). Consistent with these clinical observations, several studies have indicated that schizophrenia patients often choose concrete interpretations when asked to interpret figurative language (Chapman, 1960; Brune & Bodenstein, 2005; Kiang et al., 2007).

There have been several investigations using behavioral and/or ERP measures to test the hypothesis that patients are specifically impaired in inhibiting the literal meaning of idioms and metaphors during comprehension. Titone et al. (2002) conducted a priming experiment in which the priming context constituted idioms with both literal and figurative meanings (ambiguous idioms, e.g. "kick the bucket") or idioms with only figurative meanings (non-ambiguous idioms, e.g. "be on cloud nine"). In healthy controls, the figurative meanings of both types of idioms primed semantically related target words (e.g. "death" for the first example, and "elated" for the second example); in addition, the literal meaning of the ambiguous idioms primed semantically related target words (Titone & Connine, 1994). In patients with schizophrenia, however, only non-ambiguous idioms (without literal meanings) were effective in priming targets that were semantically related to their idiomatic meanings; ambiguous idioms only primed targets that were related to their literal meanings, suggesting that a failure to inhibit the literal meanings of these idioms prevented patients' access to their figurative meanings. Consistent findings were reported by Strandburg et al. (1997) who measured ERPs as participants judged the meaningfulness of word-pairs that were idiomatic ("pot luck"), literal ("vicious dog"), or that made no sense ("square wind"). Note that in this experiment all idiomatic expressions were unambiguous, i.e. no plausible literal interpretation was possible. Relative to healthy controls, patients took longer to respond and showed more errors and larger N400 amplitudes to the second word of the idiomatic, relative to the literal, word-pairs, suggesting that they had particular difficulty in accessing the figurative meaning of the idioms.

In contrast to these two studies, Iakimova et al. (2005) did not find specific impairments in processing metaphors in schizophrenia. Healthy adults and schizophrenia patients made meaningfulness judgments while reading metaphorical, literal and incongruous sentences. All participants showed a similar pattern of results: incongruous sentences elicited the most negative N400 amplitudes, followed by a medium-sized N400 to literal sentence endings, and the smallest amplitude N400 to metaphorical endings. However, in schizophrenia patients, there was an overall delay in the latency of both the N400 and Late Positivity components. In addition, the negativity of the N400 was greater and the amplitude of the Late Positivity was reduced. Thus, the authors concluded that patients are impaired in integrating the semantic context of sentences (both figurative and literal), rather than showing a specific deficit in metaphor processing.

One reason for these discrepancies may be differences in the symptom profiles of patients participating in these studies: some researchers have implicated delusions as being specifically related to metaphor interpretation (Rhodes & Jakes, 2004), whereas others have associated poor metaphor comprehension with negative symptoms (Langdon & Coltheart, 2004).

Sentences, ambiguity and figurative language: summary and conclusion

There is now fairly compelling evidence that patients with schizophrenia show impairments in building up sentence context, which leads to unpredictable speech and also to problems in predicting words within speech and text. Although patients appear to be able to use semantic relationships between individual words within sentences to generate some representation of meaning (leading to normal N400 effects under many circumstance), both behavioral and electrophysiological abnormalities are observed when the demands of combining the meaning of individual words with syntactic structure are high. This occurs at the final word of sentences when comprehenders usually wrap-up sentence meaning, in producing and processing syntactically complex sentences, and in comprehending sentences in which semantic relationships between individual words contradict overall meaning.

Many of these abnormalities are evident in patients without prominent positive thought disorder, although they may be more marked in thought-disordered patients. Impairments in building up context may lead to speech that is dominated by semantic associative relationships between individual words at the expense of whole meaning. It may also lead

to specific problems in resolving lexical ambiguity where context plays a particularly important role in determining whether the dominant meaning of a homonym is inhibited and the subordinate meaning is appropriately selected. Finally, there is some evidence that it may lead to specific impairments with inhibiting contextually inappropriate literal interpretations of figurative expressions (Titone *et al.*, 2002), although others have failed to find such specific deficits (Iakimova *et al.*, 2005).

Discourse

Language comprehension and production go beyond accessing the meaning of individual words and combining this with syntactic structure to build up meaning of sentences. When healthy adults produce and comprehend language, they are able to integrate ideas across multiple sentences to generate or construct a coherent discourse model. This connected discourse has two main properties: cohesion and coherence (Halliday & Hasan, 1976; Sanford & Garrod, 1994). Coherence can be established through linguistic cohesive devices that specifically link information within and across sentences (e.g. "the man," "he," "the show-off" must each be linked to a single referent). In addition we must establish logical and psychological consistency between events (e.g. through the generation of causal inferences).

Clinically, patients with schizophrenia show prominent abnormalities at the level of discourse (Andreasen *et al.*, 1995; for reviews, see Covington *et al.*, 2005; McKenna & Oh, 2005; Pavy, 1968). Indeed, tangentiality and derailment – shifts in speech from one topic to another without obvious links between them – are amongst the most common phenomena described in thought-disordered speech (Andreasen, 1979a, 1979b; Earle-Boyer *et al.*, 1986; Mazumdar *et al.*, 1995). Below we review evidence that patients with schizophrenia show abnormalities in establishing coherence during language production and processing (also see Mitchell & Crow, 2005, for a discussion of the potential role of the right hemisphere in discourse impairments, and see Ditman & Kuperberg (in press) for a framework for exploring the breakdown of links across clause boundaries in schizophrenia).

Referential coherence

In a seminal study, Rochester & Martin (1979) examined the use of cohesion markers in the speech produced by patients with schizophrenia. Irrespective of thought disorder, schizophrenia patients failed to use cohesion markers to the same degree as healthy controls and had a tendency to point to (rather than verbally identify) referents. However, more specific impairments in the use of cohesion markers did distinguish between patients with and without thought disorder. Non-TD schizophrenia patients used fewer indirect references than healthy controls, whereas TD patients used more obscure referents and were more likely to refer to information that had not been presented.

Findings of cohesion impairments in schizophrenia have been replicated and described in more detail by other researchers (Docherty et al., 1996a; Hoffman et al., 1985; Noel-Jorand et al., 1997). For example, Docherty and colleagues have developed a comprehensive measure that captures a range of referential communication failures including vague, confused and missing references. Interestingly, there is evidence that some types of referential impairments are trait markers of schizophrenia. Specifically, this evidence suggests that (1) some types of referential impairment are stable over time (Docherty et al., 2003), and (2) first-degree family members of schizophrenia patients have more referential disturbances than first-degree family members of controls (Docherty et al., 1998; Docherty & Gottesman, 2000). On the other hand, in some patients, these impairments can improve with medication (Abu-Akel, 1997).

Although there has been little work to determine whether patients with schizophrenia are specifically impaired in referential processes (linking anaphors to their antecedents) during online language comprehension, one recent ERP study provides some neural evidence that, with a sufficiently strong context, patients are able to use both semantic and contextual information to disambiguate anaphors during online comprehension, similar to healthy controls (Ditman & Kuperberg, 2008). When later asked to explicitly resolve the anaphors, however, patients were more likely than controls to erroneously resolve anaphors with contextually inappropriate, but semantically related, words. Thus, strong contextual constraints led to discourse-appropriate neural responses but later decisions were more likely guided by semantic associations. One possible explanation for this pattern of findings is that patients failed to use control mechanisms to suppress such associations, leading to their prolonged, inappropriate influence at later stages of processing.

Finally, there is some intriguing evidence for correlations between referential communication measures and performance on neuropsychological tasks indexing more general cognitive functions, such as working memory and other executive functions (discussed later in the chapter). This hypothesis could be further tested in the future using psycholinguistic paradigms that have been developed in healthy individuals to specifically tap into these working memory processes (Anderson & Holcomb, 2005; Swaab et al., 2004; van Berkum et al., 1999).

Other types of discourse coherence

One way of examining how patients construct links between sentences and concepts is to ask them to describe or recall what they see, read, or hear, and then transcribe the speech produced and examine its discourse structure in detail. Hoffman and colleagues took this approach and constructed "discourse trees" that depicted relationships between propositions within discourse. Normal discourse exhibits a systematic hierarchical structure in which propositions branch out from a central proposition. The transcripts of psychotic speech showed a more disorganized tree structure than that of controls and manic patients (Hoffman, 1986; Hoffman et al., 1982).

Another approach was taken in a study by Allen (1984) in which patients were asked to describe pictures and speech transcripts that were decomposed into "ideas" (individual sentences, semantic propositions, phrases and words), and then rated them according to whether they were appropriate to the picture or inferential. Thought-disordered patients produced significantly fewer inferences than controls, but exhibited a trend towards an increase in the number of ideas classified as inappropriate.

In a more recent study, Leroy et al. (2005) asked healthy adults and linguistically skilled patients with schizophrenia to read a story aloud and then, immediately after, to recall its contents. In healthy adults, the discourse macrostructure (the structure related to the global discourse topic) normally functions to constrain its microstructure (its more detailed structure) (Kintsch & van Dijk, 1978), so that irrelevant information is inhibited and generalizations are made. Although patients generated similar discourse plans with the same overall numbers of micro- and macro-propositions as controls, they had an increased tendency to connect micro-propositions. This was interpreted as reflecting an impairment in inhibiting irrelevant information.

Another way of probing the coherence links constructed during discourse comprehension is by examining the overall content of what is extracted and recalled. In a classic study, Bransford & Franks (1971) established that healthy adults combine propositions to extract an overall "gist." They presented healthy adults with groups of sentences, e.g. "The ants were in the kitchen. The ants ate the jelly. The jelly was sweet." On a later memory test, healthy participants misremembered (as measured by confidence ratings), encoding larger sentences, e.g. "The ant in the kitchen ate the sweet jelly." In other words, they integrated the individual propositions to create a global representation of the discourse. Knight & Sims-Knight (1979) examined whether patients with schizophrenia extracted the gist of a discourse message in a similar way. Results suggested that patients with a history of poor (or lower level) functioning (compared with controls and patients with good premorbid histories) were not able to extract the gist. However, a subsequent study using the gist paradigm by Grove & Anderson (1985) failed to find group differences between healthy adults, patients with mania and schizophrenia patients.

Healthy individuals are not only able to combine individual propositions to construct an overall gist; they can also extract messages during everyday conversations, even when normal communication norms are violated (i.e. Grice's maxim; Grice, 1975). In normal conversation, these norms may be violated under certain circumstances, requiring the comprehender to infer the intentions of the speaker to fully understand the conversation. For example, the response "Is the Pope Catholic?" to the question "Did Mike get drunk last night?" violates the maxim of relevance but indirectly communicates the speaker's opinion about Mike's drinking habits. Importantly, an inability to draw this inference would lead to a communication breakdown. Tényi et al. (2002) examined the ability of paranoid schizophrenia patients and healthy adult controls to comprehend conversational vignettes in which the maxim of relevance was flouted. Patients made more errors than controls in interpreting the true meaning intended by the characters in the vignettes, suggesting an inability to infer communicators' intentions.

Finally, one can examine whether schizophrenia patients can construct coherence links between individual sentences by determining whether they are able to benefit from such links when later asked to recall such sentences. Healthy adults' ability to recall individual sentences is improved when the encoded material is organized into a coherent discourse, relative to when it is presented as random disconnected sentences. Schizophrenia patients fail to show this improvement in recall (Harvey et al., 1986). These findings could not be attributed to poorer general memory performance. In another study, TD patients (a mixed group of mania and schizophrenia patients) showed superior recall than controls to sentences that were presented in random order during encoding (Speed et al., 1991). Schizophrenia patients have also been found to perform worse than controls when asked to organize pictures depicting various aspects of a story into a coherent discourse (Brune & Bodenstein, 2005).

Despite the evidence reviewed above that patients' speech is less coherent than that of controls, and that they are impaired in their use of coherence links to improve recall of individual sentences, there has been very little work examining whether patients can establish coherence links between sentences during online processing. Ditman & Kuperberg (2007) have some preliminary evidence supporting this hypothesis; they measured ERPs as patients and healthy controls read three-sentence discourse scenarios. While healthy controls showed a robust N400 effect to critical words within congruous sentences that were completely unrelated and intermediately related with their preceding two-sentence discourse context, patients failed to show such N400 effects. This is interesting as the N400 effect in schizophrenia is often normal to semantic anomalies within single sentences (as described above), and it therefore suggests that patients were unable to construct coherence links between sentences and build up global discourse context.

Discourse: summary and conclusion

There is now fairly robust evidence that the speech of patients with schizophrenia lacks coherence in comparison with that produced by healthy controls. Patients' speech lacks normal referential links and has an abnormal discourse structure. In addition, patients fail to benefit from coherent links between sentences to improve recall, although it remains controversial whether they are able to extract the gist of messages.

There has been very little investigation of how coherence links are established as discourse is built up during online processing in schizophrenia.

Relationship between language abnormalities and other cognitive dysfunction

Each level of language processing can be influenced by cognitive systems and processes that are used in domains other than language, such as attention, working memory and executive function. Given that schizophrenia is a disorder that affects multiple domains of cognitive function, understanding these relationships will prove essential to understanding language dysfunction in this disorder. Thus far, the approach taken to understand such links has been to correlate clinical and psychological measures of language disturbances with patients' performance in various neuropsychological tasks. Below, we review a selection of such studies.

Thought disorder

There have now been several studies reporting correlations between positive thought disorder in schizophrenia and various neuropsychological measures, including distractibility (Docherty & Gordinier, 1999; Harvey & Serper, 1990), selective attention as measured by the Stroop task (Barch et al., 1999), sustained attention as measured by the Continuous Performance Test (Nuecheterlein et al., 1986; Pandurangi et al., 1994; Strauss et al., 1993), measures of executive dysfunction (Nestor et al., 1998) and lower-level information processing deficits such as prepulse inhibition (Dawson et al., 2000; Perry & Braff, 1994). In a recent meta-analysis, Kerns & Berenbaum (2002) reported a strong association between thought disorders and impaired executive functioning.

Single words and concepts

As discussed earlier in the chapter there is some evidence that, under automatic experimental conditions, a faster and/or wider spread of activation across words within the semantic network may underlie positive thought disorder in schizophrenia. One

mechanism for this less "focused" activity may be reduced executive control. In line with this hypothesis, there have been some recent reports of significant correlations between measures of executive functioning and semantic priming. In healthy participants, Keifer et al. (2005) found that decreased working memory capacity was associated with increased semantic priming, and indirect semantic priming in particular. Poole et al. (1999) administered measures of executive dysfunction, response inhibition, motor coordination and intelligence to patients with schizophrenia, and found that only decreased response inhibition was correlated with increased automatic priming (using a short SOA and low RP). Neither motor dyscoordination nor general intelligence was associated with any measures of semantic priming. Interestingly, decreased executive functioning was associated with diminished controlled semantic priming, suggesting that different aspects of executive function may interact with automatic and controlled mechanisms of priming.

Sentences

Earlier in the chapter we discussed evidence that patients with schizophrenia are impaired in comprehending syntactically complex sentences, possibly because of difficulties in combining semantic with syntactic information to assign thematic roles. Condray et al. (1996) demonstrated that, in both patient and control groups, working memory capacity, as measured using a reading span task, predicted comprehension accuracy. The authors concluded that observed language comprehension deficits may be related to working memory impairments (see Bagner et al., 2003, for similar findings; and see Kiang et al., 2007, for similar findings with proverb comprehension).

Discourse

The most careful documentation of associations between various measures of clinical and referential language disturbances and performance on various neuropsychological tasks comes from studies by Docherty and colleagues. This group has focused on their detailed measure of referential coherence during language output (discussed above) and has demonstrated associations between referential communication disturbances and poor performance on tasks of immediate auditory memory (Docherty & Gordinier,

1999), auditory distractibility (Docherty & Gordinier, 1999; Hotchkiss & Harvey, 1990), working memory and attention (Docherty et al., 1996b). In more recent studies, they have confirmed associations between referential impairments and performance on tasks indexing sustained attention, immediate auditory memory, and conceptual sequencing (Docherty, 2005). Moreover, referential communication failures appear to be better predictors of performance on sustained attention and sequencing tasks than global "thought disorder," as measured using the Thought Language and Communication Scale or structural discourse abnormalities (Docherty, 2005; Docherty et al., 1996b).

Interestingly, a study by the same group demonstrated a more specific association between the frequency of one specific type of referential failure (missing information references) and performance on a source-monitoring task (Nienow & Docherty, 2005). The authors hypothesized that missing information references might arise from the speaker being unable to distinguish what they had just thought and what they had vocalized aloud. This finding is interesting as source memory deficits have been hypothesized to underlie other symptoms of schizophrenia such as hallucinations (Ditman & Kuperberg, 2005), and also because such deficits have been previously related to global measures of thought disorder (Harvey, 1985; Harvey & Serper, 1990) and theoretically linked to mechanisms of thought disorder (Frith, 1992).

Language abnormalities and other cognitive dysfunction: summary and conclusions

In sum, there is fairly compelling evidence that clinical and cognitive measures of language dysfunction in schizophrenia can be linked with dysfunction in domains other than language. At the word level, reduced inhibitory control has been associated with increased semantic priming under conditions which bias toward more automatic processing, both in healthy controls and patients with schizophrenia. In addition, reduced executive functioning has been related to decreased controlled semantic priming in schizophrenia patients. At the sentence level, working-memory measures predict comprehension accuracy, while at the level of discourse, measures of sustained attention and sequencing predict referential impairments.

Given these associations and our understanding of schizophrenia as a disorder that affects multiple domains of cognitive function, it becomes particularly important to understand how the mechanisms of language dysfunction in schizophrenia interact with these systems. The normal language processing system does not act in isolation, but is closely linked with working memory and executive mechanisms. There is increasing evidence that variation in working-memory function may account for individual variability in language function amongst healthy individuals, and researchers have developed a number of theories describing the nature of interactions between the language system and cognitive functions in other domains (Caplan & Waters, 1999; Just & Carpenter, 1992). More recently, neuroimaging studies have demonstrated overlaps in the neural circuitry subserving working memory, semantic memory and language function (Barde & Thompson-Schill, 2002; Thompson-Schill, 2003). The challenge now is to understand the nature of such links more precisely so as to determine how they are disturbed in disorders such as schizophrenia. This can be investigated through studies examining relationships between measures of verbal working memory and attention that are believed to specifically interact with the language system, and patients' performance on selected psycholinguistic tasks.

Implications and future directions
Clinical implications

Clinical abnormalities of language and communication in schizophrenia can be very disabling, impacting on all aspects of daily living. In schizophrenia, positive thought disorder is a strong predictor of maladaptive social and vocational functioning (Harrow & Quinlan, 1985; Hoffmann & Kupper, 1997; Norman et al., 1999). Yet there have been few attempts to alleviate it via cognitive methods. As reviewed above, the majority of evidence suggests that there is no overall loss of items stored in semantic memory; rather patients seem impaired in accessing and using items appropriately. Encouragingly, the use of strategies such as semantic cuing can improve performance in some semantic tasks, providing some hope that such deficits may be remediable. Cognitive remediation programs in schizophrenia have thus far focused on improving executive, memory and attention functions in schizophrenia, and are in their infancy.

It is also not clear how far they generalize to improving communication or quality of life. Understanding the cognitive basis of language and communication abnormalities in schizophrenia will allow the development of more specific strategies for remediation.

Implications for understanding brain dysfunction in schizophrenia

Another major implication of understanding the cognitive basis of language abnormalities in neuropsychiatric disorders is that, in combination with neuroanatomical and neurochemical measures, it may give new insights into the neurobiology of such disorders as a whole. Functional neuroimaging studies in healthy individuals have established that language and semantic processing are dependent on activity within a widespread network, distributed particularly across prefrontal, inferior parietal and temporal cortices. Many of the same regions are modulated by semantic relationships between individual words in priming paradigms (Kuperberg et al., 2008a; Rossell et al., 2003), sentences (Kuperberg et al., 2003b, 2008b) and whole discourse (Kuperberg et al., 2006b).

In schizophrenia, neuroimaging studies indicate that many of these regions are abnormally modulated during semantic processing (Kubicki et al., 2003; Ragland et al., 2004, 2005; Weiss et al., 2003). In a recent study, Kuperberg et al. demonstrated that patients, relative to controls, showed inappropriate increases in activity within temporal and prefrontal cortices to semantically associated (relative to unrelated) word pairs (Kuperberg et al., 2007). At the level of sentences, when integration demands are high, patients, relative to controls, show reduced activity within the superior dorsolateral prefrontal and parietal cortices when integration demands were particularly high (Kuperberg et al., 2008b).

In schizophrenia, there is also evidence of subtle but significant cortical gray matter thinning in many of the same temporal and prefrontal regions that show functional abnormalities (Kuperberg et al., 2003a). Finally, there is some preliminary evidence that semantic abnormalities in schizophrenia may arise from abnormalities within the dopaminergic systems and/or the glutamatergic systems. Increasing dopaminergic and glutamatergic activity can lead to reduced semantic priming under controlled conditions. Kischka et al. (1996) demonstrated a decrease in indirect semantic priming (as assessed by reaction time on a speeded lexical decision task) in healthy participants when they were administered 100 mg of L-dopa. This reduced controlled priming may be due to D1/D2 activity; Roesch-Ely reported that pergolide (a D1/D2 agonist), but not bromocriptine (a selective D2 agonist), reduced controlled semantic priming within the right hemisphere in healthy individuals (Roesch-Ely et al. 2006). Reduced controlled priming has also been reported in healthy individuals in association with the acute administration of ketamine (an NMDA receptor antagonist leading to increased glutamatergic activity) (Morgan et al., 2006). This is particularly interesting as the administration of ketamine in healthy individuals can lead to clinical language disturbances that are similar to thought disorder (Adler et al., 1998, 1999).

It remains unclear how such cognitive, functional neuroanatomical, structural neuroanatomical and neurochemical findings are related. But it is possible that widespread temporal-prefrontal cortical thinning may reflect widespread abnormalities in cortical synaptic function. This could potentially lead to an inappropriate increase in cortical activity through specific disruption of inhibitory circuitry, and in schizophrenia lead to overdependence on semantic associative links at the expense of building up context through normal modulatory activity. For example, Cohen & Servan-Schreiber (1992, 1993) have proposed that dopamine modulates the signal-to-noise ratio in cortical information processing and have suggested that increased noise in the activity of the dopamine system leads to abnormal "gating" of information into prefrontal cortex, thereby leading to impairments in both the maintenance and updating of contextual information (Braver et al., 1999).

Such relationships are currently speculative. However, with the development of theoretically grounded cognitive models of language processing in neuropsychiatric disorders, it may be possible to draw more specific links with synaptic and molecular models of brain dysfunction.

Conclusions

In this review, we have shown how paradigms at the level of words, sentences and discourse can be used to study neuropsychiatric disorders, and we have reviewed evidence suggesting that schizophrenia patients show deficits at all these levels of the language code. We are not yet at the point where we can account for all these abnormalities by postulating a single neuro-cognitive deficit. However, we can provide a broad theoretical framework to help understand the relationships between these levels of dysfunction and to help pave the way towards future theoretically motivated studies.

Abnormalities in semantic memory function and in building up linguistic context in schizophrenia have often been viewed as being distinct deficits. We suggest that they may be functionally related, reflecting two sides of the same coin. For example, in schizophrenia, patients' relative dependence on semantic relationships between individual words may contribute to their impairments in combining meaning with syntactic structure (see Kuperberg, 2007 for a more theoretical discussion). Under most circumstances, patients' relatively unimpaired ability to use semantic relationships between words within sentences would lead to an accurate representation of sentence meaning. However, impairments in combining syntactic with semantic information to build up context could lead to particular problems in selecting the most appropriate meaning of ambiguous words (e.g. homonyms) and expressions (e.g. metaphor or ambiguous idioms). It could also lead to significant problems at the level of discourse, where the build-up of an overall representation of meaning of each sentence is critical to the generation of coherent links between sentences.

Such impairments might account for the clinical observation that the meaning of sentences tends to be driven by semantic relationships between individual words, whilst the meaning of discourse tends to be driven by the meaning of individual sentences, i.e. that local context tends to inappropriately override the build-up of global context in schizophrenia. The real challenge to researchers of language dysfunction in neuropsychiatric disorders is to define the nature of these global-local contextual interactions more precisely in relation to psycholinguistic models of normal language processing, and to understand the mechanisms by which they are impacted upon by working memory, attentional, and executive dysfunction. Tackling these questions seems well worth our while as it has major implications for how we attempt to treat such language and communication disorders, as well as for linking between cognitive, neuroanatomical and neurochemical

abnormalities to understand the pathogenesis of such disorders as a whole.

Acknowledgments

Gina Kuperberg, Tali Ditman and Donna Kreher were supported by NIMH (R01 MH071635). Gina Kuperberg is also supported by NARSAD (with the Sidney Baer Trust) and a Claflin Distinguished Scholars Award from Massachusetts General Hospital. We thank Kana Okano for her help with manuscript preparation.

References

American Psychiatric Press (1990). *Diagnostic and Statistical Manual of Mental Disorders* (DSM–IV). Washington, DC: American Psychiatric Press.

Abu-Akel, A. (1997). A study of cohesive patterns and dynamic choices utilized by two schizophrenic patients in dialog, pre-and post-medication. *Language and Speech*, **40**(4), 331–351.

Adams, J., Faux, S. F., Nestor, P. G. *et al.* (1993). ERP abnormalities during semantic processing in schizophrenia. *Schizophrenia Research*, **10**(3), 247–257.

Adler, C. M., Goldberg, T. E., Malhotra, A. K., Pickar, D. & Breier, A. (1998). Effects of ketamine on thought disorder, working memory, and semantic memory in healthy volunteers. *Biological Psychiatry*, **43**(11), 811–816.

Adler, C. M., Malhotra, A. K., Elman, I. *et al.* (1999). Comparison of ketamine-induced thought disorder in healthy volunteers and thought disorder in schizophrenia. *American Journal of Psychiatry*, **156**(10), 1646–1649.

Allen, H. A. (1984). Positive and negative symptoms and the thematic organisation of schizophrenic speech. *British Journal of Psychiatry*, **144**, 611–617.

Allen, H. A. & Frith, C. D. (1983). Selective retrieval and free emission of category exemplars in schizophrenia. *British Journal of Psychology*, **74**(4), 481–490.

Allen, H. A., Liddle, P. F. & Frith, C. D. (1993). Negative features, retrieval processes and verbal fluency in schizophrenia. *British Journal of Psychiatry*, **163**, 769–775.

Aloia, M. S., Gourovitch, M. L., Missar, D. *et al.* (1998). Cognitive substrates of thought disorder, II: specifying a candidate cognitive mechanism. *American Journal of Psychiatry*, **155**(12), 1677–1684.

Aloia, M. S., Gourovitch, M. L., Weinberger, D. R. & Goldberg, T. E. (1996). An investigation of semantic space in patients with schizophrenia. *Journal of the International Neuropsychology Society*, **2**(4), 267–273.

Anand, A., Wales, R. J., Jackson, H. J. & Copolov, D. L. (1994). Linguistic impairment in early psychosis. *Journal of Nervous and Mental Diseases*, **182**(9), 488–493.

Anderson, J. & Holcomb, P. (2005). An electrophysiological investigation of the effects of coreference on word repetition and synonymy. *Brain and Language*, **94**, 200–216.

Anderson, J. R. (1983). A spreading activation theory of memory. *Journal of Verbal Learning and Verbal Behaviour*, **22**, 261–295.

Andreasen, N. C. (1979a). Thought, language and communication disorders: I. Clinical assessment, definition of terms, and evaluation of their reliability. *Archives of General Psychiatry*, **36**, 1315–1321.

Andreasen, N. C. (1979b). Thought, language and communication disorders. II. Diagnostic significance. *Archives of General Psychiatry*, **36**, 1325–1330.

Andreasen, N. C., Arndt, S., Alliger, R., Miller, D. & Flaum, M. (1995). Symptoms of schizophrenia. Methods, meanings, and mechanisms. *Archives of General Psychiatry*, **52**(5), 341–351.

Andrews, S., Shelley, A., Ward, P. B. et al. (1993). Event-related potential indices of semantic processing in schizophrenia. *Biological Psychiatry*, **34**, 443–458.

Bagner, D. M., Melinder, M. R. & Barch, D. M. (2003). Language comprehension and working memory language comprehension and working memory deficits in patients with schizophrenia. *Schizophrenia Research*, **60**(2–3), 299–309.

Balota, D. A. & Lorch, Jr., R. F. (1986). Depth of automatic spreading activation: Mediated priming effects in pronunciation but not in lexical decision. *Journal of Experimental Psychology: Learning, Memory, and Cognition*, **12**, 336–345.

Barch, D. M., Cohen, J. D., Servan-Schreiber, D. et al. (1996). Semantic priming in schizophrenia: an examination of spreading activation using word pronunciation and multiple SOAs. *Journal of Abnormal Psychology*, **105**, 592–601.

Barch, D. M., Carter, C. S., Perlstein, W. et al. (1999). Increased Stroop facilitation effects in schizophrenia are not due to increased automatic spreading activation. *Schizophrenia Research*, **39**(1), 51–64.

Barde, L. H. & Thompson-Schill, S. L. (2002). Models of functional organization of the lateral prefrontal cortex in verbal working memory: evidence in favor of the process model. *Journal of Cognitive Neuroscience*, **14**(7), 1054–1063.

Bazin, N., Perruchet, P., Hardy-Bayle, M. C. & Feline, A. (2000). Context-dependent information processing in patients with schizophrenia. *Schizophrenia Research*, **45**(1–2), 93–101.

Bearden, C. E., Glahn, D. C., Monkul, E. S. et al. (2006a). Sources of declarative memory impairment in bipolar disorder: mnemonic processes and clinical features. *Journal of Psychiatric Research*, **40**, 47–58.

Bearden, C. E., Glahn, D. C., Monkul, E. S. et al. (2006b). Patterns of memory impairment in bipolar disorder and unipolar major depression. *Psychiatry Research*, **142**, 139–150.

Becker, C. A. (1980). Semantic context effects in visual word recognition. *Memory and Cognition*, **8**, 493–512.

Benjamin, T. B. & Watt, N. F. (1969). Psychopathology and semantic interpretation of ambiguous words. *Journal of Abnormal Psychology*, **74**(6), 706–714.

Bentin, S., McCarthy, G. & Wood, C. C. (1985). Event-related potentials, lexical decision and semantic priming. *Electroencephalography and Clinical Neurophysiology*, **60**, 343–355.

Besche, C., Passerieux, C., Segui, J. et al. (1997). Syntactic and semantic processing in schizophrenic patients evaluated by lexical-decision tasks. *Neuropsychology*, **11**, 498–505.

Besche-Richard, C., Passerieux, C. & Hardy-Bayle, M. C. (2005). Double-decision lexical tasks in thought-disordered schizophrenic patients: a path towards cognitive remediation? *Brain and Language*, **95**(3), 395–401.

Blaney, P. H. (1974). Two studies on the language behavior of schizophrenics. *Journal of Abnormal Psychology*, **83**, 23–31.

Bleuler, E. (1911/1950). *Dementia Praecox, or the Group of Schizophrenias*. New York, NY: International Universities Press.

Blum, N. A. & Freides, D. (1995). Investigating thought disorder in schizophrenia with the lexical decision task. *Schizophrenia Research*, **16**(3), 217–224.

Bobes, M. A., Lei Xiao, Z., Ibanez, S., Yi, H. & Valdes-Sosa, M. (1996). Semantic matching of pictures in schizophrenia: A cross-cultural ERP study. *Biological Psychiatry*, **40**, 189–202.

Bokat, C. E. & Goldberg, T. E. (2003). Letter and category fluency in schizophrenic patients: a meta-analysis. *Schizophrenia Research*, **64**(1), 73–78.

Bransford, J. D. & Franks, J. J. (1971). The abstraction of linguistic ideas. *Cognitive Psychology*, **2**, 331–350.

Braver, T. S., Barch, D. M. & Cohen, J. D. (1999). Cognition and control in schizophrenia: a computational model of dopamine and prefrontal function. *Biological Psychiatry*, **46**(3), 312–328.

Brune, M. & Bodenstein, L. (2005). Proverb comprehension reconsidered – 'theory of mind' and the pragmatic use of language in schizophrenia. *Schizophrenia Research*, 75(2–3), 233–239.

Cameron, N. (1939). Schizophrenic thinking in a problem-solving situation. *Journal of Mental Science*, 85, 1012–1035.

Cameron, N. (1964). Experimental analysis of schizophrenia thinking. In J. Kasanin (Ed.), *Language and Thought in Schizophrenia* (pp. 50–63). Berkeley, CA: University of California Press.

Cannon, M., Caspi, A., Moffitt, T. E. *et al.* (2002). Evidence for early-childhood, pan-developmental impairment specific to schizophreniform disorder: results from a longitudinal birth cohort. *Archives of General Psychiatry*, 59(5), 449–456.

Caplan, D. & Waters, G. S. (1999). Verbal working memory and sentence comprehension. *Behavior and Brain Sciences*, 22(1), 77–94; discussion 95–126.

Carpenter, M. D. (1976). Sensitivity to syntactic structure: Good versus poor premorbid schizophrenics. *Journal of Abnormal Psychology*, 85, 41–50.

Chaika, E. (1974). A linguist looks at 'schizophrenic' language. *Brain and Language*, 1, 257–276.

Chapin, K., Vann, L. E., Lycaki, H., Josef, N. & Meyendorff, E. (1989). Investigation of the associative network in schizophrenia using the semantic priming paradigm. *Schizophrenia Research*, 2, 355–360.

Chapman, L. J. (1960). Confusion of figurative and literal usages of words by schizophrenics and brain damaged patients. *Journal of Abnormal Social Psychology*, 60, 412–416.

Chapman, L. J., Chapman, J. P. & Miller, G. A. (1964). A theory of verbal behaviour in schizophrenia. *Progress in Experimental Personality Research*, 1, 49–77.

Chen, E. Y. H., Wilkins, A. J. & McKenna, P. J. (1994). Semantic memory is both impaired and anomalous in schizophrenia. *Psychological Medicine*, 24, 193–202.

Chenery, H. J., Copland, D. A., McGrath, J. & Savage, G. (2004). Maintaining and updating semantic context in schizophrenia: an investigation of the effects of multiple remote primes. *Psychiatry Research*, 126(3), 241–252.

Chwilla, D. J. & Kolk, H. H. (2002). Three-step priming in lexical decision. *Memory and Cognition*, 30(2), 217–225.

Clare, L., McKenna, P. J., Mortimer, A. M. & Baddeley, A. D. (1993). Memory in schizophrenia: what is impaired and what is preserved? *Neuropsychologia*, 31(11), 1225–1241.

Cohen, J. D. & Servan-Schreiber, D. (1992). Context, cortex, and dopamine: a connectionist approach to behaviour and biology in schizophrenia. *Psychological Review*, 99(1), 45–77.

Cohen, J. D. & Servan-Schreiber, D. (1993). A theory of dopamine function and its role in cognitive deficits in schizophrenia. *Schizophrenia Bulletin*, 19(1), 85–104.

Cohen, J. R., Elvevaag, B. & Goldberg, T. E. (2005). Cognitive control and semantics in schizophrenia: an integrated approach. *American Journal of Psychiatry*, 162(10), 1969–1971.

Collins, A. M. & Loftus, E. F. (1975). A spreading activation theory of semantic processing. *Psychological Review*, 82, 407–428.

Condray, R., Siegle, G. J., Cohen, J. D., van Kammen, D. P. & Steinhauer, S. R. (2003). Automatic activation of the semantic network in schizophrenia: evidence from event-related brain potentials. *Biological Psychiatry*, 54(11), 1134–1148.

Condray, R., Steinhauer, S. R., Cohen, J. D., van Kammen, D. P. & Kasparek, A. (1996). Working memory capacity predicts language comprehension in schizophrenic patients. *Schizophrenia Research*, 20(1–2), 1–13.

Condray, R., Steinhauer, S. R., Cohen, J. D., van Kammen, D. P. & Kasparek, A. (1999). Modulation of language processing in schizophrenia: effects of context and haloperidol on the event-related potential. *Biological Psychiatry*, 45(10), 1336–1355.

Condray, R., Steinhauer, S. R., Cohen, J. D., van Kammen, D. P. & Kasparek, A. (2002). The language system in schizophrenia: effects of capacity and linguistic structure. *Schizophrenia Bulletin*, 28(3), 475–90.

Coulson, S., King, J. & Kutas, M. (1998). Expect the unexpected: Event-related brain responses to morphosyntactic violations. *Language and Cognitive Processes*, 13, 21–58.

Covington, M. A., He, C., Brown, C. *et al.* (2005). Schizophrenia and the structure of language: the linguist's view. *Schizophrenia Research*, 77(1), 85–98.

Craik, F. & Lockhart, R. (1971). Levels of processing: a framework for memory research. *Journal of Verbal Learning and Verbal Behavior*, 11, 671–684.

Davidson, M., Harvey, P., Welsh, K. A. *et al.* (1996). Cognitive functioning in late-life schizophrenia: a comparison of elderly schizophrenic patients and patients with Alzheimer's disease. *American Journal of Psychiatry*, 153(10), 1274–1279.

Dawson, M. E., Schell, A. M., Hazlett, E. A., Nuechterlein, K. H. & Filion, D. L. (2000). On the clinical and cognitive meaning of impaired sensorimotor gating in schizophrenia. *Psychiatry Research*, 96(3), 187–197.

de Silva, W. P. & Hemsley, D. R. (1977). The influence of context on language perception in schizophrenia. *British Journal of Social and Clinical Psychology*, 16(4), 337–345.

Deckersbach, T., Savage, C. R., Dougherty, D. D. *et al.* (2005). Spontaneous and directed application of verbal learning strategies in bipolar disorder and obsessive-compulsive disorder. *Bipolar Disorder*, 7(2), 166–175.

Deckersbach T., Savage, C. R., Reilly-Harrington, N. *et al.* (2004). Episodic memory impairment in bipolar disorder and obsessive-compulsive disorder: the role of memory strategies. *Bipolar Disorder*, 6, 233–244.

Ditman, T. & Kuperberg, G. R. (2005). A source-monitoring account of auditory verbal hallucinations in patients with schizophrenia. *Harvard Review of Psychiatry*, 13(5), 280–299.

Ditman, T. & Kuperberg, G. R. (2007). The time course of building global coherence in schizophrenia: an electrophysiological investigation. *Psychophysiology*, 44, 991–1001.

Ditman, T. & Kuperberg, G. R. (2008). An ERP examination of lexico-semantic and contextual influences across sentence boundaries in schizophrenia. Poster presented at the 15th Annual Meeting of the Cognitive Neuroscience Society (Abstract B41).

Ditman, T. & Kuperberg, G. R. (2009). Building coherence: a framework for exploring the breakdown of links across clause boundaries in schizophrenia. *Journal of Neuro-linguistics*. In press.

Docherty, N. M. (2005). Cognitive impairments and disordered speech in schizophrenia: thought disorder, disorganization, and communication failure perspectives. *Journal of Abnormal Psychology*, 114(2), 269–278.

Docherty, N. M., Cohen, A. S., Nienow, T. M., Dinzeo, T. J. & Dangelmaier, R. E. (2003). Stability of formal thought disorder and referential communication disturbances in schizophrenia. *Journal of Abnormal Psychology*, 112(3), 469–475.

Docherty, N. M., DeRosa, M. & Andreasen, N. C. (1996a). Communication disturbances in schizophrenia and mania. *Archives of General Psychiatry*, 53(4), 358–364.

Docherty, N. M. & Gordinier, S. W. (1999). Immediate memory, attention and communication disturbances in schizophrenia patients and their relatives. *Psychological Medicine*, 29(1), 189–197.

Docherty, N. M. & Gottesman, II (2000). A twin study of communication disturbances in schizophrenia. *Journal of Nervous and Mental Diseases*, 188(7), 395–401.

Docherty, N. M., Hawkins, K. A., Hoffman, R. E. *et al.* (1996b). Working memory, attention, and communication disturbances in schizophrenia. *Journal of Abnormal Psychology*, 105(2), 212–219.

Docherty, N. M., Rhinewine, J. P., Labhart, R. P. & Gordinier, S. W. (1998). Communication disturbances and family psychiatric history in parents of schizophrenic patients. *Journal of Nervous and Mental Diseases*, 186(12), 761–768.

Donchin, E. & Coles, M. G. H. (1988). Is the P300 component a manifestation of context updating? *Behavior and Brain Sciences*, 11, 355–372.

Done, D. J., Leinoneen, E., Crow, T. J. & Sacker, A. (1998). Linguistic performance in children who develop schizophrenia in adult life. Evidence for normal syntactic ability. *British Journal of Psychiatry*, 172, 130–135.

Earle-Boyer, E. A., Levinson, J. C., Grant, R. & Harvey, P. D. (1986). The consistency of thought disorder in mania and schizophrenia. II. An assessment at consecutive admissions. *Journal of Nervous and Mental Diseases*, 174(8), 443–447.

Elvevaag, B., Fisher, J. E., Gurd, J. M. & Goldberg, T. E. (2002a). Semantic clustering in verbal fluency: schizophrenic patients versus control participants. *Psychological Medicine*, 32(5), 909–917.

Elvevaag, B., Weickert, T., Wechsler, M. *et al.* (2002b). An investigation of the integrity of semantic boundaries in schizophrenia. *Schizophrenia Research*, 53(3), 187–198.

Elvevaag, B., Foltz, P. W., Weinberger, D. R. & Goldberg, T. E. (2007). Quantifying incoherence in speech: an automated methodology and novel application to schizophrenia. *Schizophrenia Research*, 93(1–3): 304–316.

Faber, R. & Reichstein, M. B. (1981). Language dysfunction in schizophrenia. *British Journal of Psychiatry*, 139, 519–522.

Fedorenko, E., Gibson, E. & Rohde, D. (2006). The nature of working memory capacity in sentence comprehension. *Journal of Memory and Language*, 54, 541–553.

Feinstein, A., Goldberg, T. E., Nowlin, B. & Weinberger, D. R. (1998). Types and characteristics of remote memory impairment in schizophrenia. *Schizophrenia Research*, 30(2), 155–163.

Fodor, J. A. & Bever, T. G. (1965). The psychological reality of linguistic segments. *Journal of Verbal Learning and Verbal Behavior*, 4, 414–420.

Ford, J. M. (1999). Schizophrenia: the broken P300 and beyond. *Psychophysiology*, 36(6), 667–682.

Frazier, L. & Rayner, K. (1982). Making and correcting errors during sentence comprehension: eye movements in the analysis of structurally-ambiguous sentences. *Cognitive Psychology*, 14, 178–210.

Frith, C. D. (1992). *The Cognitive Neuropsychology of Schizophrenia*. Hove, UK: Lawrence Erlbaum Associates.

Friedman, D., Simson, R., Ritter, W. & Rapin, I. (1975). The late positive component (P300) and information processing in sentences. *Electroencephalography and Clinical Neurophysiology*, 38, 255–262.

Fuller, R., Nopoulos, P., Arndt, S. *et al.* (2002). Longitudinal assessment of premorbid cognitive functioning in patients with schizophrenia through examination of standardized scholastic test performance. *American Journal of Psychiatry*, **159**(7), 1183–1189.

Garrett, M., Bever, T. G. & Fodor, J. (1966). The active use of grammar in speech perception. *Perception and Psycholinguistics*, **1**, 30–32.

Gold, J. M., Randolph, C. *et al.* (1992). Forms of memory failure in schizophrenia. *Journal of Abnormal Psychology*, **101**(3), 487–494.

Goldberg, T. E., Aloia, M. S., Gourovitch, M. L. *et al.* (1998). Cognitive substrates of thought disorder, I: the semantic system. *American Journal of Psychiatry*, **155**(12), 1671–1676.

Goldberg, T. E., Dodge, M., Aloia, M., Egan, M. F. & Weinberger, D. R. (2000). Effects of neuroleptic medications on speech disorganization in schizophrenia: biasing associative networks towards meaning. *Psychological Medicine*, **30**(5), 1123–1130.

Goldstein, K. (1944). Methodological approach to the study of schizophrenic thought disorder. In J. Kasanin (Ed.), *Language and Thought in Schizophrenia* (pp. 17–40). Berkeley, CA: University of California Press.

Gourovitch, M. L., Goldberg, T. E. & Weinberger, D. R. (1996). Verbal fluency deficits in patients with schizophrenia: semantic fluency is differentially impaired as compared with phonologic fluency. *Neuropsychology*, **10**(4), 573–577.

Grice, P. (1975). *Logic and Conversation*. New York, NY: Academic Press.

Grillon, C., Rezvan, A. & Glazer, W. M. (1991). N400 and semantic categorization in schizophrenia. *Biological Psychiatry*, **29**, 467–480.

Grove, W. M. & Andreasen, N. C. (1985). Language and thinking in psychosis: is there an input abnormality? *Archives of General Psychiatry*, **42**, 26–32.

Gurd, J. M., Elvevaag, B. & Cortina-Borja, M. (1997). Semantic category word search impairment in schizophrenia. *Cognitive Neuropsychiatry*, **2**, 291–302.

Halliday, M. & Hasan, R. (1976). *Cohesion in English*. London: Longman.

Harrow, M. & Quinlan, D. M. (1985). *Disordered Thinking and Schizophrenic Psychopathology*. New York, NY: Gardner.

Hart, D. S. & Payne, R. W. (1973). Language structure and predictability in overinclusive patients. *British Journal of Psychiatry*, **123**(577), 643–652.

Harvey, P. D. (1985). Reality monitoring in mania and schizophrenia: the association of thought disorder and performance. *Journal of Nervous and Mental Diseases*, **173**, 67–73.

Harvey, P. D. & Serper, M. R. (1990). Linguistic and cognitive failures in schizophrenia. *Journal of Nervous and Mental Disease*, **178**, 487–493.

Harvey, P. D., Earle-Boyer, E. A. & Wielgus, M. S. (1984). The consistency of thought disorder in mania and schizophrenia. An assessment of acute psychotics. *Journal of Nervous and Mental Diseases*, **172**(8), 458–463.

Harvey, P. D., Earle-Boyer, E. A., Wielgus, M. S. & Levinson, J. C. (1986). Encoding, memory, and thought disorder in schizophrenia and mania. *Schizophrenia Bulletin*, **12**, 252–261.

Henik, A., Nissimov, E., Priel, B. & Umansky, R. (1995). Effects of cognitive load on semantic priming in patients with schizophrenia. *Journal of Abnormal Psychology*, **104**, 576–584.

Henik, A., Priel, B. & Umansky, R. (1992). Attention and automaticity in semantic processing of schizophrenic patients. *Neuropsychiatry, Neuropsychology and Behavioural Neurology*, **5**, 161–169.

Hoff, A. L., Sakuma, M., Wieneke, M. *et al.* (1999). Longitudinal neuropsychological follow-up study of patients with first-episode schizophrenia. *American Journal of Psychiatry*, **156**(9), 1336–1341.

Hoffmann, H. & Kupper, Z. (1997). Relationships between social competence, psychopathology and work performance and their predictive value for vocational rehabilitation of schizophrenic outpatients. *Schizophrenia Research*, **23**(1), 69–79.

Hoffman, R. E. (1986). Tree structures, the work of listening, and schizophrenic discourse: a reply to Beveridge and Brown. *Brain and Language*, **27**(2), 385–392.

Hoffman, R. E., Hogben, G. L., Smith, H. & Calhoun, W. F. (1985). Message disruptions during syntactic processing in schizophrenia. *Journal of Community Disorders*, **18**(3), 183–202.

Hoffman, R. E., Kirstein, L., Stopek, S. & Cicchetti, D. V. (1982). Apprehending schizophrenic discourse: a structural analysis of the listener's task. *Brain and Language*, **15**(2), 207–233.

Hokama, H., Hiramatsu, K., Wang, J., O'Donnell, B. F. & Ogura, C. (2003). N400 abnormalities in unmedicated patients with schizophrenia during a lexical decision task. *International Journal of Psychophysiology*, **48**(1), 1–10.

Holcomb, P. J. (1993). Semantic priming and stimulus degradation: implications for the role of the N400 in language processing. *Psychophysiology*, **30**, 47–61.

Honigfeld, G. (1963). The ability of schizophrenics to understand normal, psychotic and pseudo-psychotic speech. *Diseases of the Nervous System*, **24**, 692–694.

Hotchkiss, A. P. & Harvey, P. D. (1990). Effect of distraction on communication failures in schizophrenic patients. *American Journal of Psychiatry*, **147**(4), 513–515.

Iakimova, G., Passerieux, C., Laurent, J. P. & Hardy-Bayle, M. C. (2005). ERPs of metaphoric, literal, and incongruous semantic processing in schizophrenia. *Psychophysiology*, **42**(4), 380–390.

Iddon, J. L., McKenna, P. J., Sahakian, B. J. & Robbins, T. W. (1998). Impaired generation and use of strategy in schizophrenia: evidence from visuospatial and verbal tasks. *Psychological Medicine*, **28**(5), 1049–1062.

Jung, C. G. (1981). Reaction time ratio in the association experiment. In H. Read, M. Forman & G. Alder (Eds.), *The Collected Works of C. G. Jung* (pp. 227–265). Princeton, NJ: Princeton University Press.

Just, M. A. & Carpenter, P. A. (1992). A capacity theory of comprehension: individual differences in working memory. *Psychological Review*, **99**(1), 122–149.

Kay, S. R., Fiszbein, A. & Opler, L. A. (1987). The positive and negative syndrome scale (PANSS) for schizophrenia. *Schizophrenia Bulletin*, **13**(2), 261–276.

Keifer, M., Ahlegian, M. & Spitzer, M. (2005). Working memory capacity, indirect semantic priming, and stroop interference: patterns of interindividual prefrontal performance differences in healthy volunteers. *Neuropsychology*, **19**(3), 332–344.

Kerns, J. G. & Berenbaum, H. (2002). Cognitive impairments associated with formal thought disorder in people with schizophrenia. *Journal of Abnormal Psychology*, **111**(2), 211–224.

Kiang, M., Kutas, M., Light, G. A. & Braff, D. L. (2008) An event-related brain potential study of direct and indirect semantic priming in schizophrenia. *American Journal of Psychiatry*, **165**, 74–81.

Kiang, M., Light, G. A., Prugh, J. et al. (2007). Cognitive, neurophysiological, and functional correlates of proverb interpretation abnormalities in schizophrenia. *Journal of the International Neuropsychological Society*, **13**, 653–663.

Kiefer, M., Weisbrod, M., Kern, I., Maier, S. & Spitzer, M. (1998). Right hemisphere activation during indirect semantic priming: evidence from event-related potentials. *Brain and Language*, **64**(3), 377–408.

Kintsch, W. (1968). Recognition and free recall of organised lists. *Journal of Experimental Psychology General*, **78**, 481–487.

Kintsch, W. (2000). Metaphor comprehension: a computational theory. *Psychonometric Bulletin Review*, **7**(2), 257–266.

Kintsch, W. & van Dijk, T. (1978). Toward a model of text comprehension and production. *Psychological Review*, **85**(5), 363–394.

Kischka, U., Kammer, T., Maier, S. et al. (1996). Dopaminergic modulation of semantic network activation. *Neuropsychologia*, **34**(11), 1107–1113.

Knight, R. A. & Sims-Knight, J. E. (1979). Integration of linguistic ideas in schizophrenics. *Journal of Abnormal Psychology*, **88**(2), 191–202.

Koh, S. D. & Kayton, L. (1974). Memorization of "unrelated" word strings by young nonpsychotic schizophrenics. *Journal of Abnormal Psychology*, **83**(1), 14–22.

Koh, S. D., Kayton, L. & Berry, R. (1973). Mnemonic organization in young nonpsychotic schizophrenics. *Journal of Abnormal Psychology*, **81**(3), 299–310.

Kostova, M., Passerieux, C., Laurent, J. P. & Hardy-Bayle, M. C. (2003). An electrophysiologic study: can semantic context processes be mobilized in patients with thought-disordered schizophrenia? *Canadian Journal of Psychiatry*, **48**(9), 615–623.

Kostova, M., Passerieux, C., Laurent, J. P. & Hardy-Bayle, M. C. (2005). N400 anomalies in schizophrenia are correlated with the severity of formal thought disorder. *Schizophrenia Research*, **78**(2–3), 285–291.

Koyama, S., Hokama, H., Miyatani, M. et al. (1994). ERPs in schizophrenic patients during word recognition task and reaction times. *Electroencephalography and Clinical Neurophysiology*, **92**, 546–554.

Koyama, S., Nageishi, Y., Shimokochi, M. et al. (1991). The N400 component of event-related potentials in schizophrenic patients: a preliminary study. *Electroencephalography and Clinical Neurophysiology*, **78**, 124–132.

Kraepelin, E. (1971). *Dementia Praecox and Paraphrenia*. New York, NY: Krieger.

Kravariti, E., Dixon, T., Frith, C. Murray, R. & McGuire, P. (2005). Association of symptoms and executive function in schizophrenia and bipolar disorder. *Schizophrenia Research*, **74**(2–3), 221–231.

Kreher, D. A., Holcomb, P. J., Goff, D. & Kuperberg, G. R. (2008). Neural evidence for faster and further automatic spreading activation in schizophrenic thought disorder. *Schizophrenia Bulletin*, **34**, 473–482.

Kreher, D. A., Goff, D. C. & Kuperberg, G. R. (2009). Why all the confusion? Experimental task explains discrepant semantic priming effects in schizophrenia under "automatic" conditions: evidence from event-related potentials. *Schizophrenia Research*, **111**, 174–181.

Kreher, D. A., Holcomb, P. J. & Kuperberg, G. R. (2006). An electrophysiological investigation of indirect semantic priming. *Psychophysiology*, **43**, 550–563.

Kremen, W. S., Seidman, L. J., Faraone, S. V. & Tsuang, M. T. (2003). Is there disproportionate impairment in semantic or phonemic fluency in schizophrenia? *Journal of the International Neuropsychological Society*, **9**(1), 79–88.

Kubicki, M., McCarley, R. W., Nestor, P. G. *et al.* (2003). An fMRI study of semantic processing in men with schizophrenia. *Neuroimage*, **20**(4), 1923–1933.

Kuperberg, G. R. (2007). Neural mechanisms of language comprehension: challenges to syntax. *Brain Research (Special Issue, Mysteries of Meaning)*, **1146**, 23–49.

Kuperberg, G. R. (2009). What can studying language tell us about schizophrenia (and vice versa)? *Language and Linguistics Compass*. In preparation.

Kuperberg, G. R., Broome, M. R., McGuire, P. K. *et al.* (2003a). Regionally localized thinning of the cerebral cortex in schizophrenia. *Archives of General Psychiatry*, **60**(9), 878–888.

Kuperberg, G., Caplan, D., Sitnikova, T., Eddy, M. & Holcomb, P. (2006a). Neural correlates of processing syntactic, semantic and thematic relationships in sentences. *Language and Cognitive Processes*, **21**(5), 489–530.

Kuperberg, G., Deckersbach, T., Holt, D., Goff, D. & West, W. C. (2007a). Increased temporal and prefrontal activity to semantic associations in schizophrenia. *Archives of General Psychiatry*, **64**, 138–151.

Kuperberg, G. R., Holcomb, P. J., Sitnikova, T. *et al.* (2003b). Distinct patterns of neural modulation during the processing of conceptual and syntactic anomalies. *Journal of Cognitive Neuroscience*, **15**(2), 272–293.

Kuperberg, G. R., Kreher, D. A. & Ditman, T. (2009). What can event-related potentials tell us about language, and perhaps even thought in schizophrenia? *International Journal of Psychophysiology*, In press.

Kuperberg, G. R., Kreher, D. A., Goff, D., McGuire, P. K. & David, A. S. (2006c). Building up linguistic context in schizophrenia: evidence from self-paced reading. *Neuropsychology*, **20**(4), 442–452.

Kuperberg, G., Lakshmanan, B., Caplan, D. & Holcomb, P. (2006b). Making sense of discourse: an fMRI study of causal inferencing across sentences. *Neuroimage*, **33**, 343–361.

Kuperberg, G. R., Lakshmanan, B. M. & West, W. C. (2008a). Task and semantic relationship influence both the polarity and localization of hemodynamic modulation during lexico-semantic processing. *Human Brain Mapping*, **29**(5), 544–561.

Kuperberg, G. R., McGuire, P. K. & David, A. (1998). Reduced sensitivity to linguistic context in schizophrenic thought disorder: evidence from online monitoring for words in linguistically-anomalous sentences. *Journal of Abnormal Psychology*, **107**, 423–434.

Kuperberg, G. R., McGuire, P. K. & David, A. (2000). Sensitivity to linguistic anomalies in spoken sentences: a case study approach to understanding thought disorder in schizophrenia. *Psychological Medicine*, **30**(2), 345–357.

Kuperberg, G. R., Sitnikova, T., Caplan, D. & Holcomb, P. J. (2003c). Electrophysiological distinctions in processing conceptual relationships within simple sentences. *Cognitive Brain Research*, **17**(1), 117–129.

Kuperberg, G. R., Sitnikova, T., Goff, D. & Holcomb, P. J. (2006d). Making sense of sentences in schizophrenia: electrophysiological evidence for abnormal interactions between semantic and syntactic processing. *Journal of Abnormal Psychology*, **115**(2), 243–256.

Kuperberg, G. R., West, W. C., Lakshmanan, B. M. & Goff, D. C. (2008b). fMRI reveals neuroanatomical dissociations during semantic integration in schizophrenia. *Biological Psychiatry*, **64**, 407–418.

Kutas, M. & Hillyard, S. A. (1980). Reading senseless sentences: brain potentials reflect semantic incongruity. *Science*, **207**, 203–205.

Kutas, M. & Hillyard, S. A. (1984). Brain potentials during reading reflect word expectancy and semantic association. *Nature*, **307**, 161–163.

Landauer, T. K., Foltz, P. W. & Dumais, S. T. (1998). Introduction to latent semantic analysis. *Discourse Processes*, **25**, 259–284.

Landre, N. A., Taylor, M. A. & Kearns, K. P. (1992). Language functioning in schizophrenic and aphasic patients. *Neuropsychiatry, Neuropsychology, and Behavioral Neurology*, **5**, 7–14.

Langdon, R. & Coltheart, M. (2004). Recognition of metaphor and irony in young adults: the impact of schizotypal personality traits. *Psychiatry Research*, **125**(1), 9–20.

Larson, E. R., Shear, P. K., Krikorian, R., Welge, J. & Strakowski, S. M. (2005). Working memory and inhibitory control among manic and euthymic patients with bipolar disorder. *Journal of the International Neuropsychology Society*, **11**(2), 163–172.

Laws, K. R., McKenna, P. J. & Kondel, T. K. (1998). On the distinction between access and store disorders in schizophrenia: a question of deficit severity? *Neuropsychologia*, **36**, 313–321.

Lee, J. & Park, S. (2005). Working memory impairments in schizophrenia: a meta-analysis. *Journal of Abnormal Psychology*, **114**(4), 599–611.

Leroy, F., Pezard, L., Nandrino, J. L. & Beaune, D. (2005). Dynamical quantification of schizophrenic speech. *Psychiatry Research*, **133**(2–3), 159–171.

Liddle, P. F. (1987). The symptoms of chronic schizophrenia. A re-examination of the positive-negative dichotomy. *British Journal of Psychiatry*, **151**, 145–151.

Liddle, P. F. (1992). Syndromes of schizophrenia on factor analysis. *British Journal of Psychiatry*, **161**, 861.

Maas, J. W. & Katz, M. M. (1992). Neurobiology and psychopathological states: are we looking in the right place? *Biological Psychiatry*, **31**, 757–758.

MacDonald, M. C., Pearlmutter, N. J. & Seidenberg, M. S. (1994). The lexical nature of syntactic ambiguity resolution. *Psychological Review*, **101**, 676–703.

Maher, B. A. (1983). A tentative theory of schizophrenic utterances. In B. A. Maher & W. B. Maher (Eds.), *Progress in Experimental Personality Research* (Vol. 12, pp. 1–52). San Diego, CA: Academic Press.

Manschreck, T. C., Maher, B. A., Milavetz, J. J. *et al.* (1988). Semantic priming in thought disordered schizophrenic patients. *Schizophrenia Research*, **1**, 61–66.

Manschreck, T. C., Maher, B. A., Rucklos, M. E. & White, M. T. (1979). The predictability of thought disordered speech in schizophrenic patients. *British Journal of Psychiatry*, **134**, 595–601.

Mathalon, D. H., Faustman, W. O. & Ford, J. M. (2002). N400 and automatic semantic processing abnormalities in patients with schizophrenia. *Archives of General Psychiatry*, **59**(7), 641–648.

Mazumdar, P. K., Chaturvedi, S. K. & Gopinath, P. S. (1995). A comparative study of thought disorder in acute and chronic schizophrenia. *Psychopathology*, **28**(4), 185–189.

McKenna, P. K. & Oh, T. M. (2005). *Schizophrenic Speech*. Cambridge: Cambridge University Press.

McKenna, P. K., Mortimer, A. M. & Hodges, J. R. (1994). Semantic memory and schizophrenia. In A. S. Davis & J. C. Cutting (Eds.), *The Neuropsychology of Schizophrenia* (pp. 163–178). Hove, UK: Psychology Press.

McNamara, T. P. & Altarriba, J. (1988). Depth of spreading activation revisited: semantic mediated priming occurs in lexical decisions. *Journal of Memory and Language*, **27**, 545–559.

Meyer, D. E. & Schvaneveldt, R. W. (1971). Facilitation in recognizing pairs of words: evidence of a dependence between retrieval operations. *Journal of Experimental Psychology*, **20**, 227–234.

Miller, W. K. & Phelan, J. G. (1980). Comparison of adult schizophrenics with matched normal native speakers of English as to "acceptability" of English sentences. *Journal of Psycholinguistic Research*, **9**(6), 579–593.

Minzenberg, M. J., Ober, B. A. & Vinogradov, S. (2002). Semantic priming in schizophrenia: a review and synthesis. *Journal of the International Neuropsychological Society*, **8**(5), 699–720.

Mitchell, P. F., Andrews, S., Fox, A. M. *et al.* (1991). Active and passive attention in schizophrenia: an ERP study of information processing in a linguistic task. *Biological Psychiatry*, **32**, 101–124.

Mitchell, R. L. & Crow, T. J. (2005). Right hemisphere language functions and schizophrenia: the forgotten hemisphere? *Brain*, **128**(5), 963–978.

Morgan, C. J., Rossell, S. L., Pepper, F. *et al.* (2006). Semantic priming after ketamine acutely in healthy volunteers and following chronic self-administration in substance users. *Biological Psychiatry*, **59**(3), 265–272.

Morice, R. D. & Ingram, J. C. L. (1982). Language analysis in schizophrenia: diagnostic implications. *Australian and New Zealand Journal of Psychiatry*, **16**, 11–21.

Moritz, S., Mersmann, K., Kloss, M. *et al.* (2001a). Enhanced semantic priming in thought-disordered schizophrenic patients using a word pronunciation task. *Schizophrenia Research*, **48**(2–3), 301–305.

Moritz, S., Mersmann, K., Kloss, M. *et al.* (2001b). Hyper-priming in thought-disordered schizophrenic patients. *Psychological Medicine*, **31**(2), 221–229.

Moritz, S., Woodward, T. S., Kuppers, D., Lausen, A. & Schickel, M. (2002). Increased automatic spreading of activation in thought-disordered schizophrenic patients. *Schizophrenia Research*, **59**(2–3), 181–186.

Neely, J. H. (1977). Semantic priming and retrieval from lexical memory: roles of inhibitionless spreading activation and limited-capacity attention. *Journal of Experimental Psychology: General*, **106**, 226–254.

Neely, J. H. (1991). Semantic priming effects in visual word recognition: a selective review of current findings and theories. In D. Besner & G. W. Humphreys (Eds.), *Basic Processes in Reading and Visual Word Recognition*, pp. 264–333. Hillsdale, NJ: Lawrence Erlbaum Associates.

Neely, J. H., Keefe, D. E. & Ross, K. (1989). Semantic priming in the lexical decision task: roles of prospective prime-generated expectancies and retrospective semantic matching. *Journal of Experimental Psychology: Learning, Memory and Cognition*, **15**, 1003–1019.

Nestor, P. G., Kimble, M. O., O'Donnell, B. F. *et al.* (1997). Aberrant semantic activation in schizophrenia: a neurophysiological study. *American Journal of Psychiatry*, **154**(5), 640–646.

Nestor, P. G., Shenton, M. E., Wible, C. *et al.* (1998). A neuropsychological analysis of schizophrenic thought disorder. *Schizophrenia Research*, **29**(3), 217–225.

Nienow, T. M. & Docherty, N. M. (2005). Internal source monitoring and communication disturbance in patients with schizophrenia. *Psychological Medicine*, **35**(12), 1717–1726.

Niznikiewicz, M. A., O'Donnell, B. F., Nestor, P. G. *et al.* (1997). ERP assessment of visual and auditory language processing in schizophrenia. *Journal of Abnormal Psychology*, **106**, 85–94.

Noel-Jorand, M. C., Reinert, M., Giudicelli, S. & Dassa, D. (1997). A new approach to discourse analysis in psychiatry, applied to a schizophrenic patient's speech. *Schizophrenia Research*, **25**(3), 183–198.

Norman, R. M., Malla, A. K., Cortese, L. *et al.* (1999). Symptoms and cognition as predictors of community functioning: a prospective analysis. *American Journal of Psychiatry*, **156**(3), 400–405.

Nuecheterlein, K. H., Edell, W. S., Norris, M. & Dawson, M. (1986). Attentional vulnerability indicators, thought disorder, and negative symptoms. *Schizophrenia Bulletin*, **12**, 408–426.

Ober, B. A., Vinogradov, S. & Shenaut, G. K. (1995). Semantic priming of category relations in schizophrenia. *Neuropsychology*, **9**(2), 220–228.

Ober, B. A., Vinogradov, S. & Shenaut, G. K. (1997). Automatic versus controlled semantic priming in schizophrenia. *Neuropsychology*, **11**(4), 506–513.

Ohta, K., Uchiyama, M., Matsushima, E. & Toru, M. (1999). An event-related potential study in schizophrenia using Japanese sentences. *Schizophrenia Research*, **40**(2), 159–170.

Oltmanns, T. F., Murphy, R., Berenbaum, H. & Dunlop, S. R. (1985). Rating verbal communication impairment in schizophrenia and affective disorders. *Schizophrenia Bulletin*, **11**(2), 292–299.

Osterhout, L. & Hagoort, P. (1999). A superficial resemblence does not necessarily mean you are part of the family: counterarguments to Coulson, King and Kutas (1998) in the P600/SPS-P300 debate. *Language and Cognitive Processes*, **14**, 1–14.

Ott, S. L., Allen, J. & Erlenmeyer-Kimling, L. (2001). The New York High-Risk Project: observations on the rating of early manifestations of schizophrenia. *American Journal of Medical Genetics*, **105**(1), 25–27.

Pandurangi, A. K., Sax, K. W., Pelonero, A. L. & Goldberg, S. C. (1994). Sustained attention and positive formal thought disorder in schizophrenia. *Schizophrenia Research*, **13**, 109–116.

Passerieux, C., Segui, J., Besche, C. *et al.* (1997). Heterogeneity in cognitive functioning of schizophrenic patients evaluated by a lexical decision task. *Psychological Medicine*, **27**(6), 1295–1302.

Paulsen, J. S., Romero, R., Chan, A. *et al.* (1996). Impairment of the semantic network in schizophrenia. *Psychiatry Research*, **63**(2–3), 109–121.

Pavy, D. (1968). Verbal behavior in schizophrenia: a review of recent studies. *Psychological Bulletin*, **70**(3), 164–178.

Perry, W. & Braff, D. L. (1994). Information-processing deficits and thought disorder in schizophrenia. *American Journal of Psychiatry*, **151**(3), 363–367.

Pomarol-Clotet, E, Oh, T. M., Laws, K. R. & McKenna, P. J. (2008). Semantic priming in schizophrenia: systematic review and meta-analysis. *British Journal of Psychiatry*, **192**(2), 92–97.

Poole, J. H., Ober, B. A., Shenaut, G. K. & Vinogradov, S. (1999). Independent frontal-system deficits in schizophrenia: cognitive, clinical, and adaptive implications. *Psychiatry Research*, **85**(2), 161–176.

Ragland, J. D., Gur, R. C., Valdez, J. *et al.* (2004). Event-related fMRI of frontotemporal activity during word encoding and recognition in schizophrenia. *American Journal of Psychiatry*, **161**(6), 1004–1015.

Ragland, J. D., Gur, R. C., Valdez, J. *et al.* (2005). Levels-of-Processing effect on frontotemporal function in schizophrenia during word encoding and recognition. *American Journal of Psychiatry*, **162**(10), 1840–1848.

Rhodes, J. E. & Jakes, S. (2004). The contribution of metaphor and metonymy to delusions. *Psychology and Psychotherapy*, **77**(1), 1–17.

Rochester, S. & Martin, J. R. (1979). *Crazy Talk: A Study of the Discourse of Schizophrenic Speakers*. New York, NY: Plenum Press.

Rochester, S. R., Harris, J. & Seeman, M. V. (1973). Sentence processing in schizophrenic listeners. *Journal of Abnormal Psychology*, **82**, 350–356.

Roesch-Ely, D., Weiland, S., Scheffel, H. *et al.* (2006). Dopaminergic modulation of semantic priming in healthy volunteers. *Biological Psychiatry*, **60**(6), 604–611.

Rossell, S. L. & David, A. S. (2006). Are semantic deficits in schizophrenia due to problems with access or storage? *Schizophrenia Research*, **82**(2–3), 121–134.

Rossell, S. L., Price, C. J. & Nobre, A. C. (2003). The anatomy and time course of semantic priming investigated by fMRI and ERPs. *Neuropsychologia*, **41**(5), 550–564.

Ruchsow, M., Trippel, N., Groen, G., Spitzer, M. & Kiefer, M. (2003). Semantic and syntactic processes during sentence comprehension in patients with schizophrenia: evidence from event-related potentials. *Schizophrenia Research*, **64**(2–3), 147–156.

Rugg, M. D. (1985). The effects of semantic priming and word repetition on event-related potentials. *Psychophysiology*, **22**, 642–647.

Salisbury, D. F., O'Donnell, B. F., McCarley, R. W., Nestor, P. G. & Shenton, M. E. (2000). Event-related potentials elicited during a context-free homograph task in normal versus schizophrenic subjects. *Psychophysiology*, **37**(4), 456–463.

Salisbury, D. F., Shenton, M. E., Nestor, P. G. & McCarley, R. W. (2002). Semantic bias, homograph comprehension, and event-related potentials in schizophrenia. *Clinical Neurophysiology*, **113**(3), 383–395.

Salzinger, K., Pisoni, D. B., Portnoy, S. & Feldman, R. S. (1970). The immediacy hypothesis and response-produced stimuli in schizophrenic speech. *Journal of Abnormal Psychology*, **76**, 258–264.

Salzinger, K., Portnoy, S. & Feldman, R. S. (1964). Verbal behavior of schizophrenic and normal subjects. *Annals of the New York Academy of Sciences*, **105**, 845–860.

Salzinger, K., Portnoy, S. & Feldman, R. S. (1979). The predictability of speech in schizophrenic patients [letter]. *British Journal of Psychiatry*, **135**, 284–287.

Sanford, A. & Garrod, S. (1994). *Selective Processing in Text Understanding*. San Deigo, CA: Academic Press, Inc.

Schneider, C. (1930). *Psychologie der Schizophrenie*. Leipzig.

Sitnikova, T., Salisbury, D. F., Kuperberg, G. & Holcomb, P. I. (2002). Electrophysiological insights into language processing in schizophrenia. *Psychophysiology*, **39**(6), 851–860.

Speed, M., Shugar, G. & Di Gasbarro, I. (1991). Thought disorder and verbal recall in acutely psychotic patients. *Journal of Clinical Psychology*, **47**, 735–744.

Spitzer, M. (1993). The psychopathology, neuropsychology, and neurobiology of associative and working memory in schizophrenia. *European Archives of Psychiatry and Clinical Neuroscience*, **243**, 57–70.

Spitzer, M., Braun, U., Maier, S., Hermle, L. & Maher, B. (1993). Indirect semantic priming in schizophrenic patients. *Schizophrenia Research*, **11**, 71–80.

Spitzer, M., Weisker, I., Winter, M. *et al.* (1994). Semantic and phonological priming in schizophrenia. *Journal of Abnormal Psychology*, **103**, 485–494.

Spitzer, R. L., Williams, J. B., Gibbon, M. & First, M. B. (1992). The Structured Clinical Interview for DSM–III–R (SCID) I: History, rationale and description. *Archives of General Psychiatry*, **4**, 642–649.

Strandburg, R. J., Marsh, J. T., Brown, W. S. *et al.* (1997). Event-related potential correlates of linguistic information processing in schizophrenics. *Biological Psychiatry*, **42**(7), 596–608.

Strauss, M. E., Buchanan, R. W. & Hale, J. (1993). Relations between attentional deficits and clinical symptoms in schizophrenic outpatients. *Psychiatric Research*, **47**, 205–213.

Surguladze, S., Rossell, S., Rabe-Hesketh, S. & David, A. S. (2002). Cross-modal semantic priming in schizophrenia. *Journal of the International Neuropsychology Society*, **8**(7), 884–892.

Swaab, T., Camblin, C. & Gordon, P. (2004). Electrophysiological evidence for reversed lexical repetition effects in language processing. *Journal of Cognitive Neuroscience*, **16**(5), 715–726.

Tallent, K. A., Weinberger, D. R. & Goldberg, T. E. (2001). Associating semantic space abnormalities with formal thought disorder in schizophrenia: use of triadic comparisons. *Journal of Clinical and Experimental Neuropsychology*, **23**(3), 285–296.

Taylor, W. (1953). Cloze' procedure: a new tool for measuring readability. *Journal Quarterly*, **30**, 415–433.

Tenyi, T., Herold, R., Szili, I. M. & Trixler, M. (2002). Schizophrenics show a failure in the decoding of violations of conversational implicatures. *Psychopathology*, **35**(1), 25–27.

Thomas, P., King, K., Fraser, W. I. & Kendell, R. E. (1990). Linguistic performance in schizophrenia: a comparison of acute and chronic patients. *British Journal of Psychiatry*, **156**, 204–210.

Thompson-Schill, S. L. (2003). Neuroimaging studies of semantic memory: inferring "how" from "where". *Neuropsychologia*, **41**(3), 280–292.

Titone, D. A. & Connine, C. M. (1994). Comprehension of idiomatic expressions: effects of predictability and literality. *Journal of Experimental Psychology: Learning, Memory and Cognition*, **20**(5), 1126–1138.

Titone, D., Holzman, P. S. & Levy, D. L. (2002). Idiom processing in schizophrenia: literal implausibility saves the day for idiom priming. *Journal of Abnormal Psychology*, **111**(2), 313–320.

Titone, D., Levy, D. L. & Holzman, P. S. (2000). Contextual insensitivity in schizophrenic language processing: evidence from lexical ambiguity. *Journal of Abnormal Psychology*, **109**(4), 761–767.

Ungerleider, L. G. & Haxby, J. V. (1994). 'What' and 'where' in the human brain. *Current Opinion of Neurobiology*, **4**(2), 157–165.

van Berkum, J. J., Brown, C. M. & Hagoort, P. (1999). Early referential context effects in sentence processing: evidence from event-related brain potentials. *Journal of Memory and Language*, **41**, 147–182.

Vinogradov, S., Ober, B. A. & Shenaut, G. K. (1992). Semantic priming of word pronunciation and lexical decision in schizophrenia. *Schizophrenia Research*, **8**, 171–181.

Weisbrod, M., Kiefer, M., Winkler, S. *et al.* (1999). Electrophysiological correlates of direct versus indirect semantic priming in normal volunteers. *Cognitive Brain Research*, **8**(3), 289–298.

Weisbrod, M., Maier, S., Harig, S., Himmelsbach, U. & Spitzer, M. (1998). Lateralised semantic and indirect semantic priming effects in people with schizophrenia. *British Journal of Psychiatry*, **172**, 142–146.

Weiss, A. P., Schacter, D. L., Goff, D. *et al.* (2003). Impaired hippocampal recruitment during normal modulation of memory performance in schizophrenia. *Biological Psychiatry*, **53**(1), 48–55.

Associative memory

Marc L. Seal and Anthony P. Weiss

Memory is the mother of all wisdom
Aeschylus, *Prometheus Bound* (525–456 BC)

Introduction

The formation of a memory involves the creation of new and enduring representations of our experiences. These representations contain detailed contextual information, markers of the time and place in which an event was experienced. Potentially, all elements of our experience are stored: our affective and physiological state at the time, a record of the cognitive processes occurring at that moment and, crucially, the extent to which this new experience reconciles with existing similar memories. During the encoding process, existing memories and their network of relational information may be updated and modified in the face of a new experience. The efficient storage and subsequent successful retrieval of a memory is dependent on the unique and idiosyncratic organization of contextual information that makes up a memory. These relational networks make it possible to put the right name to a familiar face or to correctly remember your passwords for your various computer accounts. Impairment in the ability to generate or access this relational information can have debilitating consequences in an individual's daily life. In this chapter we will examine the nature of associative or relational memory processes and what potential deficits in this cognitive domain can inform us about the nature of mental disorders.

Measuring associative memory

Before we commence our discussion of the application of associative memory in order to better under-

stand mental disorders, it is appropriate to review the ways in which researchers and clinicians measure this neuropsychological construct. In the broadest sense, associative memory refers to the set of processes involved in the binding of the features of a memory during encoding, in addition to the successful storage and retrieval of the memory for the event and relevant relational information. Poor performance on an associative memory task could be due to a number of causes including incomplete encoding of relational information, the compromised storage of relational information, inefficient identification of existing relational ties, incomplete retrieval of associated details or a combination of all the above factors. It is not surprising, then, that there exist different methodological techniques to measure associative memory.

First, there are tests that directly assess the ability to link information about one item with another. Typically these tasks involve the novel pairing of information during the encoding or learning phase. For example, subjects attempting a form of the Verbal Paired Associates Task (the most widely used is contained in versions of the Weschler Memory Scales; Weschler, 1987, 1997) are required to learn the pairings of combinations of words (e.g. flower – petal, crush – dark). Following the presentation of the pairs, participants are provided with the first item of each pair and asked to recall what other word was paired with it. Some versions of this task manipulate these pairings to involve words that are semantically linked, *easy pairs* (e.g. flower – petal) and other pairings which are not semantically linked, *hard pairs* (e.g. crush – dark). In general, it is easier to form and recall relational information between items that already have established contextual and semantic links. Other tasks require subjects to form more

The Neuropsychology of Mental Illness, ed. Stephen J. Wood, Nicholas B. Allen and Christos Pantelis. Published by Cambridge University Press. © Cambridge University Press 2009.

complex, abstract links across modalities, such as the pairing of unfamiliar faces with unfamiliar names, or remembering the identity of an abstract figure as well as its location/position on the presentation screen. These tasks avoid the potential confounding influence of previously learned associations. An additional, more sophisticated way of testing associative memory involves examining the phenomenon of transitive inference (see Dusek & Eichenbaum, 1997). That is, our capacity to infer possible relationships between apparently indirectly related items based on previous learning. In practice, this involves the subject learning a stimulus hierarchy $(A > B > C > D > E)$ via the presentation of a sequence of overlapping pairs (i.e. if $A > B$ and $B > C$, then $A > C$). In order to successfully complete this task subjects must form and appreciate a series of relationships between novel stimuli. Performance on this paradigm has been extensively investigated in animals (Eichenbaum, 2004), as well as via functional neuroimaging investigations involving healthy human subjects (Heckers et al., 2004). The findings of these studies suggest that there are dissociable regions in the medial temporal lobe (MTL) for recognizing relevant relational information. Recognition of previously learnt items involves widespread MTL activation with the focal point in the parahippocampal gyrus, whereas the accurate recollection of the relational information between items is centered in the hippocampus.

The second group of associative memory tasks are generally referred to as *source memory* tasks, as they attempt to assess the ability of individuals to embed an item within its context or source. The term *source* itself, refers to a set of characteristics that collectively define the conditions or context under which a memory is acquired (e.g. "Where did I read about associative memory again?"). Since our memory for such details is demonstrably fallible, the *source monitoring* framework also incorporates the set of processes underlying attributions about the origins of memories, knowledge and beliefs (for a review see Johnson et al., 1993). Well-designed source memory tasks assess memory for items and the source/context of the item memory, as well as an individual's idiosyncratic response bias to say an item was acquired in a particular context (i.e. "I must have read that in that book on Neuropsychology and Mental Disorders"). Source memory tasks can involve discriminating between memories of two externally generated events (i.e. "What did person A say that was different from what person B said?"), memories of internally generated events (i.e. What I thought or imagined and what I actually said), or memories of the actions of self and another (i.e. "Did you do that or did I?"). Accurate source monitoring relies on the quality of information associated with a memory, the effectiveness of the retrieval strategy adopted and the efficiency of post-retrieval decision processes (Johnson et al., 1993). Memories of externally generated events or perceived events are believed to have more perceptual and contextual information associated with them. That is, associated with a memory for hearing a lecture is sensory information about the tone, volume and character of the lecturer's voice, as well as information regarding what time of day and day of the week the lecture occurred. In contrast, memories of self-generated actions contain distinctive contextual cues that make them more readily identified than memories of externally or other generated events: the so-called *generation effect* (Raye et al., 1980). Simply, you are more likely to remember things said or done by you than by another, because your memory of these events is associated with privileged information; that is, your intention to act, motor information and the perceptual information related to performing the action.

The last group of associative memory tasks involves assessing associative memory via the phenomenology of the experience of recollection. One popular example of testing these phenomena, the Remember–Know paradigm, requires participants to rate the experience of recollection (see Gardiner, 2001). Subjects are asked to distinguish between memories that are accompanied with rich contextual and relational details (e.g. "I clearly remember you saying that word before") and those recollective experiences that are unaccompanied by any contextual information (e.g. "The word feels familiar but I don't remember hearing you say it before"). Individuals who have difficulties storing and retrieving relational information are less likely to describe their recollective experiences as containing rich phenomenological detail. For example, there is consistent evidence that individuals with schizophrenia are less likely to desscribe their subjective recollective experiences as like a "Remember" response, suggesting that their typical experience of recollection is accompanied by less relational information (Danion et al., 2005; Seal et al., 1997). This deficit has been interpreted as failure to form a comprehensive and stable relational network during the encoding stage (Danion et al., 1999).

Given the broad definition of associative memory, the presented information is certainly not exhaustive and there are other descriptions in the literature; however, it provides a framework for the following discussion of the assessment of associative memory.

Grounds for investigating associative memory function in mental disorders

The past decade has seen a tremendous increase in interest in the relationship between memory abnormalities and mental illness. Indeed, as seen in Figure 7.1, the number of publications on this topic has shown exponential growth. This trend has been particularly strong in the area of schizophrenia research; in 2005 one out of every seven papers published on schizophrenia focused on memory abnormalities in this disorder.

We contend that there are three overarching reasons for studying the relationship between memory and mental illness. First, the study of memory in patients with mental illness may provide clues to the underlying pathophysiological mechanisms of these disorders. This follows from the logical deduction that if memory impairment is characteristic of a particular mental illness, then those brain areas important for memory processing are somehow dysfunctional. Second, the underlying psychological processes that are involved in memory may, when abnormal, also help to explain some of the symptoms seen in individuals with mental illness. For example, individuals prone to hallucinations show impairments in recognizing the source of self-generated actions. Finally, memory dysfunction is a critical component of the overall functional impairment seen in individuals with mental illness. The level of one's memory capacity is in many ways a gauge on potential social and occupational performance, with poor memory being a significant barrier to reintegration, despite adequate symptom control.

Reason 1: Improving our understanding of underlying neuropathology

Memory is not a unitary concept, neither semantically or neurobiologically. Converging findings from

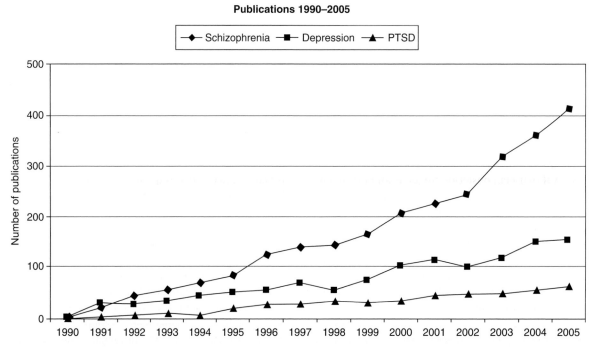

Figure 7.1. Publications over time for the intersection of memory and three major mental illnesses (schizophrenia, major depression, and post-traumatic stress disorder (PTSD)). Data obtained through a query of the ISI Web of Science (Thomson Scientific, Stamford CT) on May 2, 2006 using the terms "memory," "schizophrenia," "major depression OR depressive," and "post traumatic OR PTSD." The search was limited to English language full-length articles.

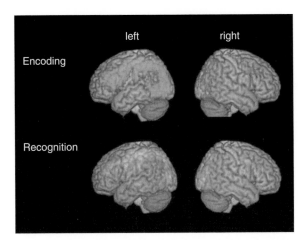

left   right

Encoding

Recognition

Figure 7.2. This figure is also reproduced in the color plate section. Brain regions involved in associative memory processes (unpublished fMR neuroimaging data from the authors). Note the important role of coordinated anterior-posterior activity associated with both encoding and retrieval processes. Data acquired from n = 17 healthy control subjects completing verbal encoding and retrieval tasks.

clinical case studies involving individuals with localized brain damage, as well as functional neuroimaging research on healthy adults indicate that there are multiple forms of memory in the brain, served by a range of cortical–subcortical–cerebellar systems (Squire, 2004). Nyberg *et al.* (2002) have characterized memory as consisting of a series of independent but interacting systems. To varying degrees, encoding and retrieval networks include: the hippocampus and surrounding medial temporal cortex, the lateral prefrontal cortex (BA 9/46), parietal cortex (BA 7, 39/40), anterior cingulate (BA 32/24) and cerebellum (see Figure 7.2). Although most work has focused on the medial temporal lobe and prefrontal cortex, Wagner *et al.* (2005) in a recent review highlight the consistent finding of posterior regions in episodic memory retrieval (parietal, posterior cingulate and precuneus), which appear to be preferentially activated when the subject is required to focus on the phenomenological experience of recollection.

Efficient and accurate memory function is dependent on the integrity of this network. Compromise of the brain structures and/or connections between these regions results in observable associative memory deficits (Squire, 2004). Eichenbaum (2004) has proposed a model of declarative memory in which the hippocampus and medial temporal lobe (MTL) receive information (sensory, affective, cognitive) from a multitude of sites in the brain. This information is indexed as "associative representational

elements" (the who, what and how of the experience), which are then "sequentially organized" in a distinctive representational network so as to preserve all the detail of the memory and to assist with accurate retrieval. Consequently, associative memory processes operate within representational networks and between separate memories.

For those mental disorders in which associative memory impairment is a significant and characteristic feature of the illness, it is reasonable to postulate that brain regions involved in the memory network detailed above are in some way dysfunctional. However, while associative memory deficits may imply that these brain regions are impaired in a particular disorder, it does not necessarily implicate them in the pathogenesis of the disorder. In order to make such a link you need to track the development of the memory deficit and the neuropathology across the course of the illness. For example, recent reviews suggest that chronic schizophrenia is characterized by a significant associative memory deficit (Aleman *et al.*, 1999) and functional neuroimaging studies have identified atypical brain activity related to episodic memory processing in schizophrenia (Achim & Lepage, 2005). In addition, while volumetric findings are variable, there is consistent and converging evidence that the hippocampus is abnormal in schizophrenia neuropathologically (Harrison, 2004), structurally (Honea *et al.*, 2005; Pantelis *et al.*, 2005; Weiss *et al.*, 2005) and functionally (Weiss *et al.*, 2003). Further, there is evidence of hippocampal volume deficits and memory deficits in individuals with first-episode psychosis.

Taken together these findings imply that hippocampal pathology is a feature of schizophrenia, but it is not clear if this pathology pre-dates the onset of psychosis. Recently this question was addressed by the largest published study to date comparing hippocampal and amygdala volumes between groups with chronic schizophrenia, first-episode psychosis and those at ultra-high risk of developing psychosis (Velakoulis *et al.*, 2006). Significantly, compared with healthy controls no structural changes were observed in the MTL until after the onset of a psychotic illness. These findings suggest that the changes to the MTL and accompanying associative memory deficits are the consequence of the brain changes involving transition to schizophrenia psychosis. Further, the pattern of structural change differed according to the type of psychosis in the first-episode psychosis (affective versus schizophrenia). Individual with non-schizophrenia psychosis had significantly enlarged amygdala but normal hippocampal volumes. Consequently it is possible to use neuroanatomical abnormalities and corresponding memory deficits to inform the onset and progression of mental disorders. This particular methodology represents the first step in developing clinically useful neuroimaging techniques to aid clinicians in diagnosis, prognosis and treatment monitoring; a substantial advance in the field of psychiatry.

Reason 2: Informing the origins of neuropsychiatric symptomatology

The application of neurocognitive models to study abnormal cognition in mental disorders has been influential in increasing our understanding of the origins of these illnesses (see Halligan & David, 2001). The systematic application of comprehensive cognitive neuropsychiatric models to mental disorders has been very useful in increasing our understanding of neurocognitive deficits, as well as the extent to which these deficits correspond to functional impairments, symptomatology and compromised brain function and structure. For example in schizophrenia neuropsychiatric models of the following cognitive domains have informed our understanding of the neurocognitive substrates of the disorder; working memory (Goldman-Rakic, 1994), semantic processing (Spitzer, 1997), motor imagery (Danckert et al., 2004), social cognition (Green & Phillips, 2004), theory of mind (Langdon et al., 1997) and olfactory memory (Pantelis & Brewer, 1995).

A salient example of this approach has been the ongoing investigation of the potential relationship between impaired associative memory function and the experience of auditory verbal hallucinations (for a recent review see Seal et al., 2004). Disturbances in associative memory processes can result in fragmented retrieval of memories, potentially causing confusion over the origin or source of a memory: "Did that really happen or did I imagine it?" The notion that disorders of self-awareness are an expression of specific cortical damage is not a new concept in neuropsychology. Johnson (1997) examined the phenomenon of confabulation in organic brain-disease patients and related it to an inability to monitor recall of experience and subsequent attribution processes. In a series of experiments McGuire and colleagues (Allen et al., 2007; Johns et al.,

2001; McGuire et al., 1995) have used increasingly sophisticated verbal self-monitoring paradigms to consistently demonstrate that hallucination-prone individuals are impaired at monitoring the generation and perception of their own speech compared with control groups. These findings suggest that from the outset there is an impairment in linking relevant relational information (the source of the speech) with the action (speaking aloud). Further, there is substantial evidence from the application of source memory paradigms ("Do you remember who said that word before?") that hallucinating subjects are selectively impaired to remember the source of a spoken item (self or other) (see Brébion et al., 2005; Keefe et al., 2002). It is important to note that amongst hallucinating subjects this relational memory deficit is often accompanied by an inappropriately liberal response bias. That is, when uncertain about the context of a memory hallucinating subjects tend to claim that they had said or done something before. It has yet to be established if this response bias represents a learnt coping mechanism in response to demonstrable poor relational memory or signifies some form of post-retrieval monitoring failure.

Reason 3: Understanding functional impairment

The final link focuses on a newly recognized connection between associative memory impairment and the overall functional level of the patient with mental illness. In schizophrenia, for example, there has been a relatively recent shift in thinking regarding the goal of treatment, away from pure symptom control and toward a more holistic concept of remission or recovery (Davidson et al., 2005). As many patients with schizophrenia demonstrate a poor functional outcome (Hegarty et al., 1994; Jobe & Harrow, 2005) despite adequate control of positive symptoms (i.e. hallucinations and delusions), other factors, including cognitive performance, have come under intense study.

Although cognitive deficits, including impairments of memory, have long been seen as a component of the schizophrenia syndrome (Hull, 1917), the link between these features of the illness and poor functional outcome was strengthened by a series of influential papers in the last decade (Green, 1996; Green et al., 2000; Green & Neuchterlein, 1999).

Of particular relevance here, the 1996 literature review by Michael Green (which has now been cited more than 750 times) described the predictive relationship between verbal memory and overall community functioning in patients with schizophrenia (Green, 1996). Subsequent to this work a number of other studies have been published substantiating this link (for a recent review see Kurtz, 2006).

As the majority of this work has been cross-sectional, it remains unclear whether the relationship between memory impairment and functional outcome is indeed a causal one. It is possible that memory impairment is simply associated with a second factor (e.g. negative symptoms) that has a more direct causal link with social functioning. That said, there is strong evidence linking memory performance to the critical skills necessary for successful social and occupational functioning (Corrigan & Toomey, 1995; Corrigan et al., 1994; Mueser et al., 1991). It is therefore likely that cognitive limitations are associated with deficiencies in skill acquisition, and thus poor functional outcome. If this were correct, improving cognition would allow patients to acquire the core skills necessary for social interaction and adequate job performance, thereby improving their overall level of well-being in society. This perspective has been adopted widely, and has propelled cognitive dysfunction (and memory in particular) into a position as a prime target for treatment in order to enhance the functional status of patients with schizophrenia (Sharma & Antonova, 2003).

The best evidence thus far is in support of cognitive remediation approaches, akin to the rehabilitation provided to patients with brain injury (Krabbendam & Aleman, 2003; Kurtz et al., 2001). This work represents a clinical extension of the findings from a handful of cognitive psychology studies showing that patients with schizophrenia can utilize novel cognitive strategies to improve memory performance (Koh et al., 1976; Kubicki et al., 2003; Ragland et al., 2005; Weiss et al., 2003). Although a 2002 review of the extant literature in this area suggested that there was no clinical benefit from this type of cognitive remediation (Pilling et al., 2002), a number of subsequent papers have shown significant cognitive improvements associated with this intervention (Bell et al., 2004; Penades et al., 2006; Sartory et al., 2005), including two studies that have demonstrated persisting benefits over a period of longitudinal follow-up (Fiszdon et al., 2004; Wykes et al.,

2003). Taken as a whole, it now appears that at least some patients with schizophrenia can benefit from intensive cognitive remediation approaches, although the degree to which the observed cognitive benefit actually leads to functional improvement remains to be seen.

At present there are no established, FDA-approved, pharmacological treatments available to reverse the memory impairment seen in schizophrenia, although the recent launch of two large-scale NIMH-funded projects MATRICS (Measurement and Treatment Research to Improve Cognition in Schizophrenia; Green & Neuchterlein, 2004; Marder & Fenton, 2004), and TURNS (Treatment Units for Research on Neurocognition and Schizophrenia, www.turns.ucla.edu/index.shtml) may serve as a harbinger of pharmacological successes to come.

Conclusion

This chapter has presented an overview of the neuropsychological construct associative memory and highlighted various ways in which measuring it can improve our understanding of mental disorders. Given the abundance of neuropsychological research associated with schizophrenia, the practical illustrations we have presented have focused on this disorder; however, we contend that that these benefits apply to all mental disorders. In fact we encourage our colleagues to explore the potential connections between associative memory and other mental illnesses, especially major depression, obsessive-compulsive and post-traumatic stress disorder. Several challenges exist for associative memory research in mental illness. The consequence of increasing the sensitivity and specificity of associative memory tasks will be a more useful tool for understanding heterogeneous presentations of mental disorders. For example, the successful completion of associative memory tasks often relies on executive processes such as post-retrieval monitoring. Accordingly, there is a need to partition out component elements of tasks to identify processes such as retrieval effort and post-retrieval monitoring (Buckner & Wheeler, 2001). Further, the application of increasingly sophisticated memory paradigms with greater selectivity of individual regions of the MTL and hippocampus will assist in understanding the specificity of neurocognitive abnormalities in the MTL (Preston et al., 2005). Finally, a recent review by Harrison & Weinberger (2005) has emphasized the role of particular candidate genes resulting in abnormal synaptogenesis and neurotransmission in schizophrenia. The next challenge for researchers is to determine which structural and functional hippocampal anomalies consistently identified in mental illness can be accounted for by a molecular and genetic mechanism.

References

Achim, A. M. & Lepage, M. (2005). Episodic memory-related activation in schizophrenia: meta-analysis. *British Journal of Psychiatry*, **187**, 500–509.

Aleman, A., Hijman, R., de Haan, E. H. F. & Kahn, R. S. (1999). Memory impairment in schizophrenia: a meta-analysis. *American Journal of Psychiatry*, **156**, 1358–1366.

Allen, P., Amaro, E., Fu, C. H. *et al.* (2007). Neural correlates of the misattribution of speech in schizophrenia. *British Journal of Psychiatry,* **190**, 162–169.

Bell, M. D., Fiszdon, J., Bryson, G. & Wexler, B. E. (2004). Effects of neurocognitive enhancement therapy in schizophrenia: normalisation of memory performance. *Cognitive Neuropsychiatry*, **9**, 199–211.

Brébion, G., David, A. S., Jones, H. & Pilowsky, L. S. (2005). Hallucinations, negative symptoms, and response bias in a verbal recognition task in schizophrenia. *Neuropsychology*, **19**(5), 612–617.

Buckner, R. L. & Wheeler, M. E. (2001). The cognitive neuroscience of remembering. *Nature Reviews Neuroscience,* **2**(9), 624–634.

Corrigan, P. W. & Toomey, R. (1995). Interpersonal problem solving and information-processing in schizophrenia. *Schizophrenia Bulletin*, **21**, 395–403.

Corrigan, P. W., Wallace, C. J., Schade, M. L. & Green, M. F. (1994). Cognitive dysfunctions and psychosocial skill learning in schizophrenia. *Behavior Therapy*, **25**, 5–15.

Danckert, J., Saoud, M. & Maruff, P. (2004). Attention, motor control and motor imagery in schizophrenia: implications for the role of the parietal cortex. *Schizophrenia Research,* **70**(2–3), 241–261.

Danion, J. M., Rizzo, L. & Bruant, A. (1999). Functional mechanisms underlying impaired recognition memory and conscious awareness in patients with schizophrenia. *Archives of General Psychiatry*, **56**(7), 639–644.

Danion, J. M., Cuervo, C., Piolino, P. *et al.* (2005). Conscious recollection in autobiographical memory: an investigation in schizophrenia. *Conscious and Cognition*, **14**(3), 535–547.

Davidson, L., Lawless, M. S. & Leary, F. (2005). Concepts of recovery, competing or complementary? *Current Opinion in Psychiatry*, **18**, 663–667.

Dusek, J. A. & Eichenbaum, H. (1997). The hippocampus and memory for orderly stimulus relations. *Proceedings of the National Academy of Sciences USA,* **94**(13), 7109–7114.

Eichenbaum, H. (2004). Hippocampus: cognitive processes and neural representations that underlie declarative memory. *Neuron,* **44**, 109–120.

Fiszdon, J. M., Bryson, G. J., Wexler, B. E. & Bell, M. D. (2004). Durability of cognitive remediation training in schizophrenia, performance on two memory tasks at 6-month and 12-month follow-up. *Psychiatry Research*, **125**, 1–7.

Gardiner, J. M. (2001). Episodic memory and autonoetic consciousness: a first-person approach. *Philosophical Transactions of the Royal Society of London Series B, Biological Sciences*, **356**(1413), 1351–1361.

Goldman-Rakic, P. S. (1994). Working memory dysfunction in schizophrenia. *Journal of Neuropsychiatry,* **6**, 348–357.

Green, M. F. (1996). What are the functional consequences of neurocognitive deficits in schizophrenia? *American Journal of Psychiatry*, **153**, 321–330.

Green, M. F. & Neuchterlein, K. H. (1999). Should schizophrenia be treated as a neurocognitive disorder? *Schizophrenia Bulletin*, **25**, 309–319.

Green, M. F. & Neuchterlein, K. H. (2004). The MATRICS initiative, developing a consensus cognitive battery for clinical trials. *Schizophrenia Research*, **72**, 1–3.

Green, M. F., Kern, R. S., Braff, D. L. & Mintz, J. (2000). Neurocognitive deficits and functional outcome in schizophrenia, are we measuring the "right stuff"? *Schizophrenia Bulletin*, **26**, 119–136.

Green, M. J. & Phillips, M. L. (2004). Social threat perception and the evolution of paranoia. *Neuroscience and Biobehavioral Reviews*, **28**(3), 333–342.

Halligan, P. W. & David, A. S. (2001). Cognitive neuropsychiatry: towards a scientific psychopathology. *Nature Reviews Neuroscience*, **2**(3), 209–215.

Harrison, P. J. (2004). The hippocampus in schizophrenia: a review of the neuropathological evidence and its pathophysiological implications. *Psychopharmacology*, **174**(1), 151–162.

Harrison, P. J. & Weinberger, D. R. (2005). Schizophrenia genes, gene expression, and neuropathology: on the matter of their convergence. *Molecular Psychiatry*, **10**(1), 40–68.

Heckers, S., Zalesak, M., Weiss, A. P., Ditman, T. & Titone, D. (2004). Hippocampal activation during transitive inference in humans. *Hippocampus*, **14**(2), 153–162.

Hegarty, J. D., Baldessarini, R. J., Tohen, M., Waternaux, C. & Oepen, G. (1994). One hundred years of schizophrenia, a meta-analysis of the outcome literature. *American Journal of Psychiatry*, **151**, 1409–1416.

Honea, R., Crow, T. J., Passingham, D. & Mackay, C. E. (2005). Regional deficits in brain volume in schizophrenia: a meta-analysis of voxel-based morphometry studies. *American Journal of Psychiatry*, **162**(12), 2233–2245.

Hull, C. L. (1917). The formation and retention of associations among the insane. *American Journal of Psychology*, **28**, 419–435.

Jobe, T. H. & Harrow, M. (2005). Long-term outcome of patients with schizophrenia, a review. *Canadian Journal of Psychiatry*, **50**, 892–900.

Johns, L. C., Rossell, S., Frith, C. *et al.* (2001). Verbal self-monitoring and auditory verbal hallucinations in patients with schizophrenia. *Psychological Medicine*, **31**(4), 705–715.

Johnson, M. K. (1997). Source monitoring and memory distortion. *Philosophical Transactions of the Royal Society of London Series B*, **352**, 1733–1745.

Johnson, M. K., Hashtroudi, S. & Lindsay, D. S. (1993). Source monitoring. *Psychological Bulletin*, **114**, 3–28.

Keefe, R. S., Arnold, M. C., Bayen, U. J., McEvoy, J. P. & Wilson, W. H. (2002). Source-monitoring deficits for self-generated stimuli in schizophrenia: multinomial modeling of data from three sources. *Schizophrenia Research*, **57**(1), 51–67.

Koh, S. D., Kayton, L. & Peterson, R. A. (1976). Affective encoding and subsequent remembering in schizophrenic young adults. *Journal of Abnormal Psychology*, **85**, 156–166.

Krabbendam, L. & Aleman, A. (2003). Cognitive rehabilitation in schizophrenia, a quantitative analysis of controlled studies. *Psychopharmacology*, **169**, 376–382.

Kubicki, M., McCarley, R. W., Nestor, P. G. *et al.* (2003). An fMRI study of semantic processing in men with schizophrenia. *Neuroimage*, **20**, 1923–1933.

Kurtz, M. M. (2006). Symptoms versus neurocognitive skills as correlates of everyday functioning in severe mental illness. *Expert Review of Neurotherapeutics*, **6**, 47–56.

Kurtz, M. M., Moberg, P. J., Gur, R. C. & Gur, R. E. (2001). Approaches to cognitive remediation of neuropsychological deficits in schizophrenia, a review and meta-analysis. *Neuropsychology Review*, **11**, 197–210.

Langdon, R., Michie, P. T., Ward, P. B. *et al.* (1997). Defective self and/or other mentalising in schizophrenia: a cognitive neuropsychological approach. *Cognitive Neuropsychiatry*, **2**, 167–193.

Marder, S. R. & Fenton, W. (2004). Measurement and Treatment Research to Improve Cognition in Schizophrenia: NIMH MATRICS initiative to support the development of agents for improving cognition in schizophrenia. *Schizophrenia Research*, **72**, 5–9.

McGuire, P. K., Silbersweig, D. A., Wright, I. *et al.* (1995). Abnormal monitoring of inner speech: a physiological basis for auditory hallucinations. *Lancet*, **346**(8975), 596–600.

Mueser, K. T., Bellack, A. S., Douglas, M. S. & Wade, J. H. (1991). Prediction of social skill acquisition in schizophrenic and major affective disorder patients from memory and symptomatology. *Psychiatry Research*, **37**, 281–296.

Nyberg, L., Forkstam, C., Petersson, K. M., Cabeza, R. & Ingvar, M. (2002). Brain imaging of human memory systems: between-systems similarities and within-system differences. *Brain Research: Cognitive Brain Research*, **13**(2), 281–292.

Pantelis, C. & Brewer, W. (1995). Neuropsychological and olfactory dysfunction in schizophrenia: relationship of frontal syndromes to syndromes of schizophrenia. *Schizophrenia Research*, **17**(1), 35–45.

Pantelis, C., Yucel, M., Wood, S. J. *et al.* (2005). Structural brain imaging evidence for multiple pathological processes at different stages of brain development in schizophrenia. *Schizophrenia Bulletin*, **31**(3), 672–696.

Penades, R., Catalan, R., Salamero, M. *et al.* (2006). Cognitive remediation therapy for outpatients with chronic schizophrenia. A controlled and randomized study. *Schizophrenia Research*, **87**(1–3), 323–331.

Pilling, S., Bebbington, P., Kuipers, E. *et al.* (2002). Psychological treatments in schizophrenia, II. Meta-analyses of randomized controlled trials of social skills training and cognitive remediation. *Psychological Medicine*, **32**, 783–791.

Preston, A. R., Shohamy, D., Tamminga, C. A. & Wagner, A. D. (2005). Hippocampal function, declarative memory, and schizophrenia: anatomic and functional neuroimaging considerations. *Current Neurology and Neuroscience Reports*, **5**(4), 249–256.

Ragland, J. D., Gur, R. C., Valdez, J. N. *et al.* (2005). Levels-of-processing effect on frontotemporal function in schizophrenia during word encoding and recognition. *American Journal of Psychiatry*, **162**, 1840–1848.

Raye, C. L., Johnson, M. K. & Taylor, T. H. (1980). Is there something special about memory for internally generated information? *Memory and Cognition*, **8**, 141–148.

Sartory, G., Zorn, C., Groetzinger, G. & Windgassen, K. (2005). Computerized cognitive remediation improves verbal learning and processing speed in schizophrenia. *Schizophrenia Research*, **75**, 219–223.

Seal, M. L., Aleman, A. & McGuire, P. K. (2004). Compelling imagery, unanticipated speech and deceptive memory: neurocognitive models of auditory verbal hallucinations in schizophrenia. *Cognitive Neuropsychiatry*, **9**(1/2); 43–72.

Seal, M. L., Crowe, S. F. & Cheung, P. (1997). Deficits in source monitoring in subjects with auditory hallucinations may be due to differences in verbal intelligence and verbal memory. *Cognitive Neuropsychiatry*, **2**(4), 273–290.

Sharma, T. & Antonova, L. (2003). Cognitive function in schizophrenia. Deficits, functional consequences, and future treatment. *Psychiatric Clinics of North America*, **26**, 25–40.

Spitzer, M. (1997). A cognitive neuroscience view of schizophrenic thought disorder. *Schizophrenia Bulletin*, **23**, 29–50.

Squire, L. R. (2004). Memory systems of the brain: a brief history and current perspective. *Neurobiology of Learning and Memory*, **82**(3), 171–177.

Velakoulis, D., Wood, S. J., Wong, M. T. *et al.* (2006). Hippocampal and amygdala volumes according to psychosis stage and diagnosis: a magnetic resonance imaging study of chronic schizophrenia, first-episode psychosis, and ultra-high-risk individuals. *Archives of General Psychiatry*, **63**(2), 139–149.

Wagner, A. D., Shannon, B. J., Kahn, I., & Buckner, R. L. (2005). Parietal lobe contributions to episodic memory retrieval. *Trends in Cognitive Sciences*, **9**(9), 445–453.

Wechsler, D. (1987). *Wechsler Memory Scale-Revised (WMS-R)*. San Antonio, TX: The Psychological Corporation.

Wechsler, D. (1997). *Wechsler Memory Scale – Third Edition (WMS–III)*. San Antonio, TX: The Psychological Corporation.

Weiss, A. P., Schacter, D. L., Goff, D. C. *et al.* (2003). Impaired hippocampal recruitment during normal modulation of memory performance in schizophrenia. *Biological Psychiatry*, **53**, 48–55.

Weiss, A. P., Dewitt, I., Goff, D., Ditman, T. & Heckers, S. (2005). Anterior and posterior hippocampal volumes in schizophrenia. *Schizophrenia Research*, **73**(1), 103–112.

Wykes, T., Reeder, C., Williams, C. *et al.* (2003). Are the effects of cognitive remediation therapy (CRT) durable? Results from an exploratory trial in schizophrenia. *Schizophrenia Research*, **61**, 163–174.

The neural basis of attention

Susan M. Ravizza, George R. Mangun and Cameron S. Carter

Introduction

The sensory world is rich in information, but our nervous system necessarily limits how much information can be processed at any given time due to intrinsic limitations on processing capacity. By enhancing the processing of relevant information and/or by inhibiting irrelevant or distracting events and actions, *selective attention* provides a means by which organisms regulate the flow of information. This attention-related prioritization in processing has been termed *selection*, a concept from cognitive psychology (Deutsch & Deutsch, 1963) that refers to the manner in which attended information is tagged (selected) for further processing while competing information is rejected. We will use the term *selection* to refer to the outcome of the attentional modulation of information processing, but without implying that unattended information has no effect or influence on cognition or behavior (Vogel *et al.*, 1998).

During the processing of information, selective attention affects how an individual perceives or experiences a stimulus, as well as how they respond to it. For example, selective attention to a location in the visual field (spatial attention) facilitates processing of stimuli appearing at the attended location: reaction times (RT) are faster and discrimination accuracy is enhanced for events at attended versus unattended locations (Downing, 1988; Handy *et al.*, 1996; Hawkins *et al.*, 1990; Heinze & Mangun, 1995; Luck *et al.*, 1994; Posner & Cohen, 1984). Recent studies have revealed that spatial attention can also alter stimulus appearance by altering the apparent contrast, spatial frequency and size of stimuli (Carrasco *et al.*, 2004; Gobell & Carrasco, 2005). It is important to note that attention can also be directed to non-spatial stimulus features and objects (Duncan, 1998) and to all sensory modalities (Macaluso & Driver, 2005 for a review).

The neural correlates of selective attention have been the focus of intense investigation and a discussion of current neural mechanisms and models of attention will be the focus of this chapter. We will first consider the neural correlates of early and late attentional selection, especially within the context of voluntary attention. Next, we will discuss how these selection processes are controlled by top-down attention networks. Finally, we will consider the neural mechanisms of reflexive attention and contrast the control of these processes with those that are involved in voluntary attention.

Levels of selection: early and late selection

For more than a century, philosophers and scientists have asked how attention affects information processing. Hermann von Helmholtz, the great physicist and sensory psychologist, suggested that when one attends selectively to a region of visual space, this somehow influences the sensory signals entering the brain (Helmholtz, 1962/1924–25). This idea permeated early studies of attention and came to be one of the key questions about selective attention: How does attention influence sensory information processing? In the 1960s this question formed the basis of a debate within psychology and neuroscience that lasted 30 years, coming to be known as the "early versus late selection debate." Some argued that attention could influence elementary sensory processing, which would lead to early attentional selection (Broadbent, 1962). Others argued for the late selection model, which proposes that sensory processing continued to completion prior to attention acting to modulate information analysis at higher stages of decision and

The Neuropsychology of Mental Illness, ed. Stephen J. Wood, Nicholas B. Allen and Christos Pantelis. Published by Cambridge University Press. © Cambridge University Press 2009.

response (Deutsch & Deutsch, 1963). Current models of attention hold that selection does not occur at any single point in the information processing stream; but rather that it can occur early, at low levels of sensory pathways, or later, including at the level of specific responses. Both the modulation of perceptual processing (early selection) and decision and action networks (late selection) ensure appropriate responses to relevant stimuli in the face of distracting information. Current research on attentional mechanisms therefore focuses more on understanding the mechanisms by which attention acts to modulate information at various stages of input and output processing, and on specifying the conditions under which early or late selection mechanisms are differentially engaged (Hopf et al., 2006).

Many functional neuroimaging studies have focused on the role attention plays in the early selection of perceptual information. Early studies using positron emission tomography (PET) provided evidence that selective attention to stimulus features (Corbetta et al., 1990) or spatial locations (Heinze et al., 1994) modulated activity in human visual cortex. More recently, using functional magnetic resonance imaging (fMRI), it has been shown in greater detail that attention to visual stimuli increases neural activation in multiple visual areas (Hopfinger et al., 2000; Kastner et al., 1998, 1999; Tootell et al., 1998), and attention to specific visual features such as motion and color selectively modulates areas associated with processing those features (Giesbrecht et al., 2003; Liu et al., 2003). Likewise, attention to auditory stimuli modulates auditory cortex (Petkov et al., 2004; Sevostianov et al., 2002). Also, attending to smell modulates frontal piriform cortex, one of two main regions involved in olfactory processing (Zelano et al., 2005).

The effects of early selection can also be observed in electrophysiological studies of attention, where the time course of information processing can be tracked on a millisecond-to-millisecond basis. Sensory-evoked event-related potentials (ERPs) recorded from electrodes placed on the human scalp are sensitive to the direction of *selective* attention. These sensory ERP components are greater in amplitude for attended-location stimuli than for the same physical stimuli at an ignored location (Van Voorhis & Hillyard, 1977). Because these sensory ERPs begin within 70–80 ms of stimulus onset and arise from visual cortical areas V1–V4 (Heinze et al., 1994; Khoe et al., 2005), the finding that spatial attention affects their amplitudes suggests that attention operates by modulating the

transmission of information in the ascending visual pathways in a spatially specific manner (reviewed in Luck et al., 2000; Mangun, 1995). Though ERP evidence for modulations of V1 with spatial attention has been inconsistent, recent studies reveal that ERPs generated in V1 can also be modulated by spatial attention under some circumstances (Khoe & Hillyard, 2005).

Consequently, most studies in awake, behaving non-human primates have also focused on attentional modulation of neural responses in sensory areas (Reynolds & Chelazzi, 2004; Salinas & Sejnowski, 2001). Attentional modulation of sensory processing in monkeys has been described at the level of single neurons in several areas of cortex, including striate (V1) (McAdams & Maunsell, 1999; McAdams & Reid, 2005) and extrastriate visual areas V2–V4 (Chelazzi et al., 1993, 2001; Maunsell & Cook, 2002; Moran & Desimone, 1985; Reynolds & Chelazzi, 2004; Treue, 2001, 2003). Selective attention has also been shown to influence higher-order perceptual processing in the ventral stream, as in inferotemporal cortex (Spitzer & Richmond, 1991), and also in dorsal stream, as in motion processing areas MT and MST (Recanzone et al., 1993; Treue & Martínez-Trujillo, 1999). Animal studies of spatial attention demonstrate that a cell's response to a stimulus presented in its receptive field is highly sensitive to where the animal is attending. For example, Moran & Desimone (1985) recorded from V4 of the macaque monkey and found that spatial attention gated the response to the cell's preferred stimulus; the response to a stimulus that was effective in driving a cell was dramatically reduced if the monkey was attending to a different stimulus within the receptive field, but only minimally reduced if the monkey was attending to a different stimulus outside the receptive field (see also Luck et al., 1997; Reynolds et al., 1999).

While many studies have explored attentional selection in primary and secondary perceptual areas, a smaller number have examined it at later stages of processing, along the perception–action continuum. Late selection processes can include attention to actions, either imminent or already partially executed, and also to the goal selection processes that govern decision-making that leads to action. In one study, Cook & Maunsell (2002) trained monkeys on a motion-detection task and measured neural activity in MT and the ventral intraparietal area (VIP) in relation to the animal's behavior. The monkeys were required to release a lever when they detected the onset of coherent random-dot motion, which could occur either at an attended or unattended location. There was some attentional modulation of the neural activity in area MT, but this modulation was insufficient to explain the behavior changes, suggesting that attention also operates at later levels of processing.

Similar to that involved in early selection, studies reveal that a fronto-parietal network is active and coupled with action representations in the motor cortex during attention to action (Rowe *et al.*, 2002, 2005). As with attentional modulation of perceptual areas, attention to action affects activity in motor cortices. For example, attending to finger movements enhances activation in motor area 4p (Binkofski *et al.*, 2002). However, it is not known whether late selection effects are topographically organized according to effectors; one study reported effector-independent activation of the intraparietal sulcus (IPS) and the frontal eye fields (Astafieve *et al.*, 2003). It is expected that activation patterns within the motor cortex during attention to action will be effector-specific, in the same way that attentional modulation in sensory cortices is modality-specific. Topographic organization of premotor and motor cortices has been clearly demonstrated during imagination (Johnson *et al.*, 2002; De Lange *et al.*, 2005) and observation (Buccino *et al.*, 2001) of action. However, direct evidence of topographical organization of attention effects during late selection is lacking to date.

The foregoing studies demonstrate that focused attention can influence the neural responses to attended and ignored stimuli. This has been likened to a gain control mechanism, which relatively increases the gain of neurons coding attended stimuli or actions, while relatively turning down the gain of neurons coding ignored events and action. What does this sort of gain control accomplish? One current concept is that it leads to a biasing in the neural responses to attended items versus ignored events. Attentional biasing is the idea that attention influences the outcome of neural competition in neural networks at a variety of stages of information processing (Desimone & Duncan, 1995). Neural competition arises from the local and global neural networks involved in sensory, cognitive or motor function, where models of attentional control propose that this competition can be biased in favor of attended inputs, thoughts and actions. In such models, the resultant biased processes and their outputs are thought to reflect attentional selection, which is the effective selection of behaviorally relevant inputs, thoughts and actions. A key question for neuroscience is to understand how these attentional selection processes are controlled in the brain and how attentional biasing processes are engaged. In the next section we consider attentional control mechanisms for voluntary attention.

Voluntary attentional control mechanisms

Models of attention have differentiated attentional control processes, and how these processes influence a site of action, such as the perceptual system (Posner & Petersen, 1990). In the preceding section, we reviewed work on the site of action (early versus late) in information processing and asked which brain systems provide the control signals that result in selective processing at early and late stages of processing. Research in animals, patients with neurological dysfunction, and healthy human subjects using ERPs and neuroimaging, suggests that the top-down control of visual spatial attention involves a complex network of widely distributed areas, including dorsolateral prefrontal cortex (DLPFC), anterior cingulate cortex, posterior parietal cortex and thalamic and midbrain structures (Bushnell *et al.*, 1981; Goldberg & Bruce, 1985; Harter *et al.*, 1989; Knight *et al.*, 1995; Mesulam, 1981; La Berge, 1997; Miller, 2000). Event-related fMRI has recently identified superior frontal, inferior parietal and superior temporal regions that are selectively activated during attentional control processing (Corbetta *et al.*, 2000; Hopfinger *et al.*, 2000). Current models hypothesize that these networks reflect top-down (voluntary) attentional influences that result in changes in levels of excitability in multiple visual cortical areas that work to achieve selective sensory processing of relevant visual targets (reviewed in Kanwisher & Wojciulik, 2000; Kastner & Ungerleider, 2000).

Goal-directed behavior in an ever-changing environment requires our brain to select relevant sensory information and flexibly link relevant stimuli to appropriate actions. The prefrontal cortex may provide the necessary attention control signals, but the actual "rewiring" of the information flow may occur in more posterior areas (Miller & Cohen, 2001). Parietal cortex would be well-suited for a key role in this function since it is located at the interface between sensory input and motor control. Non-human primate studies suggest that the parietal cortex is a collection of planning areas for goal-directed movements or shifts of visual spatial attention. However, recent evidence suggests that it might also carry signals related to "cognitive set" (Stoet & Snyder, 2004).

How the circuitry applying these signals to the sensory-motor-transformation process might work in the parietal cortex is currently unknown. It may be that "input neurons" in parietal areas carry both task-relevant and task-irrelevant sensory information (that probably already has undergone some, but insufficient, attentional modulation). The network might then be reconfigured so that task-irrelevant sensory information is filtered out and task-relevant information is linked to an appropriate action. If true, one would expect to find parietal neurons that are selective for a particular action (eye movement, etc.) and also for the sensory stimulus informing this action (similar to prefrontal or supplementary motor neurons during the learning of new stimulus-response-associations; Asaad et al., 1998; Chen & Wise, 1995). So far, parietal activity has usually been tested in experimental situations with a fixed association between stimuli and responses, and so this hypothesis has not been tested.

Functional imaging has greatly enhanced the ability to investigate widespread cortical networks participating in cognitive functions such as attentional control, but relatively little work has analyzed subcortical structures, such as the pulvinar nuclei of the thalamus, that have been implicated in attention. Rafal & Posner (1987) provided evidence of attentional-orienting deficits with thalamic infarcts that included the pulvinar in two of their three patients. La Berge (1997) proposed a role for the pulvinar in his triangular circuit model of attention, which argued that frontal and parietal cortices influence perceptual cortical processing via interactions with the pulvinar. His studies using positron emission tomography (PET) implicated the pulvinar in the filtering of distracters. Also supporting a role for the pulvinar in attention, a recent human lesion study showed deficits in attentional processing with damage to this region (Michael & Desmedt, 2004). More current models similarly implicate the pulvinar in attention (Sherman & Guillery, 2002; Shipp, 2004), but still little additional evidence has been generated for such a model.

While the pulvinar is proposed to modulate perceptual processing as a result of attentional control, it is still uncertain how the need for attentional control is initially signaled. We have argued a role for the anterior cingulate cortex (ACC) in the detection of conflict, which is used to signal the need for cognitive control (Carter et al., 1998; Kerns et al., 2004; MacDonald et al., 2000). Using the Stroop color-naming task, Kerns et al. (2004) demonstrated that activity of the ACC predicts adjustments in behavior on the next trial. Typically, activity of the ACC is not observed in studies of selective attention unless high levels of control are needed (situations in which competition among potential responses exists, and/or in speeded tasks where error rate is high). In our cued spatial attention task, ACC activity increased as difference between two cues increased in difficulty (Walsh et al., 2005). However, the ACC was not responsive to cues in general; that is, the ACC was not recruited when cues were informative as to the direction in which to shift spatial attention compared with neutral cues.

Activity of the ACC not only results in improved performance on the next trial, but activity of the DLPFC is also greater in consequence (Kerns et al., 2004a). We have proposed that the ACC signals the DLPFC to exert greater attentional control to the task at hand. One way to directly assess whether the DLPFC is involved in attentional control is to show that it is engaged in preparatory attention. The use of cueing paradigms to signal subjects to prepare and hence engage attentional control systems has a long tradition in cognitive psychology and cognitive neuroscience (Posner et al., 1980), and provides a means to dissociate attentional control from attention selection processes. In this context, cue-related activity has often been found in DLPFC and posterior parietal cortex (PPC); this has occurred in tasks in which the cue instructs participants which of several stimulus-response (S-R) mappings to use to react to a subsequent target stimulus (Barber & Carter, 2005; Corbetta et al., 2000, 2002; Corbetta & Shulman, 2002; DeSouza et al., 2003; Kincade et al., 2005; Nobre et al., 2000; Weissman et al., 2004; Woldorff et al., 2004). An effect of attentional preparation is manifested as a relative increase in activity; that is, DLPFC activation is higher when the cue tells the participant to prepare for the more demanding task. For instance, during the Stroop task, MacDonald et al. (2000) found increased DLPFC activity when a cue instructed the person to respond to the color rather than the word.

Supramodal attention

Both early and late selection appear to be modality-specific, while the implementation of goals needed to overcome more reflexive attentional adaptation may depend upon the engagement of frontal and parietal systems, which may operate in a more modality-dependent manner. Surprisingly, it is largely unknown to what extent regions involved in attentional control such as the DLPFC are dependent upon stimulus or response modality. De Souza et al. (2003) found that a cue indicating an anti-saccade response elicits greater activity in right DLPFC and the frontal eye fields (FEF). The FEF are involved with the control of overt eye movements and also with the control of covert spatial attention shifts (Corbetta et al., 1998); they are activated to cues instructing the direction of a subsequent eye movement or a covert shift of spatial attention (Kincade et al., 2005). The De Souza study shows, however, that the FEF are activated by contextual cues too, suggesting that the attention control functions supported by this region might include response modality-specific regions of the lateral PFC. Similarly, little is known about whether cue-related activation of the PFC is stimulus modality-specific. Weissman et al. (2004), using a task in which participants were instructed to respond to subsequent auditory or visual stimuli, showed that target-related activity was increased in the auditory cortex when participants were instructed to attend to auditory targets and in visual cortex following a cue to visual targets. However, no stimulus modality-specific PFC activation was observed.

Similarly, the parietal cortex has been implicated as the proximal source of attentional control across domains (Kanwisher & Wojciulik, 2000; see Behrmann et al., 2004 for a review). One neuroimaging study demonstrated that overlapping parietal regions were engaged by a variety of spatial and non-spatial tasks such as peripheral shifting, conjunction search and object matching (Kanwisher & Wojciulik, 2000). Thus, while early and late selection appear linked to the modulation of discrete, topographically organized sensory and motor systems, it is less clear that there is modality-specificity within attention-control networks.

Reflexive attention mechanisms

In contrast to the top-down processes that are engaged by the goals and intentions of the individual that we earlier reviewed, bottom-up or "stimulus-driven" mechanisms are triggered by the properties of sensory inputs. There are two general types of bottom-up influences in information processing. The first is the sensory influence of a stimulus itself, which, depending on its properties such as stimulus saliency, may bias neural competition (Robinson & Petersen, 1992). A second aspect, described as attentional in nature, occurs when bottom-up sensory signals trigger an automatic or "reflexive" orienting of attention (Hopfinger & Mangun, 1998; Klein, 2000; Posner & Cohen, 1984). Bottom-up factors and top-down influences do not act in isolation from each other, but rather interact, sometimes competing for the control of neural activity and therefore control of behavior. Indeed, top-down attentional control is most relevant when goals and strategies are in competition with bottom-up stimulus-driven influences or prepotent response tendencies (Beck & Kastner, 2005). In the following we consider the neural correlates and control mechanisms for reflexive attention.

The distinction between voluntary and reflexive attention was demonstrated in behavioral studies that established the parameters of each form of attention in terms of performance. The bottom-up attentional influences of sensory events (Jonides, 1980, 1981; Yantis, 1996) are more rapidly and transiently engaged than those associated with voluntary attention (Jonides, 1981; Posner et al., 1980). In addition, the engagement of reflexive (stimulus-driven) attention is followed by inhibition, or a relative slowing in response time at that location (Posner & Cohen, 1984). This latter effect is known as inhibition of return (IOR), and it may enable the sensory reflexive system to favor novel locations, promoting effective search of the scene (Wolfe et al., 1989).

Human ERP and fMRI studies of reflexive attention have demonstrated that when attention is reflexively captured to a visual field location, subsequent stimuli presented to that location receive enhanced cortical visual processing (Hopfinger & Mangun, 1998, 2001). Subsequent work has now shown that the earliest signs of reflexive attention in the ERPs are automatic (Hopfinger & Maxwell, 2005) and occur even when test stimuli are not task-relevant and the observers are engaged in unrelated visual tasks. Based on this sort of evidence, one can propose that reflexive attention influences early visual cortical processing as well as subcortical motor systems (Rafal & Henik, 1994; Sapir et al., 1999). Imaging research has demonstrated that these early effects of reflexive attention on visual processing occur in multiple early visual areas, including V1 (Liu *et al.*, 2005), but may involve mechanisms operating at the level of LGN via interactions of LGN and V1.

Although the attentional modulation of reflexes, social behavior and eye movements have all been studied using animal models (e.g. reflexes, Schicatano *et al.*, 2000; social behavior, Emery *et al.*, 1997 and Lorincz *et al.*, 1999; eye movements, Andersen, 1989), few single unit recording studies of reflexive attention effects on visual processing have been conducted in animals. Until recently, there was no animal study counterpart to the cognitive literature (Yantis & Jonides, 1990) or human neurophysiological literature (Hopfinger & Mangun, 1998, 2001) on reflexive attention effects on visual processing. Most work on attention in non-human primates involved voluntary (goal-driven) mechanisms (Cook & Maunsell, 2004; Moran & Desimone, 1985). There are, however, two main lines of work on reflexive attention using animal models: one in monkeys, investigating the superior colliculus (SC), and one in rats, investigating the thalamus.

Recently, in macaques, Fecteau *et al.* (2004) investigated the role of the SC in reflexive spatial attention. They demonstrated that the SC is influenced by reflexive attention in a pattern similar to that found in human behavioral and ERP studies. However, how the SC mechanisms interact with thalamo-cortical processing during reflexive attention remains unknown.

In the second study, Weese *et al.* (1999) used a variant of a non-predictive peripheral cuing paradigm to study subcortical mechanisms of attention in a rat model. Their findings suggested that reflexive attention effects in the visual pathways may be mediated by circuitry at the level of the thalamus and V1 via feedback of the cortico-thalamic afferents by the reticular nucleus of the thalamus. However, Weese *et al.* (1999) did not investigate the result on visual cortical processing, as they measured behavior following lesions restricted to subcortical sites. Nonetheless, their model suggests that reflexive cues may not engage fronto-parietal networks involved in voluntary attention, an important consideration for models of reflexive attentional control. However, the work of Weese *et al.* (1999) cannot address this question directly because they did not record from the cortex.

As noted above, the neural correlates of sensory reflexive attention are less well understood than those for voluntary attention. However, evidence suggests that partially different neural mechanisms regulate these two forms of orienting, with subcortical regions controlling reflexive orienting and cortical regions controlling voluntary orienting (Corbetta *et al.*, 1993; Posner & Peterson, 1990; Rafal & Henik, 1994). This fits with the general concept of reflexive attention being driven by "bottom-up" processes, while voluntary attention is considered a "top-down" process. However, a more likely framework involves the interaction of subcortical and cortical regulatory systems for both voluntary and reflexive attention with different regulatory networks; this interaction may be weighted more toward subcortical systems for reflexive attention (Sapir *et al.*, 1999) and cortical systems for voluntary attentional control (Coull *et al.*, 2000; Rosen *et al.*, 1999).

Several functional neuroimaging studies have suggested that voluntary and reflexive attention are regulated by largely the same neural architecture (Corbetta *et al.*, 1993; Nobre *et al.*, 1997; Peelen *et al.*, 2004; Rosen *et al.*, 1999), indicating a unitary attentional regulatory mechanism that can be engaged through somewhat different means (i.e. top-down or bottom-up). A more recent neuroimaging study (Mayer *et al.*, 2004) compared exogenous and endogenous orienting using the cue-to-target intervals expected to yield the strongest facilitation effects for each type of attention (i.e. shorter cue-target intervals for exogenous cuing). This critical aspect of the design allowed the authors to find evidence for a greater differentiation between these systems, with much of the typical attentional network (i.e. frontal eye fields, intraparietal sulcus, superior temporal gyrus, temporo-parietal junction) being activated by endogenous attention but not by exogenous attention. In addition, a recent fMRI study of overt attention similarly found distinct differences between the neural systems supporting voluntary versus reflexive saccades (Mort *et al.*, 2003). This is in line with more recent ERP evidence from how reflexive and voluntary attention affects visual information processing, which suggests that these different forms of attention are mediated by partially or wholly distinct mechanisms that act with characteristic time courses at different levels of information processing (Hopfinger & West, 2006). Further research is warranted to assess the extent to which dissociable neural control networks underlie reflexive versus voluntary attention.

Attentional deficits in psychiatric disorders

Abnormalities of attention are common subjective complaints in a range of mental disorders, including anxiety, mood and psychotic disorders. The degree to which these abnormalities have been investigated using the tools and constructs of cognitive neuroscience has varied. For example, the majority of studies of cognition in depression have used standardized batteries of clinical neuropsychological tasks that do not readily distinguish between deficits in attention versus other aspects of higher cognition, or even between specific cognitive deficits, general psychomotor slowing and/or poor motivation. The results of these studies are varied, although most report some degree of impaired performance, which is present to a degree in remitted patients, but greatest in acutely ill patients (Gualtieri et al., 2006; Den Hartog et al., 2003; Paelecke-Habermann et al., 2005). Interpretation of these studies is difficult given the variability across studies and the fact that many depressed subjects continue to experience residual symptoms after treatment. A few studies using the Stroop task generally find a lack of impairment in patients with major depression, with the possible exception of patients with the more severe melancholic subtype (Markela-Lerenc et al., 2006; Rogers et al., 2004). Several studies have used the CANTAB battery, a computerized assessment that bridges standardized neuropsychological approaches with more theoretically based experimental cognitive tasks (Purcell et al., 1997; Sweeney et al., 2000). Using this approach has produced mixed results with one study showing predominantly memory deficits (Sweeney et al., 2000) and another predominantly executive (set shifting) deficits (Purcell et al., 1997). Previous research has therefore not clarified the nature and significance of deficits in attention in depression, despite the frequency with which patients complain of these deficits. Since the numbers of subjects studied to date is small, more work is needed using a more cognitive experimental approach before we have a clearer understanding of the nature and severity of deficits, if any, in attention in major depression.

While the attention deficits per se in mood disorders is unclear and in need of further investigation, a large and consistent literature supports the fact that individuals with both depression and anxiety disorders have *content-specific attentional biases* in their orienting to emotional information in the environment, which may contribute to the development and maintenance of their symptoms. On a number of different measures, people with depression and anxiety disorders tend to selectively process negative emotional material (e.g. sad faces, angry faces, emotional words) while non-depressed or anxious individuals tend to orient away from this kind of information (Leyman et al., 2007; Mogg et al., 2000). This pattern has been seen in individuals who are in the active phases of their illness and also in remission (Joormann & Gotlib, 2007). Functional neuroimaging studies have suggested that explicit processing of emotional information in depression is associated with overactivation of the amygdala, an effect that resolves with effective treatment (Seigle et al., 2002; Sheline et al., 2001). This finding is difficult to reconcile with the observation that attentional biases in depression and anxiety are stable traits in at-risk individuals, and more research is needed to clarify what kinds of processing biases are risk factors for mood disorders and what kinds are state-related.

In contrast to mood disorders, attention in schizophrenia has been studied intensively using modern experimental methods from cognitive neuroscience. The emerging picture is that basic attentional orienting and selection mechanisms are intact in schizophrenia, while cognitive control mechanisms that are involved in detecting and overcoming conflict appear to be consistently impaired at all stages of the illness (Luck & et al., 2006). Functional neuroimaging studies suggest that these deficits in executive attention appear to be related to abnormalities in dorsolateral prefrontal and anterior cingulate cortex (Snitz et al., 2005), while more posterior attentional control systems appear to be intact. These abnormalities in attentional control have been recognized as very important since they are highly correlated with functional disability in the illness and refractory to our currently available treatments (Green, 1996). Developing effective therapies, either pharmacological or neurobehavioral, has become one of the highest priorities for modern clinical neuroscience.

Conclusion

Attentional control and selection involves a dynamic set of neural mechanisms acting at multiple stages of information processing to enable efficient stimulus analysis, decisions and response execution. The ability to control attention involves the interaction of specific cortical and subcortical neural networks that establish modulatory influences at multiple stages of information processing to bias processing in favor of attended events and actions. The modulation of attentional selection on perceptual and action systems is established dynamically, changing on a moment-to-moment basis as a function of changing goals, strategies, and stimulus and task demands. Moreover, the nature of attentional selection in perception and action is highly constrained by local neuronal and neural network properties that are specific to the sensory system or perceptual or response processes involved.

This view incorporates the idea that attentional phenomena do not rely on mechanisms acting at unitary stages of information processing or only at particular levels of neural analysis, but rather that mechanisms at the neuronal, local neuronal circuit and global neural network levels are all relevant during attentional control and selection. Therefore, to elucidate the neural mechanisms of attention it is essential to investigate and characterize attentional processes at a variety of levels of information processing. Moreover, this work can help to characterize potential attention deficits associated with psychiatric disorders that may also have a neurological basis.

Acknowledgments

Supported by NIMH grants K02MH064190 and RO1MH059883 to C.S.C. and MH55714 and MH02019 to G.R.M.

References

Andersen, R. A. (1989). Visual and eye movement functions of the posterior parietal cortex. *Annual Review of Neuroscience*, **12**, 377–403.

Asaad, W. F., Rainer, G. & Miller, E. K. (1998). Neural activity in the primate prefrontal cortex during associative learning. *Neuron*, **21**, 1399–1407.

Astafieve, S. V., Shulman, G. L., Stanley, C. M. et al. (2003). Functional organization of human intraparietal and frontal cortex for attending, looking, and pointing. *Journal of Neuroscience*, **23**, 4689–4699.

Barber, A. D. & Carter, C. S. (2005). Cognitive control involved in overcoming prepotent response tendencies and switching between tasks. *Cerebral Cortex*, **15**, 899–912.

Beck, D. M. & Kastner, S. (2005). Stimulus context modulates competition in human extrastriate cortex. *Nature Neuroscience*, **8**, 1110–1116.

Behrmann, M., Geng, J. J. & Shomstein, S. (2004). Parietal cortex and attention. *Current Opinions in Neurobiology*, **14**, 212–217.

Binkofski, F., Fink, G. R., Geyer, S. et al. (2002). Neural activity in human primary motor cortex areas 4a and 4p is modulated differentially by attention to action. *Journal of Neurophysiology*, **88**, 514–519.

Broadbent, D. E. (1962). *Attention and the Perception of Speech*. New York: W.H. Freeman and Co.

Buccino, G., Binkofski, F., Fink, G. R. et al. (2001). Action observation activates premotor and parietal areas in a somatotopic manner: an fMRI study. *European Journal of Neuroscience*, **13**, 400–404.

Bushnell, M. C., Goldberg, M. E. & Robinson, D. L. (1981). Behavioral enhancement of visual responses in monkey cerebral cortex. I. Modulation in posterior parietal cortex related to selective visual attention. *Journal of Neurophysiology*, **46**, 755–772.

Carrasco, M., Ling, S. & Read, S. (2004). Attention alters appearance. *Nature Neuroscience*, 7, 308–313.

Carter, C. S., Braver, T. S., Barch, D. M. et al. (1998). Anterior cingulate cortex, error detection and the online monitoring of performance. *Science*, **280**, 747–749.

Chelazzi, L., Miller, E. K., Duncan, J. & Desimon, R. (1993). A neural basis for visual search in inferior temporal cortex. *Nature*, **363**, 345–347.

Chelazzi, L., Miller, E. K., Duncan, J. & Desimon, R. (2001). Responses of neurons in macaque area V4 during memory-guided visual search. *Cerebral Cortex*, **11**, 345–347.

Chen, L. L. & Wise, S. P. (1995). Neuronal activity in the supplementary eye field during acquisition of conditional oculomotor associations. *Journal of Neurophysiology*, **73**, 1101–1121.

Cook, E. P. & Maunsell, J. H. (2002). Attentional modulation of behavioral performance and neuronal responses in middle temporal and ventral intraparietal areas of macaque monkey. *Journal of Neuroscience*, **22**, 1994–2004.

Cook, E. P. & Maunsell, J. H. (2004). Attentional modulation of motion integration of individual neurons in the middle temporal visual area. *Journal of Neuroscience*, **24**, 7964–7977.

Corbetta, M. & Shulman, G. (2002). Control of goal-directed and stimulus-driven attention in the brain. *Nature Reviews Neuroscience*, **3**, 201–215.

Corbetta, M., Akbudak, E., Conturo, T. E. et al. (1998). A common network of functional areas for attention and eye movements. *Neuron*, **21**, 761–773.

Corbetta, M., Kincade, J. M., Ollinger, J. M., McAvoy, M. P. & Shulman, G. L. (2000). Voluntary orienting is dissociated from target detection in human posterior parietal cortex. *Nature Reviews Neuroscience*, **3**, 292–297.

Corbetta, M., Kincade, J. M. & Shulman, G. L. (2002). Neural systems for visual orienting and their relationships to spatial working memory. *Journal of Cognitive Neuroscience*, **14**, 508–523.

Corbetta, M., Miezin, F. M., Dobmeyer, S., Shulman, G. L. & Petersen, S. E. (1990). Attentional modulation of neural processing of shape, color, and velocity in humans. *Science*, **248**, 1556–1559.

Corbetta, M., Miezin, F., Shulman, G. L. & Petersen, S. E. (1993). A PET study of visuospatial attention. *Journal of Neuroscience*, **13**, 1202–1226.

Coull, J. T., Frith, C. D., Büchel, C. & Nobre, A. C. (2000). Orienting attention in time: behavioral and neuroanatomical distinction between exogenous and endogenous shifts. *Neuropsychologia*, **38**, 808–819.

Den Hartog, H. M., Derix, M. M., Van Bemmel, A. L., Kremer, B. & Jolles, J. (2003). Cognitive functioning in young and middle-aged unmedicated out-patients with major depression: testing the effort and cognitive speed hypotheses. *Psychological Medicine*, **33**, 1443–1451.

De Lange, F. P., Hagoort, P. & Toni, I. (2005). Neural topography and content of movement representations. *Journal of Cognitive Neuroscience*, **17**, 97–112.

De Souza, J. F., Menon, R. S. & Everling, S. (2003). Preparatory set associated with pro-saccades and anti-saccades in humans investigated with event-related FMRI. *Journal of Neurophysioogy*, **89**, 1016–1023.

Desimone, R. & Duncan, J. (1995). Neural mechanisms of selective visual attention. *Annual Review Neuroscience*, **18**, 193–222.

Deutsch, J. A. & Deutsch, D. (1963). Attention: some theoretical considerations. *Psychological Review*, **70**, 51–60.

Downing, C. J. (1988). Expectancy and visual-spatial attention: effects on perceptual quality. *Journal of Experimental Psychology: Human Perception and Performance*, **14**, 188–202.

Duncan, J. (1998). Converging levels of analysis in the cognitive neuroscience of visual attention. *Philosophical Transactions of the Royal Society of London, Series B*, **353**, 1307–1317.

Emery, N., Lorincz, E., Perrett, D., Oram, M. & Baker, C. (1997). Gaze following and joint attention in rhesus monkeys (*Macaca mulatta*). *Journal of Comparative Psychology*, **111**, 286–293.

Fecteau, J. H., Bell, A. H. & Munoz, D. P. (2004). Neural correlates of the automatic and goal-driven biases in orienting spatial attention. *Journal of Neurophysiology*, **92**, 3, 1728–1737.

Gualtieri, C. T., Johnson, L. G. & Benedict, K. B. (2006). Neurocognition in depression: patients on and off medication versus healthy comparison subjects. *Journal of Neuropsychiatry and Clinical Neurosciences*, **18**, 217–225.

Giesbrecht, B., Woldorff, M. G., Song, A. W. & Mangun, G. R. (2003). Neural mechanisms of top-down control during spatial and feature attention. *Neuroimage*, **19**, 496–512.

Gobell, J. & Carrasco, M. (2005). Attention alters the appearance of spatial frequency and gap size. *Psychological Science*, **16**, 644–651.

Goldberg, M. E. & Bruce, C. J. (1985). Cerebral cortical activity associated with the orientation of visual attention in the rhesus monkey. *Vision Research*, **25**, 471–481.

Green, M. F. (1996). What are the functional consequences of neurocognitive deficits in schizophrenia? *American Journal of Psychiatry*, **153**, 321–330.

Handy, T., Kingstone A. & Mangun, G. R. (1996). Spatial distribution of visual attention: perceptual sensitivity and response latency. *Perception and Psychophysics*, **58**, 613–627.

Harter, M. R., Miller, S. L., Price, N. J., LaLonde, M. E. & Keyes, A. L. (1989). Neural processes involved in directing attention. *Journal of Cognitive Neuroscience*, **1**, 223–237.

Hawkins, H. L., Hillyard, S. A., Luck, S. J. *et al.* (1990). Visual attention modulates signal detectability. *Journal of Experimental Psychology: Human Perception and Performance*, **16**, 802–811.

Heinze, H. J. & Mangun, G. R. (1995). Electrophysiological signs of sustained and transient attention to spatial locations. *Neuropsychologia*, **33**, 889–908.

Heinze, H. J., Mangun, G. R., Burchert, W. *et al.* (1994). Combined spatial and temporal imaging of spatial selective attention in humans. *Nature*, **392**, 543–546.

Helmholtz, H. von (1962/1924–25). *Treatise on Physiological Optics* (3rd edn.). Edited by J. P. C. Southall. New York: Dover Publications.

Hopf, J., Luck, S. J., Boelmans, K. *et al.* (2006). The neural site of attention matches the spatial scale of perception. *Journal of Neuroscience*, **26**, 3532–3540.

Hopfinger, J. B. & Maxwell, J. S. (2005). Appearing and disappearing stimuli trigger a reflexive modulation of visual cortical activity. *Cognitive Brain Research*, **25**(1), 48–56.

Hopfinger, J. B. & Mangun, G. R. (1998). Reflexive attention modulates processing of visual stimuli in human extrastriate cortex. *Psychological Science*, **9**, 441–447.

Hopfinger, J. B. & Mangun, G. R. (2001). Tracking the influence of reflexive attention on sensory and cognitive processing. *Cognitive, Affective and Behavioral Neuroscience*, **1**, 56–65.

Hopfinger, J. B & West, V. M. (2006). Interactions between endogenous and exogenous attention on cortical visual processing. *Neuroimage*, **31**, 774–789.

Hopfinger, J. B., Buonocore, M. H. & Mangun, G. R. (2000). The neural mechanisms of top-down attentional control. *Nature Neuroscience*, **3**, 284–291.

Johnson, S. H., Rotte, M., Grafton, S. T. *et al.* (2002). Selective activation of a parietofrontal circuit during implicitly imagined prehension. *Neuroimage*, **17**, 1693–1704.

Jonides, J. (1980). Towards a model of the mind's eye's movement. *Canadian Journal of Psychology*, **34**, 103–112.

Jonides, J. (1981). Voluntary versus automatic control over the mind's eye movement. In J. B. Long & A. D. Baddeley (Eds.), *Attention and Performance IX* (pp. 187–203). Hillsdale, NJ: Lawrence Erlbaum Associates.

Joormann, J. & Gotlib, I. H. (2007). Selective attention to emotional faces following recovery from depression. *Journal of Abnormal Psychology*, **116**, 80–85.

Kanwisher, N. & Wojciulik, E. (2000). Visual attention: insights from brain imaging. *Nature Reviews Neuroscience*, **1**, 91–100.

Kastner, S. & Ungerleider, L. (2000). Mechanisms of visual attention in the human cortex. *Annual Review of Neuroscience*, **23**, 315–341.

Kastner, S., DeWeerd, P., Desimone, R. & Ungerleider, L. C. (1998). Mechanisms of directed attention in the human extrastriate cortex as revealed by functional MRI. *Science*, **282**, 108–111.

Kastner, S., Pinsk, M. A., De Weerd, P., Desimone, R. & Ungerleider, L. G. (1999). Increased activity in human cerebral cortex during directed attention in the absence of visual stimulation. *Neuron*, **22**, 751–761.

Kerns, J. G., Cohen, J. D., MacDonal, A. W. *et al.* (2004a). Anterior cingulate conflict monitoring and adjustments in control. *Science*, **303**, 1023–1026.

Khoe, W., Mitchell, J. F., Reynolds, J. H. & Hillyard, S. A. (2005). Exogenous attentional selection of transparent superimposed surfaces modulates early event-related potentials. *Vision Research*, **45**, 3004–3014.

Kincade, J. M., Abrams, R. A., Astafiev, S. V., Shulman, G. L. & Corbetta M. (2005). An event-related functional magnetic resonance imaging study of voluntary and stimulus-driven orienting of attention. *Journal of Neuroscience*, **18**, 4593–4604.

Klein, R. M. (2000). Inhibition of return. *Trends in Cognitive Science*, **4**, 138–147.

Knight, R. T., Grabowecky, M. F. & Scabini, D. (1995). Role of human prefrontal cortex in attention control. *Advances in Neurology*, **66**, 21–34.

La Berge, D. (1997). Attention, awareness, and the triangular circuit. *Consciousness and Cognition*, **6**, 149–181.

Leyman, L., De Raedt, R., Schacht, R. & Koster, E. H. (2007). Attentional biases for angry faces in unipolar depression. *Psychological Medicine*, **37**, 393–402.

Liu, T., Pestilli, F. & Carrasco, M. (2005). Transient attention enhances perceptual performance and FMRI response in human visual cortex. *Neuron*, **45**, 469–477.

Liu, T., Slotnick, S. D., Serences, J. T. & Yantis, S. (2003). Cortical mechanisms of feature-based attentional control. *Cerebral Cortex*, **13**, 1334–1343.

Lorincz, E. N., Baker, C. & Perrett, D. I. (1999). Visual cues for attention following in rhesus monkeys. *Cahiers de Psychologie Cognitive*, **18**, 973–1003.

Luck, S. J., Chelazzi, L., Hillyard, S. A. & Desimone, R. (1997). Neural mechanisms of spatial selective attention in areas V1, V2 and V4 of macaque visual cortex. *Journal of Neurophysiology*, **77**, 24–42.

Luck, S. J., Hillyard, S. A., Mouloua, M. *et al.* (1994). Effects of spatial cuing on luminance detectability: psychophysical and electrophysiological evidence for early selection. *Journal of Experimental Psychology: Human Perception and Performance*, **20**, 887–904.

Luck, S. J., Woodman, G. F. & Vogel, E. K. (2000). Event-related potential studies of attention. *Trends in Cognitive Science*, **4**, 432–440.

Luck, S. J., Fuller, R. L., Braun, E. L. *et al.* (2006). The speed of visual attention in schizophrenia: electrophysiological and behavioral evidence. *Schizophrenia Research*, **85**, 174–195.

Macaluso, E. & Driver, J. (2005). Multisensory spatial interactions: a window onto functional integration in the human brain. *Trends in Neuroscience*, **28**, 264–271.

MacDonald, A. W., 3rd, Cohen, J. D., Stenger, V. A. & Carter, C. S. (2000). Dissociating the role of the dorsolateral prefrontal and anterior cingulated cortex in cognitive control. *Science*, **288**, 1835–1838.

Mangun, G. R. (1995). Neural mechanisms of visual selective attention in humans. *Psychophysiology*, **32**, 4–18.

Markela-Lerenc, J., Kaiser, S., Fiedler, P., Weisbrod, M. & Mundt, C. (2006). Stroop performance in depressive patients: a preliminary report. *Journal of Affective Disorders*, **94**, 261–267.

Maunsell, J. H. & Cook, E. P. (2002). The role of attention in visual processing. *Philosophical Transactions of the Royal Society of London: Series B Biological Sciences*, **357**, 1063–1072.

Mayer, A. R., Dorflinger, J. M., Rao, S. M. & Seidenberg, M. (2004). Neural networks underlying endogenous and exogenous visual-spatial orienting. *Neuroimage*, **23**, 534–541.

McAdams, C. J. & Maunsell, J. H. (1999). Effects of attention on the reliability of individual neurons in monkey visual cortex. *Neuron*, **23**, 765–773.

McAdams, C. & Reid, C. (2005). Attention modulates the responses of simple cells in monkey primary visual cortex. *Journal of Neuroscience*, **25**(47), 11023–11033.

Mesulam, M. M. (1981). A cortical network for directed attention and unilateral neglect. *Annals of Neurology*, **10**, 309–325.

Michale, G. & Desmedt, S. (2004). The human pulvinar and attentional processing of visual distractors. *Neuroscience Letters*, **362**, 176–181.

Miller, E. K. (2000). The neural basis of top-down control of visual attention in the prefrontal cortex. In J. Driver & S. Monsell (Eds.), *Attention and Performance XVIII: The Control Over Cognitive Processes* (pp. 511–534). Cambridge, MA: MIT Press.

Miller, E. K. & Cohen, J. D. (2001). An integrative theory of prefrontal cortex function. *Annual Review Neuroscience*, **24**, 167–202.

Mogg, K., Millar, N. & Bradley, B. P. (2000). Biases in eye movements to threatening facial expressions in generalized anxiety disorder and depressive disorder. *Journal of Abnormal Psychology*, **109**, 695–704.

Moran, J. & Desimone, R. (1985). Selective attention gates visual processing in the extrastriate cortex. *Science*, **229**, 782–784.

Mort, D. J., Perry, R. J., Mannan, S. K. *et al.* (2003). Differential cortical activation during voluntary and reflexive saccades in man. *Neuroimage*, **18**, 231–246.

Nobre, A. C., Gitelman, D. R., Dias, E. C. & Mesulam, M. M. (2000). Covert visual spatial orienting and saccades: overlapping neural systems. *Neuroimage*, **11**, 210–216.

Nobre, A. C., Sebestyen, G. N., Gitelman, D. R. *et al.* (1997). Functional localization of the system for visuospatial attention using positron emission tomography. *Brain*, **120**, 515–533.

Paelecke-Habermann, Y., Pohl, J. & Leplow, B. (2005). Attention and executive functions in remitted major depression patients. *Journal of Affective Disorders*, **89**, 125–135.

Peelen, M. V., Heslenfeld, D. J. & Theeuwes, J. (2004). Endogenous and exogenous attention shifts are mediated by the same large-scale neural network. *Neuroimage*, **22**, 822–830.

Petkov, C. I., Kang, X., Alho, K. *et al.* (2004). Attentional modulation of human auditory cortex. *Nature Neuroscience*, **7**, 658–663.

Posner, M. I. (1980). Orienting of attention. *Quarterly Journal of Experimental Psychology*, **32**, 3–25.

Posner, M. I. & Cohen, Y. (1984). Components of visual orienting. In H. Bouma & D. Bouwhis (Eds.), *Attention and Performance X* (pp. 531–556). Hillsdale, NJ: Lawrence Erlbaum Associates.

Posner, M. I. & Petersen, S. E. (1990). The attention system of the human brain. *Annual Review of Neuroscience*, **13**, 25–42.

Posner, M. I., Snyder, C. R. R. & Davidson, B. J. (1980). Attention and the detection of signals. *Journal of Experimental Psychology: General*, **109**, 160–174.

Purcell, R., Maruff, P., Kyrios, M. & Pantelis, C. (1997). Neuropsychological function in young patients with unipolar major depression. *Psychological Medicine*, **27**, 1277–1285.

Rafal, R. D. & Henik, A. (1994). The neurology of inhibition. In T. Carr & D. Dagenbach (Eds.), *Inhibitory Processes in Attention, Memory and Language* (pp. 1–51). New York, NY: Academic Press.

Rafal, R. D. & Posner, M. I. (1987). Deficits in human visual spatial attention following thalamic lesions. *Proceedings of the National Academy of Sciences, USA*, **84**, 7349–7353.

Recanzone, G. H., Wurtz, R. H. & Schwarz, U. (1993). Attentional modulation of neuronal responses in MT and MST of a macaque monkey performing a visual discrimination task. *Society for Neuroscience Abstract*, **19**, 973.

Reynolds, J. H. & Chelazzi, L. (2004). Attentional modulation of visual processing. *Annual Review Neuroscience*, **27**, 611–647.

Reynolds, J. H., Chelazzi, L. & Desimone, R. (1999). Competitive mechanisms subserve attention in macaque areas V2 and V4. *Journal of Neuroscience*, **19**, 1736–1753.

Robinson, D. L. & Petersen, S. E. (1992). The pulvinar and visual salience. *Trends in Neuroscience*, **15**, 127–132.

Rogers, M. A., Bellgrove, M. A., Chiu, E., Mileshkin, C. & Bradshaw, J. L. (2004). Response selection deficits in melancholic but not nonmelancholic unipolar major depression. *Journal of Clinical Experimental Neuropsychology*, **26**, 169–179.

Rosen, A., Rao, S., Caffarra, P. *et al.* (1999). Neural basis of endogenous and exogenous spatial orienting: a functional MRI study. *Journal of Cognitive Neuroscience*, **11**, 135–152.

Rowe, J., Friston, K., Frackowiak, R. & Passingham, R. E. (2002). Attention to action: specific modulation of corticocortical interactions in humans. *Neuroimage*, **17**, 988–998.

Rowe, J. B., Stephan, K. E., Friston, K., Frackowiak, R. S. & Passingham, R. E. (2005). The prefrontal cortex shows context-specific changes in effective connectivity to motor or visual cortex during the selection of action or colour. *Cerebral Cortex*, **15**, 85–95.

Salinas, E. & Sejnowski, T. J. (2001). Gain modulation in the central nervous system: where behavior, neurophysiology, and computation meet. *Neuroscientist*, **7**, 430–440.

Sapir, A., Soroker, N., Berger, A. & Henik, A. (1999). Inhibition of return in spatial attention: direct evidence for collicular generation. *Nature Neuroscience*, **2**, 1053–1054.

Schicatano, E. J., Peshori, K. R., Gopalaswamy, R., Sahay, E. & Evinger, C. (2000). Reflex excitability regulates prepulse inhibition. *Journal of Neuroscience*, **20**, 4240–4247.

Sevostianov, A., Fromm, S., Nechaev, V., Howitz, B. & Braun, A. (2002). Effect of attention on central auditory processing: an fMRI study. *International Journal of Neuroscience*, **112**, 587–606.

Sheline, Y. I., Barch, D. M., Donnelly, J. M. et al. (2001). Increased amygdala response to masked emotional faces in depressed subjects resolves with antidepressant treatment: an fMRI study. *Biological Psychiatry*, **50**, 651–658.

Sherman, S. M. & Guillery, R. (2002). The role of the thalamus in the flow of information to the cortex. *Philosophical Transactions of the Royal Society of London: Series B Biological Sciences*, **357**(1428), 1695–1708.

Shipp, S. (2004). The brain circuitry of attention. *Trends in Cognitive Science*, **8**, 223–230.

Siegle, G. J., Steinhauer, S. R., Thase, M. E., Stenger, V. A. & Carter, C. S. (2002). Can't shake that feeling: event-related fMRI assessment of sustained amygdala activity in response to emotional information in depressed individuals. *Biological Psychiatry*, **51**, 693–707.

Snitz, B. E., MacDonald, A. 3rd, Cohen, J. D. et al. (2005). Lateral and medial hypofrontality in first-episode schizophrenia: functional activity in a medication-naive state and effects of short-term atypical antipsychotic treatment. *American Journal of Psychiatry*, **162**, 2322–2329.

Spitzer, H. & Richmond, B. J. (1991). Task difficulty: ignoring, attending to, and discriminating a visual stimulus yield progressively more activity in inferior temporal neurons. *Experimental Brain Research*, **83**, 340–348.

Stoet, G. & Snyder, L. H. (2004). Single neurons in posterior parietal cortex of monkeys encode cognitive set. *Neuron*, **42**, 1003–1012.

Sweeney, J. A., Kmiec, J. A. & Kupfer, D. J. (2000). Neuropsychologic impairments in bipolar and unipolar mood disorders on the CANTAB neurocognitive battery. *Biological Psychiatry*, **48**, 674–684.

Tootell, R. B., Hadjikhani, N., Hall, E. K. et al. (1998). The retinotopy of visual spatial attention. *Neuron*, **21**, 1409–1422.

Treue, S. (2001). Neural correlates of attention in primate visual cortex. *Trends in Neuroscience*, **24**, 295–300.

Treue, S. (2003). Visual attention: the where, what, how and why of saliency. *Current Opinion in Neurobiology*, **13**, 428–432.

Treue, S. & Martínez-Trujillo, J. C. (1999). Feature-based attention influences motion processing gain in macaque visual cortex. *Nature*, **399**, 575–579.

Van Voorhis, S. & Hillyard, S. A. (1977). Visual evoked potentials and selective attention to points in space. *Perception and Psychophysics*, **22**, 54–62.

Vogel, E. K., Luck, S. J. & Shaprio, K. L. (1998). Electrophysiological evidence for a postperceptual locus of suppression during the attentional blink. *Journal of Experimental Psychology: Human Perception and Performance*, **24**, 1656–1676.

Walsh, B. J., Fannon, S. P., Giesbrecht, B. & Mangun, G. R. (May, 2005). *Dissecting attentional control systems*. Poster presented at the Annual Meeting of the American Psychological Society, Los Angeles, CA.

Weese, G. D., Phillips, J. M. & Brown, V. J. (1999). Attentional orienting is imparied by unilateral lesions of the thalamic reticular nucleus in the rat. *Journal of Neuroscience*, **19**, 10135–10139.

Weissman, D. H., Warner, L. M. & Woldorff, M. G. (2004). The neural mechanisms for minimizing cross-modal distraction. *Journal of Neuroscience*, **24**, 10941–10949.

Woldorff, M. G., Hazlett, C. J., Fichtenholtz, H. M. et al. (2004). Functional parcellation of attentional control regions of the brain. *Journal of Cognitive Neuroscience*, **16**, 149–165.

Wolfe, J. M., Cave, K. R. & Franzel, S. L. (1989). Guided search: an alternative to the feature integration model for visual search. *Journal of Experimental Psychology: Human Perception and Performance*, **15**, 419–433.

Yantis, S. (1996). Attentional capture in vision. In A. Kramer, M. G. H. Coles & G. D. Logan (Eds.), *Converging Operations in the Study of Visual Selective Attention* (pp. 45–76). Washington, DC: American Psychiatric Association.

Yantis, S. & Jonides, J. (1990). Abrupt visual onsets and selective attention: evidence from visual search. *Journal of Experimental Psychology: Human Perception and Performance*, **16**, 121–134.

Zelano, C., Bensafi, M., Porter, J. et al. (2005). Attentional modulation in human primary olfactory cortex. *Nature Neuroscience*, **8**, 114–120.

The role of executive functions in psychiatric disorders

Renée Testa and Christos Pantelis

Introduction

Executive function (EF) deficits are the most consistently described impairments found in studies of neuro-cognition in psychiatric disorders. More recent research suggests that EF deficits are most prominent in psychiatric disorders that have their onset during the late childhood and adolescence period, including schizophrenia, bipolar disorder, obsessive-compulsive disorder (OCD) and depression. Therefore, neurodevelopmental mechanisms affecting these functions are likely to play an important role in the emergence of these psychiatric conditions or, alternatively, the emergence of these disorders may adversely affect such functions. As we discuss below, the EF system is continuing to mature into adolescence and early adulthood and we suggest that understanding the nature and extent of deficits in psychiatric disorders will depend on the interaction between the stage of brain maturation and the age of onset of psychiatric pathology.

In this chapter we first discuss issues relevant to EFs. We argue that understanding the challenges within this field can offer valuable insight to guide the assessment process. We discuss the difficulties in operationally defining EFs, and provide a brief overview of the evidence for associating EF to frontal lobe structures. Secondly, we discuss the relevance of the frontal lobe/executive system and its maturation to understanding the development of mental illness and schizophrenia in particular, and finally we suggest that this provides the context within which to understand brain–behavior relationships relevant to EF and how these are affected in mental disorders.

Defining the executive system

The frontal lobes play a pivotal role in mediating and integrating higher level, neurocognitive processes of the brain referred to as executive functions (Burgess, 2000; Chayer & Freedman, 2001). These processes are considered to act globally across all cognitive domains and impact upon all types of behavior. While there has been considerable debate about what constitutes EFs (Stuss, 2006), in the last decade there has been rapid progress in developing conceptual models of the executive system and in delineating the relevant neural networks that underlie such functions.

General descriptions of EFs as "cognitive skills required for the successful execution and completion of complex, goal-directed behaviour" are often implemented in the literature, but it has proved more difficult to identify the specific cognitive processes involved (Stuss, 2006). Although there is no comprehensive list of skills that definitively comprise the executive system, some agreement exists regarding specific situations in which this system is activated (Elliott, 2003; Salmon & Collette, 2005), and behavioral and neuropsychological observations in individuals with frontal lobe damage (Bennett et al., 2005) have helped delineate their functional outcomes. Executive deficits are most evident when an individual is confronted with complex, novel situations requiring inhibition of over-learned responses and generation of novel or non-automatic responses, necessitating an ability to be self-directed, flexible and adaptive (Spikman et al., 2000). The generation of new responses in this way is the culmination of several executive processes, including planning, decision-making, inhibitory control, cognitive

The Neuropsychology of Mental Illness, ed. Stephen J. Wood, Nicholas B. Allen and Christos Pantelis. Published by Cambridge University Press. © Cambridge University Press 2009.

flexibility, emotion regulation, reasoning and judgment (Shimamura, 2000; Stuss & Alexander, 2000; Yamasaki *et al.*, 2002). Damage to the cognitive systems underlying these abilities results in a reliance on over-learned responses, and use of inappropriate behavioral strategies that are inefficient (Bennett *et al.*, 2005; Burgess & Shallice, 1996; Stuss, 2006).

Early attempts to understand the neuroanatomical correlates of the executive system were centered upon the role of the frontal lobes as the "mediator" of these skills and were largely focused upon a localizationist viewpoint (Shimamura, 2000; Stuss, 1992; Stuss & Alexander, 2000; Yamasaki *et al.*, 2002). Recent developments demonstrate this view to be overly simplistic, with evidence from both neuropsychology and neuroimaging (e.g. functional, structural, neurochemical) (Smith & Jonides, 1999; Szameitat *et al.*, 2002; Tamm *et al.*, 2002; Taylor *et al.*, 2004; Tekin & Cummings, 2002) suggesting that more detailed conceptualizations of the executive system are required, including evidence that executive dysfunction can occur following damage to non-frontal regions (Fassbender *et al.*, 2004; Himanen *et al.*, 2005; Roth & Saykin, 2004; van der Werf *et al.*, 2000a). Such studies are also elucidating a greater range of cognitive skills as being part of the EF system through a process of fractionating and dissociating its component parts (Burgess *et al.*, 1998; Pantelis & Brewer, 1995).

The association between the frontal lobes and executive functions

There is consensus that the integrity of the frontal lobes is critical to the operation of EFs, although other brain regions are also important. This was illustrated famously in the case of Phineas Gage, a young railway foreman, who in 1848 sustained significant frontal lobe damage (Wagar & Thagard, 2004). Despite the penetrating brain injury, Gage made a rapid and apparently full recovery with little impact on his general intelligence, memory and language (Ratiu & Talos, 2004; Stuss *et al.*, 1992). However, Gage showed marked behavioral changes. Once considered a likeable, responsible and trusted person, post-injury Gage's behavior became socially inappropriate. He was rude, irresponsible and indifferent to social conformities (Bechara *et al.*, 1994) and was unable to monitor his emotional responses, resulting in marked and uncharacteristic behavioral exhibitions (Damasio *et al.*, 1994; Ratiu *et al.*, 2004). He was also incapable of making logical

decisions, which was unexpected given his premorbid abilities (Macmillan, 2000a, 2000b).

This landmark case provided important insights about functional localization within the frontal lobes, demonstrating that the integrity of the frontal lobes was critical to the operation of a collection of higher-level skills that would later be termed executive functions (Burgess, 2000; Spikman *et al.*, 2000). Gage's case also provided clues about functional specificity within subregions of the frontal cortex. In a recent study of Gage's skull, Damasio *et al.* (1994) used modern imaging techniques to accurately identify the damage. Projected trajectories of the iron bar that pierced his skull suggested that, whilst the dorsolateral region was spared, significant damage was sustained in ventromedial regions (Brodmann's areas 8 to 12, 24, 32). Such evidence implicated the ventromedial prefrontal cortex (VMPFC) in causing Gage's deficits. Reciprocal connections between the VMPFC and the amygdala and hypothalamus, which have also been implicated in these cognitive processes, support this notion (Macmillan, 2000b; Tekin & Cummings, 2002). Gage's case is also informative about regions that were spared, namely the dorsolateral prefrontal cortex (DLPFC), suggesting that those higher-level abilities that were preserved, including language and attentional abilities, may be attributable to this or other spared regions (Macmillan, 2000a, 2000b).

Subsequent research based on frontal lesion models, including work in primates, has provided further evidence to support functional specialization within frontal subregions, particularly of DLPFC and the orbitofrontal cortex (OFC) (Baddeley, 1996; Bechara *et al.*, 2000; Duncan & Owen, 2000; Levine *et al.*, 1998; Shallice & Burgess, 1991; Stuss & Levine, 2002). More recent ideas posit that these regions are differentially responsible for "cold" (DLPFC) and "hot" (OFC) cognitive processes. "Cold" cognition refers to logical decision-making processes, including judgment and reasoning abilities, whilst "hot" cognition incorporates affective processes mediating and controlling emotion, motivation and social influences (Unsworth & Engle, 2005).

Functions of the dorsolateral prefrontal cortex and orbitofrontal cortex

The DLPFC has been implicated in various cognitive abilities associated with planning, decision-making and problem-solving. Deficits commonly observed following damage to this region include difficulties in evaluating contextual information, problems in efficiently formulating and executing a plan, poor capacity to adhere to designated rules, poor ability to be flexible and adaptable within the environment, and difficulty with multitasking, organization and everyday decision-making skills (Aron *et al.*, 2004; Burgess, 2000; Shallice & Burgess, 1991). Such deficits were thought to be commonly exhibited as an inability to consider and select different behavioral strategies and to respond to environmental demands or contingencies, as well as an inability to follow time constraints, keep appointments and/or meet deadlines (Burgess, 2000; Levine *et al.*, 1998). Frith *et al.* (2000) have also demonstrated that patients with lateral PFC damage experience difficulty in assessing and placing constraints on possible strategic solutions or behavioral responses, which leads to the adoption of a trial-and-error approach (Fletcher *et al.*, 2000; Reverberi *et al.*, 2005b). In everyday situations, this type of approach is inefficient, time consuming and lacks coherence and organization (Burgess, 2000; Reverberi *et al.*, 2005a).

The mediation of attentional capacities including attentional set-shifting, selective attention and sustained attention, in addition to the strategic "use" of memory, incorporating the coordination, elaboration and interpretation of different associations within working memory, have also been attributed to this region (Stuss, 2006). Bechara and colleagues also postulated that deficits in the inhibition of inappropriate responses arise from an inability to hold and utilize internal self-representations within working memory, leading to the selection of behavioral responses with poorer long-term outcomes (Bechara *et al.*, 1994, 2000; Stuss & Levine, 2002). The relationship of the DLPFC and the executive system to working memory is currently a topic of contentious debate in the literature (Bechara *et al.*, 1998; D'Esposito *et al.*, 2006).

These skills are distinct and contrast with those attributed to the OFC, which include cognitive abilities related to social, affective, motivational and personality issues. Such skills are essential to an individual's capacity for emotional and behavioral self-regulation, in addition to the integration of subjective experiences required for self-awareness and individuality (Cicerone *et al.*, 1997; Stuss & Levine, 2002). Other skills, including the ability to regulate and select appropriate behavioral responses, reasoning and problem-solving within the social domain, the

appreciation of future consequences and the capacity to form and maintain interpersonal relationships have also been attributed to the OFC (Cicerone & Tanenbaum, 1997; Eslinger & Damasio, 1985), as have higher-level olfactory abilities (Brewer *et al.*, 2006). Impairments arising from damage to this region include a range of characteristic problems, including inability to be aware of, or to understand and integrate different social and emotional cues present in the environment, difficulty with decision-making tasks related to social and personal matters, anosmia, amnesia, disinhibition and perseveration (Damasio *et al.*, 1990; Eslinger & Damasio, 1985).

Given the strong emphasis on understanding neurocognitive processes within the prefrontal cortex, the DLPFC, which is largely responsible for more "classical" cognitive skills such as decision-making and planning abilities, has received greater attention than the OFC. This disparity is also reflected in the development of tests to assess the integrity of these regions. While various tasks have been developed to assess the DLPFC, the OFC has proved more difficult in this regard and there is still a lack of reliable and validated tests to assess OFC integrity. This is also reflected in fewer studies that assess these abilities in psychiatric disorders. More recently, work has begun to focus on the OFC in order to understand how emotion and motivation impact upon decision-making and on other cognitive processes, and how best to measure these (Happaney *et al.*, 2004). Several gambling tasks, including The Iowa Gambling Task and the Cambridge Gambling Task, have been designed specifically to examine the interaction between affective, motivational and decision-making processes, and have been used successfully to assess this region (Bechara *et al.*, 1994, 1998; Clark & Manes, 2004). Higher-level smell identification ability is attributed to the OFC and olfactory tasks have also proved useful in probing this region in psychiatric and neurological disorders (Brewer *et al.*, 2006).

As noted from the above descriptions, the DLPFC and the OFC have been largely characterized by descriptions of specific neurocognitive functions or dysfunctions that arise following damage to these regions. In addition to this approach, several authors have attempted to further elucidate the collection of reported deficits which manifest when damage is sustained to either these specific prefrontal regions or to pathways connecting these regions to subcortical areas (Cummings, 1995; Mega & Cummings, 1994;

Pantelis & Brewer, 1995; Pantelis & Maruff, 2002). Damage to the DLPFC is thought to result in a "pseudo-depressive" personality, characterized by apathetic and withdrawn behaviors, inability to engage in goal-directed behavior, and neglect for future-orientated consequences. In contrast, OFC damage, previously considered to result in a "pseudo-psychopathic" personality, has more recently been characterized and differentiated in terms of whether damage is to medial or lateral OFC. The former has been associated with personality changes including irritability, emotional lability, impulsiveness, disinhibition, lack of concern for others, marked changes in personality, environmental dependency, mood disorders (lability and mania) and obsessive-compulsive disorder (OCD), whilst lateral OFC damage results in mood disorders of depression and dysphoria, also OCD, and personality changes comprising anhedonia (Cummings, 1995; Mega & Cummings, 1994; Tekin & Cummings, 2002). Mega & Cummings (1994) argued that an increase in metabolic activity in the OFC (and caudate) could lead to OCD, whilst hypofunction (and increased amygdala activity) in the OFC was associated with depressive symptoms.

Pantelis and colleagues (Pantelis & Brewer, 1995; Pantelis et al., 2003b) argued that disturbances in fronto-striato-thalamic pathways result in different behavioral and neuropsychological syndromes of schizophrenia that are comparable to the Cummings' frontal syndromes (Curson et al., 1999). It is possible that associating different behavioral and cognitive features of psychiatric disorders to these frontal syndromes may provide insights about the underlying neural mechanisms in disorders like schizophrenia, depression, OCD and attention-deficit hyperactivity disorder (ADHD) (Barnett et al., 1999; Maruff et al., 2003; Mega & Cummings, 1994; Pantelis & Brewer, 1995; Pantelis & Maruff, 2002) Certainly, there is evidence that dysfunction of DLPFC has a significant role in depression and OCD, as evident by neuropsychological studies (Purcell et al., 1997), while deficits in smell identification implicate OFC in OCD (Barnett et al., 1999). Thus, while it may be possible to differentiate distinct neuropsychological profiles and psychiatric disorders brought about by damage to these regions, there is also considerable overlap. Further, while the notion of frontal-striatal-thalamic systems suggests a network of brain structures, a neuropsychological approach has not adequately delineated how such a network may be involved in or across various disorders.

Broadening the network of executive functions

Advances in brain-imaging technologies have provided new insights, highlighting the inadequacy of a strict localizationist approach to the study of EFs and the overly simplistic view of equating frontal lobes and EFs (Blakemore & Choudhury, 2006; Zimmerman et al., 2006). Both clinical and imaging studies in normal populations have identified that EFs also involve non-frontal regions, various neural networks and many subordinate cognitive processes (Aron et al., 2004; Carter et al., 1999; Storey et al., 1999; Stuss & Alexander, 2000). More recent work by Harrison et al. (2006) and Zakzanis & Graham (2005) has investigated the neuroanatomical correlates and possible neural networks underpinning the executive system, identifying both frontal and non-frontal (e.g. cerebellum and left middle and superior temporal gyri) regions involved. Further, reports identifying anterior cingulate cortex (ACC) activity suggest that it is an integral part of the executive system (Cohen et al., 2000; Fornito et al., 2004; Peterson et al., 1999). This is particularly relevant to morbid conditions such as schizophrenia, depression and OCD, in which morphological and functional variability of the ACC is reported (Harrison et al., 2006; Mayberg et al., 1997; Yucel et al. 2003, 2007).

The approach of clinical executive function investigations has also changed to examine patients with a range of extra-frontal cortical, subcortical, developmental and acquired injuries and, increasingly, to understand the distributed neural systems involved in various psychiatric disorders manifesting executive deficits (Collette & Van der Linden, 2002; Szameitat et al., 2002; Taylor et al., 2004). Executive deficits have been identified within different neurological groups involving both localized and diffuse injuries (Crawford & Channon, 2002; Hanninen et al., 1997; Levine et al., 1998; Paul et al., 2005; Sweeney et al., 2001), and following damage to regions connecting to the frontal lobes, including ACC (Baird et al., 2006; Fassbender et al., 2004; Rogers et al., 2004), thalamus (van der Werf et al., 2000b), hippocampus (Himanen et al., 2005), cerebellum (Collette et al., 2005; Rao et al., 1997; Riva & Giorgi, 2000; Roth & Saykin, 2004) and basal ganglia (Monchi et al., 2006).

It is noteworthy that in these investigations the additional regions identified as relevant to EFs involve structures and networks intimately linked with prefrontal cortical regions. However, it remains uncertain as to what aspects of EF are subserved by each of the nodes, and whether the frontal regions are necessarily involved in mediating or controlling such functions. Current literature has, however, demonstrated that the frontal region is a necessary component of the neural networks subserving the executive system, given that they are activated regardless of what other non-frontal regions are implicated.

The fluid nature of frontal lobe functions and relevant networks makes it difficult to identify, define or fractionate the processes involved, given that their inherent and characteristic nature is to act in a flexible and adaptable manner (Duncan & Owen, 2000). This lack of "constancy" raises questions about whether identifying the characteristic features or markers of frontal processes is feasible, as it is such a dynamic and responsive system. It also suggests that different approaches are needed in order to adequately analyze a system that changes rapidly in response to the characteristics of any given task or situation. To capture deficits of frontal processes methodological designs that can measure the temporal characteristics of these processes are required, integrating a number of imaging modalities to localize the networks involved, together with techniques to assess the temporal changes with millisecond resolution. A small number of investigations (Mathalon et al., 2003; Wolff et al., 2003) have examined measures including fMRI and ERPs; but these have been undertaken independently. To our knowledge, simultaneous, multimodal measurements of EFs are yet to be published. Further work with fMRI, offering high spatial resolution, and ERPs and MEG that provide high temporal resolution, would be informative, as would the use of transcranial magnetic stimulation (TMS) and PET, which can help to examine functional connectivity between brain regions (Banich & Weissman, 2000). Such research would provide important insights about the nature of distributed brain activations during complex cognitive processes and provide novel methods to investigate how these processes are disrupted in neuropsychiatric disorders.

What is the role of the frontal lobes?

There is continuing debate about reconciling the notion of a fractionated view of the EF system, with descriptions of the "unity" or commonality that exists between executive tasks (Burgess et al., 1998; Miyake et al., 2000; Robbins et al., 1998). Investigators (Duncan et al., 1995; Engle et al., 1999) proposing a "unitary" view argue that a common mechanism across different EFs underlies different executive components, comparable to a "domain-general" process (Stuss, 2006). This focuses upon the integrative and coordinating role of the frontal lobes to account for this unity of function, where the fluid recruitment of different cognitive processes enables the individual to successfully adapt to changing task and environmental demands (Stuss, 2006). Similarly, several researchers (Paine & Tani, 2004; Peers et al., 2005) have focused upon notions of "top-down" or "bottom-up" processes, which are related to the integration and assimilation of information that is gathered from both frontal and non-frontal cortical and subcortical regions. It is argued that the greater the system is required to be flexible and adaptable, the greater the degree of integration and assimilation from other networks that is required, which is said to be mediated by the frontal lobes (Bialystok et al. 2004, 2005). A reduced capacity to undertake this control of cognitive processes is said to lead to greater performance variability when individuals are presented with demanding tasks (West & Alain, 2000).

The capacity to integrate and coordinate multiple processes across and within different neural networks is particularly relevant to furthering our understanding of psychiatric disorders. It has been proposed that a "breakdown" in the connectivity in the brain underlies many serious psychiatric disorders, such as schizophrenia (Friston, 1998). This "disconnection hypothesis" argues that the fluid processes required for the functional integration of cortical systems necessary for cognition are dysfunctional, and that the aberrant connections should be portrayed as functional and not necessarily anatomical in nature. Therefore, it may not necessarily be specific regions that are not adequately functioning, but rather the ability to integrate functional processes across the brain that is dysfunctional. It is acknowledged that region-specific abnormalities may be evident, but these occur secondary to the dysfunctional integration (Friston, 1998). This is supported by the suggestion that the symptoms associated with schizophrenia are likely a result from aberrant interactions between different cognitive processes rather than a deficit in one specific cognitive function.

More recent literature has demonstrated alterations between specific cortical and subcortical regions, including both reductions and enhancements in functional connectivity; these include the DLPFC and the hippocampus (Meyer-Lindenberg et al., 2005), networks between the prefrontal, cerebellar and thalamic regions (Schlosser et al., 2003a, 2003b), and also the prefrontal, temporal and limbic areas (Weinberger & Lipska, 1995). A loss of "synchrony" may also result from white-matter abnormalities often reported in schizophrenia; this may cause a slowing of neural transmission speed and efficiency required to support the integration of neural networks (Bartzokis, 2002). Another possibility is presented by Callicott et al. (2003) who argue that given patients with schizophrenia require greater prefrontal resources and are more inefficient when undertaking working-memory tasks, deficits may result from an inability to maintain the network of activity and undertake neural strategies for managing or dealing with information that require DLPFC involvement.

Tasks such as those of new learning and memory (Friston et al., 1998), and spatial working-memory and inhibition tasks (Sweeney et al., 2007; Wood et al., 2003) that call upon a widely distributed network of cortical activity, may consequently provide some insight into an individual's capacity to perform such cognitive (or functional) acts. Indeed, functional connectivity in the brain may never develop adequately in patients, and may be the cause of their failure on such demanding tasks, even in the early stages of illness or pre-illness onset (Brewer et al., 2005; Wood et al., 2003). Given this, the need to better understand these fluid and interactive processes in the normally developing and functioning brain is vital, in order to understand how these processes may break down or inappropriately develop in psychiatric illnesses.

Working memory

Investigation into components and processes involved in working memory and its maturational trajectory is important in understanding the cognitive mechanisms underlying several psychiatric disorders, such as schizophrenia, bipolar disorder, OCD and ADHD, which have neurodevelopmental origins and manifest throughout adolescence. Working-memory deficits are a consistent and robust finding in such disorders, particularly schizophrenia. Working memory is a central component to the development and functioning of many other cognitive processes including attention, language and executive functioning. Therefore, understanding the basis for working-memory deficits may explain deficits in cognition and behavior and their impact on daily functioning in these disorders. Further, because different processes and domains of working memory develop throughout the lifespan from early childhood to early adulthood, disorders manifesting at different ages will likely manifest different profiles of impairment, including differences at different illness stages. Thus, documenting the growth trajectory of these deficits in concert with the development of illness will provide a better understanding of the nature and extent of the observed impairments and the mechanisms underlying them.

In order to ascertain how these processes become dysfunctional in psychiatric populations, a working definition and a comparative "normal" model of working memory is required. Working memory is commonly regarded as the process of holding and manipulating incoming, task-relevant information. This also permits the integration of other information from long-term memory or "working on memory" during the performance of cognitive tasks (Baddeley, 1996; Baddeley & Della Sala, 1996; Moscovitch, 1992). Perhaps because of this link to memory systems, the status of working memory as part of the executive domain has been the subject of considerable debate. However, given that working memory is effortful and places considerable demands on an individual's cognitive resources, requiring the individual to have direct intent and the strategic or controlled allocation of attentional resources to perform working-memory tasks, executive function skills are arguably required. Further, given the complexity of working-memory processes within different domains (verbal, visual, visuospatial etc.), there has been much debate regarding its conceptualization. Several different processes have been proposed, including a storage capacity, a rehearsal or maintenance process, and a controller process that permits mental coordination and manipulation of information (Bayliss et al., 2003; Rypma & D'Esposito, 1999). Storage components are considered responsible for domain-specific processes (visual, verbal, spatial) (D'Esposito et al., 2006; Ravizza et al., 2006; Smith & Jonides, 1999; Ventre-Dominey *et al.*, 2005), while higher-level manipulative and integrative functions of working memory involve domain-general processes (Bayliss *et al.*, 2003; Engle *et al.*, 1999; Smith *et al.*, 1996).

The evidence regarding the dissociability of storage and manipulation components of working memory demonstrates that the more attentionally demanding and effortful components required for active rehearsal, integration and coordination involves primarily frontal, executive processes. Neuroimaging investigations consistently demonstrate activations within the frontal regions, including the DLPFC, when participants are engaged in working-memory tasks, and that these activations can be differentiated (in level of activation and regions) from those of simpler short-term memory tasks that predominantly engage posterior cortices including the right middle and right inferior parietal lobe (Ackerman *et al.*, 2005; Collette *et al.*, 1999; D'Esposito *et al.*, 2006; Duncan & Owen, 2000; Gerton *et al.*, 2004; Passingham & Sakai, 2004; Wager & Smith, 2003). Primate work (Castner *et al.*, 2004; Fuster, 2000; Levy & Goldman-Rakic, 1999) has also demonstrated differentiation between short-term memory and working-memory systems, with working-memory tasks activating distributed networks including and beyond that of the frontal lobe region, while short-term memory activates predominantly regions in the parietal lobe.

The relevance of spatial working memory to psychiatric disorders

As discussed earlier, examining abilities that develop at the time of illness onset may also offer some insight into the underlying mechanisms that take place at the time of its emergence. Spatial working memory (SWM) has often been studied in individuals at high risk for, and with first-episode and/or chronic schizophrenia, with consistent findings of significant deficits in comparison with controls. Indeed, poor performance on SWM tasks may represent a precursor to the development of psychosis (Lencz *et al.*, 2006; Saperstein *et al.*, 2006; Wood *et al.*, 2003).

Spatial working memory requires a good ability to integrate and coordinate multiple cognitive processes from and across different cognitive networks, with involvement of the frontal lobes to control the integration of multiple processes simultaneously (Fuster, 1991). Maturation of this ability is not established until adulthood, which suggests that best performance in SWM tasks would not be possible until this time, when frontal lobe and associated networks are fully developed (De Luca *et al.*, 2003; Luna & Sweeney, 2001). In line with this Schweinsburg *et al.* (2005) reported that younger teenagers rely more on spatial rehearsal rather than engaging encoding processes in a SWM task, and therefore are not as efficient in using strategies to optimize performance (Scherf *et al.*, 2006). Sweeney *et al.* (2007) also suggested that there is a developmental transition from reliance on striatal regions in childhood when performing this task, to a more widely distributed and efficient circuitry including prefrontal, premotor and posterior parietal regions in adolescence. Poor performance on SWM tasks may then reflect an inability to efficiently integrate and coordinate cognitive processes in a specialized and organized fashion.

These notions regarding the late development of SWM provide some insight into mechanisms underlying the nature and severity of deficits in schizophrenia and other psychiatric disorders including ADHD and OCD. The finding that in schizophrenia clinically high-risk adolescents show deficits on a SWM task, before onset of illness (Smith *et al.*, 2006; Wood *et al.*, 2003), suggests that aberrant networks are present before the illness manifests. As SWM is not fully matured until early adulthood (De Luca *et al.*, 2003), this skill may never fully develop as onset of the disorder or its prodrome may interfere with maturation leading to "developmental arrest." Studies investigating child and adult ADHD (Martinussen & Tannock, 2006; Rhodes *et al.*, 2006; Vance *et al.*, 2007) and/or OCD (Barnett *et al.*, 1999; Purcell *et al.*, 1998a, 1998b; van der Wee *et al.*, 2007) have reported SWM deficits in these groups, but not in those with major depression (Purcell *et al.*, 1997, 1998b) or, surprisingly, in Tourette's syndrome (Watkins *et al.*, 2005). Interestingly, only bipolar patients who also present with psychosis exhibit SWM deficits (Badcock *et al.*, 2005; Glahn *et al.*, 2007; Pirkola *et al.*, 2005). This questions what comparable neurodevelopmental mechanisms are occurring in these disorders that do not permit and/or hinder the networks required for SWM to fully develop appropriately. A comprehensive understanding of brain maturational processes relevant to EFs is required in order to better understand such impairments.

Brain development and the maturation of executive functions: a hypothesis for the emergence of executive function deficits in neuropsychiatric disorders

Features that characterize many of the psychiatric disorders discussed in this volume include onset during adolescence or young adulthood and the presence of EF deficits, often associated with brain functional and structural abnormalities involving prefrontal brain regions. For example, deficits in EF are reported in schizophrenia (Barnett *et al.*, 2007a; Pantelis *et al.*, 1997; Simon *et al.*, 2006; Tan *et al.*, 2006), depression (Herrmann *et al.*, 2007; Porter *et al.*, 2007; Purcell *et al.*, 1997; Westheide *et al.*, 2007), bipolar disorder (Glahn *et al.*, 2007; Stoddart *et al.*, 2007), OCD (Bannon *et al.*, 2006; Purcell *et al.*, 1998a,b; Roth *et al.*, 2005; van der Wee *et al.*, 2007) and ADHD (Barnett *et al.*, 2001; Biederman *et al.*, 2004, 2007; Doyle, 2006; Wodka *et al.*, 2007). In this context, an understanding of the nature, severity and progression of EF deficits in these disorders should take account of the developmental (maturational) trajectory of EF abilities and examine this in relation to other brain changes occurring developmentally (e.g. changes in cortical gray matter. The *growth curves* in individuals developing psychiatric disorders can be compared with those in normal young people, and will provide evidence as to whether abnormalities (a) result from failed or arrested development, (b) represent a normal trajectory that is below average or (c) are indicative of progressive deterioration (see Figure 9.1). An informative longitudinal study by Shaw *et al.* (2006) characterized the relationship between cortical development and intelligence in a large group of children and adults who ranged between 3.8–29 years of age. Results demonstrated that level of intelligence during childhood and adolescence was related to the pattern of growth, including increases and decreases, in cortical thickness. Furthermore, an interaction between age and level (Average, High Average and Superior) of intelligence was noted in relation to the trajectories of change in cortical thickness, most notably within the prefrontal cortex. Whilst the Superior intelligent children initially demonstrated thinner cortex that markedly increased at approximately 11 years of age, and then rapidly declined from early adolescence, the High Average

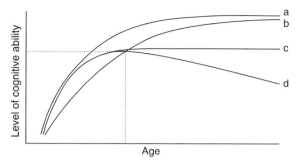

Figure 9.1. Graph depicting possible neurodevelopmental trajectories of cognitive abilities during maturation. (a) normal development; (b) neurodevelopmental lag; (c) neurodevelopmental arrest; (d) neurodegeneration. At the point of intersection of dotted lines, individuals with very different developmental trajectories have the same degree of impairment.

and Average intelligent children only showed a slower but comparable decline that commenced from early to late childhood. These results not only demonstrate that level of intelligence is related to dynamic changes in cortical thickness, but also that the adoption of a longitudinal, as opposed to cross-sectional approach provides greater insight into developmental patterns of cortical change and the fluid nature of the relationships between cognitive and cortical measures.

The benefit of adopting such an approach was illustrated in a study by Gochman *et al.* (2005) investigating IQ in childhood-onset schizophrenia (COS). Early notions considered that intelligence declined in both child- and adult-onset groups, consistent with a deterioration of cognitive skills over the illness period; however, Gochman *et al.* (2005) examined raw scores from the Wechsler Intelligence Scale within a longitudinal framework, as opposed to age-scaled scores that can obscure the nature of changes occurring during a dynamic period of normal growth. They reported that IQ does not decrease and actually stabilizes from approximately 2 years post illness onset. These findings are consistent with "neurodevelopmental arrest," where cognitive abilities that have already matured are not "lost" via neurodegenerative processes, but rather there is failure of further maturation (see Figure 9.1).

The identification of whether cognitive deficits manifest as a result of "neurodevelopmental arrest" or "neurodegeneration" requires comment about how the frontal lobe develops neuroanatomically and functionally.

The frontal region is one of the last brain structures to develop, with maturation progressing from posterior to anterior cerebral regions from childhood to adulthood (Segalowitz & Rose-Krasnor, 1992). Thus, cerebral processes that take place throughout development including dendritic arborization, myelination, synaptogenesis and cortical synapse elimination (i.e. synaptic pruning) occur later in the frontal lobes than in other brain regions (Bartzokis *et al.*, 2001; Fuster, 1993; Jernigan & Tallal, 1990; Kolb, 1989; Paus *et al.*, 1999). The morphological maturation of the frontal cortex, including cell differentiation and division into sublayers is considered to reach completion when an individual approaches puberty, yet developmental changes continue into early adulthood (Orzhekhovskaya, 1981). Myelination begins during the second trimester of gestation, continuing well into the third decade of life (Benes *et al.*, 1994), progressing in a graded fashion from inferior to superior and posterior to anterior, with the cerebellum developing first and the frontal lobes last (Yakovlev & Lecours, 1967). The apoptotic elimination of excess synapses results in remodeling and refinement of the neural circuitry, which is thought to strengthen the remaining functional connections and reduce competition from suboptimal associations. While the result of this essentially Darwinian process is improved and more efficient neuronal communication, it is important to note that this also leads to reduced redundancy available in the brain. This may be particularly relevant to understanding the longitudinal trajectory of behavioral and neuropsychological features observed in young people developing psychopathology (Brewer *et al.*, 2006; Pantelis *et al.*, 2005).

These processes of myelination and synaptic pruning that occur later in frontal regions are consistent with the observed changes on MRI that have illustrated maturational changes in vivo during adolescence (Giedd, 2004; Giedd *et al.*, 1999; Gogtay *et al.*, 2004; Reiss *et al.*, 1996). Using diffusion tensor imaging to examine axonal integrity in the frontal lobes of children and adults, Klingberg *et al.* (1999) found that white matter continues to increase into the second decade of life in this region, with the white matter increase located in dorsal prefrontal rather than orbitofrontal cortex (Reiss *et al.*, 1996). While both these prefrontal regions are implicated in early-onset disorders, such as autistic spectrum disorders, ADHD, OCD and schizophrenia (Barnett *et al.*, 1999; Brewer *et al.*, 1996, 2001, 2006; Kopala *et al.*, 1989, 1993, 1994; Moberg *et al.*, 1999;

Pantelis *et al.*, 1997), the impact on DLPFC versus OFC in these disorders may be dependent on the developmental stage of the brain at the time of their onset (Brewer *et al.*, 2006). Structurally, OFC matures later than DLPFC, although myelination occurs earlier than that occurring in DLPFC (Yakovlev & Lecours, 1967; Gogtay *et al.*, 2004). Such differential rates of change across brain development may have implications for the nature and extent of functional abnormalities observed, depending on the age of onset of psychiatric disorders along this trajectory (Pantelis *et al.*, 2003b).

Normative investigations have established that the development of executive functions follows a multi-stage process, with different EFs emerging throughout childhood and adolescence at various stages. Accelerated growth periods, thought to reflect underlying cortical maturation (Levin *et al.*, 1991), have been reported in the frontal region between birth and 2 years of age, 7–9 years, 11–13 years, 14–16 years and finally at 18–20 years (Hudspeth & Pribram, 1992; Thatcher, 1992; Thatcher *et al.*, 1987). The initial and last growth periods are greatest in magnitude and are associated with an increase in cognitive functioning (Thatcher, 1992), so that maturation of the EF system parallels development of the frontal region. Neuropsychological literature supports this and has identified that the emergence of executive abilities follows a timeline, with some skills coming "online" considerably earlier than others (Anderson *et al.*, 2001; Brewer *et al.*, 2006; De Luca *et al.*, 2003; Levin *et al.*, 1991). The higher-level cognitive changes apparent in adolescence also occur in concert with maturation of social interaction and increase in risk-taking behavior (Spear, 2000) and are accompanied by improved capacity in social cognition, response inhibition, monitoring, emotion regulation and the capacity for abstract, reflective and hypothetical thinking (Nelson *et al.*, 2005; Paus, 2005).

Smith *et al.* (1992) supported these notions in their study demonstrating incremental improvement on frontal-lobe tasks between age 10–13 years, including the obtainment of a number of executive functions similar to that of an adult. At this age children start to develop the cognitive capabilities to maximize executive functioning, to deal with situations requiring novel strategies, and capacity for independent and purposeful behavior. In their investigation of EF maturation, Levin *et al.* (1991) found significant age-related increments in ability between age 9–12 years, specifically in the ability to problem solve, plan, form concepts, verbal reasoning and strategy use. Anderson et al. (2001) also noted that cognitive flexibility and monitoring had reached adult levels of maturity by 11 years, that planning and goal-setting skills showed some maturation around 12 years of age, but that attentional control and processing speed demonstrated the most rapid growth spurts between 7–9 years and 15 years of age.

Conklin et al. (2007) specifically investigated working memory development and also noted a protracted trajectory, with forward digit and spatial span (13–15 years and 11–12 years) developing earlier than backward conditions of these tasks (16–17 years and 13–15 years), due to the more demanding manipulation requirements. Age-related developments were however noted on SWM tasks until 16–17 years of age, possibly due to strategic and planning demands requiring greater cognitive maturity. The authors noted that the order in which these skills developed closely paralleled the development of the neural substrates thought to underlie these cognitive skills. In their cross-sectional study across the life span from age 8–65, De Luca et al. (2003) found that ability on a SWM task gradually improved during adolescence and early adulthood, with optimal performance in early adulthood (mid-20s), and a gradual deterioration after age 30. A significant gender effect was also found, with males outperforming females at all ages on this spatial task. Taking account of such gender effects and changes across the life span is relevant to assessing patients at different developmental stages and at different phases of illness.

Despite the above-mentioned studies, there are inconsistencies in the literature as to when a number of executive abilities are fully developed. This reflects the multifaceted nature of the system and the methodological issues in their assessment, given that executive function tests differ in their complexity and the degree to which they require other executive and non-executive type skills. Further, there may be discrepancies between documenting when an EF skill emerges and is identifiable via a child's ability to complete a test, versus the time at which it is fully matured. Luna et al. (2004) describe a useful "change point" analysis technique that documents the time at which improvement in performance plateaus. Such developments may be difficult to detect on standardized tests and may require different tests (or versions of) relevant to various developmental

stages. Executive functions will also depend on the development of several other cognitive processes, such as attentional control and processing speed, which are closely aligned and necessary for good executive performance (Luna et al., 2004; Luna & Sweeney, 2004). Thus, during adolescence and early adulthood individuals undertake and coordinate such abilities more efficiently, allowing greater mastery of increasingly complex executive skills (Tamm et al., 2002).

Additionally, EF maturation may be better assessed by measuring the neural system changes relevant to undertaking such skills with greater efficiency, as demonstrated by recent fMRI studies examining inhibitory control in subjects from childhood to adulthood (Luna et al., 2004; Tamm et al., 2002). In the study by Tamm et al. (2002), whilst there were no behavioral differences identified in performance, with all ages (8–20 years) making relatively few errors, the younger age group activated greater regions of the prefrontal cortex to perform the same task as their older counterparts, who demonstrated increasingly selective activation in distinct regions implicated in response inhibition. The greater cortical involvement seen in the younger group was considered to result from inefficient recruitment of cortical regions and poor management of multiple demands. Luna et al. (2004) found comparable results, reporting that although the ability to inhibit a response could be observed in very young children, efficiency at performing this skill was not achieved until late adolescence, supporting the notion of parallel development in cognition and cortical (neural) maturation. Documenting the growth curves that map the emergence and maturation (to adult levels) of cognitive skills together with longitudinal imaging to assess changes at the neural level will help future studies that seek to understand the emergence of deficits in psychiatric disorders and the neural systems that underpin them.

The relevance to psychiatric disorders is that these disorders often have their onset during adolescence at a time when the brain is showing considerable change, particularly in the prefrontal cortex and in maturation of EF abilities. It is likely that the onset of disorder at this stage of maturation disrupts the normal developmental trajectory and may disturb the developmental processes at a neural as well as functional level. Plotting the growth curves of brain structure and function in these disorders and identifying the nature of the disruption in brain maturation caused by or preceding the onset of psychiatric conditions may help explain the severity of the executive function deficits observed in such conditions. Thus, in schizophrenia, functions that mature early in life when the brain is more adaptable show fewer deficits in comparison with functions that develop later, such as executive abilities (Pantelis *et al.*, 2003b, 2005). Therefore, in order to understand the deficits in executive function in psychiatric disorders, it is important to consider these in the context of brain maturational changes affecting the executive system and their neural substrate.

The notion that the emergence of a psychiatric or neurological disorder at a critical stage of development is associated with "developmental arrest" of key functions that should be emerging at particular maturational stages has a number of implications. First, it would suggest that deficits in those cognitive domains that have yet to develop would be observed across a range of disorders that have their onset early during critical developmental stages. There is evidence to support this notion, for example, deficits in SWM are observed at all stages of schizophrenia (Brewer *et al.*, 2006; Pantelis *et al.*, 1997; Wood *et al.*, 2003), in OCD (Purcell *et al.*, 1998), and in ADHD (Barnett *et al.*, 1999). Second, earlier age of onset would be associated with more profound deficits, though there is limited evidence to support this as yet, and this may depend upon whether the neural substrate has already been damaged at earlier developmental stages, such that patients "grow into deficit" (Lipska & Weinberger, 2000; Lipska *et al.*, 1993; Weinberger, 1987). Third, as already suggested, the dynamic interplay of the emergence of illness and brain maturation during childhood and adolescence suggests that the approach to early-onset disorders, like schizophrenia, should be to examine whether the disorder is a consequence of anomalous trajectories in brain maturation, both structurally and functionally, from childhood through to adulthood. If this is the case, it raises interesting questions about the factors driving such anomalous development, including genetic and non-genetic influences on brain development.

Genetic influences on executive functions

Studies have begun to examine the relevance of genetic factors to the development of the frontal lobes and executive functions and the relevance of these

genes to psychiatric disorders. For example, evidence of an association between genes and performance on neuropsychological measures associated with frontal-subcortical networks has generated interest in psychiatric disorders in which these networks are dysfunctional, such as schizophrenia and depressive disorder. Further, gene–environment interactions have differing effects on various brain regions at specific developmental stages (Cannon, 2005; Winterer & Goldman, 2003), suggesting a complex interplay between developmental stage, brain region, type of disorder and time of onset. Given disorders such as schizophrenia have been proposed to be neurodevelopmental in nature, this has significant implications for understanding the emergence of different cognitive deficits at different stages of the illness.

Current research aims to identify genes that increase susceptibility to schizophrenia and/or contribute to the observed cognitive deficits. Evidence for the heritability of cognitive deficits in schizophrenia is demonstrated in familial studies showing that non-affected relatives manifest comparable deficits to patients (Weinberger *et al.*, 2001). Such evidence has been used to suggest that schizophrenia-relevant genes also disrupt cognition and, therefore, greater severity of such deficits will be observed in those at greater genetic risk for the disorder (Faraone *et al.*, 2000; Johnson *et al.*, 2003). Given that such a genetic basis has been found, it should be possible to identify the specific genes mediating this relationship.

A number of genes are being examined in assessing the relationship between cognition and genetic vulnerability to schizophrenia, including COMT (Barnett *et al.*, 2007b, 2007c; Harrison, 2007; MacDonald *et al.*, 2007), TRAX (Cannon *et al.*, 2005; Thomson *et al.*, 2005; Zhang *et al.*, 2005), MAO-A (Norton *et al.*, 2002; Zammit *et al.*, 2004) and MTHFR (Roffman *et al.*, 2007a, 2007b). However, interest has primarily centered on the COMT gene, which plays a significant role in the uptake, processing and catabolism of dopamine in the frontal lobe region. Dopamine has been strongly implicated in cognition, including working-memory processes (Ho *et al.*, 2005; Sawaguchi & Goldman-Rakic, 1991), and the degree of heritability for short-term memory and working memory capacity (verbal and spatial) has been reported to be almost 50% (Shah & Miyake, 1996). The transmission of a specific allele of the COMT gene (*Val*) has been related to poorer prefrontal cortex functioning; in contrast, the *Met* allele confers a lower level of activity and therefore a reduced level of dopamine catabolism, leading to better bioavailability of dopamine and better cognitive performance (Weinberger *et al.*, 2001).

While promising, however, the majority of studies fail to find a significant relationship to support the COMT gene as a susceptibility locus for schizophrenia (Egan *et al.*, 2001; Goldberg *et al.*, 2003; Joober *et al.*, 2002; Strous *et al.*, 1997). Further, studies examining the relationship between COMT and EF performance have been mixed. The most consistent evidence shows that patients with the *Val* allele perform more poorly on EF tasks, including WCST and working-memory tasks, although the effect size has been small (Egan *et al.*, 2001; Goldberg *et al.*, 2003; Joober *et al.*, 2002). This may result from poorer prefrontal cortical efficiency due to the higher dopamine catabolism produced by this genotype. Interestingly, this relationship is reported irrespective of diagnosis, suggesting that the influence of COMT is generic. Therefore, COMT does not appear related to the risk for schizophrenia, although it may play a role in mediating cognitive activity associated with the PFC via its influence on dopamine.

Further, a number of studies have failed to demonstrate a relationship between COMT and EF neuropsychological performance. For example, Ho *et al.* (2005) found no significant relationship between COMT genotype and clinical diagnosis, no relationship between COMT and EFs, and no significant interaction between COMT genotype, EF performance and clinical diagnosis. However, using more sensitive electrophysiological measures of EF, Ehlis *et al.* (2007) recently found a strong relationship between COMT genotype and cognition in schizophrenia. Thus, more sensitive measures of cortical activity may be required to elucidate this relationship (Winterer & Goldman, 2003).

As above, it may be relevant to examine the genetics of schizophrenia from a developmental (brain maturational) perspective. Recent work (Tunbridge *et al.*, 2007a, 2007b; Weickert *et al.*, 2007) has examined the expression of specific dopamine-related genes or dopamine markers across the postnatal period. Weickert *et al.* (2007) found changes in different pre- and postsynaptic dopamine markers in the frontal lobe during postnatal development ranging from early infancy to old age. In particular, a peak found in the dopamine D1 receptor in early adulthood/adolescence may be relevant to the emergence

of psychiatric disorders. Tunbridge *et al.* (2007b) has similarly mapped changes in COMT activity in comparable age groups and reported a significant increase in COMT enzyme activity from the neonate to adulthood period, with a specific increase or peak occurring at approximately adulthood (31–43 years of age) and a further non-significant decrease between 68–86 years of age. Further, Barnett *et al.* (2007b) in a study of male children showed that COMT had a significant effect on EF and IQ tests, particularly when stage of pubertal development was considered.

These data suggest that protracted developmental changes in dopamine activity are occurring in the prefrontal cortex during this postnatal period. Further investigation of dopamine and COMT on the maturation of the frontal lobe region is clearly warranted, especially considering that other dopaminergic markers have been found to reach adult levels prior to adolescence, suggesting that this gene may play a specific role in the maturation of these later-developing executive skills (Tunbridge *et al.*, 2007a).

We suggest that a better understanding of the relationship between onset of a psychiatric disorder, executive functions and genetics, requires examination of a gene's influence on the development of the frontal lobe and maturation of different executive skills at different stages of childhood and adulthood. This will provide greater insight into how vulnerability to a particular disorder, such as predisposition for schizophrenia, interacts or disrupts this relationship at a critical developmental stage, resulting in aberrant maturational and neurobiological processes that lead to the features of the illness, including neuropsychological deficits.

Conclusions

Despite the uncertainty regarding the underlying components comprising the EF system, the available evidence supports its fractionation into subcomponents, with different executive tests assessing unique cognitive abilities (Duncan *et al.*, 1997; Miyake *et al.*, 2000). These abilities may be differentially affected in different psychiatric disorders, and we suggest that the nature and extent of the EF deficits observed may depend on the timing of the onset of the disorder in the context of the stage of maturation of such functions. This is particularly the case for psychiatric disorders of childhood and adolescence, which develop during a critical period when EFs and their neural substrates are still maturing; with different EFs maturing at different rates and stages over this time. The onset of disorder at a critical stage of such maturation may result in "developmental arrest" of such ability; this is exemplified most profoundly for spatial working memory in patients developing schizophrenia. Further, an understanding of the genetics relevant to such abilities needs to take account of how genes relevant to brain maturation interact with ability development; this is needed before examining how such genes may relate to the genes that code specific disorders.

To conclude, the following should be considered in understanding the relevance of the executive system in psychiatric disorders:

(1) The need to use a developmental and longitudinal framework to understand psychiatric illness; examination of "growth curves" in comparison with healthy individuals will provide important information about how deficits arise.

(2) Understanding the differential development of EF skills is likely to be relevant to the nature and progression of deficits in psychiatric illness. We propose that functions developing early may be relatively spared, at least initially, while late-developing abilities will be more severely affected.

(3) The diagnostic specificity of EF deficits may depend on the nature of the disorder, and the timing of its onset in relation to maturational stage.

(4) A maturational perspective may also be relevant to understanding the genetics of various psychiatric disorders, particularly when examining the relationship to the EF system.

Acknowledgments

We thank David Griffiths for help in generating the Figure on neurodevelopmental trajectories. This work was supported by grants from the NHMRC Australia (350241 & 566529).

References

Ackerman, P. L., Beier, M. E. & Boyle, M. O. (2005). Working memory and intelligence: the same or different constructs? *Psychological Bulletin*, **131**, 30–60.

Anderson, V. A., Anderson, P., Northam, E., Jacobs, R. & Catroppa, C. (2001). Development of executive functions through late childhood and adolescence in an Australian sample. *Developmental Neuropsychology*, **20**(1), 385–406.

Aron, A. R., Robbins, T. W. & Poldrack, R. A. (2004). Inhibition and the right inferior frontal cortex. *Trends in Cognitive Science*, **8**(4), 170–177.

Badcock, J. C., Michiel, P. T. & Rock, D. (2005). Spatial working memory and planning ability: contrasts between schizophrenia and bipolar I disorder. *Cortex*, **41**(6), 753–763.

Baddeley, A. (1996). The fractionation of working memory. *Proceedings of the National Academy of Sciences USA*, **93**(24), 13468–13472.

Baddeley, A. & Della Sala, S. (1996). Working memory and executive control. *Philosophical Transactions of the Royal Society London Series B Biological Sciences*, **351**(1346), 1397–1403; discussion 1403–1394.

Baird, A., Dewar, B. K., Critchley, H. *et al.* (2006). Cognitive functioning after medial frontal lobe damage including the anterior cingulate cortex: a preliminary investigation. *Brain and Cognition*, **60**(2), 166–175.

Banich, M. T. & Weissman, D. H. (2000). One of twenty questions for the twenty-first century: how do brain regions interact and integrate information? *Brain and Cognition*, **42**(1), 29–32.

Bannon, S., Gonsalvez, C. J., Croft, R. J. & Boyce, P. M. (2006). Executive functions in obsessive-compulsive disorder: state or trait deficits? *Australian and New Zealand Journal of Psychiatry*, **40**(11–12), 1031–1038.

Barnett, J. H., Croudace, T. J., Jaycock, S. *et al.* (2007a). Improvement and decline of cognitive function in schizophrenia over one year: a longitudinal investigation using latent growth modelling. *British Medical Council Psychiatry*, **7**, 16.

Barnett, J. H., Heron, J., Ring, S. M. *et al.* (2007b). Gender-specific effects of the catechol-O-methyltransferase Val108/158Met polymorphism on cognitive function in children. *American Journal of Psychiatry*, **164**(1), 142–149.

Barnett, J. H., Jones, P. B., Robbins, T. W. & Muller, U. (2007c). Effects of the catechol-O-methyltransferase Val158Met polymorphism on executive function: a meta-analysis of the Wisconsin Card Sort Test in schizophrenia and healthy controls. *Molecular Psychiatry*, **12**(5), 502–509.

Barnett, R., Maruff, P., Purcell, R. *et al.* (1999). Impairment of olfactory identification in obsessive-compulsive disorder. *Psychological Medicine*, **29**(5), 1227–1233.

Barnett, R., Maruff, P., Vance, A. *et al.* (2001). Abnormal executive function in attention deficit hyperactivity disorder: the effect of stimulant medication and age on spatial working memory. *Psychological Medicine*, **31**(6), 1107–1115.

Bartzokis, G. (2002). Schizophrenia: breakdown in the well-regulated lifelong process of brain development and maturation. *Neuropsychopharmacology*, **27**(4), 672–683.

Bartzokis, G., Beckson, M., Lu, P. H. *et al.* (2001). Age-related changes in frontal and temporal lobe volumes in men: a magnetic resonance imaging study. *Archives of General Psychiatry*, **58**(5), 461–465.

Bayliss, D. M., Jarrold, C., Gunn, D. M. & Baddeley, A. D. (2003). The complexities of complex span: explaining individual differences in working memory in children and adults. *Journal of Experimental Psychology: General*, **132**(1), 71–92.

Bechara, A., Damasio, A. R., Damasio, H. & Anderson, S. W. (1994). Insensitivity to future consequences following damage to human prefrontal cortex. *Cognition*, **50**(1–3), 7–15.

Bechara, A., Damasio, H., & Damasio, A. R. (2000). Emotion, decision making and the orbitofrontal cortex. *Cerebral Cortex*, **10**(3), 295–307.

Bechara, A., Damasio, H., Tranel, D. & Anderson, S. W. (1998). Dissociation of working memory from decision making within the human prefrontal cortex. *Journal of Neuroscience*, **18**(1), 428–437.

Benes, F. M., Turtle, M., Khan, Y. & Farol, P. (1994). Myelination of a key relay zone in the hippocampal formation occurs in the human brain during childhood, adolescence and adulthood. *Archives of General Psychiatry*, **51**, 477–484.

Bennett, P., Ong, B. & Ponsford, J. (2005). Assessment of executive dysfunction following traumatic brain injury: comparison of the BADS with other clinical neuropsychological measures. *Journal of the International Neuropsychological Society*, **11**(5), 606–613.

Bialystok, E., Craik, F. I., Grady, C. et al. (2005). Effect of bilingualism on cognitive control in the Simon task: evidence from MEG. *Neuroimage*, **24**(1), 40–49.

Bialystok, E., Craik, F. I., Klein, R. & Viswanathan, M. (2004). Bilingualism, aging, and cognitive control: evidence from the Simon task. *Psychology and Aging*, **19**(2), 290–303.

Biederman, J., Monuteaux, M. C., Doyle, A. E. et al. (2004). Impact of executive function deficits and attention-deficit/hyperactivity disorder (ADHD) on academic outcomes in children. *Journal of Consulting Clinical and Psychology*, **72**(5), 757–766.

Biederman, J., Petty, C. R., Fried, R. et al. (2007). Stability of executive function deficits into young adult years: a prospective longitudinal follow-up study of grown up males with ADHD. *Acta Psychiatrica Scandinavica*, **116**(2), 129–136.

Blakemore, S. J. & Choudhury, S. (2006). Development of the adolescent brain: implications for executive function and social cognition. *Journal of Child Psychology and Psychiatry*, **47**(3–4), 296–312.

Brewer, W. J., Edwards, J., Anderson, V., Robinson, T. & Pantelis, C. (1996). Neuropsychological, olfactory, and hygiene deficits in men with negative symptom schizophrenia. *Biological Psychiatry*, **40**(10), 1021–1031.

Brewer, W. J., Francey, S. M., Wood, S. J. et al. (2005). Memory impairments identified in people at ultra-high risk for psychosis who later develop first-episode psychosis. *American Journal of Psychiatry*, **162**(1), 71–78.

Brewer, W. J., Pantelis, C., Anderson, V. et al. (2001). Stability of olfactory identification deficits in neuroleptic-naive patients with first-episode psychosis. *American Journal of Psychiatry*, **158**(1), 107–115.

Brewer, W. J., Wood, S. J., Phillips, L. J. et al. (2006). Generalized and specific cognitive performance in clinical high-risk cohorts: a review highlighting potential vulnerability markers for psychosis. *Schizophrenia Bulletin*, **32**(3), 538–555.

Burgess, P. W. (2000). Strategy application disorder: the role of the frontal lobes in human multitasking. *Psychological Research*, **63**(3–4), 279–288.

Burgess, P. W. & Shallice, T. (1996). Bizarre responses, rule detection and frontal lobe lesions. *Cortex*, **32**(2), 241–259.

Burgess, P. W., Alderman, N., Evans, J., Emslie, H. & Wilson, B. A. (1998). The ecological validity of tests of executive function. *Journal of the International Neuropsychology Society*, **4**(6), 547–558.

Callicott, J. H., Mattay, V. S., Verchinski, B. A. et al. (2003). Complexity of prefrontal cortical dysfunction in schizophrenia: more than up or down. *American Journal of Psychiatry*, **160**(12), 2209–2215.

Cannon, T. D. (2005). The inheritance of intermediate phenotypes for schizophrenia. *Current Opinion in Psychiatry*, **18**(2), 135–140.

Cannon, T. D., Hennah, W., van Erp, T. G. et al. (2005). Association of DISC1/TRAX haplotypes with schizophrenia, reduced prefrontal gray matter, and impaired short- and long-term memory. *Archives of General Psychiatry*, **62**(11), 1205–1213.

Carter, C. S., Botvinick, M. M. & Cohen, J. D. (1999). The contribution of the anterior cingulate cortex to executive processes in cognition. *Reviews in Neuroscience*, **10**(1), 49–57.

Castner, S. A., Goldman-Rakic, P. S. & Williams, G. V. (2004). Animal models of working memory: insights for targeting cognitive dysfunction in schizophrenia. *Psychopharmacology (Berlin)*, **174**(1), 111–125.

Chayer, C. & Freedman, M. (2001). Frontal lobe functions. *Current Neurology and Neuroscience Report*, **1**(6), 547–552.

Cicerone, K. D. & Tanenbaum, L. N. (1997). Disturbance of social cognition after traumatic orbitofrontal brain injury. *Archives of Clinical Neuropsychology*, **12**(2), 173–188.

Clark, L. & Manes, F. (2004). Social and emotional decision-making following frontal lobe injury. *Neurocase*, **10**(5), 398–403.

Cohen, J. D., Botvinick, M. & Carter, C. S. (2000). Anterior cingulate and prefrontal cortex: who's in control? *Nature Neuroscience*, **3**(5), 421–423.

Collette, F. & Van der Linden, M. (2002). Brain imaging of the central executive component of working memory. *Neuroscience and Biobehavioral Review*, **26**(2), 105–125.

Collette, F., Salmon, E., Van der Linden, M. *et al.* (1999). Regional brain activity during tasks devoted to the central executive of working memory. *Brain Research: Cognitive Brain Research*, **7**(3), 411–417.

Collette, F., Van der Linden, M., Laureys, S. *et al.* (2005). Exploring the unity and diversity of the neural substrates of executive functioning. *Human Brain Mapping*, **25**(4), 409–423.

Conklin, H. M., Luciana, M., Hooper, C. J. & Yarger, R. S. (2007). Working memory performance in typically developing children and adolescents: behavioral evidence of protracted frontal lobe development. *Developmental Neuropsychology*, **31**(1), 103–128.

Crawford, S. & Channon, S. (2002). Dissociation between performance on abstract tests of executive function and problem solving in real-life-type situations in normal aging. *Aging and Mental Health*, **6**(1), 12–21.

Cummings, J. L. (1995). Anatomic and behavioral aspects of frontal-subcortical circuits. *Annals of the New York Academy of Science*, **769**, 1–13.

Curson, D. A., Duke, P. J., Harvey, C. A., Pantelis, C. & Barnes, T. R. (1999). Four behavioural syndromes of schizophrenia: a replication in a second inner-London epidemiological sample. *Schizophrenia Research*, **37**(2), 165–176.

D'Esposito, M., Cooney, J. W., Gazzaley, A., Gibbs, S. E. & Postle, B. R. (2006). Is the prefrontal cortex necessary for delay task performance? Evidence from lesion and FMRI data. *Journal of the International Neuropsychology Society*, **12**(2), 248–260.

Damasio, A. R., Tranel, D. & Damasio, H. (1990). Individuals with sociopathic behavior caused by frontal damage fail to respond autonomically to social stimuli. *Behavior and Brain Research*, **41**(2), 81–94.

Damasio, H., Grabowski, T., Frank, R., Galaburda, A. M. & Damasio, A. R. (1994). The return of Phineas Gage: clues about the brain from the skull of a famous patient. *Science*, **264**(5162), 1102–1105.

De Luca, C. R., Wood, S. J., Anderson, V. *et al.* (2003). Normative data from the CANTAB. I: development of executive function over the lifespan. *Journal of Clinical and Experimental Neuropsychology*, **25**(2), 242–254.

Doyle, A. E. (2006). Executive functions in attention-deficit/hyperactivity disorder. *Journal of Clinical Psychiatry*, **67** (Suppl 8), 21–26.

Duncan, J. & Owen, A. M. (2000). Common regions of the human frontal lobe recruited by diverse cognitive demands. *Trends in Neuroscience*, **23**(10), 475–483.

Duncan, J., Burgess, P. & Emslie, H. (1995). Fluid intelligence after frontal lobe lesions. *Neuropsychologia*, **33**(3), 261–268.

Duncan, J., Johnson, R., Swales, M. & Freer, C. (1997). Frontal lobe deficits after head injury: unity and diversity of function. *Cognitive Neuropsychology*, **14**(5), 713–741.

Egan, M. F., Goldberg, T. E., Kolachana, B. S. *et al.* (2001). Effect of COMT Val108/158 Met genotype on frontal lobe function and risk for schizophrenia. *Proceedings of the National Academy of Sciences USA*, **98**(12), 6917–6922.

Ehlis, A. C., Reif, A., Herrmann, M. J., Lesch, K. P. & Fallgatter, A. J. (2007). Impact of catechol-O-methyltransferase on prefrontal brain functioning in schizophrenia spectrum disorders. *Neuropsychopharmacology*, **32**(1), 162–170.

Elliott, R. (2003). Executive functions and their disorders. *British Medical Bulletin*, **65**, 49–59.

Engle, R. W., Tuholski, S. W., Laughlin, J. E. & Conway, A. R. (1999). Working memory, short-term memory, and general fluid intelligence: a latent-variable approach. *Journal of Experimental Psychology: General*, **128**(3), 309–331.

Eslinger, P. J. & Damasio, A. R. (1985). Severe disturbance of higher cognition after bilateral frontal lobe ablation: patient EVR. *Neurology*, **35**(12), 1731–1741.

Faraone, S. V., Seidman, L. J., Kremen, W. S. *et al.* (2000). Neuropsychologic functioning among the nonpsychotic relatives of schizophrenic patients: the effect of genetic loading. *Biological Psychiatry*, **48**(2), 120–126.

Fassbender, C., Murphy, K., Foxe, J. J. *et al.* (2004). A topography of executive functions and their interactions revealed by functional magnetic resonance imaging. *Brain Research Cognitive Brain Research*, **20**(2), 132–143.

Fletcher, P. C., Shallice, T. & Dolan, R. J. (2000). "Sculpting the response space" – an account of left prefrontal activation at encoding. *Neuroimage*, **12**(4), 404–417.

Fornito, A., Whittle, S., Wood, S. J. *et al.* (2006). The influence of sulcal variability on morphometry of the human anterior cingulate and paracingulate cortex. *Neuroimage*, **33**(3), 843–854.

Fornito, A., Yucel, M., Wood, S. *et al.* (2004). Individual differences in anterior cingulate/paracingulate morphology are related to executive functions in healthy males. *Cerebral Cortex*, **14**(4), 424–431.

131

Friston, K. J. (1998). The disconnection hypothesis. *Schizophrenia Research*, **30**(2), 115–125.

Friston, K. J., Fletcher, P., Josephs, O. *et al.* (1998). Event-related fMRI: characterizing differential responses. *Neuroimage*, **7**(1), 30–40.

Frith, C. D., Blakemore, S. J. & Wolpert, D. M. (2000). Abnormalities in the awareness and control of action. *Philosophical Transactions of the Royal Society London Series B Biological Science*, **355**(1404), 1771–1788.

Fuster, J. M. (1991). The prefrontal cortex and its relation to behavior. *Progress in Brain Research*, **87**, 201–211.

Fuster, J. M. (1993). Frontal lobes. *Current Opinion in Neurobiology*, **3**(2), 160–165.

Fuster, J. M. (2000). Prefrontal neurons in networks of executive memory. *Brain Research Bulletin*, **52**(5), 331–336.

Gerton, B. K., Brown, T. T., Meyer-Lindenberg, A. *et al.* (2004). Shared and distinct neurophysiological components of the digits forward and backward tasks as revealed by functional neuroimaging. *Neuropsychologia*, **42**(13), 1781–1787.

Giedd, J. N. (2004). Structural magnetic resonance imaging of the adolescent brain. *Annals of the New York Academy of Sciences*, **1021**, 77–85.

Giedd, J. N., Blumenthal, J., Jeffries, N. O. *et al.* (1999). Brain development during childhood and adolescence: a longitudinal MRI study. *Nature Neuroscience*, **2**(10), 861–863.

Glahn, D. C., Bearden, C. E., Barguil, M. *et al.* (2007). The neurocognitive signature of psychotic bipolar disorder. *Biological Psychiatry*, **62**(8), 910–916.

Gochman, P. A., Greenstein, D., Sporn, A. *et al.* (2005). IQ stabilization in childhood-onset schizophrenia. *Schizophrenia Research*, **77**(2–3), 271–277.

Gogtay, N., Giedd, J. N., Lusk, L. *et al.* (2004). Dynamic mapping of human cortical development during childhood through early adulthood. *Proceedings of the National Academy of Sciences USA*, **101**(21), 8174–8179.

Goldberg, T. E., Egan, M. F., Gscheidle, T. *et al.* (2003). Executive subprocesses in working memory: relationship to catechol-O-methyltransferase Val158Met genotype and schizophrenia. *Archives of General Psychiatry*, **60**(9), 889–896.

Hanninen, T., Hallikainen, M., Koivisto, K. *et al.* (1997). Decline of frontal lobe functions in subjects with age-associated memory impairment. *Neurology*, **48**(1), 148–153.

Happaney, K., Zelazo, P. D. & Stuss, D. T. (2004). Development of orbitofrontal function: current themes and future directions. *Brain and Cognition*, **55**(1), 1–10.

Harrison, B. J., Yucel, M., Shaw, M. *et al.* (2006). Dysfunction of dorsolateral prefrontal cortex in antipsychotic-naive schizophreniform psychosis. *Psychiatry Research*, **148**(1), 23–31.

Harrison, P. J. (2007). Schizophrenia susceptibility genes and neurodevelopment. *Biological Psychiatry*, **61**(10), 1119–1120.

Herrmann, L. L., Goodwin, G. M. & Ebmeier, K. P. (2007). The cognitive neuropsychology of depression in the elderly. *Psychological Medicine*, **37**, 1–10.

Himanen, L., Portin, R., Isoniemi, H. *et al.* (2005). Cognitive functions in relation to MRI findings 30 years after traumatic brain injury. *Brain Injury*, **19**(2), 93–100.

Ho, B. C., Wassink, T. H., O'Leary, D. S. *et al.* (2005). Catechol-O-methyl transferase Val158Met gene polymorphism in schizophrenia: working memory, frontal lobe MRI morphology and frontal cerebral blood flow. *Molecular Psychiatry*, **10**(3), 229, 287–298.

Hudspeth, W. J. & Pribram, K. H. (1992). Psychophysiological indices of cerebral maturation. *International Journal of Psychophysiology*, **12**(1), 19–29.

Jernigan, T. L. & Tallal, P. (1990). Late childhood changes in brain morphology observable with MRI. *Developmental Medicine and Child Neurology*, **32**(5), 379–385.

Johnson, J. K., Tuulio-Henriksson, A., Pirkola, T. *et al.* (2003). Do schizotypal symptoms mediate the relationship between genetic risk for schizophrenia and impaired neuropsychological performance in co-twins of schizophrenic patients? *Biological Psychiatry*, **54**(11), 1200–1204.

Joober, R., Gauthier, J., Lal, S. *et al.* (2002). Catechol-O-methyltransferase Val-108/158-Met gene variants associated with performance on the Wisconsin Card Sorting Test. *Archives of General Psychiatry*, **59**(7), 662–663.

Klingberg, T., Vaidya, C. J., Gabrieli, J. D. E., Moseley, M. E. & Hedehus, M. (1999). Myelination and organization of the frontal white matter in children: a diffusion tensor MRI study. *Neuroreport*, **10**, 2817–2821.

Kolb, B. (1989). Brain development, plasticity, and behavior. *American Psychologist*, **44**(9), 1203–1212.

Kopala, L., Clark, C. & Hurwitz, T. A. (1989). Sex differences in olfactory function in schizophrenia. *American Journal of Psychiatry*, **146**(10), 1320–1322.

Kopala, L. C., Clark, C. & Hurwitz, T. (1993). Olfactory deficits in neuroleptic naive patients with schizophrenia. *Schizophrenia Research*, **8**(3), 245–250.

Kopala, L. C., Good, K. P. & Honer, W. G. (1994). Olfactory hallucinations and olfactory identification ability in patients with schizophrenia and other psychiatric disorders. *Schizophrenia Research*, **12**(3), 205–211.

Lencz, T., Smith, C. W., McLaughlin, D. *et al.* (2006). Generalized and specific neurocognitive deficits in prodromal schizophrenia. *Biological Psychiatry*, **59**(9), 863–871.

Levin, H., Culhane, K. A., Hartmann, J. *et al.* (1991). Developmental changes in performance on tests of purported frontal lobe functioning. *Developmental Neuropsychology*, **7**(3), 377–395.

Levine, B., Stuss, D. T., Milberg, W. P. *et al.* (1998). The effects of focal and diffuse brain damage on strategy application: evidence from focal lesions, traumatic brain injury and normal aging. *Journal of the International Neuropsychology Society*, **4**(3), 247–264.

Levy, R. & Goldman-Rakic, P. S. (1999). Association of storage and processing functions in the dorsolateral prefrontal cortex of the nonhuman primate. *Journal of Neuroscience*, **19**(12), 5149–5158.

Lipska, B. & Weinberger, D. (2000). To model a psychiatric disorder in animals: schizophrenia as a reality test. *Neuropsychopharmacology*, **23**(3), 223–239.

Lipska, B. K., Jaskiw, G. E. & Weinberger, D. R. (1993). Postpubertal emergence of hyperresponsiveness to stress and to amphetamine after neonatal excitotoxic hippocampal damage: a potential animal model of schizophrenia. *Neuropsychopharmacology*, **9**(1), 67–75.

Luna, B. & Sweeney, J. A. (2001). Studies of brain and cognitive maturation through childhood and adolescence: a strategy for testing neurodevelopmental hypotheses. *Schizophrenia Bulletin*, **27**(3), 443–455.

Luna, B. & Sweeney, J. A. (2004). The emergence of collaborative brain function: FMRI studies of the development of response inhibition. *Annals of the New York Academy of Sciences*, **1021**, 296–309.

Luna, B., Garver, K. E., Urban, T. A., Lazar, N. A. & Sweeney, J. A. (2004). Maturation of cognitive processes from late childhood to adulthood. *Child Development*, **75**(5), 1357–1372.

MacDonald, A. W., 3rd, Carter, C. S., Flory, J. D., Ferrell, R. E. & Manuck, S. B. (2007). COMT val158Met and executive control: a test of the benefit of specific deficits to translational research. *Journal of Abnormal Psychology*, **116**(2), 306–312.

Macmillan, M. (2000a). Nineteenth-century inhibitory theories of thinking: Bain, Ferrier, Freud (and Phineas Gage). *History of Psychology*, **3**(3), 187–217.

Macmillan, M. (2000b). Restoring Phineas Gage: a 150th retrospective. *Journal of the History of Neuroscience*, **9**(1), 46–66.

Martinussen, R. & Tannock, R. (2006). Working memory impairments in children with attention-deficit hyperactivity disorder with and without comorbid language learning disorders. *Journal of Clinical and Experimental Neuropsychology*, **28**(7), 1073–1094.

Maruff, P., Wilson, P. & Currie, J. (2003). Abnormalities of motor imagery associated with somatic passivity phenomena in schizophrenia. *Schizophrenia Research*, **60**(2–3), 229–238.

Mathalon, D. H., Bennett, A., Askari, N. *et al.* (2003). Response-monitoring dysfunction in aging and Alzheimer's disease: an event-related potential study. *Neurobiology of Aging*, **24**(5), 675–685.

Mayberg, H. S., Brannan, S. K., Mahurin, R. K. *et al.* (1997). Cingulate function in depression: a potential predictor of treatment response. *Neuroreport*, **8**(4), 1057–1061.

Mega, M. S. & Cummings, J. L. (1994). Frontal-subcortical circuits and neuropsychiatric disorders. *Journal of Neuropsychiatry and Clinical Neuroscience*, **6**(4), 358–370.

Meyer-Lindenberg, A. S., Olsen, R. K., Kohn, P. D. *et al.* (2005). Regionally specific disturbance of dorsolateral prefrontal-hippocampal functional connectivity in schizophrenia. *Archives of General Psychiatry*, **62**(4), 379–386.

Miyake, A., Friedman, N. P., Emerson, M. J. *et al.* (2000). The unity and diversity of executive functions and their contributions to complex "Frontal Lobe" tasks: a latent variable analysis. *Cognitive Psychology*, **41**(1), 49–100.

Moberg, P. J., Agrin, R., Gur, R. E. *et al.* (1999). Olfactory dysfunction in schizophrenia: a qualitative and quantitative review. *Neuropsychopharmacology*, **21**(3), 325–340.

Monchi, O., Ko, J. H. & Strafella, A. P. (2006). Striatal dopamine release during performance of executive functions: a [(11)C] raclopride PET study. *Neuroimage*, **33**(3), 907–912.

Moscovitch, M. (1992). Memory and working with memory: A component process model based on modules and central systems. *Journal of Cognitive Neuroscience*, **4**, 257–267.

Nelson, E. E., Leibenluft, E., McClure, E. B. & Pine, D. S. (2005). The social re-orientation of adolescence: a neuroscience perspective on the process and its relation to psychopathology. *Psychological Medicine*, **35**(2), 163–174.

Norton, N., Kirov, G., Zammit, S. *et al.* (2002). Schizophrenia and functional polymorphisms in the MAOA and COMT genes: no evidence for association or epistasis. *American Journal of Medical Genetics*, **114**(5), 491–496.

Orzhekhovskaya, N. S. (1981). Fronto-striatal relationships in primate ontogeny. *Neuroscience and Behavioral Physiology*, **11**(4), 379–385.

Paine, R. W. & Tani, J. (2004). Motor primitive and sequence self-organization in a hierarchical recurrent neural network. *Neural Networks*, **17**(8–9), 1291–1309.

Pantelis, C. & Brewer, W. (1995). Neuropsychological and olfactory dysfunction in schizophrenia: relationship of frontal syndromes to syndromes of schizophrenia. *Schizophrenia Research*, **17**(1), 35–45.

Pantelis, C. & Maruff, P. (2002). The cognitive neuropsychiatric approach to investigating the neurobiology of schizophrenia and other disorders. *Journal of Psychosomatic Research*, **53**(2), 655–664.

Pantelis, C., Barnes, T. R., Nelson, H. E. *et al.* (1997). Frontal-striatal cognitive deficits in patients with chronic schizophrenia. *Brain*, **120**(10), 1823–1843.

Pantelis, C., Velakoulis, D., McGorry, P. D. (2003a). Neuroanatomical abnormalities before and after onset of psychosis: a cross-sectional and longitudinal MRI comparison. *Lancet*, **361**(9354), 281–288.

Pantelis, C., Yucel, M., Wood, S. J., McGorry, P. D. & Velakoulis, D. (2003b). Early and late neurodevelopmental disturbances in schizophrenia and their functional consequences. *Australia and New Zealand Journal of Psychiatry*, **37**(4), 399–406.

Pantelis, C., Yucel, M., Wood, S. J. *et al.* (2005). Structural brain imaging evidence for multiple pathological processes at different stages of brain development in schizophrenia. *Schizophrenia Bulletin*, **31**(3), 672–696.

Passingham, D. & Sakai, K. (2004). The prefrontal cortex and working memory: physiology and brain imaging. *Current Opinion in Neurobiology*, **14**(2), 163–168.

Paul, R. H., Clark, C. R., Lawrence, J. *et al.* (2005). Age-dependent change in executive function and gamma 40 Hz phase synchrony. *Journal of Integrated Neuroscience*, **4**(1), 63–76.

Paus, T. (2005). Mapping brain maturation and cognitive development during adolescence. *Trends in Cognitive Science*, **9**(2), 60–68.

Paus, T., Zijdenbos, A., Worsley, K. *et al.* (1999). Structural maturation of neural pathways in children and adolescents: in vivo study. *Science*, **283**(5409), 1908–1911.

Peers, P. V., Ludwig, C. J., Rorden, C. *et al.* (2005). Attentional functions of parietal and frontal cortex. *Cerebral Cortex*, **15**(10), 1469–1484.

Peterson, B. S., Skudlarski, P., Gatenby, J. C. *et al.* (1999). An fMRI study of Stroop word-color interference: evidence for cingulate subregions subserving multiple distributed attentional systems. *Biological Psychiatry*, **45**(10), 1237–1258.

Pirkola, T., Tuulio-Henriksson, A., Glahn, D. *et al.* (2005). Spatial working memory function in twins with schizophrenia and bipolar disorder. *Biological Psychiatry*, **58**(12), 930–936.

Porter, R. J., Bourke, C. & Gallagher, P. (2007). Neuropsychological impairment in major depression: its nature, origin and clinical significance. *Australian and New Zealand Journal of Psychiatry*, **41**(2), 115–128.

Purcell, R., Maruff, P., Kyrios, M. & Pantelis, C. (1997). Neuropsychological function in young patients with unipolar major depression. *Psychological Medicine*, **27**(6), 1277–1285.

Purcell, R., Maruff, P., Kyrios, M. & Pantelis, C. (1998a). Cognitive deficits in obsessive-compulsive disorder on tests of frontal-striatal function. *Biological Psychiatry*, **43**(5), 348–357.

Purcell, R., Maruff, P., Kyrios, M. & Pantelis, C. (1998b). Neuropsychological deficits in obsessive-compulsive disorder: a comparison with unipolar depression, panic disorder, and normal controls. *Archives of General Psychiatry*, **55**(5), 415–423.

Rao, S. M., Harrington, D. L., Haaland, K. Y. *et al.* (1997). Distributed neural systems underlying the timing of movements. *Journal of Neuroscience*, **17**(14), 5528–5535.

Ratiu, P. & Talos, I. F. (2004). Images in clinical medicine. The tale of Phineas Gage, digitally remastered. *New England Journal of Medicine*, **351**(23), e21.

Ratiu, P., Talos, I. F., Haker, S., Lieberman, D. & Everett, P. (2004). The tale of Phineas Gage, digitally remastered. *Journal of Neurotrauma*, **21**(5), 637–643.

Ravizza, S. M., McCormick, C. A., Schlerf, J. E. *et al.* (2006). Cerebellar damage produces selective deficits in verbal working memory. *Brain*, **129**(2), 306–320.

Reiss, A. L., Abrams, M. T., Singer, H. S., Ross, J. L. & Denckla, M. B. (1996). Brain development, gender and IQ in children: a volumetric imaging study. *Brain*, **119**, 1763–1774.

Reverberi, C., Lavaroni, A., Gigli, G. L., Skrap, M. & Shallice, T. (2005a). Specific impairments of rule induction in different frontal lobe subgroups. *Neuropsychologia*, **43**(3), 460–472.

Reverberi, C., Toraldo, A., D'Agostini, S. & Skrap, M. (2005b). Better without (lateral) frontal cortex? Insight problems solved by frontal patients. *Brain*, **128**(12), 2882–2890.

Rhodes, S. M., Coghill, D. R. & Matthews, K. (2006). Acute neuropsychological effects of methylphenidate in stimulant drug-naive boys with ADHD II – broader executive and non-executive domains. *Journal of Child Psychology and Psychiatry*, **47**(11), 1184–1194.

Riva, D. & Giorgi, C. (2000). The cerebellum contributes to higher functions during development: evidence from a series of children surgically treated for posterior fossa tumours. *Brain*, 123(5), 1051–1061.

Robbins, T. W., James, M., Owen, A. M. *et al.* (1998). A study of performance on tests from the CANTAB battery sensitive to frontal lobe dysfunction in a large sample of normal volunteers: implications for theories of executive functioning and cognitive aging. Cambridge Neuropsychological Test Automated Battery. *Journal of the International Neuropsychology Society*, 4(5), 474–490.

Roffman, J. L., Weiss, A. P., Deckersbach, T. *et al.* (2007a). Effects of the methylenetetrahydrofolate reductase (MTHFR) C677T polymorphism on executive function in schizophrenia. *Schizophrenia Research*, 92(1–3), 181–188.

Roffman, J. L., Weiss, A. P., Purcell, S. *et al.* (2007b). Contribution of methylenetetrahydrofolate reductase (MTHFR) polymorphisms to negative symptoms in schizophrenia. *Biological Psychiatry*, 63(1), 43–48.

Rogers, M. A., Kasai, K., Koji, M. *et al.* (2004). Executive and prefrontal dysfunction in unipolar depression: a review of neuropsychological and imaging evidence. *Neuroscience Research*, 50(1), 1–11.

Roth, R. M., Milovan, D., Baribeau, J. & O'Connor, K. (2005). Neuropsychological functioning in early- and late-onset obsessive-compulsive disorder. *Journal of Neuropsychiatry and Clinical Neuroscience*, 17(2), 208–213.

Roth, R. M. & Saykin, A. J. (2004). Executive dysfunction in attention-deficit/hyperactivity disorder: cognitive and neuroimaging findings. *Psychiatric Clinics of North America*, 27(1), 83–96, ix.

Rypma, B. & D'Esposito, M. (1999). The roles of prefrontal brain regions in components of working memory: effects of memory load and individual differences. *Proceedings of the National Academy of Sciences USA*, 96(11), 6558–6563.

Salmon, E. & Collette, F. (2005). Functional imaging of executive functions. *Acta Neurologica Belgica*, 105(4), 187–196.

Saperstein, A. M., Fuller, R. L., Avila, M. T. *et al.* (2006). Spatial working memory as a cognitive endophenotype of schizophrenia: assessing risk for pathophysiological dysfunction. *Schizophrenia Bulletin*, 32(3), 498–506.

Sawaguchi, T. & Goldman-Rakic, P. S. (1991). D1 dopamine receptors in prefrontal cortex: involvement in working memory. *Science*, 251(4996), 947–950.

Scherf, K. S., Sweeney, J. A. & Luna, B. (2006). Brain basis of developmental change in visuospatial working memory. *Journal of Cognitive Neuroscience*, 18(7), 1045–1058.

Schlosser, R., Gesierich, T., Kaufmann, B. *et al.* (2003a). Altered effective connectivity during working memory performance in schizophrenia: a study with fMRI and structural equation modeling. *Neuroimage*, 19(3), 751–763.

Schlosser, R., Gesierich, T., Kaufmann, B., Vucurevic, G. & Stoeter, P. (2003b). Altered effective connectivity in drug free schizophrenic patients. *Neuroreport*, 14(17), 2233–2237.

Schweinsburg, A. D., Nagel, B. J. & Tapert, S. F. (2005). fMRI reveals alteration of spatial working memory networks across adolescence. *Journal of the International Neuropsychology Society*, 11(5), 631–644.

Segalowitz, S. J. & Rose-Krasnor, L. (1992). The construct of brain maturation in theories of child development. *Brain and Cognition*, 20(1), 1–7.

Shah, P. & Miyake, A. (1996). The separability of working memory resources for spatial thinking and language processing: an individual differences approach. *Journal of Experimental Psychology: General*, 125(1), 4–27.

Shallice, T. & Burgess, P. W. (1991). Deficits in strategy application following frontal lobe damage in man. *Brain*, 114(2), 727–741.

Shaw, P., Greenstein, D., Lerch, J. *et al.* (2006). Intellectual ability and cortical development in children and adolescents. *Nature*, 440(7084), 676–679.

Shimamura, A. P. (2000). Toward a cognitive neuroscience of metacognition. *Conscious Cognition*, 9(2), 313–323; discussion 324–316.

Simon, A. E., Berger, G. E., Giacomini, V., Ferrero, F. & Mohr, S. (2006). Insight, symptoms and executive functions in schizophrenia. *Cognitive Neuropsychiatry*, 11(5), 437–451.

Smith, C. W., Park, S. & Cornblatt, B. (2006). Spatial working memory deficits in adolescents at clinical high risk for schizophrenia. *Schizophrenia Research*, 81(2–3), 211–215.

Smith, E. E. & Jonides, J. (1999). Storage and executive processes in the frontal lobes. *Science*, 283(5408), 1657–1661.

Smith, E. E., Jonides, J. & Koeppe, R. A. (1996). Dissociating verbal and spatial working memory using PET. *Cerebral Cortex*, 6(1), 11–20.

Smith, M., Kates, J. & Vriezen, E. R. (1992). The development of frontal-lobe functions. In S. J. Segalowitz & J. Rapin (Eds.), *Handbook of Neuropsychology* (Vol. 7). Amsterdam: Elsevier.

Spear, L. P. (2000). The adolescent brain and age-related behavioral manifestations. *Neuroscience and Biobehavior Review*, 24(4), 417–463.

Spikman, J. M., Deelman, B. G. & van Zomeren, A. H. (2000). Executive functioning, attention and frontal lesions in patients with chronic CHI. *Journal of Clinical and Experimental Neuropsychology*, 22(3), 325–338.

Stoddart, S. D., Craddock, N. J. & Jones, L. A. (2007). Differentiation of executive and attention impairments in affective illness. *Psychological Med*, 37, 1–11.

Storey, E., Forrest, S., Shaw, J., Mitchell, P. & Gardner, R. M. (1999). Spinocerebellar ataxia type 2: clinical features of a pedigree displaying prominent frontal-executive dysfunction. *Archives of Neurology*, 56(1), 43–50.

Strous, R. D., Bark, N., Woerner, M. & Lachman, H. M. (1997). Lack of association of a functional catechol-O-methyltransferase gene polymorphism in schizophrenia. *Biological Psychiatry*, 41(4), 493–495.

Stuss, D. T. (1992). Biological and psychological development of executive functions. *Brain and Cognition*, 20(1), 8–23.

Stuss, D. T. (2006). Frontal lobes and attention: processes and networks, fractionation and integration. *Journal of the International Neuropsychology Society*, 12(2), 261–271.

Stuss, D. T. & Alexander, M. P. (2000). Executive functions and the frontal lobes: a conceptual view. *Psychological Research*, 63(3–4), 289–298.

Stuss, D. T. & Levine, B. (2002). Adult clinical neuropsychology: lessons from studies of the frontal lobes. *Annual Review of Psychology*, 53, 401–433.

Stuss, D. T., Gow, C. A. & Hetherington, C. R. (1992). "No longer Gage": frontal lobe dysfunction and emotional changes. *Journal of Consulting and Clinical Psychology*, 60(3), 349–359.

Sweeney, J. A., Luna, B., Keedy, S. K., McDowell, J. E. & Clementz, B. A. (2007). fMRI studies of eye movement control: investigating the interaction of cognitive and sensorimotor brain systems. *Neuroimage*, 36 (Suppl. 2), T54–T60.

Sweeney, J. A., Rosano, C., Berman, R. A. & Luna, B. (2001). Inhibitory control of attention declines more than working memory during normal aging. *Neurobiology of Aging*, 22(1), 39–47.

Szameitat, A. J., Schubert, T., Muller, K. & Von Cramon, D. Y. (2002). Localization of executive functions in dual-task performance with fMRI. *Journal of Cognitive Neuroscience*, 14(8), 1184–1199.

Tamm, L., Menon, V. & Reiss, A. L. (2002). Maturation of brain function associated with response inhibition. *Journal of the American Academy of Child and Adolescent Psychiatry*, 41(10), 1231–1238.

Tan, H. Y., Sust, S., Buckholtz, J. W. *et al.* (2006). Dysfunctional prefrontal regional specialization and compensation in schizophrenia. *American Journal of Psychiatry*, 163(11), 1969–1977.

Taylor, S. F., Welsh, R. C., Wager, T. D. *et al.* (2004). A functional neuroimaging study of motivation and executive function. *Neuroimage*, 21(3), 1045–1054.

Tekin, S. & Cummings, J. L. (2002). Frontal-subcortical neuronal circuits and clinical neuropsychiatry: an update. *Journal of Psychosomatic Research*, 53(2), 647–654.

Thatcher, R. W. (1992). Cyclic cortical reorganization during early childhood. *Brain and Cognition*, 20(1), 24–50.

Thatcher, R. W., Walker, R. A. & Giudice, S. (1987). Human cerebral hemispheres develop at different rates and ages. *Science*, 236(4805), 1110–1113.

Thomson, P. A., Wray, N. R., Millar, J. K. *et al.* (2005). Association between the TRAX/DISC locus and both bipolar disorder and schizophrenia in the Scottish population. *Molecular Psychiatry*, 10(7), 657–668, 616.

Tunbridge, E. M., Lane, T. A. & Harrison, P. J. (2007a). Expression of multiple catechol-o-methyltransferase (COMT) mRNA variants in human brain. *American Journal of Medical Genetics Part B (Neuropsychiatric Genetics)*, 144B(6), 834–839.

Tunbridge, E. M., Weickert, C. S., Kleinman, J. E. *et al.* (2007b). Catechol-o-methyltransferase enzyme activity and protein expression in human prefrontal cortex across the postnatal lifespan. *Cerebral Cortex*, 17(5), 1206–1212.

Unsworth, N. & Engle, R. W. (2005). Individual differences in working memory capacity and learning: evidence from the serial reaction time task. *Memory and Cognition*, 33(2), 213–220.

Van der Wee, N. J., Ramsey, N. F., van Megen, H. J. *et al.* (2007). Spatial working memory in obsessive-compulsive disorder improves with clinical response: a functional MRI study. *European Journal of Neuropsychopharmacology*, 17(1), 16–23.

Van der Werf, S. P., Prins, J. B., Jongen, P. J., van der Meer, J. W. & Bleijenberg, G. (2000a). Abnormal neuropsychological findings are not necessarily a sign of cerebral impairment: a matched comparison between chronic fatigue syndrome and multiple sclerosis. *Neuropsychiatry, Neuropsychology and Behavioral Neurology*, 13(3), 199–203.

Van der Werf, Y. D., Witter, M. P., Uylings, H. B. & Jolles, J. (2000b). Neuropsychology of infarctions in the thalamus: a review. *Neuropsychologia*, 38(5), 613–627.

Vance, A., Silk, T. J., Casey, M. *et al.* (2007). Right parietal dysfunction in children with attention deficit hyperactivity disorder, combined type: a functional MRI study. *Molecular Psychiatry*, 12, 826–832.

Ventre-Dominey, J., Bailly, A., Lavenne, F. *et al.* (2005). Double dissociation in neural correlates of visual working memory: a PET study. *Brain Research: Cognitive Brain Research*, 25(3), 747–759.

Wagar, B. M. & Thagard, P. (2004). Spiking Phineas Gage: a neurocomputational theory of cognitive-affective integration in decision making. *Psychological Review*, **111**(1), 67–79.

Wager, T. D. & Smith, E. E. (2003). Neuroimaging studies of working memory: a meta-analysis. *Cognitive and Affective Behavioral Neuroscience*, **3**(4), 255–274.

Watkins, L. H., Sahakian, B. J., Robertson, M. M. *et al.* (2005). Executive function in Tourette's syndrome and obsessive-compulsive disorder. *Psychological Medicine*, **35**(4), 571–582.

Weickert, C. S., Webster, M. J., Gondipalli, P. *et al.* (2007). Postnatal alterations in dopaminergic markers in the human prefrontal cortex. *Neuroscience*, **144**(3), 1109–1119.

Weinberger, D. R. (1987). Implications of normal brain development for the pathogenesis of schizophrenia. *Archives of General Psychiatry*, **44**(7), 660–669.

Weinberger, D. R., Egan, M. F., Bertolino, A. *et al.* (2001). Prefrontal neurons and the genetics of schizophrenia. *Biological Psychiatry*, **50**(11), 825–844.

West, R. & Alain, C. (2000). Evidence for the transient nature of a neural system supporting goal-directed action. *Cerebral Cortex*, **10**(8), 748–752.

Westheide, J., Wagner, M., Quednow, B. B. *et al.* (2007). Neuropsychological performance in partly remitted unipolar depressive patients: focus on executive functioning. *European Archive of Psychiatry and Clinical Neuroscience*, **257**(7), 389–395.

Winterer, G. & Goldman, D. (2003). Genetics of human prefrontal function. *Brain Research: Brain Research Review*, **43**(1), 134–163.

Wodka, E. L., Mahone, E. M., Blankner, J. G. *et al.* (2007). Evidence that response inhibition is a primary deficit in ADHD. *Journal of Clinical and Experimental Neuropsychology*, **29**(4), 345–356.

Wolff, M., Benhassine, N., Costet, P. *et al.* (2003). Delay-dependent working memory impairment in young-adult and aged 5-HT1BKO mice as assessed in a radial-arm water maze. *Learning and Memory*, **10**(5), 401–409.

Wood, S. J., Pantelis, C., Proffitt, T. *et al.* (2003). Spatial working memory ability is a marker of risk-for-psychosis. *Psychological Medicine*, **33**(7), 1239–1247.

Yakovlev, P. & Lecours, A. (1967). The myelogenetic cycles of regional maturation of the brain. In A. Minkowski (Ed.), *Regional Development of the Brain in Early Life* (pp. 3–70). Oxford: Blackwell.

Yamasaki, H., LaBar, K. S. & McCarthy, G. (2002). Dissociable prefrontal brain systems for attention and emotion. *Proceedings of the National Academy of Sciences USA*, **99**(17), 11447–11451.

Yucel, M., Lubman, D. I., Harrison, B. J. *et al.* (2007). A combined spectroscopic and functional MRI investigation of the dorsal anterior cingulate region in opiate addiction. *Molecular Psychiatry*, **12**(7), 611, 691–702.

Yucel, M., Wood, S. J., Fornito, A. *et al.* (2003). Anterior cingulate dysfunction: implications for psychiatric disorders? *Journal of Psychiatry and Neuroscience*, **28**(5), 350–354.

Zakzanis, K. K., Mraz, R. & Graham, S. J. (2005). An fMRI study of the Trail Making Test. *Neuropsychologia*, **43**(13), 1878–1886.

Zammit, S., Jones, G., Jones, S. J. *et al.* (2004). Polymorphisms in the MAOA, MAOB, and COMT genes and aggressive behavior in schizophrenia. *American Journal of Medical Genetics Part B (Neuropsychiatric Genetics)*, **128**(1), 19–20.

Zhang, X., Tochigi, M., Ohashi, J. *et al.* (2005). Association study of the DISC1/TRAX locus with schizophrenia in a Japanese population. *Schizophrenia Research*, **79**(2–3), 175–180.

Zimmerman, M. E., Brickman, A. M., Paul, R. H. *et al.* (2006). The relationship between frontal gray matter volume and cognition varies across the healthy adult lifespan. *American Journal of Geriatric Psychiatry*, **14**(10), 823–833.

Decision-making

Luke Clark and Trevor W. Robbins

Introduction: relevance of decision-making to neuropsychiatry

Decision-making is a collection of processes that allow humans to adopt flexible goal-directed behavior in an ever-changing environment. Impairments in decision-making are central features of a number of psychiatric and neurological disorders, and are often referred to specifically in the diagnostic (DSM–IV) criteria. Within the affective disorders, difficulty and slowness in decision-making characterize clinical depression, whereas bipolar manic patients show a tendency to make decisions associated with the potential for painful consequences (e.g. excessive spending or sexual indiscretions) (American Psychiatric Association, 2000). Substance-use disorders, and other forms of addictive behavior like pathological gambling, can be formulated as the persistent choice of an option (drug administration, gambling) with the potential for negative long-term effects on health, finances and personal relationships (Elster & Skog, 1999; Vuchinich & Heather, 2003). Substance users may persist in drug taking despite insight into these negative consequences. Obsessive-compulsive disorder (OCD) may also relate to pathology in decision-making processes: the obsessive component may relate to prolonged deliberation, whereas the compulsive component may arise from repeated selection of a response option long after that option has ceased to be beneficial or contextually appropriate. Characterization of decision-making at a neuropsychological level may indicate novel forms of treatment for these disorders, and may provide an objective marker for quantifying treatment response.

The relationship between psychology and economics in decision-making

To refine our psychological definition, the term *decision-making* refers to the processes that govern choice behavior when the individual is confronted with situations that have multiple response options. In this chapter, we will focus on *affective* aspects of decision-making, where the response options differ in their potential to cause positive and negative outcomes. These options may vary along at least three dimensions: (1) the magnitude of expected gain or loss, (2) the probability of gain or loss, and (3) the delay between choosing the option and receipt of the gain or loss (Ho *et al.*, 1999). In economic approaches to decision-making, the expected value (EV) of a given option is calculated from the magnitude of that option, weighted by the probability of that outcome occurring. By this account, choice is based on the straightforward selection of the option that maximizes EV. Similar models have been developed to account for choice behavior between options that differ in delay (reviewed by Frederick *et al.*, 2002). In a widely used scenario, the subject is given the choice between a small reward available soon (e.g. $10 delivered tomorrow) versus a larger reward available in the future ($30 delivered in one month). Humans and other animals (e.g. rats, pigeons) typically discount future rewards. The degree of temporal discounting has been found to follow a hyperbolic function, where discounting is steeper at short delays compared with long delays (Mazur, 1987; Rachlin *et al.*, 1991). This hyperbolic model can explain the phenomenon of preference reversal (Kirby & Herrnstein, 1995), where a conservative decision

The Neuropsychology of Mental Illness, ed. Stephen J. Wood, Nicholas B. Allen and Christos Pantelis. Published by Cambridge University Press. © Cambridge University Press 2009.

made far in advance (e.g. preferring $11 in 366 days over $10 in 365 days) may be reversed as the point of delivery draws close ($10 now versus $11 tomorrow).

The concept of *risk* can be introduced to decision-making scenarios in a number of guises. The subject could be offered a choice between a certain $10 win and a gamble with 0.5 probability of winning $50 or a 0.5 probability of losing $30. The EV of these two options is identical $(($50 \times 0.5) - ($30 \times 0.5) = $10)$, and therefore a strictly rational model might predict equal choice behavior. The gamble may be considered the more risky option for two distinct reasons: first, the outcome variance is greater, and second, there is potential for monetary loss (or other aversive consequences) (see Lopes, 1987; Mellers *et al.*, 1999). Healthy subjects do not display equal choice in these circumstances, and consistently select the safe secure win, a phenomenon known as loss aversion (Tversky & Kahneman, 1991). There are also consistent differences in risk preference depending on whether the gamble has a winning or losing context (more commonly known as a positive or negative *frame*) (Gonzalez *et al.*, 2005; Tversky & Kahneman, 1981). When offered the choice between a certain small win ($10) and a gamble that may yield a large win ($20) or no win ($0), subjects typically prefer the small certain option. Hence, in these positive frames (where there is no capacity for losing points), healthy subjects can be described as risk averse. In a negative frame, given the choice between a certain loss ($10) and the chance of losing a larger amount ($20) or losing nothing ($0), subjects are typically risk preferent: they are prepared to take a chance to avoid a loss.

The economic literature also emphasizes a distinction between decision-making under *risk* and decision-making under *uncertainty* (Camerer & Weber, 1992; Ellsberg, 1961). This refers to the level of knowledge about the outcome probabilities at the point of decision: when these probabilities are explicit, this is known as decision-making under risk, whereas if the outcome probabilities are unknown, this is known as decision-making under uncertainty. Decision-makers are typically risk averse when probabilities are unknown, which is labeled the ambiguity effect (Ellsberg, 1961). In most decision-making contexts, there is a middle ground where the subject has an estimate of the probabilities involved, which is continually adjusted on the basis of ongoing feedback. We refer to this situation as decision-making under ambiguity.

The examples reviewed above demonstrate a number of situations where human behavior deviates from strict models of rationality based on mathematical utility. Fundamentally, in many real-world situations it may be better to make a suboptimal decision rapidly than to slowly reach a perfect decision. Moreover, the concept of value in the standard economic framework is inherently subjective (i.e. expected utility), and many real-life decisions require the comparison of options that represent value on different scales; for example, how do we decide between the pleasures of eating luxurious foods versus the costs of being overweight (e.g. in terms of health or social evaluation)? To compare apples and oranges, an intuitive hypothesis is that the brain must convert these values into an "independent metric" (Sanfey *et al.*, 2006). The integration of economics theory with ideas from psychology and neuroscience represents a burgeoning field of research that has recently been labeled "neuroeconomics" (Glimcher & Rustichini, 2004; Sanfey *et al.*, 2006).

The neuropsychology of decision-making

Damage to the ventromedial and orbitofrontal aspects of the prefrontal cortex (PFC) is associated with a complex behavioral syndrome in humans that includes gross alterations in social and emotional behavior. Other cognitive domains including perception, language, memory and even certain aspects of executive functions may be preserved in these patients. The core changes in the orbitofrontal syndrome include emotional lability, impulsivity, socially inappropriate behavior and poor judgment in everyday life (Malloy *et al.*, 1993). The syndrome is sometimes known as frontal disinhibition syndrome or acquired sociopathy (Damasio *et al.*, 1990). Deficits in decision-making have been proposed to lie at the core of this syndrome (Damasio, 1994). In single case studies, these patients display a consistent tendency to make financial, occupational and interpersonal decisions based on short-term benefits, without considering (or caring about) the long-term ramifications (Cato *et al.*, 2004; Damasio, 1994; Dimitrov *et al.*, 1999; Eslinger & Damasio, 1985).

The precise anatomical substrates of the orbitofrontal syndrome remain somewhat unclear. The ventral portion of the prefrontal cortex represents a large and anatomically heterogeneous region (Ongur

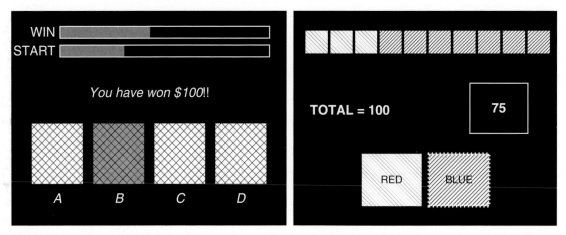

Figure 10.1. In the Iowa Gambling Task (left), the subject makes 100 card choices from four decks. Decks A and B offer high rewards ($100 per choice) but higher losses. Decks C and D offer only $50 per choice, but small losses resulting in profit over time. Patients with ventromedial prefrontal lesions persist in selecting from the risky decks despite accruing high debts. In the Cambridge Gamble Task (right; see www.camcog.com), the subject must decide if a hidden token is under a red or blue box (there are always 10 boxes in total). On this trial, the subject has selected blue, the most likely outcome. After making this probabilistic judgment they must place a bet on their confidence in their decision.

et al., 2003). The orbitofrontal cortex covers the lower surface of the frontal lobe above the orbits of the eyes (Brodmann Area (BA) 10, 11, 12, 13, 11/47). It extends from the medial wall to the lateral surface. Elsewhere in the literature, groups refer to the ventromedial PFC (Bechara *et al.*, 2000; Fellows & Farah, 2003; Shamay-Tsoory *et al.*, 2003), which includes the medial part of the orbitofrontal region (BA 10, 11, 12) and the more ventral sectors of the anterior cingulate cortex and the medial PFC (BA 25 and lower 24, 32). This region also includes the so-called "sub-genual" anterior cingulate region (BA 25) implicated in the neuroanatomy of depression (Drevets *et al.*, 1997). It is increasingly likely that the inferior frontal gyrus (IFG; BA 44 and 45), particularly in the right hemisphere, also contributes to the frontal disinhibition syndrome. This region is reliably activated in functional imaging studies using Go–No Go and Stop Signal tasks of response inhibition (Horn *et al.*, 2003; Rubia *et al.*, 2003), and the volume of damage in right (but not left) IFG in lesion cases has been shown to correlate with deficits on the Stop Signal test of response inhibition (Aron *et al.*, 2003; Clark *et al.*, 2007).

The Iowa Gambling Task and somatic marker hypothesis

Extensive neuropsychological evaluation of Damasio's case EVR showed remarkably intact performance on many measures of executive function (e.g. working memory and cognitive flexibility) and knowledge of social conventions (Eslinger & Damasio, 1985; Saver & Damasio, 1991). The Iowa Gambling Task (IGT) (Bechara *et al.*, 1994) was developed by this group in an effort to quantify the deficits in real-life judgment that were displayed by patients like EVR. During this task, the subject makes a series of 100 choices from four card decks (decks A, B, C, D). Each card choice results in a monetary win, but occasional choices also result in monetary loss, and the four decks differ in the profile of wins and losses (see Figure 10.1). At the start of the task, the subject has no information about the four decks, and must learn to choose advantageously based on trial-by-trial feedback. Decks A and B are "risky" decks, associated with high immediate wins ($100 per choice) but dramatically large occasional penalties that result in net loss over time. Decks C and D are "safe" decks, associated with smaller immediate wins ($50 per choice) but negligible long-term losses, such that subjects accumulate gradual profit from choosing these decks. Healthy subjects typically develop a preference for the safe decks during the task, whereas ventromedial PFC lesion patients maintain a preference for the risky decks throughout the task, despite accruing significant debt (Bechara *et al.*, 1994, 2000).

By monitoring autonomic responses during performance of the IGT, Bechara *et al.* (1996) identified an "anticipatory" skin conductance response (SCR) in healthy subjects in the 5-second window prior to choice. These anticipatory responses developed throughout the task and were greater before risky decisions. These somatic responses were argued to reflect the accumulating knowledge about the long-term negative consequences of these decisions. Patients with ventromedial PFC lesions did not show anticipatory SCRs, but exhibited intact verbal "appraisal" responses to winning and losing feedback. In summary, Bechara, Damasio and colleagues argued that the behavior of the ventromedial PFC patients was driven by the short-term benefits associated with the risky decks, rather than the long-term punishments. This profile was labeled "myopia for the future" (Bechara *et al.*, 1994).

The early studies with the IGT formed the cornerstone of the somatic marker hypothesis (Damasio, 1994). In essence, this theory proposes that decision-making is covertly biased by visceral and emotional signals. When faced with a decision, visceral and emotional responses that have previously been associated with each option are re-activated. Options that have previously yielded reward are promoted, and options that have previously yielded punishment are suppressed. In this manner, the overall number of available options is narrowed down, and deliberation time could be greatly reduced relative to a purely economic cost–benefit analysis. The ventromedial PFC was proposed to be the crucial structure that integrates the cognitive representations of the various response options with their associated somatic markers. Thus, patients with ventromedial PFC lesions are unable to retrieve the emotional consequences of their prior decisions. As a result, their decision-making may become driven by the information held in working memory ("Deck A won $100 the last time").

In addition to the ventromedial PFC, the somatic marker hypothesis proposed an extended neural circuit supporting decision-making, which also includes the amygdala and the somatosensory cortex/insula region. The amygdala was proposed to process "primary inducers": innate or learned stimuli that directly trigger pleasurable or aversive states. In contrast, the ventromedial PFC was argued to process "secondary inducers"; thoughts or memories that, once re-activated, can trigger emotional experiences. Amygdala lesion patients also showed impaired performance on the IGT, but their autonomic signature was distinct: the feedback (appraisal) autonomic

responses to decision outcomes (wins and losses) were also disrupted (Bechara *et al.*, 1999). These appraisal responses were intact in ventromedial PFC patients, but they were unable to re-evoke these responses to guide future behavior.

As a further component of the decision-making circuit, the somatosensory cortex/insula region was proposed to hold the visceral and emotional representations that were associated with secondary inducers. These representations are accessed by the ventromedial PFC during decision-making, and the ventromedial PFC integrates this information with the cognitive representations of the decision-making option. By this account, patients with damage to the somatosensory cortex/insula region should also display quantitatively similar decision-making impairments and problems with emotional behavior to ventromedial PFC lesion patients (Bar-On *et al.*, 2003; Shiv *et al.*, 2005). Whilst any distinct contributions of somatosensory/insula cortex and the ventromedial PFC have yet to be confirmed, a number of functional-imaging studies have reported insula activations during risky decisions (Kuhnen & Knutson, 2005; Paulus *et al.*, 2003). Insula activity has also been reported during the "Ultimatum Game," where the participant and an illusory second player are asked to split a sum of money. On any given trial, the second player may propose a "fair" (e.g. 50:50) or an "unfair" (e.g. 10% to you, 90% to them) split, and the participant must decide whether to accept or reject the offer. By accepting the offer, both players receive their cut, but by rejecting the offer, both players receive nothing. In this manner, all rejections may be viewed as economically irrational, as acceptance will always yield a win of some magnitude. Sanfey *et al.* (2003b) reported insula activity during receipt of unfair offers, and particularly during rejection of unfair offers. These data are consistent with an emotional response, perhaps mediated by visceral signals, which may be able to over-ride more rational routes to effective decision-making.

The IGT is currently the most widely used measure of decision-making in neuropsychiatric studies (see Dom *et al.*, 2005; Dunn *et al.*, 2006 for review). However, the IGT and the somatic marker hypothesis have both attracted criticism on a number of grounds. With regard to the task itself, a number of distinct mechanisms have been proposed to explain IGT impairments, such as impaired reversal learning (Fellows & Farah, 2005b), impaired inhibition (Dunn *et al.*, 2006), impaired working memory (Hinson *et al.*, 2002) and increased risk preference (Rogers *et al.*, 1999). The use of a fixed pseudo-random trial sequence ensures that early in the IGT, the risky decks actually have a higher expected utility until the initial punishments have been received. In this short time, the subject may develop a response "set" to the risky decks, and thus may have to perform a response reversal to the safe decks in order to display advantageous decision-making. Impaired reversal learning, exemplified by perseveration to the previously reinforced stimulus, has been reported in several studies in patients with ventral prefrontal lesions (Fellows & Farah, 2003; Hornak *et al.*, 2004; Rolls *et al.*, 1994). By shuffling the order of cards in the early trials so that penalties were introduced very early on, Fellows & Farah (2005a) showed that the impairment in ventromedial PFC patients was alleviated, consistent with a deficit in reversal learning rather than decision-making per se.

The anatomical specificity of the IGT to the ventral PFC has also been questioned. Several lesion studies have demonstrated IGT impairments in patients with focal dorsolateral PFC lesions (Clark *et al.*, 2003; Fellows & Farah, 2005b; Manes *et al.*, 2002), and functional imaging studies using the IGT have implicated a large frontal network supporting optimal performance (Adinoff *et al.*, 2003; Bolla *et al.*, 2004; Ernst *et al.*, 2002). There is evidence for lateralization of decision-making processes to the right frontal cortex (Clark *et al.*, 2003; Tranel *et al.*, 2002), although this laterality effect may be gender-dependent (Bolla *et al.*, 2004; Tranel *et al.*, 2005). Studies using a dual-task methodology, where IGT performance has been combined with an executive working-memory task (random sequence generation), have suggested that executive processes may interfere with development of advantageous decision-making (Hinson *et al.*, 2002; Jameson *et al.*, 2004). As such, the dorsolateral PFC involvement in the IGT may be linked to working memory representations for the four card decks.

Preference for risk

In the somatic marker hypothesis, patients may make apparently 'risky' choices because they are unaware of the potential negative consequences that have been associated previously with those options. An alternative account is that patients may prefer decks A and B because of a more conscious, explicit preference towards high-risk alternatives. This is similar to ideas from personality theory of sensation-seeking and venturesomeness (Eysenck & Eysenck, 1978; Zuckerman, 1979). For example, a driver may take a blind corner on the wrong side of the road, in full awareness that this maneuver is dangerous, in order to derive an illicit thrill from the experience. In a neuropsychological context, a subject may prefer high-risk options for a number of ancillary reasons, including an increased sensitivity to reward, a reduced sensitivity to punishment or an attenuation of naturally conservative decision-making biases such as loss aversion.

It is difficult to isolate risk preference on the IGT because of the emphasis on learning, which is central to the somatic marker hypothesis. The Cambridge Gamble Task (CGT) was developed to assess decision-making without placing such a demand on learning. On each trial on the CGT, the subject is presented with an array of 10 red and blue boxes. A token is hidden underneath one of the 10 boxes, and the subject must decide whether the token is hidden under a red box or a blue box. This initial decision is a relatively simple probability judgment that does not entail risk processing. Following this judgment, the subject is invited to bet a number of points on their red/blue decision. If their judgment of box color was correct, their bet is added to their total score, enabling a higher bet to be placed on the next trial. If their red/blue judgment is incorrect, the bet is subtracted from their total score. Analysis of betting behavior provides a more direct index of risk-taking, and by displaying the probability information (i.e. the ratio of red to blue boxes) on each trial, the CGT does not place any demands on working memory or learning mechanisms. In choosing the bet, the subject is offered a sequence of fixed bets, presented in either an ascending or descending order (e.g. in the Ascending condition, the presented bets are 5%, 25%, 50%, 75% and 90% of the current points total). Comparison of Ascend and Descend blocks enables the separation of risk-preferent behavior from an effect of motor impulsivity or delay aversion. Impulsive or delay-averse subjects would be expected to select a high bet in the Descend condition (where the bets start at the maximum), but a low bet in the Ascend condition (where the bets start very small). Healthy subjects make the majority of probability judgments towards the box color in the majority, and their betting behavior is moderated by the ratio of red to blue boxes, such that subjects place higher bets at a 9:1 ratio compared with a 6:4 ratio.

A number of studies have shown abnormal CGT performance in patient groups with pathology affecting the ventral PFC. In the initial study (Rogers et al., 1999), a small group of patients with orbito-frontal cortex lesions showed impaired probability judgment (i.e. reduced preference for the box color in the majority) coupled with reduced betting behavior. Several subsequent studies have found *increases* in betting behavior (i.e. larger bets), coupled with intact probability judgment, in patients with large frontal lesions including the orbitofrontal cortex (Manes et al., 2002), in patients with subarachnoid hemorrhage of the anterior communicating artery (the major blood vessel supplying the ventral and medial aspects of the frontal lobes) (Mavaddat et al., 2000), and in patients with fronto-temporal dementia (Rahman et al., 1999) (see below). In each of these three examples, it is likely that the damage extends outside the ventral PFC. However, in a recent dataset (Clark et al., 2008), we have shown that betting behavior is increased in a group of patients with selective ventromedial PFC lesions, but not in a group of lesion controls with dorsolateral PFC damage. The ventromedial PFC group again displayed intact probability judgment. The increase in betting could not be explained by changes in impulsivity or delay aversion (the ventromedial PFC patients placed higher bets in both the ascending and descending conditions). The ventromedial PFC group also experienced more "bankruptcies" during the CGT, where the block is terminated if the points score reaches zero (see also Mavaddat et al., 2000). This latter effect confirms that increased betting on the CGT is "risky" and dysfunctional, and results in overall loss.

Comparison of the CGT and IGT also highlights the distinction between decision-making under risk and decision-making under uncertainty. In the CGT, the outcome probabilities are indicated explicitly by the ratio of red to blue boxes, and hence this task primarily assesses decision-making under risk. At the start of the IGT, participants' decisions are made from a point of complete uncertainty, as there is no information provided about the probabilities of winning and losing on the four decks. During the course of the task, the participant develops subjective estimates for the probability distributions of the four decks, best described as decision-making under ambiguity. Preliminary evidence suggests that this distinction may be significant at a neuropsychological level. Using functional magnetic resonance imaging

(fMRI), Hsu et al. (2005) found that the level of ambiguity during decision-making correlated positively with the neural response in the amygdala and the lateral orbitofrontal cortex. In the same study, patients with orbitofrontal cortex lesions (n = 5) showed attenuated aversion to both ambiguous and risky decisions. Using a similar fMRI design, Huettel et al. (2006) found that activity within the lateral prefrontal cortex predicted the degree of preference to uncertain gambles. The response in this region was negatively correlated with a questionnaire measure of impulsivity, suggesting that this region may implement control over impulsive responses. In the Huettel study, the degree of preference to explicitly risky gambles was predicted by activity in the posterior parietal cortex. It remains unclear whether patients with lesions to this area show actual changes in affective decision-making. The lack of orbitofrontal cortex activity is surprising in the Huettel experiment and may relate to signal drop-out from the orbitofrontal cortex region due to inhomogeneities in the magnetic field.

Risk-taking may also be considered in terms of outcome variance (Lopes, 1987). Sanfey et al. (2003a) tested a group of ventromedial PFC patients and healthy controls on a modified version of the IGT where the four decks were equated for EV but varied in outcome variance. The healthy subjects showed strong risk aversion, preferring the decks with low outcome variance. Performance in the ventromedial PFC patients was heterogeneous, and patients could be divided into two subgroups: one subgroup who behaved like controls, and another who preferred the high variance decks. There were no observable differences in lesion location between the two subgroups. A study by Tomb et al. (2002) further highlighted the potential importance of outcome variance. Tomb et al. (2002) initially replicated the anticipatory SCR effect reported by Bechara et al. (1996), but were concerned that the effect may relate to the higher immediate benefits of the risky decks rather than the long-term negative consequences. They measured autonomic responses on a variant of the IGT where the safe decks produced greater magnitude wins and losses compared with the risky decks. Here, healthy subjects showed relatively greater anticipatory responses to the safe decks, even though this was now the advantageous strategy. It is difficult to disentangle the causal nature of the anticipatory SCR effect, but from this study it is possible that the anticipatory

143

SCRs signal the riskiness of the response in terms of outcome variance (see Dunn *et al.*, 2006 for other explanations).

A number of other decision-making tasks have been developed to assess riskiness. Shiv *et al.* (2005) used an investment task based on a simplified stock market. Across each of 20 trials, the subject had to decide whether to invest in a coin-toss gamble, or to not invest and skip the go. Although the EV of investing was positive, healthy subjects displayed loss aversion on the task, and became more conservative after both winning and losing on investment gambles. A combined group of lesion patients with ventromedial PFC or somatosensory cortex/insula damage made more profit than controls, after investing for a greater number of trials. Shiv *et al.* argued that in healthy subjects, somatic signals may interfere with a rational cost–benefit analysis in some circumstances, and these situations may enable ventromedial PFC lesion patients to show superior performance to controls. Other tasks have measured risk-taking as the persistence of a response with incrementing degrees of reward and punishment, such as in the Balloon Analogue Risk Task (Lejuez *et al.*, 2003) or Risky Gains procedure (Paulus *et al.*, 2003). Tasks of this type are discussed below in relationship to substance-use disorders and alcoholism.

Choice between delayed rewards

The IGT and CGT primarily emphasize the processing of probability and magnitude of loss/reward in decision-making. Decision processes between delayed outcomes have received less attention in neuropsychological research at the present time, despite a large body of work investigating intertemporal choice in various forms of addiction (for review, see Bickel & Marsch, 2001). Temporal discounting tasks have also been widely used in rodents, where preference for a small immediate reward can be treated as an index of impulsivity. The delay to the large reinforcer can be varied across blocks of the task to ascertain the *indifference point*, where the two options are valued equally (Mazur, 1987). Orbitofrontal cortex lesions (using quinolinic acid administered before task training) increased preference for small immediate rewards over large delayed rewards in rodents (Mobini *et al.*, 2002). This effect generalized to a probability discounting procedure, increasing preference for a small certain reward over a larger

uncertain reinforcer (Mobini *et al.*, 2002). In contrast, Winstanley *et al.* (2004) found that lesions of the rat orbitofrontal cortex made after training produced enhanced choice for the large delayed reward. However, lesions of the basolateral amygdala (projecting to the core region of the nucleus accumbens) also induced impulsive choice, as did lesions to the nucleus accumbens (Cardinal *et al.*, 2001). This latter effect contrasted with unchanged performance following lesions to the anterior cingulate cortex, and a possible effect on temporal discrimination following medial PFC lesions (Cardinal *et al.*, 2001). These data suggest that choice between delayed rewards may be supported by a limbic fronto-striatal circuit comprising the amygdala, the orbitofrontal cortex and the nucleus accumbens.

An fMRI study in human volunteers is broadly consistent with these data. McClure *et al.* (2004) presented subjects with a series of choices between imaginary delayed rewards during scanning. In an event-related analysis, choice of the small immediate reward was associated with a response in the ventral striatum (subsuming the nucleus accumbens), and also in the medial and the orbitofrontal cortex. A second circuit, comprising the dorsolateral PFC and posterior parietal cortex was activated during delayed choice regardless of the delay interval, and was argued to reflect reasoning and logical processing. Comparison of the two systems showed relatively greater activity in the dorsolateral PFC, with the parietal network predicting choice of the large reward. However, a single study in human lesion cases has failed to substantiate orbitofrontal (or dorsolateral PFC) involvement. Fellows & Farah (2005a) found intact temporal discounting functions in ventromedial PFC lesion and dorsolateral PFC lesion groups, with the patients with ventromedial PFC lesions displaying shortened time perspectives on a questionnaire measure. Impaired orienting to the future may contribute to everyday difficulties in ventromedial PFC patients, although this deficit was associated with ratings of apathy and not impulsivity.

Information sampling and 'reflection impulsivity'

The majority of tests used to assess decision-making present an array of information at the start of each trial, from which the subject is expected to make a response. In many real-life situations, it is necessary to gather and evaluate information over a period of time, before making a decision (for example, when buying a car, renting a flat or simply deciding whether to take an umbrella out in the morning). In these scenarios, inadequate sampling of information will have an inevitable impact on the accuracy of the eventual decision (Evenden, 1999). Other recent data suggest that some complex decisions involving multiple attributes may be performed better in situations where the subject is distracted from cogitating or reflecting on the decision (Dijksterhuis *et al.*, 2006). The construct of "reflection impulsivity" was developed by Kagan (1966) to refer to consistent individual differences in information-gathering behavior and the speed–accuracy relationship. In the Matching Familiar Figures Test (MFFT), subjects are presented with a template picture (e.g. a bicycle) and six variants. Of the variants, only one is a perfect match, and the other five pictures vary subtly along a number of dimensions (e.g. number of spokes, shape of handle-bars, tire thickness). Healthy children displayed a bimodal pattern of performance on the MFFT, where some children consistently responded very rapidly but with poor accuracy, whereas the other subgroup took much longer over each decision and were very accurate. The first group was labeled "impulsive" and the second group "reflective" (Kagan, 1966). The impulsive style has been associated with attention-deficit hyperactivity disorder (Messer, 1976) and responds to psychostimulant treatment (Brown & Sleator, 1979). However, interpretation of MFFT findings can be problematic given the task's substantial demands on perception and working memory.

Several recent studies have suggested that orbitofrontal and ventromedial PFC lesions may disrupt information-gathering behavior and create an impulsive decision-making style. Dimitrov *et al.* (1999) reported a single case study of a Vietnam war veteran (MGS) who was retired from service after a shrapnel wound to the right orbitofrontal region. On return home, MGS's personality changed dramatically and he was married and divorced three times in the space of several years to a runaway, a drug addict and a prostitute. On neuropsychological assessment, MGS showed a consistent shift in the speed–accuracy relationship across several different tests, towards rapid but low-accuracy decisions. In a group study of 23 orbitofrontal cortex lesion patients, increased MFFT impulsivity was seen in the OFC group compared with both healthy controls and non-OFC frontal lobe

lesions, mainly affecting the dorsolateral PFC (Berlin *et al.*, 2004). Fellows (2006) has recently examined information-gathering behavior on a more complex decision-making task where the subject must decide which of six apartments to rent by gathering information on several different attributes (e.g. the rent payment, space and noise level). Healthy subjects and patients with dorsolateral PFC lesions showed an "attribute-based" strategy on the task where they focused on specific attributes in turn and compared the six apartments. Whilst the ventromedial PFC patients sampled a similar total amount of information, they employed a qualitatively different strategy for acquiring information by assessing several attributes for each apartment, before moving to the next apartment (i.e. an "alternative-based" strategy). In more open-ended and uncertain contexts, this difference in acquisition style may have concomitant effects on decision-making accuracy.

Decision-making in neuropsychiatric patient groups
Frontal variant fronto-temporal dementia

Frontal variant fronto-temporal dementia (fvFTD) is one of the most prevalent forms of early-onset dementia (Ratnavalli *et al.*, 2002). Patients typically present with a florid disinhibition syndrome that can profoundly affect interpersonal function. Neurocognitive testing has revealed a pattern of impairment in fvFTD comparable with patients with ventromedial PFC lesions. For example, Rahman *et al.* (1999) originally reported impaired reversal learning on the IDED attentional shifting task, and increased betting (coupled with intact probability judgment) on the CGT. Torralva *et al.* (2007) have confirmed that fvFTD patients are also impaired on the IGT, as well as on measures of social cognition and Theory of Mind, although these deficits are not intercorrelated (see also Gregory *et al.*, 2002). Neuroanatomical evidence for orbitofrontal cortex dysfunction has been borne out in subsequent neuroimaging studies (Diehl *et al.*, 2004; Ibach *et al.*, 2004). For example, a European multicenter PET study showed that the ventromedial frontopolar cortex was critically affected in every one of 29 fvFTD cases (Salmon *et al.*, 2003).

We have recently explored the neurochemical substrates of the increased betting effect in frontal dementia cases. In a placebo-controlled crossover

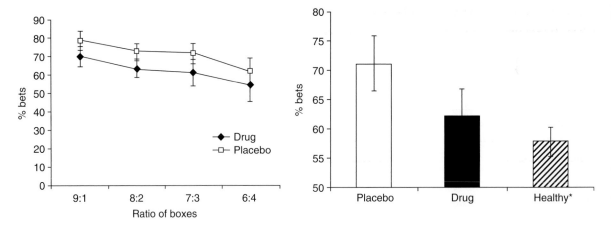

Figure 10.2. Betting behavior on the Cambridge Gamble Task is significantly increased in patients with frontal variant fronto-temporal dementia (Rahman *et al.*, 1999). Single dose treatment with methylphenidate (40 mg) significantly reduced betting behavior and effectively normalized the impairment. *Healthy data from the placebo condition of Turner *et al.* (2003) *Psychopharmacology*, **168**, 455–464. Data reproduced from Rahman *et al.* (2006).

design, an acute dose of methylphenidate (Ritalin; 40 mg) significantly reduced betting in eight cases with frontal dementia, to the level of healthy elderly controls (Rahman *et al.*, 2006) (see Figure 10.2). A similarly designed study found no effects of acute paroxetine, a selective serotonin reuptake inhibitor (SSRI) (Deakin *et al.*, 2004). Methylphenidate is a psychostimulant drug that increases extracellular levels of dopamine and noradrenaline via blockade of the reuptake transporters. How this beneficial effect of methylphenidate is mediated is presently unclear. It is possible that methylphenidate acts to replenish depleted catecholamine levels in patients with fvFTD (Sjogren *et al.*, 1998). However, this account would predict remediation of other neurocognitive measures, like executive function, which was not seen in the Rahman *et al.* study. The specific effect on decision-making may be explained by an action on reward signaling, or the stimulation of central somatic markers carried by the ascending catecholamine projections.

Substance abuse and alcoholism

Addictive disorders appear to reflect a breakdown of rational decision-making processes. Patients with substance-abuse disorders continue to select the short-term reward of drug administration above the long-term negative consequences for their health, finances and interpersonal relationships. Research aiming to characterize the profile of abnormal decision-making in substance abuse has received

further impetus from studies implicating orbitofrontal cortex circuitry in drug craving and drug expectancy (Goldstein & Volkow, 2002 for review). A wealth of research has demonstrated deficient decision-making on the IGT in drug users dependent upon a variety of substances including stimulants, opiates, alcohol and marijuana (see Dom *et al.*, 2005 for review). For example, Bechara & Damasio (2002) examined IGT performance in 46 individuals attending drug rehabilitation at an inpatient center. Most subjects abused multiple substances ("poly-drug" users) but there were similar numbers of subjects whose preferred drug was cocaine, amphetamine or alcohol. Performance on the IGT showed a bimodal distribution in the substance users, with 63% of subjects preferring the risky decks, and the remaining 37% behaving similarly to controls. Task impairment did not covary with drug of choice, and psychophysiological recording confirmed the absence of anticipatory SCRs in the behavioraly impaired subgroup.

Although these studies with the IGT demonstrate reliable statistically significant differences between substance-user groups and healthy controls, not all studies found an actual preference for the risky decks in the substance users (Goudriaan *et al.*, 2005; Mazas *et al.*, 2000; Stout *et al.*, 2005). Risk-preferent biases in decision-making have been explored with a variety of other tasks. The CGT was used to demonstrate qualitative differences in decision-making quality in groups of stimulant and opiate abusers. Deficits in this measure correlated significantly with the

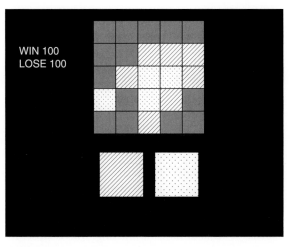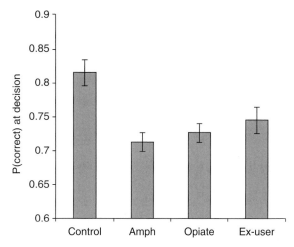

Figure 10.3. The Information Sampling Task (see www.camcog.com). Each trial commences (left) with presentation of 25 gray boxes arranged in a 5 × 5 matrix, covering a random assortment of two colors of squares; these two colors are displayed on panels at the foot of the screen. When the subject touches a box (middle), it opens to reveal its color. The subject must decide which of the two colors lies in the majority on the board. They are told they can open as many boxes as they wish in order to make this decision. They are told to touch the corresponding panel at the foot of the screen (bottom right) once they have decided which color is in the majority. Amphetamine-dependent (Amph) subjects, opiate-dependent subjects, and ex-users of amphetamines or opiates opened fewer boxes than non-drug-using controls, and tolerate a lower probability of making a correct response at the time of decision. This is thought to indicate altered reflection impulsivity in current and former drug users. Reproduced from Clark *et al.* (2006) *Biological Psychiatry*, **60**, 512–522, with permission. Copyright © 2006 Society of Biological Psychiatry.

duration of substance use (Rogers *et al.*, 1999). However, neither group of drug users showed evidence of increased betting, motor impulsivity or delay aversion on the CGT.

In the Risky Gains procedure (Paulus *et al.*, 2003), the numbers 20, 40 and 80 appear on a computer screen in an ascending order. Selection of the 20 guarantees a 20-point gain (the safe option). By waiting to select 40 or 80, the subject may win more points (40 or 80). However, there is also a risk of punishment: if 40 or 80 appear in an alternative color, these points are deducted (the risky option). Recreational stimulant users selected more risky responses than stimulant-naïve controls (Leland & Paulus, 2005). The Balloon Analogue Risk Task (BART) is a similar procedure, where the subject may continue pumping air into the balloon to attain more points, but if the balloon explodes, all points are lost. Lejuez *et al.* (2003) showed that the BART – but not the IGT – was able to discriminate current cigarette smokers from never-smokers. Increased risky responses were also demonstrated in alcohol-dependent subjects on a similar task (Bjork *et al.*, 2004).

Substance use has also been associated with impulsive choice on measures of delayed reward and temporal discounting, where drug users consistently prefer small rewards available at short delays over

larger rewards available in the future (see Bickel & Marsch, 2001 for review). Steeper rates of temporal discounting have been seen with hypothetical monetary rewards or quantities of drug-of-choice, and also with abstract rewards like health or freedom (Baker *et al.*, 2003; Johnson & Bickel, 2002; Madden *et al.*, 1997). This preference was correlated with the number of disadvantageous decisions on the IGT in a group of cocaine users (Monterosso *et al.*, 2001). Preference for small immediate reward has also been demonstrated on a delayed reward task with genuine "experiential" delays (e.g. 5 cents in 5 seconds, versus 15 cents after 15 seconds) (Allen *et al.*, 1998; Moeller *et al.*, 2002). As an important demonstration of ecological validity, steeper rates of temporal discounting have been associated with shared needle use in opiate users (Odum *et al.*, 2000).

Substance users may show consistent differences in the gathering and evaluation of information at the pre-decisional stage. Work on recreational MDMA ("Ecstasy") users has shown impulsive patterns of performance on the Matching Familiar Figures Test (Morgan, 1998; Morgan *et al.*, 2002, 2005), putatively related to the neurotoxic effects on MDMA on serotonergic neurons. We developed a novel task (see Figure 10.3) of information-sampling behavior to minimize the visual search and strategic demands of the MFFT, which may be independently impaired in substance users (Fox *et al.*, 2002). We administered this test as part of a neuropsychological assessment to chronic stimulant and opiate users (Clark *et al.*, 2006). Current and former substance users both sampled less information on the task than healthy controls and tolerated a lower probability of making a correct decision. These effects were seen regardless of drug preference (stimulants or opiates). As a consequence of reduced information sampling, the substance users also made more errors on the task, suggesting that a tendency to make decisions based on inadequate pre-decisional processing may have concomitant effects on real-life decision accuracy.

Decision-making impairments in drug users are mirrored in abnormal patterns of frontal lobe activity during decision-making performance. Ersche *et al.* (2005) employed a variant of the CGT (the Risk Task) adapted for PET imaging. In the Risk Task, a fixed bet is associated with either box color, and on each trial the subject is offered a choice between a small but more likely reward, and a larger but less likely reward. During decision-making blocks (compared against a visuo-motor control condition), current opiate users and current amphetamine users displayed altered patterns of blood flow between the left and right orbitofrontal cortex, coupled with decreased blood flow in dorsolateral PFC (Ersche *et al.*, 2005). These changes appear to persist across long periods of abstinence from drug use: ex-users of opiates or amphetamines who had been abstinent from all illicit drugs for at least one year also differed from healthy controls and showed a similar pattern of brain activation to the current users. Somewhat similar effects were reported in abstinent cocaine users (Bolla *et al.*, 2003). Detoxified alcoholics who were abstinent for over 6 years on average also still displayed robust impairments on the IGT (Fein *et al.*, 2004).

It remains unclear whether these changes in decision-making occur as an irreversible consequence of chronic drug use, or whether these changes in fact pre-date drug-taking and are associated with the vulnerability to addiction. There is evidence that both pathways are at least plausible. Structural imaging studies have shown gray matter reductions in the frontal cortex of stimulant, opiate and alcohol users (Franklin *et al.*, 2002; Lyoo *et al.*, 2006; Wilson *et al.*, 1996), presumably related to long-term neurotoxicity. However, there is also evidence that impaired behavioral inhibition (Tarter *et al.*, 2004) and increased

trait impulsivity (Vitaro *et al.*, 1999) may pre-date addictive disorders, and that impaired decision-making (on the IGT and temporal discounting tasks) may be present in pathological gamblers where neurotoxic and neuroadaptive effects seem unlikely (Cavedini *et al.*, 2002b; Petry, 2001). The separation of cause and effect in addiction may be studied more directly through research on experimental animals (Perry *et al.*, 2005).

In summary, a wealth of research has demonstrated impairments in decision-making ability in substance users with a variety of preferred drugs of abuse (including stimulants, opiates and alcohol). Recent studies have begun to investigate specific subcomponents of decision-making, where substance users again display robust impairments in multiple processes, including choice of delayed rewards, processing of probability and risk, and pre-decisional reflection. Functional imaging studies have implicated PFC abnormalities in these behavioral deficits. These data are consistent with neurobiological theories of addiction that highlight the loss of inhibitory control over reward-driven behavior, governed in the healthy brain by the frontal cortex (Goldstein & Volkow, 2002; Jentsch & Taylor, 1999).

Obsessive-compulsive disorder

Decision-making processes have been less widely studied in relation to other neuropsychiatric disorders. Choice behavior and response selection are clearly relevant to the symptomatology of OCD, and imaging data have implicated orbitofrontal cortex and ventral striatal circuitry in the pathophysiology of this condition (Chamberlain *et al.*, 2005). Moreover, ventromedial frontal leucotomy is an effective treatment for severe and refractory OCD (Irle *et al.*, 1998). However, decision-making processes have been examined in only a handful of studies in OCD to date. Performance on the IGT was examined in 34 OCD patients, 34 healthy controls and a smaller group of panic disorder patients (n = 16) to control for anxiety levels (Cavedini *et al.*, 2002a). The OCD group were impaired relative to both control groups, and significantly preferred the risky decks over the safe decks. In this study, disadvantageous decision-making also predicted a poor response to a 10-week course of SSRI treatment, demonstrating the potential clinical benefits of neuropsychological assessment in guiding treatment selection. However, a similarly powered study published at the same time reported no significant difference in IGT performance between OCD patients and controls (Nielen *et al.*, 2002), and a later study found similar performance in patients with schizophrenia, with and without obsessive symptoms (Whitney *et al.*, 2004). A single study using the CGT also reported no impairment in an OCD group (Watkins *et al.*, 2005). At the present time, studies assessing decision-making in OCD using complex tasks like the IGT have yielded equivocal results. Future research may benefit from fractionating specific components of the decision-making process, including aspects of inhibitory control and (compulsive) perseveration of previously reinforced choices. These studies will also need to control carefully for comorbid depression and anxiety levels, and SSRI medication status.

Schizophrenia and affective disorders

The research on decision-making is similarly inconsistent in schizophrenia, where the extent of orbitofrontal cortex dysfunction remains controversial. On the CGT, first-episode patients and chronic patients with schizophrenia displayed slower deliberation times and attenuated risk adjustment (i.e. betting behavior was less affected by the ratio of boxes). The chronic patients showed an additional impairment in probability judgment, where they selected the unlikely box color more often (Hutton *et al.*, 2002). Studies employing the IGT in groups of patients with schizophrenia have reported mixed results including preference for the risky decks (Bark *et al.*, 2005; Ritter *et al.*, 2004), no overall impairment (Wilder *et al.*, 1998), increased preference for infrequent punishment (i.e. decks B and D over decks A and C) (Shurman *et al.*, 2005), and performance dependent upon medication status (Beninger *et al.*, 2003). Given the generalized pattern of background neuropsychological impairment in schizophrenia, combined with the demands for learning and cognitive flexibility that are inherent to the IGT, it is likely that more specific measures may be necessary to elucidate the subcomponents of decision-making in schizophrenia.

In affective illness, decision-making has been examined mainly in relation to the manic phase of bipolar disorder. Some of the cardinal symptoms of mania, like socially inappropriate remarks, impulsivity and poor judgment, bear a strong resemblance to the orbitofrontal cortex lesion syndrome (Clark &

Sahakian, 2006). Patients with affective disorder may also show structural brain abnormalities in the medial and orbital aspects of the PFC (Drevets *et al.*, 1997; Lacerda *et al.*, 2004). An assessment of IGT performance in a group of manic patients yielded equivocal findings: the manic group were significantly impaired relative to controls but did not clearly prefer either the risky decks or the safe decks (Clark *et al.*, 2001). As such, the deficit did not fully resemble the ventromedial PFC profile, and their poor performance could be attributable to deficient learning or inattention. On the CGT, manic patients showed approximately normal betting behavior on the task, although they were less able to adjust their betting according to the ratio of boxes compared with controls (Murphy *et al.*, 2001). Further, the manic group showed impaired probability judgment and increased deliberation times, and the deficit in probability judgment correlated with manic symptom ratings on the Young scale. Probability judgment was intact in a control group of patients with unipolar depression (Murphy *et al.*, 2001) and in remitted patients with bipolar disorder (Rubinsztein *et al.*, 2000), suggesting that the deficit in probability judgment is a state-related abnormality specific to mania. A subsequent PET imaging experiment measured regional cerebral blood flow in manic patients during the CGT variant (Risk) task used in the Ersche *et al.* (2005) study (described above). In the manic group, brain activations associated with decision-making were increased in the anterior cingulate cortex (BA 32) but reduced in the inferior frontal gyrus (BA 47), suggesting a dysregulation of medial and ventral prefrontal circuitry in mania.

There are currently a paucity of studies examining decision-making in unipolar depression (Major Depressive Illness), despite the listing of "indecisiveness" as one of the key cognitive symptoms of depression in the DSM–IV. A control group of unipolar depressed patients included in the Murphy *et al.* (2001) study showed longer deliberation times than healthy controls on the CGT, although this could relate to generalized psychomotor slowing rather than a specific decision-making impairment. Overall, given the quantity of neuropsychological research investigating executive function in affective and psychotic illnesses, it is perhaps surprising that measures of decision-making have received so little examination. Preliminary evidence of decision-making abnormalities in bipolar mania are particularly intriguing, given the core tendency of manic patients to make "risky" decisions with the potential for painful consequences, and the clear similarities between mania and the orbitofrontal lesion syndrome.

Conclusions

This chapter has reviewed the increasing evidence of impaired decisional processes following frontal brain damage and in a number of neuropsychiatric disorders in which prefrontal cortical pathology is suspected. The major advance has been the introduction of a number of well-designed tests of human decision-making that take into account the multiple dimensions that contribute to performance, including, for example, the utility of the decisions and their framing. Pioneering and still prominent among these tests is the IGT (Bechara *et al.* 1994), which has a rich structure and considerable ecological validity. This test can be exquisitely sensitive to orbitofrontal cortex deficits, and coupled with psychophysiological recording, such as skin conductance responses, has led to novel hypotheses of decision-making based upon "somatic markers" (Damasio, 1994). However, the IGT is a complex task and has a strong loading on learning and working-memory functions, which may confound the assessment of decision-making per se. Researchers have also questioned the extent to which deficits on the IGT can be synthesized from other component impairments commonly produced by frontal damage, such as reversal learning, response inhibition, and aspects of delay discounting and reinforcement sensitivity.

Consequently, there has been much recent activity directed at isolating subcomponents of decision-making with a variety of new instruments. For example, the CGT (Rogers *et al.*, 1999) presents explicit choices with defined contingencies that minimizes learning across the task. The CGT also incorporates measures of decisional quality, as well as the propensity to gamble, but its measures of reward-driven and loss-avoidant processing are somewhat conflated. Other tests of risk-preferent biases include the Risky Gains procedure (Leland & Paulus 2005; Paulus *et al.*, 2003) and the Balloon Analogue Risk Task (Lejuez *et al.*, 2003). Temporal discounting paradigms are also becoming increasingly popular because of their clear implications for framing decisions about future health status, for example, in substance abuse. These methods have the advantage of quantitative

theoretical models that relate salient task variables such as magnitude and delay of reward to the value of each response option. However, it now seems likely that "prospective" discounting, typically involving long delays stretching into the future (days to weeks), and "experiential" discounting, involving real delays over much shorter timeframes (typically under one minute), may depend on distinct neural circuitry and may reflect different components of complex processing that are somehow integrated to provide apparently orderly "discounting" behavior. The majority of this research involves discounting of the former type, typically tested using questionnaires ("Would you prefer $10 today or $30 in 7 days?") (Kirby *et al.*, 1999). More recent studies using experiential delays are more comparable with the extensive literature on experimental animals (Cardinal *et al.*, 2001; Mazur, 1987; Winstanley *et al.*, 2004). It can, however, be difficult to implement these experiential discounting tasks in human subjects, because of strategy use and the potentially confounding effects of abnormal delay processing.

It has also been recognized that information gathering is an important precondition for effective decision-making, and that deficits in "reflection" can lead to impulsive decision-making (Evenden, 1999; Fellows, 2006; Kagan, 1966). The traditional test of reflection impulsivity, the MFFT, has been another classic instrument, especially for testing impulsivity in children; however, possible confounding factors such as perceptual and attentional processing may potentially produce inflated indices of impulsivity. A novel measure of reflection impulsivity (Clark *et al.*, 2006) overcomes many of these difficulties, but like many of the newer tasks described above, it requires further refinement and validation in key patient groups like ventromedial PFC lesion cases.

An over-arching difficulty with these "objective" tests of decision-making is the relationship with subjective evaluation of traits such as impulsivity. Thus the well-known and useful Barratt Impulsivity Scale (Patton *et al.*, 1995) contains a subscale of "non-planning impulsivity" (see also Whiteside & Lynam, 2001), which should be closely related to some of the variables measured objectively in the tests we have described. However, correlations between laboratory tests and trait self-report measures are notoriously erratic (Carrillo-de-la-Pena *et al.*, 1993; Lijffijt *et al.*, 2004; Swann *et al.*, 2002). Future research must focus on the reasons for this, and enable the further development of such scales as well as tests of decision-making cognition.

Impaired decision-making, impulsivity and loss of inhibitory control are fundamental concepts in current descriptions of a number of neuropsychiatric disorders. Neuropsychological analysis of these complex multifactorial processes, and detailed description of the underlying neural circuitry, promises to have implications for psychological and pharmacological treatments. Within this chapter, we have focused primarily on the relevance of decision-making to substance abuse, frontal dementia, OCD and affective disorders, but these principles may be applied equally to other conditions including ADHD, personality disorders and eating disorders, where the research in these areas is currently in its infancy. It is also critical to acknowledge the neurodevelopmental changes in these cognitive abilities, where the relatively late development of prefrontal cortical control mechanisms (which do not reach full maturity until early adulthood) may be able to explain the typical onset of several forms of psychopathology during the period of adolescence (Chambers *et al.*, 2003). Identification of the environmental and biological factors that convey vulnerability to – and resilience against – these forms of psychopathology will represent a formidable challenge for the coming period.

Acknowledgments

This work was funded by a Wellcome Trust programme grant to T.W.R., B.J. Sahakian, B.J. Everitt and A.C. Roberts, and completed within the University of Cambridge Behavioural and Clinical Neuroscience Institute supported by a consortium award from the Wellcome Trust and Medical Research Council. L.C. and T.W.R. consult for Cambridge Cognition plc (www.camcog.com) who distribute several of the tasks described, including the Cambridge Gamble Task and Information Sampling Task.

References

Adinoff, B., Devous, M. D., Sr., Cooper, D. B. *et al.* (2003). Resting regional cerebral blood flow and gambling task performance in cocaine-dependent subjects and healthy comparison subjects. *American Journal of Psychiatry*, **160**, 1892–1894.

Allen, T. J., Moeller, F. G., Rhoades, H. M. & Cherek, D. R. (1998). Impulsivity and history of drug dependence. *Drug and Alcohol Dependence*, **50**, 137–145.

American Psychiatric Association (2000). *Diagnostic and Statistical Manual of Mental Disorders – Text Revision* (5th edn.). Washington, DC: APA.

Aron, A. R., Fletcher, P. C., Bullmore, E. T., Sahakian, B. J. & Robbins, T. W. (2003). Stop-signal inhibition disrupted by damage to right inferior frontal gyrus in humans. *Nature Neuroscience*, **6**, 115–116.

Baker, F., Johnson, M. W. & Bickel, W. K. (2003). Delay discounting in current and never-before cigarette smokers: similarities and differences across commodity, sign, and magnitude. *Journal of Abnormal Psychology*, **112**, 382–392.

Bark, R., Dieckmann, S., Bogerts, B. & Northoff, G. (2005). Deficit in decision making in catatonic schizophrenia: an exploratory study. *Psychiatry Research*, **134**, 131–141.

Bar-On, R., Tranel, D., Denburg, N. L. & Bechara, A. (2003). Exploring the neurological substrate of emotional and social intelligence. *Brain*, **126**, 1790–1800.

Bechara, A. & Damasio, H. (2002). Decision-making and addiction (part I): impaired activation of somatic states in substance dependent individuals when pondering decisions with negative future consequences. *Neuropsychologia*, **40**, 1675–1689.

Bechara, A., Damasio, A. R., Damasio, H. & Anderson, S. W. (1994). Insensitivity to future consequences following damage to human prefrontal cortex. *Cognition*, **50**, 7–15.

Bechara, A., Damasio, H., Damasio, A. R. & Lee, G. P. (1999). Different contributions of the human amygdala and ventromedial prefrontal cortex to decision-making. *Journal of Neuroscience*, **19**, 5473–5481.

Bechara, A., Tranel, D. & Damasio, H. (2000). Characterization of the decision-making deficit of patients with ventromedial prefrontal cortex lesions. *Brain*, **123**, 2189–2202.

Bechara, A., Tranel, D., Damasio, H. & Damasio, A. R. (1996). Failure to respond autonomically to anticipated future outcomes following damage to prefrontal cortex. *Cerebral Cortex*, **6**, 215–225.

Beninger, R. J., Wasserman, J., Zanibbi, K. *et al.* (2003). Typical and atypical antipsychotic medications differentially affect two nondeclarative memory tasks in schizophrenic patients: a double dissociation. *Schizophrenia Research*, **61**, 281–292.

Berlin, H. A., Rolls, E. T. & Kischka, U. (2004). Impulsivity, time perception, emotion and reinforcement sensitivity in patients with orbitofrontal cortex lesions. *Brain*, **127**, 1108–1126.

Bickel, W. K. & Marsch, L. A. (2001). Toward a behavioral economic understanding of drug dependence: delay discounting processes. *Addiction*, **96**, 73–86.

Bjork, J. M., Hommer, D. W., Grant, S. J. & Danube, C. (2004). Impulsivity in abstinent alcohol-dependent patients: relation to control subjects and type 1-/type 2-like traits. *Alcohol*, **34**, 133–150.

Bolla, K. I., Eldreth, D. A., London, E. D. *et al.* (2003). Orbitofrontal cortex dysfunction in abstinent cocaine abusers performing a decision-making task. *Neuroimage*, **19**, 1085–1094.

Bolla, K. I., Eldreth, D. A., Matochik, J. A. & Cadet, J. L. (2004). Sex-related differences in a gambling task and its neurological correlates. *Cerebral Cortex*, **14**, 1226–1232.

Brown, R. T. & Sleator, E. K. (1979). Methylphenidate in hyperkinetic children: differences in dose effects on impulsive behavior. *Pediatrics*, **64**, 408–411.

Camerer, C. & Weber, M. (1992). Recent developments in modelling preferences: uncertainty and ambiguity. *Journal of Risk and Uncertainty*, **5**, 325–370.

Cardinal, R. N., Pennicott, D. R., Sugathapala, C. L., Robbins, T. W. Everitt, B. J. (2001). Impulsive choice induced in rats by lesions of the nucleus accumbens core. *Science*, **292**, 2499–2501.

Carrillo-de-la-Pena, M. T., Otero, J. M. & Romero, E. (1993). Comparison among various methods of assessment of impulsiveness. *Perceptual and Motor Skills*, **77**, 567–575.

Cato, M. A., Delis, D. C., Abildskov, T. J. & Bigler, E. (2004). Assessing the elusive cognitive deficits associated with ventromedial prefrontal damage: a case of a modern-day Phineas Gage. *Journal of the International Neuropsychological Society*, **10**, 453–465.

Cavedini, P., Riboldi, G., D'Annucci, A. *et al.* (2002a). Decision-making heterogeneity in obsessive-compulsive disorder: ventromedial prefrontal cortex function predicts different treatment outcomes. *Neuropsychologia*, **40**, 205–211.

Cavedini, P., Riboldi, G., Keller, R., D'Annucci, A. & Bellodi, L. (2002b). Frontal lobe dysfunction in pathological gambling patients. *Biological Psychiatry*, **51**, 334–341.

Chamberlain, S. R., Blackwell, A. D., Fineberg, N. A., Robbins, T. W. Sahakian, B. J. (2005). The neuropsychology of obsessive compulsive disorder: the importance of failures in cognitive and behavioural inhibition as candidate endophenotypic markers. *Neuroscience and Biobehavioral Reviews*, **29**, 399–419.

Chambers, R. A., Taylor, J. R. & Potenza, M. N. (2003). Developmental neurocircuitry of motivation in adolescence: a critical period of addiction vulnerability. *American Journal of Psychiatry*, **160**, 1041–1052.

Clark, L. & Sahakian, B. J. (2006). Neuropsychological and biological approaches to understanding bipolar disorder. In S. Jones and R. P. Bentall (Eds.), *The Psychology of Bipolar Disorder* (pp. 139–178) Oxford: Oxford University Press.

Clark, L., Bechara, A., Damasio, H. *et al.* (2008). Differential effects of insula and ventromedial prefrontal cortex lesions on risky decision-making. *Brain*, **131**, 1311–1322.

Clark, L., Blackwell, A. D., Aron, A. R. *et al.* (2007). Association between response inhibition and working memory in adult ADHD: a link to right frontal cortex pathology. *Biological Psychiatry*, **61**, 1395–1401.

Clark, L., Iversen, S. D. & Goodwin, G. M. (2001). A neuropsychological investigation of prefrontal cortex involvement in acute mania. *American Journal of Psychiatry*, **158**, 1605–1611.

Clark, L., Manes, F., Antoun, N., Sahakian, B. J. & Robbins, T. W. (2003). The contributions of lesion laterality and lesion volume to decision-making impairment following frontal lobe damage. *Neuropsychologia*, **41**, 1474–1483.

Clark, L., Robbins, T. W., Ersche, K. D. & Sahakian, B. J. (2006). Reflection impulsivity in current and former substance users. *Biological Psychiatry*, **60**, 512–522.

Damasio, A. (1994). *Descartes' Error: Emotion, Reason and the Human Brain*. New York, NY: G.P. Putnam.

Damasio, A. R., Tranel, D. & Damasio, H. (1990). Individuals with sociopathic behavior caused by frontal damage fail to respond autonomically to social stimuli. *Behavioral Brain Research*, **41**, 81–94.

Deakin, J. B., Rahman, S., Nestor, P. J., Hodges, J. R. & Sahakian, B. J. (2004). Paroxetine does not improve symptoms and impairs cognition in frontotemporal dementia: a double-blind randomized controlled trial. *Psychopharmacology (Berlin)*, **172**, 400–408.

Diehl, J., Grimmer, T., Drzezga, A. *et al.* (2004). Cerebral metabolic patterns at early stages of frontotemporal dementia and semantic dementia. A PET study. *Neurobiology of Aging*, **25**, 1051–1056.

Dijksterhuis, A., Bos, M. W., Nordgren, L. F. & van Baaren, R. B. (2006). On making the right choice: the deliberation-without-attention effect. *Science*, **311**, 1005–1007.

Dimitrov, M., Phipps, M., Zahn, T. P. & Grafman, J. (1999). A thoroughly modern Gage. *Neurocase*, **5**, 345–354.

Dom, G., Sabbe, B., Hulstijn, W. & van den Brink, W. (2005). Substance use disorders and the orbitofrontal cortex: systematic review of behavioural decision-making and neuroimaging studies. *British Journal of Psychiatry*, **187**, 209–220.

Drevets, W. C., Price, J. L., Simpson, J. R., Jr. *et al.* (1997). Subgenual prefrontal cortex abnormalities in mood disorders. *Nature*, **386**, 824–827.

Dunn, B. D., Dalgleish, T. & Lawrence, A. D. (2006). The somatic marker hypothesis: a critical evaluation. *Neuroscience and Biobehavioral Reviews*, **30**, 239–271.

Ellsberg, D. (1961). Risk, ambiguity and the Savage axioms. *Quarterly Journal of Economics*, **75**, 643–669.

Elster, J. & Skog, O.-J. (Eds.) (1999). *Getting Hooked: Rationality and Addiction*. Cambridge: Cambridge University Press.

Ernst, M., Bolla, K., Mouratidis, M. *et al.* (2002). Decision-making in a risk-taking task: a PET study. *Neuropsychopharmacology*, **26**, 682–691.

Ersche, K. D., Fletcher, P. C., Lewis, S. J. *et al.* (2005). Abnormal frontal activations related to decision-making in current and former amphetamine and opiate dependent individuals. *Psychopharmacology (Berlin)*, **180**, 612–623.

Eslinger, P. J. & Damasio, A. R. (1985). Severe disturbance of higher cognition after bilateral frontal lobe ablation: patient EVR. *Neurology*, **35**, 1731–1741.

Evenden, J. L. (1999). The pharmacology of impulsive behaviour in rats V: the effects of drugs on responding under a discrimination task using unreliable visual stimuli. *Psychopharmacology (Berlin)*, **143**, 111–122.

Eysenck, S. B. & Eysenck, H. J. (1978). Impulsiveness and venturesomeness: their position in a dimensional system of personality description. *Psychological Reports*, **43**, 1247–1255.

Fein, G., Klein, L., Finn, P. (2004). Impairment on a simulated gambling task in long-term abstinent alcoholics. *Alcohol: Clinical and Experimental Research*, **28**, 1487–1491.

Fellows, L. K. (2006). Deciding how to decide: ventromedial frontal lobe damage affects information acquisition in multi-attribute decision making. *Brain*, **129**, 944–952.

Fellows, L. K. & Farah, M. J. (2003). Ventromedial frontal cortex mediates affective shifting in humans: evidence from a reversal learning paradigm. *Brain*, **126**, 1830–1837.

Fellows, L. K. & Farah, M. J. (2005a). Dissociable elements of human foresight: a role for the ventromedial frontal lobes in framing the future, but not in discounting future rewards. *Neuropsychologia*, **43**, 1214–1221.

Fellows, L. K. & Farah, M. J. (2005b). Different underlying impairments in decision-making following ventromedial and dorsolateral frontal lobe damage in humans. *Cerebral Cortex*, **15**, 58–63.

Fox, H. C., McLean, A., Turner, J. J. *et al.* (2002). Neuropsychological evidence of a relatively selective profile of temporal dysfunction in drug-free MDMA ("ecstasy") polydrug users. *Psychopharmacology (Berlin)*, **162**, 203–214.

Franklin, T. R., Acton, P. D., Maldjian, J. A. *et al.* (2002). Decreased gray matter concentration in the insular, orbitofrontal, cingulate, and temporal cortices of cocaine patients. *Biological Psychiatry*, **51**, 134–142.

Frederick, S., Loewenstein, G. & O'Donaghue, T. (2002). Time discounting and time preference: a critical review. *Journal of Economic Literature*, **40**, 351–401.

Glimcher, P. W. & Rustichini, A. (2004). Neuroeconomics: the consilience of brain and decision. *Science*, **306**, 447–452.

Goldstein, R. Z. & Volkow, N. D. (2002). Drug addiction and its underlying neurobiological basis: neuroimaging evidence for the involvement of the frontal cortex. *American Journal of Psychiatry*, **159**, 1642–1652.

Gonzalez, C., Dana, J., Koshino, H. & Just, M. (2005). The framing effect and risky decisions: examining cognitive functions with fMRI. *Journal of Economic Psychology*, **26**, 1–20.

Goudriaan, A. E., Oosterlaan, J., de Beurs, E. & van den Brink, W. (2005). Decision making in pathological gambling: a comparison between pathological gamblers, alcohol dependents, persons with Tourette syndrome, and normal controls. *Brain Research: Cognitive Brain Research*, **23**, 137–151.

Gregory, C., Lough, S., Stone, V. *et al.* (2002). Theory of mind in patients with frontal variant frontotemporal dementia and Alzheimer's disease: theoretical and practical implications. *Brain*, **125**, 752–764.

Hinson, J. M., Jameson, T. L. & Whitney, P. (2002). Somatic markers, working memory, and decision making. *Cognitive, Affective and Behavioral Neuroscience*, **2**, 341–353.

Ho, M. Y., Mobini, S., Chiang, T. J., Bradshaw, C. M. & Szabadi, E. (1999). Theory and method in the quantitative analysis of "impulsive choice" behaviour: implications for psychopharmacology. *Psychopharmacology (Berlin)*, **146**, 362–372.

Horn, N. R., Dolan, M., Elliott, R., Deakin, J. F. & Woodruff, P. W. (2003). Response inhibition and impulsivity: an fMRI study. *Neuropsychologia*, **41**, 1959–1966.

Hornak, J., O'Doherty, J., Bramham, J. *et al.* (2004). Reward-related reversal learning after surgical excisions in orbito-frontal or dorsolateral prefrontal cortex in humans. *Journal of Cognitive Neuroscience*, **16**, 463–478.

Hsu, M., Bhatt, M., Adolphs, R., Tranel, D. & Camerer, C. F. (2005). Neural systems responding to degrees of uncertainty in human decision-making. *Science*, **310**, 1680–1683.

Huettel, S. A., Stowe, C. J., Gordon, E. M., Warner, B. T. & Platt, M. L. (2006). Neural signatures of economic preferences for risk and ambiguity. *Neuron*, **49**, 765–775.

Hutton, S. B., Murphy, F. C., Joyce, E. M. *et al.* (2002). Decision making deficits in patients with first-episode and chronic schizophrenia. *Schizophrenia Research*, **55**, 249–257.

Ibach, B., Poljansky, S., Marienhagen, J. *et al.* (2004). Contrasting metabolic impairment in frontotemporal degeneration and early onset Alzheimer's disease. *Neuroimage*, **23**, 739–743.

Irle, E., Exner, C., Thielen, K., Weniger, G. & Ruther, E. (1998). Obsessive-compulsive disorder and ventromedial frontal lesions: clinical and neuropsychological findings. *American Journal of Psychiatry*, **155**, 255–263.

Jameson, T. L., Hinson, J. M. & Whitney, P. (2004). Components of working memory and somatic markers in decision making. *Psychonomic Bulletin and Reviews*, **11**, 515–520.

Jentsch, J. D. & Taylor, J. R. (1999). Impulsivity resulting from frontostriatal dysfunction in drug abuse: implications for the control of behavior by reward-related stimuli. *Psychopharmacology (Berlin)*, **146**, 373–390.

Johnson, M. W. & Bickel, W. K. (2002). Within-subject comparison of real and hypothetical money rewards in delay discounting. *Journal of the Experimental Analysis of Behavior*, **77**, 129–146.

Kagan, J. (1966). Reflection-impulsivity: the generality and dynamics of conceptual tempo. *Journal of Abnormal Psychology*, **71**, 17–24.

Kirby, K. N. & Herrnstein, R. J. (1995). Preference reversals due to myopic discounting of delayed reward. *Psychological Science*, **6**, 83–89.

Kirby, K. N., Petry, N. M. & Bickel, W. K. (1999). Heroin addicts have higher discount rates for delayed rewards than non-drug-using controls. *Journal of Experimental Psychology: General*, **128**, 78–87.

Kuhnen, C. M. & Knutson, B. (2005). The neural basis of financial risk taking. *Neuron*, **47**, 763–770.

Lacerda, A. L., Keshavan, M. S., Hardan, A. Y. *et al.* (2004). Anatomic evaluation of the orbitofrontal cortex in major depressive disorder. *Biological Psychiatry*, **55**, 353–358.

Lejuez, C. W., Aklin, W. M., Jones, H. A. *et al.* (2003). The Balloon Analogue Risk Task (BART) differentiates smokers and nonsmokers. *Experimental and Clinical Psychopathology*, **11**, 26–33.

Leland, D. S. & Paulus, M. P. (2005). Increased risk-taking decision-making but not altered response to punishment in stimulant-using young adults. *Drug and Alcohol Dependence*, **78**, 83–90.

Lijffijt, M., Bekker, E. M., Quik, E. H. *et al.* (2004). Differences between low and high trait impulsivity are not associated with differences in inhibitory motor control. *Journal of Attention Disorders*, **8**, 25–32.

Lopes, L. L. (1987). Between fear and hope: the psychology of risk. In L. Berkowitz (Ed.), *Advances in Experimental Social Psychology* (pp. 255–295) New York, NY: Academic Press.

Lyoo, I. K., Pollack, M. H., Silveri, M. M. *et al.* (2006). Prefrontal and temporal gray matter density decreases in opiate dependence. *Psychopharmacology (Berlin)*, **184**, 139–144.

Madden, G. J., Petry, N. M., Badger, G. J. & Bickel, W. K. (1997). Impulsive and self-control choices in opioid-dependent patients and non-drug-using control participants: drug and monetary rewards. *Experimental and Clinical Psychopharmacology*, **5**, 256–262.

Malloy, P., Bihrle, A., Duffy, J. & Cimino, C. (1993). The orbitomedial frontal syndrome. *Archives of Clinical Neuropsychology*, **8**, 185–201.

Manes, F., Sahakian, B., Clark, L. *et al.* (2002). Decision-making processes following damage to the prefrontal cortex. *Brain*, **125**, 624–639.

Mavaddat, N., Kirkpatrick, P. J., Rogers, R. D. & Sahakian, B. J. (2000). Deficits in decision-making in patients with aneurysms of the anterior communicating artery. *Brain*, **123**, 2109–2117.

Mazas, C. A., Finn, P. R. & Steinmetz, J. E. (2000). Decision-making biases, antisocial personality, and early-onset alcoholism. *Alcohol: Clinical and Experimental Research*, **24**, 1036–1040.

Mazur, J. (1987). An adjusting procedure for studying delayed reinforcement. In M. L. Commons, J. E. Mazur, J. A. Nevin & H. Rachlin (Eds.), *Quantitative Analysis of Behavior. The effect of Delay and of Intervening Events on Reinforcement Value* (vol. **5**, pp. 55–74). Hillsdale, NJ: Lawrence Erlbaum Associates.

McClure, S. M., Laibson, D. I., Loewenstein, G. & Cohen, J. D. (2004). Separate neural systems value immediate and delayed monetary rewards. *Science*, **306**, 503–507.

Mellers, B. A., Schwartz, A. & Ritov, I. (1999). Emotion-based choice. *Journal of Experimental Psychology: General*, **128**, 332–345.

Messer, S. B. (1976). Reflection-impulsivity: a review. *Psychological Bulletin*, **83**, 1026–1052.

Mobini, S., Body, S., Ho, M. Y. *et al.* (2002). Effects of lesions of the orbitofrontal cortex on sensitivity to delayed and probabilistic reinforcement. *Psychopharmacology (Berlin)*, **160**, 290–298.

Moeller, F. G., Dougherty, D. M., Barratt, E. S. *et al.* (2002). Increased impulsivity in cocaine dependent subjects independent of antisocial personality disorder and aggression. *Drug and Alcohol Dependence*, **68**, 105–111.

Monterosso, J., Ehrman, R., Napier, K. L., O'Brien, C. P. & Childress, A. R. (2001). Three decision-making tasks in cocaine-dependent patients: do they measure the same construct? *Addiction*, **96**, 1825–1837.

Morgan, M. J. (1998). Recreational use of "ecstasy" (MDMA) is associated with elevated impulsivity. *Neuropsychopharmacology*, **19**, 252–264.

Morgan, M. J., McFie, L., Fleetwood, H. & Robinson, J. A. (2002). Ecstasy (MDMA): are the psychological problems associated with its use reversed by prolonged abstinence? *Psychopharmacology (Berlin)*, **159**, 294–303.

Morgan, M. J., Impallomeni, L. C., Pirona, A. & Rogers, R. D. (2005). Elevated impulsivity and impaired decision-making in abstinent Ecstasy (MDMA) users compared to polydrug and drug-naive controls. *Neuropsychopharmacology*, **31**(7), 1562–1573.

Murphy, F. C., Rubinsztein, J. S., Michael, A. *et al.* (2001). Decision-making cognition in mania and depression. *Psychological Medicine*, **31**, 679–693.

Nielen, M. M., Veltman, D. J., de Jong, R., Mulder, G. & den Boer, J. A. (2002). Decision making performance in obsessive compulsive disorder. *Journal of Affective Disorders*, **69**, 257–260.

Odum, A. L., Madden, G. J., Badger, G. J. & Bickel, W. K. (2000). Needle sharing in opioid-dependent outpatients: psychological processes underlying risk. *Drug and Alcohol Dependence*, **60**, 259–266.

Ongur, D., Ferry, A. T. & Price, J. L. (2003). Architectonic subdivision of the human orbital and medial prefrontal cortex. *Journal of Comparative Neurology*, **460**, 425–449.

Patton, J. H., Stanford, M. S. & Barratt, E. S. (1995). Factor structure of the Barratt impulsiveness scale. *Journal of Clinical Psychology*, **51**, 768–774.

Paulus, M. P., Rogalsky, C., Simmons, A., Feinstein, J. S. & Stein, M. B. (2003). Increased activation in the right insula during risk-taking decision making is related to harm avoidance and neuroticism. *Neuroimage*, **19**, 1439–1448.

Perry, J. L., Larson, E. B., German, J. P., Madden, G. J. & Carroll, M. E. (2005). Impulsivity (delay discounting) as a predictor of acquisition of IV cocaine self-administration in female rats. *Psychopharmacology (Berlin)*, **178**, 193–201.

Petry, N. M. (2001). Pathological gamblers, with and without substance use disorders, discount delayed rewards at high rates. *Journal of Abnormal Psychology*, **110**, 482–487.

Rachlin, H., Raineri, A. & Cross, D. (1991). Subjective probability and delay. *Journal of the Experimental Analysis of Behavior*, **55**, 233–244.

Rahman, S., Robbins, T. W., Hodges, J. R. *et al.* (2006). Methylphenidate ('Ritalin') can ameliorate abnormal risk-taking behavior in the frontal variant of frontotemporal dementia. *Neuropsychopharmacology*, **31**, 651–658.

Rahman, S., Sahakian, B. J., Hodges, J. R., Rogers, R. D. & Robbins, T. W. (1999). Specific cognitive deficits in mild frontal variant frontotemporal dementia. *Brain*, **122**, 1469–1493.

Ratnavalli, E., Brayne, C., Dawson, K. & Hodges, J. R. (2002). The prevalence of frontotemporal dementia. *Neurology*, **58**, 1615–1621.

Ritter, L. M., Meador-Woodruff, J. H. & Dalack, G. W. (2004). Neurocognitive measures of prefrontal cortical dysfunction in schizophrenia. *Schizophrenia Research*, **68**, 65–73.

Rogers, R. D., Everitt, B. J., Baldacchino, A. *et al.* (1999). Dissociable deficits in the decision-making cognition of chronic amphetamine abusers, opiate abusers, patients with focal damage to prefrontal cortex, and tryptophan-depleted normal volunteers: evidence for mono-aminergic mechanisms. *Neuropsychopharmacology*, **20**, 322–339.

Rolls, E. T., Hornak, J., Wade, D. & McGrath, J. (1994). Emotion-related learning in patients with social and emotional changes associated with frontal lobe damage. *Journal of Neurology, Neurosurgery and Psychiatry*, **57**, 1518–1524.

Rubia, K., Smith, A. B., Brammer, M. J. & Taylor, E. (2003). Right inferior prefrontal cortex mediates response inhibition while mesial prefrontal cortex is responsible for error detection. *Neuroimage*, **20**, 351–358.

Rubinsztein, J. S., Michael, A., Paykel, E. S. & Sahakian, B. J. (2000). Cognitive impairment in remission in bipolar affective disorder. *Psychological Medicine*, **30**, 1025–1036.

Salmon, E., Garraux, G., Delbeuck, X. *et al.* (2003). Predominant ventromedial frontopolar metabolic impairment in frontotemporal dementia. *Neuroimage*, **20**, 435–440.

Sanfey, A. G., Hastie, R., Colvin, M. K. & Grafman, J. (2003a). Phineas gauged: decision-making and the human prefrontal cortex. *Neuropsychologia*, **41**, 1218–1229.

Sanfey, A. G., Loewenstein, G., McClure, S. M. & Cohen, J. D. (2006). Neuroeconomics: cross-currents in research on decision-making. *Trends in Cognitive Science*, **10**, 108–116.

Sanfey, A. G., Rilling, J. K., Aronson, J. A., Nystrom, L. E. & Cohen, J. D. (2003b). The neural basis of economic decision-making in the Ultimatum Game. *Science*, **300**, 1755–1758.

Saver, J. L. & Damasio, A. R. (1991). Preserved access and processing of social knowledge in a patient with acquired sociopathy due to ventromedial frontal damage. *Neuropsychologia*, **29**, 1241–1249.

Shamay-Tsoory, S. G., Tomer, R., Berger, B. D. & Aharon-Peretz, J. (2003). Characterization of empathy deficits following prefrontal brain damage: the role of the right ventromedial prefrontal cortex. *Journal of Cognitive Neuroscience*, **15**, 324–337.

Shiv, B., Loewenstein, G., Bechara, A., Damasio, H. & Damasio, A. R. (2005). Investment behavior and the negative side of emotion. *Psychological Science*, **16**, 435–439.

Shurman, B., Horan, W. P. & Nuechterlein, K. H. (2005). Schizophrenia patients demonstrate a distinctive pattern of decision-making impairment on the Iowa Gambling Task. *Schizophrenia Research*, **72**, 215–224.

Sjogren, M., Minthon, L., Passant, U., Blennow, K. & Wallin, A. (1998). Decreased monoamine metabolites in frontotemporal dementia and Alzheimer's disease. *Neurobiology of Aging*, **19**, 379–384.

Stout, J. C., Rock, S. L., Campbell, M. C., Busemeyer, J. R. & Finn, P. R. (2005). Psychological processes underlying risky decisions in drug abusers. *Psychology of Addictive Behavior*, **19**, 148–157.

Swann, A. C., Bjork, J. M., Moeller, F. G. & Dougherty, D. M. (2002). Two models of impulsivity: relationship to personality traits and psychopathology. *Biological Psychiatry*, **51**, 988–994.

Tarter, R. E., Kirisci, L., Habeych, M., Reynolds, M. & Vanyukov, M. (2004). Neurobehavior disinhibition in childhood predisposes boys to substance use disorder by young adulthood: direct and mediated etiologic pathways. *Drug and Alcohol Dependence*, **73**, 121–132.

Tomb, I., Hauser, M., Deldin, P. & Caramazza, A. (2002). Do somatic markers mediate decisions on the gambling task? *Nature Neuroscience*, **5**, 1103–1104.

Torralva, T., Kipps, C., Hodges, J. R. *et al.* (2007). The relationship between affective decision-making and theory of mind in frontal variant frontotemporal dementia. *Neuropsychologia*, **45**, 342–349.

Tranel, D., Bechara, A. & Denburg, N. L. (2002). Asymmetric functional roles of right and left ventromedial prefrontal cortices in social conduct, decision-making, and emotional processing. *Cortex*, **38**, 589–612.

Tranel, D., Damasio, H., Denburg, N. L. & Bechara, A. (2005). Does gender play a role in functional asymmetry of ventromedial prefrontal cortex? *Brain*, **128**, 2872–2881.

Turner, D. C., Robbins, T. W., Clark, L. *et al.* (2003). Relative lack of cognitive effects of methylphenidate in elderly male volunteers. *Psychopharmacology*, **168**, 455–464.

Tversky, A. & Kahneman, D. (1981). The framing of decisions and the psychology of choice. *Science*, **211**, 453–458.

Tversky, A. & Kahneman, D. (1991). Loss aversion in riskless choice: a reference dependent model. *Quarterly Journal of Economics*, **106**, 1039–1061.

Vitaro, F., Arseneault, L. & Tremblay, R. E. (1999). Impulsivity predicts problem gambling in low SES adolescent males. *Addiction*, **94**, 565–575.

von Neumann, J. & Morganstern, O. (1944). *Theory of Games and Economic Behavior*. Princeton, NJ: Princeton University Press.

Vuchinich, R. E. & Heather, N. (Eds.) (2003). *Choice, Behavioural Economics and Addiction*. Amsterdam: Elsevier.

Watkins, L. H., Sahakian, B. J., Robertson, M. M. *et al.* (2005). Executive function in Tourette's syndrome and obsessive-compulsive disorder. *Psychological Medicine*, **35**, 571–582.

Whiteside, S. P. & Lynam, D. R. (2001). The five factor model and impulsivity: using a structural model of personality to understand impulsivity. *Personality and Individual Differences*, **30**, 669–689.

Whitney, K. A., Fastenau, P. S., Evans, J. D. & Lysaker, P. H. (2004). Comparative neuropsychological function in obsessive-compulsive disorder and schizophrenia with and without obsessive-compulsive symptoms. *Schizophrenia Research*, **69**, 75–83.

Wilder, K. E., Weinberger, D. R. & Goldberg, T. E. (1998). Operant conditioning and the orbitofrontal cortex in schizophrenic patients: unexpected evidence for intact functioning. *Schizophrenia Research*, **30**, 169–174.

Wilson, J. M., Kalasinsky, K. S., Levey, A. I. *et al.* (1996). Striatal dopamine nerve terminal markers in human, chronic methamphetamine users. *Nature Medicine*, **2**, 699–703.

Winstanley, C. A., Theobald, D. E., Cardinal, R. N. & Robbins, T. W. (2004). Contrasting roles of basolateral amygdala and orbitofrontal cortex in impulsive choice. *Journal of Neuroscience*, **24**, 4718–4722.

Zuckerman, M. (1979). *Sensation Seeking: Beyond the Optimal level of Arousal*. New York, NY: Lawrence Erlbaum Associates.

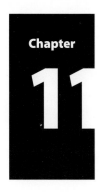

Chapter

11

The neuropsychology of social cognition: implications for psychiatric disorders

Tamara A. Russell and Melissa J. Green

Social cognition in an evolutionary framework

Social cognition refers to cognitive processes necessary for the accurate perception and interpretation of information conveyed by conspecifics (other individuals of the same species). This is particularly relevant to higher cognitive processes that underpin the formulation of appropriate and flexible behavioral responses that are required in everyday social interactions (Adolphs, 1999; Ostrom, 1984).

Social information is distinct from non-social information in several ways. Non-social cognitive stimuli are most commonly of neutral valence (e.g. auditory tones, visual shapes, letters or numbers), while social cognitive stimuli are often personally relevant and take the form of dynamic bi-directional interactions, insofar as each participant's responses can influence the social exchange (Fiske, 1991). Also, social inferences are often based upon the perception of fleeting information (i.e. dynamic displays of facial emotion), or the perception of unobservable characteristics requiring inference from subtle behavioral displays (e.g. judgments about personality characteristics may be based on the observation of interpersonal behavior, but cannot be observed per se); these types of inference are not as common in non-social cognition (Fiske, 1991). Social cognition may also be seen as distinct from non-social cognition given that adequate skills in this domain are required for efficient social behavior and social functioning (Pinkham et al., 2003). Given these distinctions, social cognitive skills are not typically assessed by standard neuropsychological tools. However, effective social cognition may certainly rely upon effective functioning in

domain-general cognitive domains (e.g. attention, memory, working memory, executive functioning; this issue is addressed in later discussion).

In a seminal review, Brothers proposed an evolutionary argument for the existence of distinct neural architecture subserving specific social cognitive functions that developed in response to the demands of living in large social groups (Brothers, 1990). Furthermore, primate neocortex volume is argued to have evolved in direct proportion to the size of the social group. As the size of the social group increased, so did the cognitive demands of living within a complex social order, requiring a brain capable of responding to subtle social cues (such as eye gaze and facial displays of emotion) and representing the intentions of others. Indeed, neocortex size in primates is correlated with five separate indices of social complexity, including social group size, grooming clique size, the extent to which social skills are used in male mating strategies, the frequency of tactical deception and the frequency of social play (Byrne & Corp, 2004; Dunbar, 2003). Thus, evolutionary approaches to social cognition predict the existence of specialized neural networks facilitating prosocial behaviors such as cooperation and altruism (thereby increasing access to reliable food sources, security from predators and better mate choice), as well as manipulative behaviors such as coercion and deception of conspecifics in response to the increased competition for food and mates. The existence of cognitive mechanisms facilitating the manipulation of one's own and others' behavior for the effective negotiation of the social environment is evident in many primates, including *Homo sapiens* (Dunbar, 2003). Furthermore, these mechanisms range from low-level perceptual skills

The Neuropsychology of Mental Illness, ed. Stephen J. Wood, Nicholas B. Allen and Christos Pantelis. Published by Cambridge University Press. © Cambridge University Press 2009.

Table 11.1 DSM–IV and ICD–10 criteria related to social functioning for different psychiatric diagnoses.

Disorder	Emotion-related symptoms related to social functioning*
Conduct disorder	Criteria A: repetitive and persistent pattern of behavior in which the basic rights of others or major age-appropriate societal norms or rules are violated. Criteria B: behavior causes clinically significant impairment in social, academic or occupational functioning
Schizophrenia, schizoaffective disorder, schizophreniform disorder	Affective flattening, anhedonia
Major depressive disorder	Depressed mood, anhedonia
Social phobia	Marked and persistent fear, anxious anticipation (related to interpersonal or social situations)
Obsessive-compulsive disorder	Marked anxiety or distress
Post-traumatic stress disorder	Irritability, anger, physiological reactivity, distress, anhedonia, restricted range of affect
Acute stress disorder	Symptoms of anxiety or increased arousal
Generalized anxiety disorder	Excessive anxiety and worry, irritability
Paranoid personality disorder	Quick to react angrily
Schizoid personality disorder	Emotional coldness, detachment, flattened affectivity
Schizotypal personality disorder	Inappropriate or constricted affect, excessive social anxiety
Antisocial personality disorder	Lack of remorse, irritability
Borderline personality disorder	Affective instability due to marked reactivity of mood, inappropriate intense anger, or difficulty controlling anger
Histrionic personality disorder	Rapidly shifting and shallow expressions of emotions
Narcissistic personality disorder	Lacks empathy
Avoidant personality disorder	Fear of criticism, disapproval or rejection
Dependent personality disorder	Fear of being unable to care for self, being left alone

Note: Parts of this table have been adapted from Kring & Werner (2004).

(such as gaze direction detection), which may be common to all social species, to high-level species-specific processes (such as belief representation) that may be unique to humans.

In humans, specific social cognitive skills include the recognition of a relative or friend (through the analysis of facial features and/or gait), decoding displays of emotion (facial and vocal affect processing), and inferring what someone believes about the state of the world in order to predict and explain behavior ("Theory of Mind," ToM; Premack & Woodruff, 1978). It is usually apparent when an individual has difficulties in the social domain. Individuals with autism and Aspergers' syndrome may be seen to represent a particularly salient example of the abnormal social brain, showing profound deficits in social cognition, exemplified by the inability to represent the mental states of others as distinct from their own representation of the world (Baron-Cohen, 1995). Various social cognitive impairments have also been demonstrated in schizophrenia (Corrigan & Penn, 2001), bipolar disorder (Kerr et al., 2003) and unipolar depression (Suslow et al., 2001) and some of the more severe personality disorders (Skodol et al., 2002). Impairments in moral reasoning and decision-making are evident in socially deviant individuals (Blair, 1997). Indeed, it is notable that some form of decline in social functioning forms part of the diagnostic criteria for the majority of severe psychiatric illnesses (Table 11.1). Also, in some disorders (e.g.

schizophrenia), social problems are likely to pre-date the manifestation of overt symptoms. The investigation of various psychiatric disorders from a social cognitive perspective may therefore aid in elucidating the cause of some symptoms of mental disorder (Brune, 2001; Brune & Brune-Cohrs, 2006).

In the following sections of this chapter, we explore evidence from neuropsychology and neuroscience regarding the sovereignty of social cognition. That is, the question of whether social cognition can be regarded as comprising a range of specialized cognitive processes devoted to the performance of social tasks (domain-specific processes) or whether social-cognitive skills depend upon basic neuropsychological processes such as attention, executive functioning or memory (domain-general processes). To assume the domain-specificity of social cognition one would need to show a dissociation between these two types of processes in a single individual, by demonstrating the existence of either (a) impairments in social-cognitive skills alongside intact domain-general neuropsychological skills, or (b) intact social cognition alongside specific neuropsychological deficits. We thus explore evidence for dissociation between cognitive and social-cognitive performance in individuals with specific neurological abnormalities or psychiatric disorders, following a brief review of the evidence from social-cognitive neuroscience regarding the role of specialized neural networks for the processing of social information (such as facial emotion and ToM skills). While there exists specialized neuroanatomy and cognitive architecture to subserve some aspects of social information processing, the evidence regarding the domain-specificity of higher order social-cognitive skills such as ToM remains equivocal. Thus, we conclude that it is unlikely that social-cognitive skills can be presumed to function adequately without intact domain-general cognitive capacities.

The neural basis of social cognition in healthy humans

Evidence from lesion, neuroimaging and electrophysiological studies converges to support the existence of distributed "social brain" networks that involve the primary visual cortices, amygdala, superior temporal sulcus, medial frontal cortex, orbitofrontal cortex and right parietal and anterior cingulate cortices (Adolphs, 2003). This network guides our perception and interpretation of social behavior, including the perception of biological motion,[1] facial identity and emotion recognition, right through to complex attributions, personality judgments and inferences about the mental states of others. In this section we review the evidence from recent brain-imaging studies to examine the notion of specialized neural circuits for the processing of social information.

Face perception

Face perception is mediated by a widely distributed neural system in humans that consists of multiple, bilateral regions of the ventral temporal and association cortices (Haxby et al., 2002). The functional organization of this system includes the representation of invariant aspects of faces that, as compared to houses and other classes of objects, is the basis for recognizing individuals, and which is located in a region of the posterior temporal and extrastriate cortex (fusiform face area, FFA; Kanwisher et al., 1997).[2] It has been shown, however, that activation of the (ventral) temporal cortex in response to the representation of faces and object categories extends beyond regions that demonstrate category-related response preferences (such as the FFA) and includes regions that respond both maximally and submaximally, as well as other cortical areas (Haxby et al., 2001). In contrast, the representation of changeable aspects, such as eye gaze, expression and lip movement, which underlies the perception of information that facilitates social communication, is located in the lateral temporal cortex, including the superior temporal sulcus (STS) (Beauchamp et al., 2003; Haxby et al., 2004).

However, convergent evidence suggests that these regions are not limited to the processing of such information from faces, given their role in broader biological motion processing. Early visual analysis of faces is mediated by a core system comprising occipito-temporal regions in extrastriate visual cortex, while an extended system of regions including neural systems involved in other cognitive functions acts in concert with the core system to extract meaning from faces. Within the extended system for face perception, the amygdala plays a central role in processing the social relevance of information gleaned from faces, particularly when that information may signal a potential threat (Haxby et al., 2002).

Facial emotion recognition

Despite early studies implying a greater involvement of the non-dominant (usually right) hemisphere, including the somatosensory cortices, for the detection, recognition and representation of facial expressions of emotion (Adolphs *et al.*, 2000; see Borod *et al.*, 2002 for a review), recent neuroimaging studies suggest that facial emotion is processed bilaterally (Phan *et al.*, 2004; Phillips *et al.*, 2003a) or may be predominantly processed in the left hemisphere of right-handed people (Stone *et al.*, 1996). The disparity of findings from neuropsychology and neuroimaging studies regarding the laterality of emotion processing may be due to task-related performance demands, such as verbal labeling. For example, in a patient with a severed corpus collosum it has been demonstrated that verbal catagorization of emotion was better when stimuli were presented to the right visual hemi-field (stimulating the left hemisphere), while presentations to the left visual hemi-field (stimulating the right hemisphere) resulted in improved performance on an association task (Stone *et al.*, 1996). Similarly, field potentials recorded with MEG during explicit verbal catagorization have been shown to engage the left posterior temporal lobe (Liu *et al.*, 1999), while covert emotion-recognition tasks (requiring participants to attend to gender rather than facial emotion) engage the right posterior temporal lobe (Krolak-Salmon *et al.*, 2001). Differences in performance demands may also influence the distribution of brain responses to emotional faces in neuroimaging studies. For example, explicit (verbal emotion-labeling) tasks result in activation of a wider network (including the ventral frontal cortex and temporal cortex), while implicit (gender- or age-discrimination) tasks maximally activate subcortical structures such as the hippocampus and amygdala (Critchley *et al.*, 2000; Hariri *et al.*, 2000; Lange *et al.*, 2003).

Recent studies exploring the recognition of specific emotions implicate a primary, but by no means exclusive, role for the amygdala in the detection of negative emotions (Adolphs, 2001; Adolphs *et al.*, 1999), particularly fear (Morris *et al.*, 1998; Phillips *et al.*, 1997). The amygdala is believed to operate at both an unconscious level of awareness for rapid, automatic evaluation of threat, and at a conscious level for the effortful reappraisal of a threat stimulus once it is detected (Adolphs, 2003; LeDoux, 1998). These proposals build upon a long tradition of animal studies exploring the role of the amygdala in fear conditioning. Animals with amygdala lesions demonstrate impaired fear conditioning alongside a profile of abnormal social behaviors, including social disinhibition and inappropriate approach/avoidance responses alongside otherwise healthy functioning (Bauman *et al.*, 2004; Diergaarde *et al.*, 2004). While it has been argued that the amygdala plays a key role in learning via positive/negative reinforcement and the "tagging" of emotional significance to a particular context (via feedback loops with other limbic network structures such as the ventromedial frontal cortex), the temporal dynamics of this complex interplay are yet to be fully elucidated (Damasio, 1996). Other brain regions have been implicated for the recognition of specific facial emotions: for example, the insula in response to facial and vocal expressions of disgust (Phillips *et al.*, 1997, 1998), the OFC and ACC for facial expressions of anger (Blair *et al.*, 1999), and the amygdala, insula and ACC in response to facial expressions of fear (Morris *et al.*, 1996).

Theory of Mind

Considerable evidence suggests that ToM abilities in humans involve a network of regions within the medial prefrontal cortex, the temporal poles and the temporo-parietal junction (Frith & Frith, 2003). For example, early studies implicated a role for the medial frontal lobes in the appreciation of stories requiring the understanding of the story protagonist's mental state (Fletcher *et al.*, 1995), or simple mental state inferences (Goel *et al.*, 1995). More recent studies using both verbal and non-verbal ToM tasks have revealed support for the role of the medial prefrontal cortex (Castelli *et al.*, 2000; Gallagher *et al.*, 2000; McCabe *et al.*, 2001; Vogeley *et al.*, 2001).

The study of brain responses during ToM tasks in individuals with known social-cognitive difficulties has corroborated the above findings. For example, activation of the medial prefrontal cortex has been shown to be absent in individuals with autism and Asperger's syndrome, compared with healthy controls, when performing mentalizing conditions of Happé's cartoon task (Happé *et al.*, 1996). Similarly, a study of mentalizing using Baron-Cohen's Eyes Task in individuals with Asperger's syndrome revealed an absence of activity in the amygdala and superior temporal gyrus (structures that would normally be activated in healthy controls in the comparison of mentalizing and non-mentalizing conditions; Baron-Cohen *et al.*, 1999). Using this task in a study of schizophrenia patients, a reduction in activation in a region of the left frontal lobe, as well as the left superior temporal gyrus, was observed (Russell *et al.*, 2000).

Social cognition: distinct from traditional neuropsychology?

Inferences about the feelings and intentions of other agents may be crucially dependent upon the adequate development of non-social cognitive processing capacities. One example of these domain-general processes is context-dependent information processing, as a function of working memory. In particular, deficits in representing others' mental states may reflect difficulty maintaining representations of context derived from verbal information, and/or difficulty constructing an appropriate representation of context from abstract visual information (such as gestures or facial expressions). For example, a classic paradigm for the investigation of ToM ability is the "Sally Anne Task" (Baron-Cohen *et al.,* 1985). In this task, subjects must correctly interpret the meaning of visually presented drawings of social scenes, in order to represent and maintain the beliefs of two characters separately, and then use this information to coordinate the actual state of affairs. The correct inference in this task therefore relies on the accurate formation and maintenance of contextual information, held in working memory, in the form of each character's belief about the particular situation. This relatively simple task reflects the complex interaction between the appreciation of other minds and working-memory requirements that are necessary for accurate ToM performance.

In this section we will review the evidence for dissociation of cognitive processes subserving social and non-social cognition. Evidence will be drawn from neuropsychological investigations of individuals with focal brain lesions, and the study of disordered populations known to exhibit deficits in specific domain-general cognitive domains (including the genetic disorder William's syndrome and psychiatric disorders such as autism, schizophrenia and bipolar disorder). We will be particularly concerned with issues surrounding experimental design and the implications of findings from particular diagnostic categories for distinguishing the cognitive architecture of social and non-social cognition. What is critical in these studies is the ability to separate the contribution of domain-general processes (such as language or executive function) with regard to their impact on social-cognitive task *performance* and *competence*. For example, patients with impaired working memory might fail false-belief tasks (used to tap ToM ability) because they cannot maintain and update crucial social information that is necessary to perform the task (i.e. performance demands). Alternatively, if belief reasoning is carried out by a domain-general reasoning system, impaired working memory would necessarily lead to impaired competence on the task even if performance demands are adequately controlled (Apperly *et al.*, 2005). Furthermore, if components of ToM are carried out by domain-specific processes (Leslie & Thaiss, 1992), then there should be no effect of impairments in working memory on belief-reasoning tasks if performance demands are adequately controlled. Clarification of the cognitive basis of social-information processing thus requires methods that allow clear separation of performance and competence demands, as well as sufficiently precise measures of competence (Apperly *et al.*, 2005). A summary of the tasks used to measure specific social-cognitive abilities and the domain-general processes implicated in each is presented in Table 11.2.

Dissociation of social and non-social cognitive function

One line of evidence in support for the relative independence of social cognition from basic non-social cognition (or neurocognition) comes from the dissociation of specific cognitive skills in single case studies with focal brain damage. For example, individuals with selective brain damage to the prefrontal cortex (Anderson *et al.*, 1999) or amygdala (Fine *et al.*, 2001) demonstrate aberrant social behavior and impaired social functioning alongside intact cognitive skills such as memory and language. Furthermore, in further single case studies reporting a dissociation between ToM abilities and executive function (Bird *et al.*, 2004; Fine *et al.*, 2001; Rowe *et al.*, 2001), impaired executive functioning did not necessarily *predict* difficulties with ToM tasks (Bird *et al.*, 2004), and gross impairments in ToM were seen in the context of normal performance on tests of executive functioning (Fine *et al.*, 2001). In addition, one study

Table 11.2 Theory of mind tasks.

Task	Description of task	Control condition	Non-social-cognitive components
Sally Anne Task (Wimmer & Perner, 1983)	The experimenter uses two dolls, "Sally" and "Anne." Sally has a basket; Anne has a box. Experimenters show the participants (usually children) a simple skit, in which Sally puts a marble in her basket and then leaves the scene. While Sally is away, Anne takes the marble out of Sally's basket and puts it into her box. Sally then returns and the participant is asked where they think Sally will look for her marble. A child is said to "pass" the test if they understand that Sally will first look inside her basket (on the basis of her false belief) before realizing that her marble isn't there. The participant has to understand that even though Anne has moved the ball, Sally still has in mind the original location of the object and will therefore look in the wrong place	Control questions can be used to determine how well the basics of the situation have been grasped (i.e. by asking who moved the ball, or what object was moved)	Context-dependent processing: working memory, holding in mind two conflicting beliefs
Happé story task (Happé et al., 1999)	Written stories which require either a mental or physical state inference in order for a correct response to be given. Correct response normally relates to how a particular character will act and includes an explanation of why the character acts that way – usually need to understand that someone has a false belief about something and therefore may behave in a particular way on the basis of that false belief.	Matched control stories requiring a physical inference for their understanding. Control questions to check memory and understanding can also be incorporated	Verbal/reading ability, working memory (although the latter depends on how the task is administered).

Task	Description	Control condition	Skills/confounds required
Happé cartoon task (Happé et al., 1999)	A task based on cartoons taken from American newspapers. There are two conditions – one set of cartoons requires a mental state inference and one requires a physical state inference. Responses are marked according to whether or not the person 'got' the joke, scoring criteria are provided	Matched control cartoons requiring inference of physical as opposed to mental states	Visual attention and visual search, intact visual grouping (early stage context processing), perspective taking
Eyes Task (Baron-Cohen et al., 1997) Revised version (Baron-Cohen et al., 2001).	Individuals have to determine the mental state expressed by an eye pair from one of four complex mental state terms displayed alongside the eye image. A glossary of word meanings is provided. Adult and child versions are available	A control task has sometimes been included in this assessment in which individuals have to determine the gender of the eyes	Knowledge of complex emotions and mental states
Hinting Task (Corcoran et al., 1995)	A verbal task in which one character drops a verbal hint to another person in order to get them to do something	No specific control condition although prompting questions could additionally be given to the participant	Verbal (reading ability), working memory (if written information does *not* remain in front of the individual), knowledge of social norms
Picture arrangement tasks Original Version: Baron-Cohen et al. (1986). Other versions: Langdon et al. (1997); Sarfati et al. (1997); Brunet et al. (2003)	In this task participants typically have to arrange 3 or 4 pictures so that they make a coherent story. Some of these stories or situations will require the individual to have an understanding of the intention or desire/goal/belief of a character in order to sequence the cards correctly. Variations on this task have been used by a number of authors with different populations (including Langdon et al., Sarfati et al. and Brunet et al.)	Physical, non-social or mechanical picture arrangement tasks have been used as matched within-task controls	Logical reasoning, visual attention (visual search; attention to detail; intact visual grouping/ early stage context processing), knowledge of social norms

has demonstrated the statistical independence of social and non-social cognitive skills even when performance in both domains was impaired (Rowe *et al.*, 2001). Similarly, individuals with prosopagnosia show a selective impairment in their ability to recognize familiar faces despite the retention of other non-social perceptual abilities, suggesting that face processing recruits domain-specific neural mechanisms (Haxby *et al.*, 2001; Kanwisher, 2000).

Further evidence for the independence of social cognition comes from the comparison of the neuro-cognitive and social-cognitive profiles of genetic disorders such as William's syndrome and autism. On the one hand, high-functioning individuals with autism and Asperger's syndrome display dysfunctional social behavior and impaired social cognition that is not associated with general cognitive capacity. In contrast, individuals with Williams' syndrome (who tend to be socially extroverted, displaying enhanced empathy and hyposociality) demonstrate a relative sparing of social-cognitive skills (such as the ability to recognize other people's mental states and emotions from information contained in their eyes), while at the same time showing impairments in tasks requiring spatial cognition and fine motor control (Bellugi *et al.*, 1999; Tager-Flusberg *et al.*, 1998). These findings provide evidence for distinct social processing networks in the form of a dissociation of social and non-social cognitive function across two clinical conditions.

Correlations with neuropsychological performance

In order to determine the relative contribution of domain-general processes to social cognition, one can statistically account for any concomitant neuropsychological impairment when analysing social-cognitive performance. Using this strategy, significant correlations were revealed between scores on a mentalizing task and executive function in a sample of patients with anterior and posterior lobe damage (Channon & Crawford, 2000) while, in contrast, fewer correlations of this kind were found in the healthy IQ-matched control sample. This raises the interesting question of whether the potential links between social and non-social cognitive processes are likely to be strengthened in individuals whose pathology may have resulted in (or indeed been caused by) the development of aberrant connectivity between particular

brain regions. Further evidence for this proposal comes from the finding of modest correlations between performance on a ToM task (Happé's cartoon task) and executive function in fronto-temporal dementia (Snowden *et al.*, 2003). However, using the strategy of covarying for executive functioning in the performance of fronto-temporal dementia patients on the same task, Lough *et al.* (2006) concluded that the influence of executive functioning was not specific to mentalizing ability. Opposing findings have been reported in a group of patients with frontal lobe epilepsy (Farrant *et al.*, 2005), where no significant correlations between neuropsychological test variables and a range of social cognitive tasks (including Happé's cartoons and stories, the *faux pas* test and Baron-Cohen's Eyes Task) were reported in the clinical group, but moderate correlations were found between executive function, non-mental state inference cartoons and performance on the Eyes Task in the control group.

The relative contribution of working memory, language demands and inferential capabilities to ToM performance (using Happé's cartoons and stories tasks) has also been examined in patients with various forms of traumatic brain injury (TBI) (Bibby & McDonald, 2005). In this study, neuropsychological factors did contribute to (and in some cases predict) performance on the ToM tasks, but they did not completely explain the impairment in the TBI group. Similarly, modest correlations between social and non-social tasks have been reported in individuals with amygdala damage and healthy controls, yet the majority of group differences in social cognitive tasks remained when executive function, logical memory and general intelligence were included as covariates (Shaw *et al.*, 2005). Lastly, a single case study of an individual with orbitofrontal damage reports that ToM and affect-processing abilities were independent of executive functioning (Bach *et al.*, 2000).

Recent studies of ToM and neurocognitive performance in schizophrenia similarly suggest that executive function and verbal working memory are associated with impaired social perception and cognition, but that deficits in executive functioning and memory can only partially account for impaired social cognition in schizophrenia (Brune, 2005; Greig *et al.*, 2004; Lancaster *et al.*, 2003). For example, Lancaster *et al.* (2003) report that performance on the Wisconsin Card Sort Test (WCST) accounted for only 35% of the variance in social-cue perception in schizophrenia, while memory contributed to only

8% of the variance in social cognition in the study by Greig and colleagues. Using a different method of analysis, Brune (2005) showed that social-cognitive performance was the strongest predictor of schizophrenia group membership (94.4% correctly classified by ToM), over WCST performance (70%) and other measures of executive function, whereas by contrast an earlier study (Brune, 2003) reported that no differences in ToM performance were found between schizophrenia and control subjects after controlling for IQ. A study of bipolar affective disordered patients has also revealed an association between executive functioning deficits and ToM impairments during the euthymic phase of illness (Olley et al., 2005).

A further strategy adopted by some authors is to examine the role of general intellectual functioning (assessed by IQ tests) in relation to social cognitive performance. This is particularly important in populations (such as schizophrenia) where there are likely to be group differences in general intellectual functioning. A strong correlation between IQ and scores on the Hinting task has been reported in schizophrenia but not in controls (Corcoran et al., 1995), although group differences on ToM tasks have been shown to remain after controlling for IQ (Corcoran et al., 1995; Sarfati et al., 1997). In a later study, after controlling for IQ, ToM deficits were found in separate comparisons between control subjects and particular subgroups of schizophrenia patients defined in terms of a hierarchical classification of symptoms (i.e. paranoid, behavioral signs, and passivity phenomena; Corcoran et al., 1997). However, two studies which have explored the role of IQ in ToM performance in schizophrenia report no differences between control and patient groups when the groups are matched for IQ (Brune, 2003; Pickup & Frith, 2001).

Use of this strategy in affective-disordered patients has yielded mixed results. A study by Inoue et al. (2004) reports no association between IQ and ToM in a large mixed sample of patients with both unipolar and bipolar depression; the affective disordered group showed clear impairments in ToM using a picture sequencing task. In contrast, ToM deficits revealed in another study of bipolar-disordered patients were significantly correlated with IQ, although this relationship disappeared when those in the manic phase of the illness were excluded from the analyses (Kerr et al., 2003). Since the manic patients in this sample had significantly lower IQ than those in the euthymic phase of illness, the original association between IQ

and ToM impairment was considered to be due to the low IQ scores in the manic group.

These studies converge to suggest that while executive processes or general intellectual functioning may play a role in social cognitive skills, deficits in these domain-general abilities cannot completely account for ToM dysfunction in disordered populations. It is notable that this pattern of findings appears in both neuropsychological investigations of brain-damaged patients and studies of patients with psychiatric disorder.

Within-task non-social control conditions

In some ToM studies, the inclusion of a non-ToM (or non-mental state inference) control question or condition (matched for all elements of processing bar the mental state inference) is used to isolate ToM skills. Demonstration of difficulties on the ToM condition alone, with intact performance on the matched control condition, implies that a relatively selective ToM mechanism has been affected by the damage, while domain-general cognitive processes required for the overall comprehension and interpretation of the stimulus are spared. Tasks such as Happé's cartoon task and Happé's stories fall into this category as they include matched, non-mental state inference conditions. Disproportionate impairment on cartoons that require mental state inference (as opposed to those requiring physical inference) has been identified in different patients including those with right hemisphere damage (Happé et al., 1999), a single case study of an individual who underwent stereotactic anterior capsulotomy (Happé et al., 2001), individuals with fronto-temporal dementia (Lough et al., 2006), and paranoid patients with schizophrenia (Corcoran et al., 1997). Note that this last study used a set of cartoon stimuli created by Corcoran, while the other studies used Happé's cartoon task. Furthermore, performance on Happé's task by a patient with left amygdala damage revealed scores within the normal range for the cartoons requiring physical inference, but well below the normal range on the mental state inference cartoons; this suggests specificity of the mentalizing deficit (Fine et al., 2001). In another study (Pickup & Frith, 2001) 'mentalizing' and 'non-mentalizing' versions of other first-order and second-order ToM tasks were administered to a group of individuals with schizophrenia. Using composite scores of the mental and non-mental data across tasks, there was no significant difference between psychiatric and healthy controls on the non-mental composite, but highly significant group differences for the mentalizing composite scores.

Using Happé's cartoons, Bibby & McDonald (2005) found no evidence for specific ToM impairment in subjects with traumatic brain injury; that is, performance on the mental state and physical state cartoons was impaired to the same degree (Bibby & McDonald, 2005). A failure to demonstrate a specific ToM impairment using this task has also been reported in studies of patients with epilepsy (Snowden et al., 2003), fronto-temporal dementia group (Lough et al., 2006), anorexia nervosa (Tchanturia et al., 2004) and a group of individuals with paranoid schizophrenia (Russell, 2002). While poor performance on both cartoon conditions suggests that these groups have no specific mentalizing impairment, these findings may also be due to methodological shortcomings of the task itself. That is, individuals may find both physical and mental state inferences difficult due to common task demands that are not directly related to mental state inference (for example, low-level visual perceptual abilities e.g. related to visual grouping, or context processing; controlled visual attention; or problems with "metarepresentation" itself). To address this point, Russell (2002) prompted paranoid individuals to attend to the relevant aspects of the cartoons as a means to ensure that they were taking in the correct information from the stimulus. This method improved performance, however, mental state cartoons were still less well understood than physical state cartoons. This pattern fits with the suggestion above that while underlying cognitive processes may help to solve social cognitive problems, they do not provide the whole picture. A further suggestion is that the very nature of cartoons (i.e. the cartoonist intends the joke to be funny) results in both conditions involving an element of mentalizing (i.e. interpreting intentions).

Cartoon-type stimuli (in the form of picture arrangement tasks) have also been utilized to study the ToM performance of individuals with schizophrenia (Brunet et al., 2003; Langdon et al., 1997; Sarfati & Hardy-Baylé, 1999; Sarfati et al., 1997, 1999). These studies followed on from Baron-Cohen's earlier work demonstrating that children with autism show impaired performance when sequencing cards that require the inference of mental states compared with near normal performance arranging picture stimuli requiring physical-state inference (Baron-Cohen et al., 1986). Langdon et al. (1997) used a picture-sequencing task that included physical, causal and mentalizing conditions in order to isolate the ability to infer causal mental states. Selective mentalizing deficits were found in some schizophrenia patients, while others (e.g. those with severe thought disorder) made general sequencing errors in both types of stories. A similar approach was taken by Brunet et al. (2003) in contrasting performance on sequencing tasks requiring either attribution of intention or attribution of physical causality (for example reasoning about the weight, location or speed of an object), in stories with and without human characters. Overall individuals with schizophrenia showed impairments in the attribution of intention condition; this result was found even when only participants with good performance on the physical logic condition were included for analysis and verbal IQ was covaried. These studies suggest a specific deficit in mental state inference/attribution in schizophrenia. However, this specificity may not be as clearly apparent in patients with more generalized cognitive deficits, such as those with chronic negative symptoms (see Langdon et al., 1997). A set of studies by Sarfati and colleagues (1997, 1999) has demonstrated an impaired ability to sequence cards referring mental-state inference in thought-disordered schizophrenia patients, however, these studies did not include appropriate physical or mechanical comparisons, and are therefore limited in their capacity to reveal specific ToM deficits.

Finally, a study by Pickup & Frith (2001) found that ToM deficits remain in schizophrenia patients, even after controlling for their poor recall performance in relation to items on Corcoran's Hinting Task. The use of additional items to probe memory for details of the ToM task is a useful test of the ability to meet performance demands that may interfere with competence on the ToM task. This method has similarly been employed in other studies of patients with fronto-temporal dementia (Rowe et al., 2001) and bipolar affective disorder (Kerr et al., 2003). In these studies, ToM performance was found to be impaired in each of the clinical groups after memory was controlled for.

In regards to the use of within-task control conditions in the face-processing literature, it is common for non-emotional face-processing tasks (such as identity, age or gender discrimination) to be employed alongside emotion-recognition tasks in order to delineate specific difficulties in the recognition of emotions within the context of intact recognition of other facial features. Studies of patients with focal brain lesions provide evidence that impaired recognition of emotional facial expressions may exist alongside intact processing of other facial characteristics such as identity recognition, and inferences of gender or age (Adolphs *et al.*, 1994, 1996; Bowers *et al.*, 1985; Calder *et al.*, 1996; Sprengelmeyer *et al.*, 1996; Tranel *et al.*, 1988; Young *et al.*, 1993). Furthermore, single case studies have shown that patients with bilateral damage to the amygdala or insula have specific difficulties in recognizing facial displays of emotion (fear and disgust, respectively) alongside intact recognition of other emotions and spared function in other cognitive domains (Adolphs *et al.*, 1994; Calder *et al.*, 1996, 2000). For example, Case SM (who has bilateral calcification of the amygdalae) demonstrates intact recognition of all emotions except fear, and to a lesser extent surprise, alongside entirely normal neuropsychological and executive functioning (Adolphs *et al.*, 2005).

A particularly noteworthy and challenging strategy for delineating the neurocognitive basis of specific emotion-processing deficits is to examine the performance tasks of psychiatric and lesioned subject groups on various face-processing tasks (Adolphs *et al.*, 2001). For example, Adolphs *et al.* (2001) examined individuals with autism and a group with amygdala damage on a number of face-processing tasks (including face recognition, emotion labeling, emotional intensity discrimination, social judgment from faces and social judgment from lexical stimuli). In general the autistic individuals had no difficulty in the identification of faces, emotions or in rating the intensity of emotional expressions, nor in social judgments from lexical stimuli. The group with amygdala damage showed impairments in emotion-processing tasks but not facial identity recognition or social judgments from the lexical task. However, both groups were very impaired in their judgment of trustworthiness from faces, suggesting that cognitive processes for both emotion recognition and facial identity are distinct from those used to make more ambiguous social judgments such as "trustworthiness" from faces. One recent study has also conducted a comparison of patients with right-brain damage, chronic schizophrenia and healthy controls on tasks of emotion labeling, emotion recognition and facial identity recognition (Kucharska-Pietura & Klimkowski, 2002). In this

study, schizophrenia and brain-damaged groups were impaired on all tasks relative to controls, with no difference in performance between the two clinical groups after controlling for face-recognition performance. Some individuals with schizophrenia have also shown impairments on tests sensitive to amygdala damage, such as fear perception, to a degree that distinguishes them from depressed individuals (Evangeli & Broks, 2000).

Several studies have examined whether difficulties in facial-affect perception in schizophrenia stem from a more generalized face-processing dysfunction (Kerr & Neale, 1993). Some studies have revealed evidence for an affect-specific deficit (Bryson *et al.*, 1997; Heimberg *et al.*, 1992; Morrison *et al.*, 1988; Walker *et al.*, 1984), while others report generalized face-processing impairments in schizophrenia (Addington & Addington, 1998; Archer *et al.*, 1994; Borod *et al.*, 1993; Feinberg *et al.*, 1986; Gessler *et al.*, 1989; Kerr & Neale, 1993; Mueser *et al.*, 1997; Novic *et al.*, 1984; Salem *et al.*, 1996; Schneider *et al.*, 1995). In some studies, affect-specific deficits have been shown to remain robust even when controlling for identity recognition (Borod *et al.*, 1993; Novic *et al.*, 1984), while other evidence suggests that facial-affect recognition deficits are related to specific neurocognitive dysfunctions in visual attention (Kee *et al.*, 1998), memory and language abilities (Addington & Addington, 1998; Kohler *et al.*, 2000; Mandal & Palchoudhury, 1989; Schneider *et al.*, 1995).

Social cognition: implications for psychiatry

In the previous sections we have reviewed evidence from the neuropsychological and neuroscience literature that provides support for the relative independence of social cognition from non-social cognition. The elucidation of the neural networks subserving social cognition may prove to be particularly important for identifying the neuropathology of major psychiatric disorders such as autism and schizophrenia, and will be pertinent to the formulation of effective treatments for social-cognitive disturbances in these individuals. With respect to schizophrenia, a number of models pertaining specifically to social-cognitive dysfunction have been offered in recent years to account for the symptoms of psychosis (Bentall *et al.*, 2001; Burns, 2004; Green & Phillips, 2004; Grossberg, 2000; Lee *et al.*, 2004). It is notable that abnormal neural circuitry in schizophrenia has been reported in regions corresponding with those implicated in social cognition, such as dysfunctional prefrontal-thalamic and temporo-limbic or cerebellar connections (Andreasen *et al.*, 1998; Weinberger *et al.*, 1992), as well as abnormalities in cells and functional integrity of temporo-limbic structures (e.g. amygdala, thalamus, hippocampus, parahippocampal gyri) and the orbitofrontal and anterior cingulate cortex (Andreasen *et al.*, 1999; Benes, 1999; Bogerts *et al.*, 1993; Chua *et al.*, 1997; Gray *et al.*, 1995; Liddle *et al.*, 1992). A comprehensive review of the structural and functional abnormalities in schizophrenia within regions important for emotion processing and social cognition has recently been provided elsewhere (Phillips *et al.*, 2003b). Similar conceptualizations of autism as a disorder of social-cognitive functioning have been dominant in recent decades (Baron-Cohen, 1995; Baron-Cohen *et al.*, 1985). Furthermore, following recent reports of impairments in ToM ability during both the affective and euthymic phases of bipolar disorder (Inoue *et al.*, 2004; Kerr *et al.*, 2003; Olley *et al.*, 2005), specific social-cognitive dysfunction may soon also feature in etiological models of the affective disorders (see Green & Malhi, 2006; Nelson *et al.*, 2005).

We turn now to a final discussion of specific findings from the study of social-cognitive disturbances with reference to their implications for the major psychiatric disorders. Beginning with face processing, as outlined above, the Fusiform Face Area (FFA) has been delineated in studies of healthy individuals as a region responding preferentially (but not exclusively) to faces. It is notable that this region is less active in autistic individuals when they are passively viewing facial expressions of emotion (Pierce *et al.*, 2001; Schultz *et al.*, 2003). This has led to the suggestion that individuals with autism fail to become face "experts," insofar as the key brain regions of the social network are not activated when processing human faces. Whilst this proposal may be taken to suggest that the functional integrity of specific social-processing regions (such as the FFA) are impaired in autism, a recent case study of an autistic child who demonstrates expertise with specific cartoon characters revealed that his fusiform area responded to cartoon images but not human faces, implying that the cognitive architecture underlying high-level expertise is in fact intact and highly plastic (Grelotti *et al.*, 2005). Clearly this finding suggests that a more complex problem underlies the autistic problem with facial emotion perception.

In schizophrenia, a number of neuroimaging studies have explored face processing (reviewed in Russell *et al.*, 2007a), most commonly within an emotion-specific deficit framework. Brain regions of interest in these studies have usually included only those related to the processing of emotion-specific stimuli (such as the amygdala in studies of fear perception). However, two recent imaging studies in schizophrenia that included face-processing regions in their analyses reported reduced activity in the occipital face area and the FFA in response to emotion and gender discrimination from faces (Johnston *et al.*, 2005; Quintana *et al.*, 2003). This implies that emotion-specific deficits may be secondary to early visual-processing difficulties, which may themselves be influenced by domain-general processes such as attention. It is here that we come full circle, with the implication that despite the existence of specific brain regions or networks specialized for social material, these networks may still be modulated by domain-general processes (see Pessoa *et al.*, 2005 for commentary on the role of attention). Further understanding of these complex reciprocal interactions will be important for those studies making tentative steps toward remediation of social-cognitive skills in clinical populations (Frommann *et al.*, 2003; Russell *et al.*, 2006).

Abnormalities in facial emotion perception (Bozikas *et al.*, 2006; George *et al.*, 1998; Getz *et al.*, 2003; Lembke & Ketter, 2002; Lennox *et al.*, 2004; McClure *et al.*, 2003) and Theory of Mind (Bora *et al.*, 2005; Inoue *et al.*, 2004; Kerr *et al.*, 2003; Olley *et al.*, 2005) have been recently demonstrated in bipolar affective disorder, and may comprise the first stages of dysfunction in the regulation of emotion (see Green & Malhi, 2006). For example, over-reactive limbic responses during appraisal of emotional material such as facial expressions (Chen *et al.*, 2006), or abnormal inhibitory processing of emotional material (Murphy *et al.*, 1999) in bipolar disorder may contribute to the generation of extreme emotional responses that are difficult to regulate. In support of this proposal, abnormal neural responses during the generation of affect in bipolar disorder have been associated with both periods of depression (Malhi *et al.*, 2004b) and mania (Malhi *et al.*, 2004a). Current theoretical accounts of major depressive disorder as an adaptive response to the threat of social exclusion also highlight the importance of social cognitive processes in affective disorder (Allen & Badcock, 2006).

It is clear from the evidence reviewed in this chapter that the issue of domain specificity with respect to social cognitive processes has yet to be definitively determined. Whilst neuropsychological studies suggest that social cognition cannot be fully accounted for by the domain-general processes (such as attention, memory or executive functioning) assessed in previous studies, this does not warrant an overarching conclusion that social cognition is completely independent of domain-specific processes (see Apperly et al., 2005). In a recent evaluation of the contribution of domain-general processes to ToM abilities, Apperly and colleagues note that although belief reasoning may withstand known impairments in grammar, verbal fluency or planning, there may be other forms of executive function that impair ToM performance, but which have not so far been assessed adequately. Furthermore, these authors suggest that there may be multiple domain-general processes that contribute to the ability to reason about other minds, such that "standard measures designed to test aspects of executive function in isolation are likely to be blunt instruments for testing whether belief reasoning is independent of domain-general processes. A more powerful approach might be to look for dissociations between performance on false-belief tasks and other reasoning tasks that demand a similar *combination* of domain-general processing demands but not belief reasoning" (Apperly et al., 2005, p. 576). An alternative approach would be to define and isolate the subcomponents of a specific social cognitive process, and then test the domain specificity of each of these processes independently. When considering these speculations in light of obvious neuropsychological impairment in psychiatric disorders such as schizophrenia and autism, it is likely that previous studies have not adequately assessed the possible combination of domain-general processes that may contribute to social cognitive dysfunction in this population. Further research is required to be undertaken with these methodological issues in mind.

Other notable caveats for research into social cognition include the failure of many current tasks to take into account the dynamic nature of most interpersonal interactions, particularly the bi-directionality of social encounters. Faces and their movement also convey much more than emotion. For example,

decisions about trustworthiness, morality and friendliness are often made on the basis of a fleeting glance at a novel face. These less tangible aspects of social cognition may be seen to be evading experimental techniques designed to measure cognition within the social domain. Future progress on the delineation of the social brain depends crucially upon the development of tasks that allow social-cognitive processes to be distinguished from the demands of general cognitive function, and will undoubtedly be important in the elucidation of the neuropathology of severe psychiatric disturbances.

Endnotes

1. The representation of intentional movement has been proposed as a precursor to the development of theory of mind abilities (Baron-Cohen et al., 1985).

2. The specificity of the FFA has been questioned on the basis of evidence suggesting it may be employed during the classification of objects with which humans have certain expertise (Gauthier et al., 2005), but see also Kanwisher et al. (1999).

References

Addington, J. & Addington, D. (1998). Facial affect recognition and information processing in schizophrenia and bipolar disorder. *Schizophrenia Research*, **32**(3), 171–181.

Adolphs, R. (1999). Social cognition and the human brain. *Trends in Cognitive Sciences*, **3**(12), 469–479.

Adolphs, R. (2001). The neurobiology of social cognition. *Current Opinion in Neurobiology*, **11**(2), 231–239.

Adolphs, R. (2003). Cognitive neuroscience of human social behaviour. *Nature Reviews Neuroscience*, **4**(3), 165–178.

Adolphs, R., Damasio, H., Tranel, D., Cooper, G. & Damasio, A. R. (2000). A role for somatosensory cortices in the visual recognition of emotion as revealed by three-dimensional lesion mapping. *Journal of Neuroscience*, **20**(7), 2683–2690.

Adolphs, R., Damasio, H., Tranel, D. & Damasio, A. R. (1996). Cortical systems for the recognition of emotion in facial expressions. *Journal of Neuroscience*, **16**(23), 7678.

Adolphs, R., Gosselin, F., Buchanan, T. W. et al. (2005). A mechanism for impaired fear recognition after amygdala damage. *Nature*, **433**(7021), 68–72.

Adolphs, R., Russell, J. A. & Tranel, D. (1999). A role for the human amygdala in recognizing emotional arousal from unpleasant stimuli. *Psychological Science*, **10**(2), 167–171.

Adolphs, R., Sears, L. & Piven, J. (2001). Abnormal processing of social information from faces in autism. *Journal of Cognitive Neuroscience*, **13**(2), 232–240.

Adolphs, R., Tranel, D., Damasio, H. & Damasio, A. (1994). Impaired recognition of emotion in facial expressions following bilateral damage to the human amygdala. *Nature*, **372**(6507), 669–672.

Allen, N. B. & Badcock, P. B. (2006). Darwinian models of depression: a review of evolutionary accounts of mood and mood disorders. *Progress in Neuro-Psychopharmacology and Biological Psychiatry*, **30**(5), 815–826.

Anderson, S. W., Bechara, A., Damasio, H., Tranel, D. & Damasio, A. R. (1999). Impairment of social and moral behavior related to early damage in human prefrontal cortex. *Nature Neuroscience*, **2**(11), 1032–1037.

Andreasen, N. C., Nopoulos, P., O'Leary, D. S. *et al.* (1999). Defining the phenotype of schizophrenia: cognitive dysmetria and its neural mechanisms. *Biological Psychiatry*, **46**(7), 908–920.

Andreasen, N. C., Paradiso, S. & O'Leary, D. S. (1998). "Cognitive dysmetria" as an integrative theory of schizophrenia: a dysfunction in cortical-subcortical-cerebellar circuitry? *Schizophrenia Bulletin*, **24**(2), 203–218.

Apperly, I. A., Samson, D. & Humphreys, G. W. (2005). Domain-specificity and theory of mind: evaluating neuropsychological evidence. *Trends in Cognitive Sciences*, **9**(12), 572–577.

Archer, J., Hay, D. C. & Young, A. W. (1994). Movement, face processing, and schizophrenia: evidence of a differential deficit in expression analysis. *British Journal of Clinical Psychology*, **33**(4), 517–528.

Bach, L. J., Happé, F., Fleminger, S. & Powell, J. (2000). Theory of mind: independence of executive function and the role of the frontal cortex in acquired brain injury. *Cognitive Neuropsychiatry*, **5**(3), 175–192.

Baron-Cohen, S. (1995). *Mindblindness: An Essay on Autism and Theory of Mind*. Boston, MA: MIT Press.

Baron-Cohen, S., Leslie, A. M. & Frith, U. (1985). Does the autistic child have a "theory of mind"? *Cognition*, **21**(1), 37.

Baron-Cohen, S., Leslie, A. M. & Frith, U. (1986). Mechanical, behavioural and intentional understanding of picture stories in autistic children. *British Journal of Developmental Psychology*, **4**(2), 113–125.

Baron-Cohen, S., Ring, H. A., Wheelwright, S. *et al.* (1999). Social intelligence in the normal and autistic brain: an fMRI study. *European Journal of Neuroscience*, **11**(6), 1891–1898.

Baron-Cohen, S., Wheelwright, S. & Jolliffe, T. (1997). Is there a "language of the eyes"? Evidence from normal adults, and adults with autism or Asperger syndrome. *Visual Cognition*, **4**(3), 311–331.

Baron-Cohen, S., Wheelwright, S., Hill, J., Raste, Y. & Plumb, I. (2001). The "reading the mind in the eyes" test revised version: a study with normal adults, and adults with Asperger syndrome or high-functioning autism. *Journal of Child Psychology and Psychiatry*, **42**(2), 241–251.

Bauman, M. D., Lavenex, P., Mason, W. A., Capitanio, J. P. & Amaral, D. G. (2004). The development of mother–infant interactions after neonatal amygdala lesions in rhesus monkeys. *Journal of Neuroscience*, **24**(3), 711–721.

Beauchamp, M. S., Lee, K. E., Haxby, J. V. & Martin, A. (2003). FMRI responses to video and point-light displays of moving humans and manipulable objects. *Journal of Cognitive Neuroscience*, **15**(7), 991–1001.

Bellugi, U., Adolphs, R., Cassady, C. & Chiles, M. (1999). Towards the neural basis for hypersociability in a genetic syndrome. *Neuroreport: For Rapid Communication of Neuroscience Research*, **10**(8), 1653–1657.

Benes, F. M. (1999). Evidence for altered trisynaptic circuitry in schizophrenic hippocampus. *Biological Psychiatry*, **46**(5), 589–599.

Bentall, R., Corcoran, R., Howard, R., Blackwood, N. & Kinderman, P. (2001). Persecutory delusions: a review and theoretical integration. *Clinical Psychology Review*, **21**(8), 1143–1192.

Bibby, H. & McDonald, S. (2005). Theory of mind after traumatic brain injury. *Neuropsychologia*, **43**(1), 99.

Bird, C., Castelli, F., Malik, O., Frith, U. & Husain, M. (2004). The impact of extensive medial frontal lobe damage on 'theory of mind' and cognition. *Brain*, **127**, 914–928.

Blair, J. R. (1997). Moral reasoning and the child with psychopathic tendencies. *Personality and Individual Differences*, **22**, 731–739.

Blair, R. J. R., Morris, J. S., Frith, C. C., Perrett, D. I. & Dolan, R. J. (1999). Dissociable neural responses to facial expressions of sadness and anger. *Brain*, **122**(5), 883–893.

Bogerts, B., Lieberman, J. A., Ashtari, M. *et al.* (1993). Hippocampus-amygdala volumes and psychopathology in chronic schizophrenia. *Biological Psychiatry*, **33**(4), 236–246.

Bora, E., Vahip, S., Gonul, A. *et al.* (2005). Evidence for theory of mind deficits in euthymic patients with bipolar disorder. *Acta Psychiatrica Scandinavica*, **112**(2), 110–116.

Borod, J. C., Bloom, R. L., Brickman, A. M., Nakhutina, L. & Curko, E. A. (2002). Emotional processing deficits in individuals with unilateral brain damage. *Applied Neuropsychology*, **9**(1), 23.

Borod, J. C., Martin, G. C., Alpert, M., Brozgold, A. & Welkowitz, J. (1993). Perception of facial emotion in schizophrenic and right brain-damaged patients. *Journal of Nervous and Mental Disease*, **181**(8), 494.

Bowers, D., Bauer, R., Coslett, H. & Heilman, K. (1985). Processing of faces by patients with unilateral hemisphere lesions. I. Dissociation between judgments of facial affect and facial identity. *Brain and Cognition*, **4**, 258–272.

Bozikas, V. P., Tonia, T., Fokas, K., Karavatos, A. & Kosmidis, M. H. (2006). Impaired emotion processing in remitted patients with bipolar disorder. *Journal of Affective Disorders*, **91**(1), 53–56.

Brothers, L. (1990). The social brain: a project for integrating primate behaviour and neurophysiology in a new domain. *Concepts in Neuroscience*, **1**, 27–51.

Brune, M. (2001). Social cognition and psychopathology in an evolutionary perspective. *Psychopathology*, **34**(2), 85–94.

Brune, M. (2003). Theory of mind and the role of IQ in chronic disorganized schizophrenia. *Schizophrenia Research*, **60**(1), 57.

Brune, M. (2005). Emotion recognition, 'theory of mind,' and social behavior in schizophrenia. *Psychiatry Research*, **133**(2–3), 135–147.

Brune, M. & Brune-Cohrs, U. (2006). Theory of mind – evolution, ontogeny, brain mechanisms and psychopathology. *Neuroscience and Biobehavioural Reviews*, **30**(4), 437–455.

Brunet, E., Sarfati, Y., Hardy-Bayle, M.-C. & Decety, J. (2003). Abnormalities of brain function during a nonverbal theory of mind task in schizophrenia. *Neuropsychologia*, **41**(12), 1574.

Bryson, G., Bell, M. & Lysaker, P. (1997). Affect recognition in schizophrenia: a function of global impairment or a specific cognitive deficit. *Psychiatry Research*, **71**(2), 105–113.

Burns, J. (2004). An evolutionary theory of schizophrenia: cortical connectivity, metarepresentation, and the social brain. *Behavioural and Brain Sciences*, **27**, 831–885.

Byrne, R. & Corp, N. (2004). Neocortex size predicts deception in primates. *Proceedings of the Royal Society of London Series B: Biological Sciences*, **271**, 1693–1699.

Calder, A., Keane, J., Manes, F., Antoun, N. & Young, A. (2000). Impaired recognition and experience of disgust following brain injury. *Nature Neuroscience*, **3**, 1077–1078.

Calder, A., Young, A., Rowland, D. *et al.* (1996). Facial emotion recognition after bilateral amygdala damage: differentially severe impairment of fear. *Cognitive Neuropsychology*, **13**(5), 699–745.

Castelli, F., Happé, F., Frith, U. & Frith, C. (2000). Movement and mind: a functional imaging study of perception and interpretation of complex intentional movement patterns. *Neuroimage*, **12**(3), 314.

Channon, S. & Crawford, S. (2000). The effects of anterior lesions on performance on a story comprehension test: left anterior impairment on a theory of mind-type task. *Neuropsychologia*, **38**(7), 1006–1017.

Chen, C. H., Lennox, B., Jacob, R. *et al.* (2006). Explicit and implicit facial affect recognition in manic and depressed states of bipolar disorder: a functional magnetic resonance imaging study. *Biological Psychiatry*, **59**(1), 31–39.

Chua, S. E., Wright, I. C., Poline, J. B. *et al.* (1997). Grey matter correlates of syndromes in schizophrenia. A semi-automated analysis of structural magnetic resonance images. *British Journal of Psychiatry*, **170**, 406–410.

Corcoran, R., Cahill, C. & Frith, C. D. (1997). The appreciation of visual jokes in people with schizophrenia: a study of 'mentalizing' ability. *Schizophrenia Research*, **24**(3), 319–327.

Corcoran, R., Mercer, G. & Frith, C. D. (1995). Schizophrenia, symptomatology and social inference: investigating "theory of mind" in people with schizophrenia. *Schizophrenia Research*, **17**(1), 5.

Corrigan, P. & Penn, D. L. (2001). *Social Cognition and Schizophrenia*. Washington, DC: American Psychological Association.

Critchley, H., Daly, E., Phillips, M. *et al.* (2000). Explicit and implicit neural mechanisms for processing of social information from facial expressions: a functional magnetic resonance imaging study. *Human Brain Mapping*, **9**(2), 93.

Damasio, A. R. (1996). The somatic marker hypothesis and the possible functions of the prefrontal cortex. *Philosophical Transactions of the Royal Society of London, Series B: Biological Sciences*, **351**(1346), 1413.

Diergaarde, L., Gerriis, M., Stuy, A., Spruijt, B. & van Ree, J. (2004). Neonatal amygdala lesions and juvenile isolation in the rat: differential effects on locomotor and social behavior later in life. *Behavioral Neuroscience*, **118**(2), 298–306.

Dunbar, R. (2003). Social brain: mind, language and society in evolutionary perspective. *Annual Review of Anthropology*, **32**, 163–181.

Evangeli, M. & Broks, P. (2000). Face processing in schizophrenia: parallels with the effects of amygdala damage. *Cognitive Neuropsychiatry*, **5**(2), 81–104.

Farrant, A., Morris, R. G., Russell, T. *et al.* (2005). Social cognition in frontal lobe epilepsy. *Epilepsy and Behavior*, **7**(3), 506.

Feinberg, T. E., Rifkin, A., Schaffer, C. & Walker, E. (1986). Facial discrimination and emotional recognition in schizophrenia and affective disorders. *Archives of General Psychiatry*, **43**(3), 276–279.

Fine, C., Lumsden, J. & Blair, R. (2001). Dissociation between "theory of mind" and executive functions in a patient with early left amygdala damage. *Brain: A Journal of Neurology*, **124**(2), 287–298.

Fiske, S. T. (1991). *Social Cognition* (2nd edn.). New York, NY: McGraw-Hill.

Fletcher, P. C., Happé, F., Frith, U. *et al.* (1995). Other minds in the brain: a functional imaging study of "theory of mind" in story comprehension. *Cognition*, **57**(2), 109.

Frith, U. & Frith, C. (2003). Development and neurophysiology of mentalising. *Philosophical Transactions of the Royal Society of London, Series B: Biological Sciences*, **358**, 459–473.

Frommann, N., Streit, M. & Woelwer, W. (2003). Remediation of facial affect recognition impairments in patients with schizophrenia: a new training program. *Psychiatry Research*, **117**(3), 281–284.

Gallagher, H. L., Happé, F., Brunswick, N. *et al.* (2000). Reading the mind in cartoons and stories: an fMRI study of "theory of mind" in verbal and nonverbal tasks. *Neuropsychologia*, **38**(1), 11.

Gauthier, I., Curby, K. M., Skudlarski, P. & Epstein, R. A. (2005). Individual differences in FFA activity suggest independent processing at different spatial scales. *Cognitive, Affective and Behavioral Neuroscience*, **5**(2), 222–234.

George, M. S., Huggins, T., McDermut, W. *et al.* (1998). Abnormal facial emotion recognition in depression: serial testing in an ultra-rapid-cycling patient. *Behavior Modification*, **22**(2), 192–204.

Gessler, S., Cutting, J., Frith, C. D. & Weinman, J. (1989). Schizophrenic inability to judge facial emotion: a controlled study. *British Journal of Clinical Psychology*, **28**(1), 19–29.

Getz, G. E., Shear, P. K. & Strakowski, S. M. (2003). Facial affect recognition deficits in bipolar disorder. *Journal of the International Neuropsychological Society*, **9**(4), 623–632.

Goel, V., Grafman, J., Sadato, N. & Hallett, M. (1995). Modeling other minds. *Neuroreport*, **6**(13), 1741–1746.

Gray, J. A., Joseph, M. H., Hemsley, D. R. *et al.* (1995). The role of mesolimbic domapinergic and retrohippocampal afferents to the nucleus accumbens in latent inhibition: implications for schizophrenia. *Behavioural Brain Research*, **71**, 19–31.

Green, M. J. & Malhi, G. S. (2006). Neural mechanisms of the cognitive control of emotion. *Acta Neuropsychiatrica*, **18**, 144–153.

Green, M. J. & Phillips, M. L. (2004). Social threat perception and the evolution of paranoia. *Neuroscience and Biobehavioral Reviews*, **28**(3), 333–342.

Greig, T. C., Bryson, G. J. & Bell, M. D. (2004). Theory of mind performance in schizophrenia: diagnostic, symptom, and neuropsychological correlates. *Journal of Nervous and Mental Disease*, **192**(1), 12–18.

Grelotti, D. J., Klin, A. J., Gauthier, I. *et al.* (2005). FMRI activation of the fusiform gyrus and amygdala to cartoon characters but not to faces in a boy with autism. *Neuropsychologia*, **43**(3), 373–385.

Grossberg, S. (2000). The imbalanced brain: from normal behavior to schizophrenia. *Biological Psychiatry*, **48**(2), 81–98.

Happé, F., Brownell, H. & Winner, E. (1999). Acquired 'theory of mind' impairments following stroke. *Cognition*, **70**(3), 211.

Happé, F., Ehlers, S., Fletcher, P. C. *et al.* (1996). 'Theory of mind' in the brain. Evidence from a PET scan study of Asperger syndrome. *Neuroreport*, **20**(8), 197–201.

Happé, F., Malhi, G. S. & Checkley, S. (2001). Acquired mind-blindness following frontal lobe surgery? A single case study of impaired 'theory of mind' in a patient treated with stereotactic anterior capsulotomy. *Neuropsychologia*, **39**(1), 83.

Hariri, A. R., Bookheimer, S. Y. & Mazziotta, J. C. (2000). Modulating emotional responses: effects of a neocortical network on the limbic system. *Neuroreport*, **11**(1), 43.

Haxby, J. V., Gobbini, M., Furey, M. L. *et al.* (2001). Distributed and overlapping representations of faces and objects in ventral temporal cortex. *Science*, **293**(5539), 2425–2430.

Haxby, J. V., Gobbini, M. & Montgomery, K. (2004). Spatial and temporal distribution of face and object representations in the human brain. In M. S. Gazzaniga (Ed.), *The Cognitive Neurosciences* (3rd edn.), (pp. 889–904). Boston, MA: MIT Press.

Haxby, J. V., Hoffman, E. A. & Gobbini, M. (2002). Human neural systems for face recognition and social communication. *Biological Psychiatry*, **51**(1), 59–67.

Heimberg, C., Gur, R. E., Erwin, R. J., Shtasel, D. L. & Gur, R. C. (1992). Facial emotion discrimination: Iii. Behavioural findings in schizophrenia. *Psychiatry Research*, **42**(3), 253–265.

Inoue, Y., Tonooka, Y., Yamada, K. & Kanba, S. (2004). Deficiency of theory of mind in patients with remitted mood disorder. *Journal of Affective Disorders*, **82**(3), 403–409.

Johnston, P. J., Stojanov, W., Devir, H. & Schall, U. (2005). Functional MRI of facial emotion recognition deficits in schizophrenia and their electrophysiological correlates. *European Journal of Neuroscience*, **22**(5), 1221–1232.

Kanwisher, N. (2000). Domain specificity in face perception. *Nature Neuroscience*, **3**(8), 759–763.

Kanwisher, N., McDermott, J. & Chun, M. M. (1997). The fusiform face area: a module in human extrastriate cortex specialized for face perception. *Journal of Neuroscience*, **17**(11), 4302–4311.

Kanwisher, N., Stanley, D. & Harris, A. (1999). The fusiform face area is selective for faces not animals. *Neuroreport*, **10**, 183–187.

Kee, K. S., Kern, R. S. & Green, M. F. (1998). Perception of emotion and neurocognitive functioning in schizophrenia: what's the link? *Psychiatry Research*, **81**(1), 57–65.

Kerr, N., Dunbar, R. I. M. & Bentall, R. P. (2003). Theory of mind deficits in bipolar affective disorder. *Journal of Affective Disorders*, **73**(3), 253.

Kerr, S. L. & Neale, J. M. (1993). Emotion perception in schizophrenia: specific deficit or further evidence of generalised poor performance? *Journal of Abnormal Psychology*, **102**(2), 312–318.

Kohler, C. G., Bilker, W., Hagendoorn, M., Gur, R. E. & Gur, R. C. (2000). Emotion recognition deficit in schizophrenia: association with symptomatology and cognition. *Biological Psychiatry*, **48**, 127–136.

Kring, A. M. & Werner, K. H. (2004). Emotion regulation and Psychopathology. In P. Philippot & R. S. Feldman (Eds), *The Regulation of Emotion* (pp. 359–385). Hove, UK: Lawrence Erlbaum Associates.

Krolak-Salmon, P., Fischer, C., Vighetto, A. & Mauguiere, F. (2001). Processing of facial emotional expression; spatio-temporal data as assessed by scalp event-related potentials. *European Journal of Neuroscience*, **13**(5), 987–994.

Kucharska-Pietura, K. & Klimkowski, M. (2002). Perception of facial affect in chronic schizophrenia and right brain damage. *Acta Neurobiologiae Experimentalis*, **62**(1), 33–43.

Lancaster, R. S., Evans, J. D., Bond, G. R. & Lysaker, P. H. (2003). Social cognition and neurocognitive deficits in schizophrenia. *Journal of Nervous and Mental Disease*, **191**(5), 295–299.

Langdon, R., Michie, P. T., Ward, P. B. *et al.* (1997). Defective self and/or other mentalising in schizophrenia: a cognitive neuropsychological approach. *Cognitive Neuropsychiatry*, **2**(3), 167–193.

Lange, K., Williams, L., Young, A. *et al.* (2003). Task instructions modulate neural responses to fearful facial expressions. *Biological Psychiatry*, **53**, 226–232.

LeDoux, J. (1998). *The Emotional Brain*. London: Phoenix.

Lee, K. H., Farrow, T. F. D., Spence, S. A. & Woodruff, P. W. R. (2004). Social cognition, brain networks and schizophrenia. *Psychological Medicine*, **34**(3), 391–400.

Lembke, A. & Ketter, T. A. (2002). Impaired recognition of facial emotion in mania. *American Journal of Psychiatry*, **159**(2), 302–304.

Lennox, B., Jacob, R., Calder, A., Lupson, V. & Bullmore, E. (2004). Behavioural and neurocognitive responses to sad facial affect are attenuated in patients with mania. *Psychological Medicine*, **34**(5), 795–802.

Leslie, A. M. & Thaiss, L. (1992). Domain specificity in conceptual development: neuropsychological evidence from autism. *Cognition*, **43**(3), 225–251.

Liddle, P. F., Friston, K. J., Frith, C. D. *et al.* (1992). Patterns of cerebral blood flow in schizophrenia. *British Journal of Psychiatry*, **160**, 179–186.

Liu, L., Ioannades, A. & Streit, M. (1999). Single trial analysis of neurophysiological correlates of the recognition of complex objects and facial expressions of emotion. *Brain Topography*, **11**(4), 291–303.

Lough, S., Kipps, C. M., Treise, C. *et al.* (2006). Social reasoning, emotion and empathy in frontotemporal dementia. *Neuropsychologia*, **44**(6), 950.

Malhi, G. S., Lagopoulos, J., Sachdev, P. (2004a). Cognitive generation of affect in hypomania: an fMRI study. *Bipolar Disorders*, **6**(4), 271–285.

Malhi, G. S., Lagopoulos, J., Ward, P. B. *et al.* (2004b). Cognitive generation of affect in bipolar depression: an fMRI study. *European Journal of Neuroscience*, **19**(3), 741–754.

Mandal, M. K. & Palchoudhury, S. (1989). Identifying the components of facial emotion and schizophrenia. *Psychopathology*, **22**(6), 295–300.

McCabe, K., Houser, D., Ryan, L., Smith, V. & Trouard, T. (2001). A functional imaging study of cooperation in two-person reciprocal exchange. *Proceedings of the National Academy of Sciences USA*, **98**(20), 11832–11835.

McClure, E. B., Pope, K., Hoberman, A. J., Pine, D. S. & Leibenluft, E. (2003). Facial expression recognition in adolescents with mood and anxiety disorders. *American Journal of Psychiatry*, **160**(6), 1172–1174.

Morris, J. S., Friston, K. J., Buchel, C. *et al.* (1998). A neuromodulatory role for the human amygdala in processing emotional facial expressions. *Brain*, **121**(1), 47–57.

Morris, J. S., Frith, C. D., Perrett, D. I. *et al.* (1996). A differential neural response in the human amygdala to fearful and happy facial expressions. *Nature*, **383**(31), 812–815.

Morrison, R. L., Bellack, A. S. & Bashore, T. R. (1988). Perception of emotion among schizophrenic patients. *Journal of Psychopathology and Behavioral Assessment*, **10**(4), 319–332.

Mueser, K. T., Penn, D. L., Blanchard, J. J. & Bellack, A. S. (1997). Affect recognition in schizophrenia: a synthesis of findings across three studies. *Psychiatry: Interpersonal and Biological Processes*, **60**(4), 301–308.

Murphy, F. C., Sahakian, B. J., Rubinsztein, J. S. *et al.* (1999). Emotional bias and inhibitory control processes in mania and depression. *Psychological Medicine*, **29**(6), 1307–1321.

Nelson, E. E., Leibenluft, E., McClure, E. & Pine, D. S. (2005). The social re-orientation of adolescence: a neuroscience perspective on the process and its relation to psychopathology. *Psychological Medicine*, **35**(2), 163–174.

Novic, J., Luchins, D. J. & Perline, R. (1984). Facial affect recognition in schizophrenia: is there a differential deficit? *British Journal of Psychiatry*, **144**, 533–537.

Olley, A. L., Malhi, G. S., Bachelor, J. *et al.* (2005). Executive functioning and theory of mind in euthymic bipolar disorder. *Bipolar Disorders*, 7(Suppl. 5), 43–52.

Ostrom, T. M. (1984). The sovereignty of social cognition. In R. S. Wyer & T. K. Srull (Eds), *Handbook of Social Cognition* (Vol. 1, pp. 1–37). Hillsdale, NJ: Lawrence Erlbaum Associates.

Pessoa, L., Padmala, S. & Morland, T. (2005). Fate of unattended fearful faces in the amygdala is determined by both attentional resources and cognitive modulation. *Neuroimage*, **28**(1), 249–255.

Phan, K., Wager, T., Taylor, S. & Liberzon, M. (2004). Functional neuroimaging studies of human emotions. *CNS Spectrums*, **9**(4), 258–266.

Phillips, M., Drevets, W., Rauch, S. & Lane, R. (2003a). Neurobiology of emotion perception i: The neural basis of normal emotion perception. *Biological Psychiatry*, **54**, 504–514.

Phillips, M., Drevets, W., Rauch, S. & Lane, R. (2003b). Neurobiology of emotion perception ii: Implications for major psychiatric disorders. *Biological Psychiatry*, **54**, 515–528.

Phillips, M. L., Young, A. W., Scott, S. K. *et al.* (1998). Neural responses to facial and vocal expressions of fear and disgust. *Proceedings of the Royal Society of London, Series B: Biological Sciences*, **265**(1408), 1809–1817.

Phillips, M. L., Young, A. W., Senior, C. *et al.* (1997). A specific neural substrate for perceiving facial expressions of disgust. *Nature*, **389**(6650), 495.

Pickup, G. J. & Frith, C. D. (2001). Theory of mind impairments in schizophrenia: symptomatology, severity and specificity. *Psychological Medicine*, **31**, 207–220.

Pierce, K., Muller, R., Ambrose, J., Allen, G. & Courchesne, E. (2001). Face processing occurs outside the fusiform 'face area' in autism: evidence from functional MRI. *Brain*, **124**(10), 2059–2073.

Pinkham, A. E., Penn, D. L., Perkins, D. O. & Lieberman, J. (2003). Implications for the neural basis of social cognition for the study of schizophrenia. *American Journal of Psychiatry*, **160**(5), 815–824.

Premack, D. & Woodruff, G. (1978). Does the chimpanzee have a theory of mind? *Behavioral and Brain Sciences*, **1**(4), 515–526.

Puce, A., Allison, T., Bentin, S., Gore, J. C. & McCarthy, G. (1998). Temporal cortex activation in humans viewing eye and mouth movements. *Journal of Neuroscience*, **18**(6), 2188–2199.

Quintana, J., Wong, T., Ortiz-Portillo, E., Marder, S. R. & Mazziotta, J. C. (2003). Right lateral fusiform gyrus dysfunction during facial information processing in schizophrenia. *Biological Psychiatry*, **53**(12), 1099–1112.

Rowe, A. D., Bullock, P. R., Polkey, C. E. & Morris, R. G. (2001). Theory of mind' impairments and their relationship to executive functioning following frontal lobe excisions. *Brain*, **124**(3), 600–616.

Russell, T. A. (2002). An exploration of theory of mind in schizophrenia: a symptom-based approach. Unpublished PhD thesis, Institute of Psychiatry, University of London.

Russell, T. A., Chu, E. & Phillips, M. (2006). A pilot study to investigate the effectiveness of emotion recognition remediation in schizophrenia using the micro-expression training tool. *British Journal of Clinical Psychology*, **45**, 579–583.

Russell, T., Reynaud, E., Pietura, K. *et al.* (2007). Neural responses to dynamic expressions of fear in schizophrenia. *Neuropsychologia*, **45**(1), 107–123.

Russell, T. A., Rubia, K., Bullmore, E. T. *et al.* (2000). Exploring the social brain in schizophrenia: left prefrontal underactivation during mental state attribution. *American Journal of Psychiatry*, **157**(12), 2040–2042.

Salem, J. E., Kring, A. M. & Kerr, S. L. (1996). More evidence for generalized poor performance in facial emotion perception in schizophrenia. *Journal of Abnormal Psychology*, **105**(3), 480–483.

Sarfati, Y. & Hardy-Bayle, M.-C. (1999). How do people with schizophrenia explain the behaviour of others? A study of theory of mind and its relationship to thought and speech disorganization in schizophrenia. *Psychological Medicine*, **29**(3), 613–620.

Sarfati, Y., Hardy-Bayle, M., Besche, C. & Widlocher, D. (1997). Attribution of intentions to others in people with schizophrenia: a non-verbal exploration with comic strips. *Schizophrenia Research*, **25**, 199–209.

Sarfati, Y., Hardy-Bayle, M.-C., Brunet, E. & Widlocher, D. (1999). Investigating theory of mind in schizophrenia: influence of verbalization in disorganized and non-disorganized patients. *Schizophrenia Research*, **37**(2), 183.

Schneider, F., Gur, R. C., Gur, R. E. & Shtasel, D. L. (1995). Emotional processing in schizophrenia: neurobehavioral probes in relation to psychopathology. *Schizophrenia Research*, **17**(1), 67–75.

Schultz, R. T., Grelotti, D. J., Klin, A. *et al.* (2003). The role of the fusiform face area in social cognition: implications for the pathobiology of autism. In U. Frith & E. Hill (Eds.), *Autism: Mind and Brain* (pp. 267–294). Oxford: Oxford University Press.

Shaw, P., Bramham, J., Lawrence, E. *et al.* (2005). Differential effects of lesions of the amygdala and prefrontal cortex on recognizing facial expressions of complex emotions. *Journal of Cognitive Neuroscience*, **17**(9), 1410–1419.

Skodol, A. E., Gunderson, J. G., McGlashan, T. H. *et al.* (2002). Functional impairment in patients with schizotypal, borderline, avoidant, or obsessive-compulsive personality disorder. *American Journal of Psychiatry*, **159**(2), 276–283.

Snowden, J. S., Gibbons, Z. C., Blackshaw, A. *et al.* (2003). Social cognition in frontotemporal dementia and Huntington's disease. *Neuropsychologia*, **41**(6), 688.

Sprengelmeyer, R., Young, A., Calder, A. *et al.* (1996). Loss of disgust: perception of faces and emotions in Huntington's disease. *Brain*, **119**, 1647–1665.

Stone, V. E., Nisenson, L., Eliassen, J. & Gazzaniga, M. (1996). Left hemisphere representations of emotional facial expressions. *Neuropsychologia*, **34**, 23–29.

Suslow, T., Junghanns, K. & Arolt, V. (2001). Detection of facial expressions of emotions in depression. *Perceptual and Motor Skills*, **92**, 857–868.

Tager-Flusberg, H., Boshart, J. & Baron-Cohen, S. (1998). Reading the windows to the soul: evidence of domain-specific sparing in Williams syndrome. *Journal of Cognitive Neuroscience*, **10**(5), 631–639.

Tchanturia, K., Happé, F., Godley, J. *et al.* (2004). 'Theory of mind' in anorexia nervosa. *European Eating Disorders Review*, **12**, 361–366.

Tranel, D., Damasio, A. & Damasio, H. (1988). Intact recognition of facial expression, gender and age inpatients with impaired recognition of face identity. *Neurology*, **38**, 690–696.

Vogeley, K., Bussfeld, P., Newen, A. *et al.* (2001). Mind reading: neural mechanisms of theory of mind and self-perspective. *Neuroimage*, **14**, 170–181.

Walker, E., McGuire, M. & Bettes, B. (1984). Recognition and identification of facial stimuli by schizophrenics and patients with affective disorders. *British Journal of Clinical Psychology*, **23**(1), 37–44.

Weinberger, D. R., Berman, K. F., Suddath, R. & Torrey, E. F. (1992). Evidence of dysfunction of a prefrontal-limbic network in schizophrenia: a magnetic resonance imaging and regional cerebral blood flow study of discordant monozygotic twins. *American Journal of Psychiatry*, **149**(7), 890–897.

Wimmer, H. & Perner, J. (1983). Beliefs about beliefs: representation and constraining function of wrong beliefs in young children's understanding of deception. *Cognition*, **13**(1), 103–128.

Young, A., Newcombe, F., de Haan, E., Small, M. & Hay, D. (1993). Face perception after brain injury: selective impairments affecting identity and expression. *Brain*, **116**, 941–959.

Section 2

The importance of methods

It is self evident that before one can draw intelligent conclusions from one's data, one's methods must be of the highest standard. However, even when following the best practice of the age, methodology can still be flawed. In this section, both the strengths and limitations of methods used in the study of neuropsychological processes within mental illness are explored.

The issue of primary importance to the field is diagnosis. Jackson & McGorry argue that although reliability was improved with the publication of the DSM–III, validity remains a major concern. They attempt to bring together the competing approaches to psychopathology, one clinical and one biological, using a clinical staging model that combines these phenomena. One result of this is to return the focus of diagnosis to the guidance of treatment and prediction of outcome.

Of course, neuropsychological study of mental illness is critically dependent on the quality of the assessment. Woods *et al.* address issues of study design and test selection in studying the epidemiology, mechanisms and functional impact of cognitive impairment in mental disorders, as well as how demographic factors, test-taking effort, disease characteristics and data-analytic strategies can influence the interpretation of neuropsychological research in these populations.

The following chapter, by Savage *et al.*, examines the study of emotion and its interaction with cognition. They evaluate some of the batteries that have been used to assess emotion, and provide an overview of methodologies that have been applied to test the impact of emotional state on attention, memory and learning. They also point to the roles that functional neuroimaging and electrophysiology have played in furthering our understanding of the neuropsychology of emotion.

A more detailed appraisal of neurophysiology is given in the next chapter by Ford & Mathalon. Using the example of studying auditory hallucinations in schizophrenia, they demonstrate how neurophysiological approaches can provide a window into the pathophysiology of mental disorders. This is followed by a chapter on neuroimaging techniques by Fusar-Poli & McGuire. They outline the basic principles of various imaging modalities, including magnetic resonance imaging, positron emission tomography and magnetic resonance spectroscopy, and highlight their potential uses and limitations. Importantly, they discuss the integration of these modalities to take advantage of their complementary strengths – an approach which has only rarely been adopted.

In Chapter 17, Honey discusses pharmacological models of psychiatric disorders and how they can be used to investigate cognitive function. This is done with particular reference to ketamine, a non-competitive NMDA receptor antagonist that is known to be psychotomimetic. He argues for the advantage of this approach in terms of both investigating individual differences and fractionating the cognitive processes, although he also acknowledges its limitations – most prominently the uncertain clinical validity of the models.

In the final chapter of this section, Bilder *et al.* discuss cognitive phenomics – essentially the attempt to systematically understand cognitive phenotypes and their genetic basis. These phenotypes include neuronal elements, neural systems, cognitive phenotypes and cognitive syndromes, a massive task which the authors point out will need novel informatics strategies that enable the representation, visualization and modeling of complex relations among measured variables and theoretical concepts. Nevertheless, this approach offers the promise of more tractable phenotypic targets relative to the psychiatric syndromes, and therefore may provide a way to deal with the diagnostic problems raised in the opening chapter of this section.

Psychiatric diagnoses: purposes, limitations and an alternative approach

Henry J. Jackson and Patrick D. McGorry

Introduction

A major purpose of diagnosis is to indicate the type of treatment that is required for the presenting patient. Other purposes of diagnosis identified by Kendell (1975) include predicting course and prognosis, understanding etiology and factors leading to the condition, and in the calculation of prevalence and incidence rates in epidemiological research. The latter indicates the "health" of the nation and aids in determining the allocation of mental health infrastructure and resources to specific geographic regions with the greatest unmet need.

Issues of reliability and, to a lesser extent, the validity of diagnoses dominate the study of psychopathology. These issues led to the publication of DSM–III (American Psychiatric Association, 1980). They are of the utmost importance; however, we have shored up reliability without impacting on validity. Indeed, validity has largely weakened over the past 20 years as treatments diffuse across diagnostic boundaries, e.g. antidepressants being prescribed for both major depressive disorder (MDD) and obsessive-compulsive disorder (OCD) (Palmer & Benfield, 1994).

Philosophical differences revolve around the role of psychopathology as the basis for reaching a diagnosis. Two approaches – one clinical and one biological – represent the major differences. The clinical approach posits clinical pictures as being of paramount importance in defining psychopathology, i.e. the observations of clinicians, the reports of patients and of others – including family members. Proponents of the clinical perspective place great emphasis on the clinician's acumen in judging the presence or absence of phenomena and in grading those phenomena. This was a dominant approach to characterizing and diagnosing psychiatric illness in the middle of the last century and the phenomenological movement flourished in Europe and the UK.

Critics of this approach are more likely to stress the importance of less directly observable factors and rely on results yielded by neuropsychological, neurological, psychophysiological, biochemical, genetic and neuroradiological data. A greater sense of security is derived from focusing on the results of biological tests. These tests are perceived as being more valid – more objective and less open to the vagaries of subjective perception and interpretation. The philosophical differences are further highlighted when an attempt is made to link these biological variables with clinical phenotypes. This linkage is not necessarily straightforward. Proponents of the biological viewpoint argue that the linkage is poor due to the fact that the phenotypes are so numerous, poorly operationalized and unstable over time, to be of any value. Instead of trying to identify neurocognitive variables underpinning phenotypes, they argue a superior strategy would be to focus initially on neurocognitive and biological biases or deficits and then link them to phenotypes. In this chapter we will argue for a conciliation of these two approaches.

In the first part of this chapter we discuss definitional issues and briefly review reliability issues. In the second section we examine the concept of phenotypes within the psychometric framework adopted by the nosologies of ICD–10 (World Health Organization, 1992) and DSM–III and subsequent editions. We indicate problems to date with this approach. In the third section, we examine the relationship of neurocognitive and biological "markers" to the phenotypes. We selectively review the area of biological and neuropsychological variables and point out limitations to this approach to diagnosis. Finally, and

The Neuropsychology of Mental Illness, ed. Stephen J. Wood, Nicholas B. Allen and Christos Pantelis. Published by Cambridge University Press. © Cambridge University Press 2009.

as foreshadowed above, we argue for an alternative diagnostic approach that combines both "clinical descriptions" and "biological" variables, is phase-of-disorder[1] focused and treatment oriented. Moreover, in this fourth section we examine a framework to achieve this ambition.

Definitions and phenomenology: the clinician as assessor

In some ways, "psychopathology" and "psychiatric disorder" are terms still in search of comprehensive definitions. A well-known textbook extensively prescribed for undergraduate psychology classes describes "psychopathology" as including three core elements: psychological impairment in the behavioral, cognitive or emotional domains, causing personal distress, and the fact that the phenomenology is atypical as regards to culture, i.e. not commensurate with cultural concepts and expectations of "normality" (Barlow & Durand, 2005). These factors are all considered important in determining whether or not a person suffers from "a disorder." We would add two other factors – the construct of disability or *dysfunction*, meaning that the psychological impairments detrimentally interfere with the person's daily social, family, occupational and leisure functioning, and the "perceived need for care" by the patient. All five factors appear useful and possess face validity, although all five may not be operative for all "disorders." For example, people with antisocial personality disorder usually do not experience personal distress nor perceive a need for care.

Nevertheless, much of the literature has focused on the concept of impairment, i.e. in the cognitive, emotional and behavioral domains. One of the most fundamental dilemmas facing the clinician is in deciding whether the phenomena the patient experiences are abnormal or not. This in turn raises a number of issues. The first is whether a symptom is dimensionally distributed or not. The general assumption is that most phenomena are normally distributed and although this needs to be empirically tested, it does possess face validity. The point at issue then, is where one draws the cut-off point between normality and abnormality as regards a specific phenomenon. At the endpoint of this distribution, agreements appear to be easier, e.g. the person has severe sleep deprivation. But with milder forms of sleep disturbance, i.e. around the mid-point of severity,

the agreement may be less than convincing and the decision becomes more reliant on the internal threshold of each individual clinician, including their tolerance of "deviance." Of course, there may be inherent differences among clinicians as to whether they consider a symptom abnormal or not. To take a second example, clinicians' "lived in" experience may lead one clinician to assess a personality feature as evidence that the person is "confident" whilst a second clinician assesses the same personality characteristic as evidence the person is "entitled." Given the dichotomous nature of all the diagnostic criteria (present/not present), which do not incorporate rating gradations of severity, individual clinicians may not rate the symptom sufficiently severe to warrant endorsement (i.e. the threshold effect).

The problem is further amplified when one moves from a single phenomenon to multiple phenomena, as is the case in deciding whether or not one is confronted by a syndrome, i.e. a group of say five or more phenomena, each of which needs to be judged as being abnormal or not in its own right. This may be difficult enough, but there is yet another component to this consideration. This is the issue of discounting other phenomena, not seen to be part and parcel of the focal syndrome. So, the clinician is required to assess and judge other phenomena as not being present and as not being abnormal. One can see that implicit in the above discussion are issues reflecting the dimensional versus categorical debate about descriptive psychopathology, clinician judgment, and "formal" measurement of aspects of syndromes. In fact, psychometric investigations of aspects of syndromes have been a major research activity over the past 30 years. Table 12.1 indicates key aspects of psychiatric syndromes investigated by researchers. We briefly describe and comment on two of these aspects: inter-rater reliability and test-retest reliability.

Inter-rater reliability

One way of attempting to deal with the issue of clinician judgment is to request two or more clinicians to assess a phenomenon. Inter-rater reliability appears optimized when two clinicians contemporaneously observe and rate the patient (another method is to involve multiple clinicians independently observing a videotaped patient or patient vignette). This notion of inter-rater reliability has occurred infrequently at the level of a single phenomenon, whether

Table 12.1. Key psychometric aspects of syndromes.

Aspect	Question
Content validity	Do the signs and symptoms appear to measure the "known" construct, e.g. depression?
Inter-rater reliability	Is the syndrome reliably assessed by two or more clinicians?
Test-retest reliability	Is the syndrome reliably measured (stable) over time?
Convergent validity	How correlated are the signs and symptoms of the syndrome with one another?
Divergent validity	Can the syndrome be distinguished from other so-called "neighborhood" syndromes?

behavioral, cognitive or emotional in nature, but has occurred commonly at the level of a syndrome. For example, the DSM–III was totally focused around inter-rater reliability for syndromes and to a lesser extent, convergent and divergent validity. DSM–III stipulated operationalized criteria and required patients to meet a specified number of those criteria, plus it required duration criteria that in themselves need to be questioned for their arbitrariness.

Further complications arise when two or more clinicians observe and assess the patient at different times, but within a limited time envelope of hours to a few days. One clinician may fail to inquire about a specific symptom or is not sufficiently observant of a sign. Additionally, a patient may fail to report symptoms because of genuine oversight on their part or dissemble because of mistrust of the clinician.

Test-retest reliability

Stability of symptoms and syndromes over time is problematic because some symptoms may genuinely resolve and disappear while others may emerge, unrelated to the disorder of interest. This is worsened because of the dichotomous nature (yes/no; present/absent) of the criteria as set out in the two major nosologies of DSM and ICD. Symptoms may fluctuate over time even without treatment, so a person may meet the criteria for a diagnosis on one occasion and not on a second occasion because the symptoms have faded; but they may return on a third occasion and the person meets the diagnostic threshold once again.

Naturally, on a fourth occasion, a person may meet additional criteria.

Comment

Our reading of the literature is that inter-rater reliability and test-retest reliability appear better for some diagnoses than others, and the literature suggests inconsistent results even within diagnostic categories (see Butler, 1999a).[2]

We would argue that whilst inter-rater reliability and test-retest reliability may have improved with the DSM and ICD under research conditions using structured or semi-structured instruments, reliability remains poor under ordinary clinical conditions (see Butler, 1999a for some examples). Further, McGorry *et al.* (1995) found that despite holding the diagnostic criteria constant, using differential diagnostic instruments led to a significant degree of differential diagnostic classification or misclassification, i.e. "spurious precision." Another point is that reliability acts as a ceiling for validity, so if the syndrome has poor inter-rater reliability, this casts into question the validity of the syndrome (Kendell, 1975; McGorry *et al.*, 1989).

Defining the phenotype?

In addition to the issues briefly covered above, we propose four issues that are of critical importance in thinking about phenomenologically focused diagnoses. The first is of paramount importance, as it refers to the switch that has occurred over the last 30 years away from "classic" categories. In "classic" or monothetic categories, for a given diagnosis *all* stipulated criteria must be present; that is, all are necessary and no one single criterion is sufficient. DSM–IV (American Psychiatric Association, 1994) is based on the notion of "polythetic" categories, meaning *all* stipulated criteria are of equal value, but only a specific number are needed for the diagnosis. In some DSM diagnostic categories the disorder is fully "polythetic," such as the specific personality disorders, where all stipulated criteria are accorded equal value in making the diagnosis. Conversely, in some other disorders, there may be one or more essential criteria that the person must meet, such as having depressed mood, but then the person must meet a specific number of criteria from the remaining symptom list. Such disorders, such as major depression, might be considered "part-polythetic." The assumption is that all people labeled with depression are the same, because they have been diagnosed as such. Yet the polythetic criteria produce many phenotypes – some of which are relatively non-overlapping with one another. Consider the example of borderline personality disorder: nine criteria are specified by DSM–IV, but to meet diagnostic "caseness" one only needs any five out of the nine criteria. This leads to many possible combinations of criteria – 126 to be precise!

The second major issue is that "wastebasket" categories are required in nosologies such as DSM, e.g. depressive disorder Not Otherwise Specified (NOS) or psychotic disorder NOS, because a given person may not meet all the necessary criteria for a diagnosis. They may fall one criterion short of reaching the threshold for a diagnosis of Major Depressive Disorder (MDD). Instead they receive a diagnosis of depressive disorder NOS, yet in all other ways they are identical to another person with the MDD phenotype. It may be the case that two people each have the same *type* of symptoms, but one has one less symptom. In the former case, the person receives a diagnosis of MDD, the other depressive disorder NOS.

A third issue pertains to the endurance and differentiation of signs and symptoms. As a general rule, in the early stages of a disorder, people may experience signs and symptoms – many of which are non-specific and non-enduring. With time, these symptoms may wax and wane – some drop out and disappear – others emerge and endure with greater clarity. They may begin to converge, crystallize and become distinguishable from other so-called syndromes (discriminant validity) (see Eaton *et al.*, Melton, 1995). The essential point is that nosologies such as DSM or ICD are based on crystallized forms of disorders with clear symptom pictures and with built-in duration criteria. They assume that a syndrome is "concrete" and stable across all phases of a disorder, and this is not necessarily the case. Such "classic" prototypes may not be accurate depictions or representations of disorders at the earliest stages where symptoms may be undifferentiated and non-specific. If one follows patients forward in time then the symptoms may or may not coalesce, consolidate and differentiate from non-specific symptom mixtures. But even with the emergence of a florid episode, i.e. where the person meets "caseness" for a given disorder for the first time, this does not necessarily guarantee that the symptomatology will remain stable over time. If relapse occurs, the patient may not necessarily present with the same phenotype and may deserve another

diagnostic label. It is only with repeated episodes and time (i.e. chronicity) that the features may become more or less concretized and stable. The problem, however, is that such chronic "cases" represent end stages of a disorder and are not typical. Many of our diagnoses are based on chronic patient populations. Here, prognosis and diagnosis have become confused, leading to pessimism about the power to intervene and change the shape, course and outcomes of a disorder.

A fourth and final problem pertains to the notion of additional symptoms. A given person may meet the criterion for MDD but have some anxiety symptoms sufficient in number and coherence to be considered a "syndrome." Yet, these anxiety symptoms are discounted by the application of the diagnostic system. It seems the case that DSM has reified "syndromes" which naturally may be poorly defined at the boundaries and merge with other syndromes.

Another approach: focusing on biological and cognitive factors as prime determinants of making a diagnosis

Some researchers argue that one should put more faith in biological or neurocognitive factors in making a diagnosis – that such variables are more valid. Others go further and suggest that those factors could be a marker of, or indicate, the genesis of the disorder (Gould & Gottesman, 2006). They would argue that phenotypes have outlived their usefulness and that instead of identifying a phenotype and then identifying a biological or cognitive marker, the roles should be completely reversed, i.e. we should identify potentially "hot" markers, e.g. reduced hippocampal volume or dorsal lateral frontal atrophy in psychosis, and then identify the clinical pictures or phenotypes that are associated with those. Of course, this approach has a long and venerable history as outlined by Millon in his history of psychiatry (Millon, 2005). The approach is most useful once *a definitive lesion of etiology* has been identified, e.g. Huntington's disease. In Huntington's disease the presence of the gene determines the diagnosis regardless of the heterogeneous presentation across different patients, particularly at different illness stages and ages.

We argue that the available germane evidence does not allow us to feel confident that the extant biological or neurocognitive data are more or less valid than phenomenological data. There are several reasons for reaching this conclusion. The first pertains to the nature of the designs used in most studies; the second is that the same biological or neurocognitive deficits are found across a range of disorders; the third is the stability of neurocognitive factors over time, the predictive value of the same, and their strength of association with the syndrome; the fourth relates to the size of the differences found between pathological and control groups, and interpretation of their meaningfulness; and the fifth pertains to the stage at which the differences emerge.

To elaborate, cross-sectional designs have been employed in the majority of studies which have reported frequency counts, correlations or simple comparisons between one group and another. For example, studies found that patients with schizophrenia had impaired olfactory thresholds, quality discrimination, and identification compared with controls, and that these patients also had reduced hippocampus, amygdala and/or perirhinal and entorhinal volumes (Rupp et al., 2005; Turetsky et al., 2003). However, these results are associations; they are not predictive and one does not know whether one is dealing with cause or consequence, with these neurocognitive and biological factors presaging functional deterioration, symptom intensification or poorer course or end-states.

A second reason for being skeptical about assigning pride of place to biological or neurocognitive factors is that certain factors are found in a range of disorders; that is, they are not specific to one disorder. Table 12.2 provides details of studies investigating these factors and illustrates the point that the same biological or neurocognitive variables have been found in different conditions. So, for example, hyperactivity of the hypothalamic-pituitary-adrenal (HPA)-axis is implicated in depersonalization disorder (Simeon et al., 2001), dementia (Gottfries et al., 1994; Spada et al., 2001), anorexia nervosa (Gross et al., 1994) and depression (Landro et al., 2001), and working memory deficits have been identified in schizophrenia (Pantelis et al., 1997; Park & Holzman, 1992), OCD (Purcell et al., 1998b), attention-deficit hyperactivity disorder (ADHD) (Barnett et al., 2005; Westerberg et al., 2004) and bipolar disorder (Doyle et al., 2005).

A third issue relates to the stability and predictive validity of biological and neurocognitive factors and their strength of association with the syndrome in question. In the case of psychosis there is some evidence for the stability of cognitive deficits over time, e.g. executive function impairment in schizophrenia (Rund, 1998; Tyson et al., 2004). Nevertheless, there are inconsistent findings regarding the relationship between these persisting deficits and the syndrome itself. For example, Hughes et al. (2003) found that in a group of patients with schizophrenia and schizoaffective disorder, the severity of negative symptoms at baseline predicted poor performance on a range of neuropsychological tasks; however, improvement in positive and negative symptoms at 6-month follow-up did not predict improvements in cognitive functioning, where the cognitive deficits remained relatively stable. In contrast, baseline deficits in attention and memory were found to significantly predict poor outcome at 2-year follow-up in patients with first-episode psychosis (Keshavan et al., 2003). To take another example, relative to healthy controls, deficits in sustained attention have been found in individuals at risk of developing psychosis, but this was not predictive of subsequent transition to psychosis (Francey et al., 2005). Most critically, we do not know whether these deficits were present prior to the development of the clinical picture or emerged contemporaneously with the clinical symptoms.

A fourth reason is the method used in deciding whether the change in a neurocognitive variable or another biological variable is meaningful. How is this assessed? Typically, it is accomplished by comparing mean scores on a specific test – say a test of working memory – obtained from a patient group of interest with those from another comparison patient or "healthy control" group. Now there may be statistical differences using ANOVAs, but we need to know how clinically important these differences are between the groups.

Related to this, however, is the issue of difference versus prediction. Just because there is a mean difference at the 0.05 or 0.01 level does not imply in itself that the cognitive variable is the prime driver of differences in symptom levels between the two groups, for example. If it is a true vulnerability or trait marker, then it should be present in some people who are not symptomatic at all, exhibit increased prevalence in those considered at risk, and be present in all those who meet the criteria for diagnostic caseness for a specific mental disorder. So correlation or mean differences between groups are no substitute for prediction.

Table 12.2. Potential neurocognitive and biological markers.

Biological variable studied	Identified in which conditions	Studies
Working memory	Schizophrenia (1–3)	(1) Park & Holzman (1992)
	Depression (4–6)	(2) Pantelis et al. (1997)
	Attention-deficit hyperactivity disorder (7–8)	(3) Mathes et al. (2005)
	Bipolar disorder (9)	(4) O'Brien et al. (2004)
	Obsessive-compulsive disorder (10)	(5) Landro et al. (2001)
	Borderline personality disorder (11)	(6) Stordal et al. (2004)
	Schizotypal personality disorder (12)	(7) Westerberg et al. (2004)
		(8) Barnett et al. (2005)
		(9) Doyle et al. (2005)
		(10) Purcell et al. (1998b)
		(11) Stevens et al. (2004)
		(12) Farmer et al. (2000)
Executive functioning (e.g. planning, problem-solving, set-shifting, etc.)	Depression (1–5)	(1) O'Brien et al. (2004)
	Borderline personality disorder (4)	(2) Stordal et al. (2004)
	Antisocial personality disorder (6)	(3) Purcell et al. (1997)
	Adult attention-deficit hyperactivity disorder (7–8)	(4) Kilcher et al. (2000)
	Schizophrenia (9–10)	(5) Kaviani et al. (2005)
	Obsessive-compulsive disorder (11)	(6) Dolan & Park (2002)
		(7) Boonstra et al. (2005)
		(8) Murphy et al. (2001)
		(9) Tyson et al. (2004)
		(10) Pantelis et al. (1997)
		(11) Purcell et al. (1998a, 1998b)

Table 12.2. (cont.)

Biological variable studied	Identified in which conditions	Studies
Olfactory identification	Schizophrenia (1–5)	(1) Rupp et al. (2005)
	Obsessive-compulsive disorder (6)	(2) Turetsky et al. (2003)
	Asperger's disorder (7)	(3–5) Brewer et al. (2001, 2003, 2007)
	Adult attention-deficit hyperactivity disorder (8)	(6) Barnett et al. (1999)
	Personality disorders, depression, dysthymia, other Axis I disorders (9)	(7) Suzuki et al. (2003)
		(8) Murphy et al. (2001)
		(9) Hirsch & Trannel (1996)
HPA activity	Attention-deficit hyperactivity disorder/oppositional-defiant disorder (1)	(1) Kariyawasam et al. (2002)
	Depersonalization disorder (2)	(2) Simeon et al. (2001)
	Dementia (3–4)	(3) Spada et al. (2001)
	Anorexia nervosa (5)	(4) Gottfries et al. (1994)
	Depression (6)	(5) Gross et al. (1994)
	Alcohol dependent, and alcohol and stimulant dependent (7)	(6) O'Brien et al. (2004)
	Psychosis (8)	(7) Lovallo et al. (2000)
		(8) Garner et al. (2005)
Temporal lobe limbic deficits (e.g. hippocampal and amygdala volume)	Schizophrenia (1–6)	(1) Rupp et al. (2005)
	Bipolar disorder (6–8)	(2) Turetsky et al. (2003)
	Schizotypal personality disorder (9)	(3) Blennow et al. (1999)
	Borderline personality disorder (10)	(4) Montoya et al. (2005)
	Depression (11)	(5–6) Velakoulis et al. (1999, 2006)
		(7) Frazier et al. (2005)
		(8) Hajek et al. (2005)
		(9) Voglmaier et al. (1997)

Category	Disorder	Reference
		(10) van Elst et al. (2003)
		(11) O'Brien et al. (2004)
Attentional problems	Depression (1)	(1) Landro et al. (2001)
	Schizophrenia (2)	(2) Tyson et al. (2004)
Skin conductance	Depersonalization disorder (1)	(1) Sierra et al. (2002)
	Depression (2)	(2) Miquel et al. (1999)
	Schizotypal personality disorder (3)	(3) Raine et al. (1997)
	Schizophrenia (4)	(4) Katsanis & Iacono (1994)
Stress hormones	Alcohol dependent, and alcohol and stimulant dependent (1)	(1) Lovallo et al. (2000)
	Social phobia (2)	(2) Condren et al. (2002)
	Anorexia nervosa (3)	(3) Gross et al. (1994)

Table 12.3. Types of neurocognitive and biological markers and stages of disorder.

Marker	Premorbid and first-degree relatives	Prodrome	First episode	Remission	Chronic	Relapse
Vulnerability/trait	☞	☞	☞	☞	☞	☞
State	X	☞ / X	☞	X	X / ?	☞
Consequences	X	X	X	☞ / ?	☞	☞ / X

Note: ☞ = present; X = absent; ? = not known/unsure.

A more current approach to biological or neuro-cognitive variables is the notion of "endophenotypes," described as "quantifiable components in the genes-to-behaviors pathways, distinct from psychiatric symptoms, which make genetic and biological studies for disease categories more manageable" (Gould & Gottesman, 2006, p. 113). In other words, endophenotypes are intermediate between genes and the phenotypes and "they can be neurophysiological, biochemical, endocrine, neuroanatomical, cognitive or neuropsychological" (Gould & Gottesman, 2006, p. 113). They are associated with a disorder and are heritable, state independent and co-segregate within families, and are found in some unaffected relatives (Gould & Gottesman, 2006). Some examples of putative endophenotypes in bipolar disorder are early onset white-matter abnormalities, attention deficits, reduced anterior cingulate volume, abnormal regulation of circadian instability, and response to psychostimulants (Gould & Gottesman, 2006; Lenox et al., 2002).

Comments

Our view is that reversing and putting neurocognitive or biological markers first and defining clinical pictures on that basis may turn out to be appropriate for a subset of cases, but we would speculate that for the rest they would need to be diagnosed as "Not Otherwise Specified" or "Atypical."

As regards "endophenotypes," we find this is an interesting approach but remain somewhat skeptical. Although the DSM model has led to a proliferation of diagnoses ("splitting"), the endophenotypic approach will probably lead to a lumping of phenotypes. For example, as previously noted, working-memory deficits are found in a range of disorders and so appear to be relatively non-specific (see Table 12.2), and we still need to be convinced of the stability and state independence of these endophenotypes, and especially whether or not they are present at the earliest stages of illness. Most attempts at identifying endophenotypes have occurred in cross-sectional studies, so in our view they are too weak or "subthreshold" to qualify as the basis for a diagnosis or "disease entity." Most critically, we need to be persuaded of the value of endophenotypes for treatment, remembering that the selection of appropriate treatments is a major function of diagnosis.

Parenthetically, from our perspective, "risk factors" and "markers" require more careful elucidation, as does their relationship to outcome. We need to take into account the temporal sequence of each risk factor; whether or not one risk factor dominates; and whether risk factors are proxies, overlapping, independent, or mediators or moderators (see Kraemer et al., 2001). Our approach is somewhat simpler than Kraemer et al. (2001). We need to be clear about the onset and offset dimension and distinguish between vulnerability and trait markers, state markers, and the consequences of the "disorder". Table 12.3 shows examples of the three types. With *vulnerability and trait markers*, they should be found in asymptomatic cases, in symptomatic cases, in remitted, relapsing and chronic cases – at all stages. As regards to causation, these markers may be necessary but not sufficient to "cause" a disorder, *or* neither necessary nor sufficient, i.e. a contributing cause, *or* they could be a single casual risk factor. In regards to *state factors*, biological or neurocognitive factors may neither be necessary or sufficient, but may be present at the stage of symptom intensification (i.e. the prodrome), be present in the first episode, disappear with remission and re-appear with relapse. Such state factors may not be predictive of the "disorder," but may or may not add to impairment by contributing to daily dysfunction, e.g. poor executive functioning. Finally, factors such as impaired executive functioning may appear only in the wake of a first episode and not during or before that episode; that is, as a *consequence* of a "disorder." Such factors may make a contribution to daily functioning somewhat independently of phase of illness and severity of symptomatology.

Another approach to psychiatric diagnosis: a Staging Model

The key driver behind the staging approach is to prevent progression of an "illness" to a subsequent severe stage.

In Table 12.4 we outline the principles underpinning a staging model – one which combines phenomenological pictures with cognitive and biological factors and adds a temporal dimension (McGorry *et al.*, 2003). Although the phenomenological approach and the biological approach each put greater or lesser emphasis on certain features in reaching a diagnosis, in reality, the features emphasized in both approaches are flawed and indiscriminate. We argue for refraining from endless debates about whether biological variables or phenomenological features are more or less accurate components of a syndrome. Rather, we should adopt a clinical heuristic stance, acknowledge the importance of using both sets of features, and retain the concept of syndrome as a somewhat crude but useful heuristic in clinical practice; but, continue to improve on it with further research.

The first and second principles stated in Table 12.4 are general and overarching principles that state that diagnosis should be treatment focused and outcome focused, i.e. on improving functioning not just symptoms. The third principle states that in making a diagnosis we need to tolerate a degree of ambiguity and uncertainty; clearly, certainty of diagnosis may vary from one stage to another, i.e. the temporal dimension. If we wish to develop an early intervention model then we need to move to earlier stages of disorder where the symptoms are vague, less fixed and may appear to be relatively non-specific.

The fourth principle states that biological and cognitive variables may be associated with changes

Table 12.4. Principles underpinning a staging model: a manifesto.

1. Diagnosis should be treatment focused.
2. Diagnosis should be outcome focused, i.e. on improving functioning not just symptoms.
3. In making a diagnosis we need to tolerate a degree of ambiguity and uncertainty and this is most true at the earliest stages of disorder.
4. Biological and cognitive variables may be associated with changes in stage and/or presage symptom intensification and syndrome clarification.
5. Biological and cognitive variables – irrespective of whether or not they are endophenotypes – may have a direct or indirect relationship to functioning.
6. Treatment should have wider applicability to larger populations and be less expensive at the earliest stages.
7. Treatments should be milder, more benign and have fewer side-effects at the earliest stages of disorder.
8. Treatment must focus not only on symptoms but on improvement, if not full restoration, of functioning.
9. Some biological and cognitive variables are potentially modifiable and should be a target for intervention, if remediation is thought to improve functioning, distress, or prevent progression to a more severe stage of illness.

in stage and/or presage symptom intensification and syndrome clarification. For example, Pantelis *et al.* (2003) found evidence of this in people who were at ultra-high risk for psychosis. At baseline, his group examined MRI scans and found less gray matter in the right medial temporal, lateral temporal, and inferior frontal cortex, and in the cingulate cortex bilaterally in those who eventually became psychotic compared with those who did not. But, most critically, in the longitudinal component of the study they found additional neuroanatomical differences that occurred in those who became psychotic. A reduction in gray matter in the left parahippocampal, fusiform, orbitofrontal and cerebellar cortices and bilaterally in the cingulate gyri was found. In those who did not become psychotic, longitudinal changes were found only in the cerebellum.

In accordance with our fifth principle, we assert that biological and neurocognitive changes and impairments may have a strong relationship with day-to-day functioning and contribute to dysfunction at least somewhat independently of symptoms. An example of this could be deficits in problem-solving and abstract reasoning related to problems in dealing with tradespeople, or governmental agencies. This relationship could be mediated through negative symptoms of schizophrenia, but could have a direct relationship as well. For instance, Green (1996) found verbal reasoning to be consistently and directly associated with all types of functional outcome and vigilance with social problem-solving and skill acquisition.

Principles 6 to 9 in Table 12.4 pertain to treatment/ intervention. The implications for treatment are different according to the specific stage. So, at an early stage when non-specific symptoms are manifested, the level of risk is low and the percentage of natural remission is high and widespread. At this early stage we do not know whether these symptoms will resolve or harden, or even transmute into more malignant subthreshold phenotypic forms. So interventions at the earliest stage need to be easily delivered and benign (no side-effects) because of the potentially very large numbers of false positives (Principles 6 and 7). This could take the form of public health information messages and mental health literacy, e.g. leaflets, television advertisements and billboard messages for people to exercise, observe sleep hygiene and engage in positive activities involving mastery and pleasure (Jorm, 2000; Jorm et al., 2003). Such treatments are benign since they do not involve the ingestion of medications, and are relatively cost-effective since they do not involve intensive one-to-one intervention requiring high levels of clinical expertise or equipment (Principles 6 and 7). They are also non-stigmatizing.

A later stage would involve those individuals who are distressed, have manifested a drop in functioning, and are seeking treatment. They may not meet "caseness" for mood disorder, i.e. they have three symptoms which have endured for 2 weeks and they report a family history of depression. They are worthy of treatment; for example, targeted cognitive-behavioral therapy (CBT) and perhaps low dose medication of some type. Moreover, functioning is equally worthy of intervention, e.g. skills training, structured activities and CBT aimed at return to school or vocational placement (Principle 8). Now at this stage, one has to weigh up the costs

and benefits in terms of side-effects. Some of these people will not go on to develop a full diagnostic mood or related disorder. The argument is that one is unnecessarily exposing some people to potentially serious side-effects of treatment. This means that the benefits to the group as a whole must be significant and the risks to the entire group comparatively low (McGorry et al., 2002).

We have already noted that biological features are to be found at different phases of the disorder and may or may not presage a change in the phase of disorder, that is, from one stage to another. We would argue that the marker may itself be amenable to intervention, e.g. cognitive remediation might focus on addressing problem-solving and working-memory deficits underpinning the negative symptoms of schizophrenia (Principle 9).

We would argue for a combinatorial approach which takes into account symptom severity, intensity, coherence and duration, functioning, and cognitive and biological variables (McGorry et al., 2006). Table 12.5 shows a worked through example with regard to psychosis and severe mood disorders. Some general comments are that this 4-stage model assumes that the phenotype is not necessarily stable or even coherent at a very early stage (Stage 1a), and leaves open the notion that the phenotype, or a portion thereof, may be altered by treatment. Progression of the person from, say, Stage 1 to Stage 2 could therefore be prevented. From Stage 0 to Stage 1b would see the emergence of non-differentiated symptoms, the intensification of existing features, the accretion of more features and a decrease in functioning (representing a smaller number of people at Stage 1b than at Stages 1a and 0). By Stage 1b there would be evidence of a subthreshold syndrome with reduction in functioning. Stage 2 would represent the onset of a coherent florid phenotype (the first episode), Stages 3a to 3c incomplete remission, single and multiple relapses, and Stage 4 severe, persistent or unrelenting illness.

Although Fava & Kellner (1993) deserve credit for first discussing a staging approach to psychiatric classification, it has received little empirical attention outside of the psychosis field where it is increasing in credibility with regard to "at risk" and prodromal conditions (McGorry et al., 2003). Clearly, more work needs to be done, but we believe staging models have great relevance to a whole array of psychiatric disorders.

Table 12.5. Clinical staging model framework for psychotic and severe mood disorders.

Clinical stage	Definition	Target populations for recruitment	Potential interventions	Indicative biological and endophenotypic markers
0	Increased risk of psychotic or severe mood disorder No symptoms currently	First-degree teenage relatives of probands	Improved mental health literacy; family education, drug education; brief cognitive skills training	Trait marker candidates and endophenotypes, e.g. smooth pursuit eye movements, P50, niacin sensitivity, binocular rivalry, prepulse inhibition, mismatch negativity, olfactory deficits
1a	Mild or non-specific symptoms, including neurocognitive deficits, of psychosis or severe mood disorder. Mild functional change or decline	Screening of teenage populations; referral by primary care physicians; referral by school counsellors	Formal mental health literacy; family psychoeducation; formal CBT; active substance abuse reduction	Trait and state candidates where feasible according to sample size
1b	Ultra high risk: moderate but subthreshold symptoms, with moderate neurocognitive changes and functional decline to caseness (GAF < 70)	Referral by educational agencies, primary care physicians, emergency departments, welfare agencies	Family psychoeducation; formal CBT; active substance abuse reduction; atypical antipsychotic agents for episode; antidepressant agents or mood stabilizers	Niacin sensitivity; folate status; MRI and MRS changes; HPA axis dysregulation
2	First episode of psychotic or severe mood disorder. Full threshold disorder with moderate-severe symptoms, neurocognitive deficits and functional decline (GAF 30–50)	Referral by primary care physicians, emergency departments, welfare agencies; specialist care agencies; drug and alcohol services	Family psychoeducation; formal CBT; active substance abuse reduction; atypical antipsychotic agents for episode; antidepressant agents or mood stabilizers; vocational rehabilitation	Continue with markers of illness state, trait and progression
3a	Incomplete remission from FE of care. Could be linked or fast-tracked to stage 4	Primary and specialist care services	As for "2" with additional emphasis on medical and psychosocial strategies to achieve full remission	Continue with markers of illness state, trait and progression
3b	Recurrence or relapse of psychotic or mood disorder which stabilizes with treatment at a level of GAF, residual symptoms, or neurocognition below the	Primary and specialist care services	As for "3a" with additional emphasis on relapse prevention and "early warning signs" strategies	Continue with markers of illness state, trait and progression

Table 12.5. (cont.)

Clinical stage	Definition	Target populations for recruitment	Potential interventions	Indicative biological and endophenotypic markers
	best level achieved following remission from first episode			
3c	Multiple relapses, provided worsening in clinical extent and impact of illness is objectively present	Specialist care services	As for "3b" with emphasis on long-term stabilization	Continue with markers of illness state, trait and progression
4	Severe, persistent OR unremitting illness as judged on symptoms, neurocognition and disability criteria Note: could fast track to this stage at first presentation through specific clinical and functional criteria (from stage 2) or alternatively by failure to respond to treatment (from stage 3a)	Specialized care services	As for "3c" but with emphasis on clozapine, other tertiary treatments, social participation despite ongoing disability	Continue with markers of illness state, trait and progression

Adapted with permission from McGorry et al. (2006).

Note: The clinical staging model provides greater utility for testing efficacy, cost-effectiveness, risk–benefit ratios and feasibility of available interventions; clinicopathological correlates and predictors of illness stages can also be introduced within a neurodevelopmental framework.

Conclusions

The purpose of this chapter has been to argue that we have lost sight of a major primary purpose of diagnosis, which is to guide treatment and predict outcome. We believe there has been too much of a focus on reliability of signs and symptoms at the expense of validity. We have set out two apparently diametrically opposed approaches – one which gives phenomenology pride of place in determining diagnosis, and the second which assigns primacy to biological or neurocognitive variables. We argue both approaches have limitations and propose that a combinatorial approach represents a way forward. Additionally, we argue for a staging model in which symptoms at the earliest stages may lack the coherence and clarity they do at later stages, but are still deserving of treatment. We outline nine principles underlining the staging model and provide a worked-through-example for psychotic and severe mood disorders.

Acknowledgments

The authors want to express their great appreciation to Angie Jackman and Kelly Allott for their valuable assistance in researching the material for this chapter. The work in this chapter is in part supported by a National Health and Medical Research Council (NH&MRC) Program Grant (2004–2008) held by Patrick McGorry, Christos Pantelis, Ian Hickie, Henry Jackson and Alison Yung.

Endnotes

1. We use the terms "syndrome" and "disorder" interchangeably. We believe "disorder" is a misnomer because of the lack of discriminant validity and large overlap between "syndromes." Of course, "disorder" is the term used in DSM, but it connotes a notion of immutability and concretization.

2. Parenthetically, readers might find interest in the debate about the DSM–III system between Butler (1999a, 1999b) and Parker

(1999). Issues are not confined to reliability but the political and socio-cultural processes influencing, and according to Butler (1999a) compromising, the science underpinning the DSM system.

References

American Psychiatric Association (1980). *Diagnostic and Statistical Manual of Mental Disorders* (3rd edn.). Washington, DC: APA.

American Psychiatric Association (1994). *Diagnostic and Statistical Manual of Mental Disorders* (4th edn.). Washington, DC: APA.

Barlow, D. H. & Durand, V. M. (2005). *Abnormal Psychology: An Integrative Approach*. Belmont, CA: Thomson/Wadsworth.

Barnett, R., Maruff, P., Purcell, R. *et al.* (1999). Impairment of olfactory identification in obsessive-compulsive disorder. *Psychological Medicine*, 29, 1227–1233.

Barnett, R., Maruff, P. & Vance, A. (2005). An investigation of visuospatial memory impairment in children with attention deficit hyperactivity disorder (ADHD), combined type. *Psychological Medicine*, 35, 1433–1443.

Blennow, K., Bogdanovic, N., Gottfries, C.-G. & Davidsson, P. (1999). The growth-associated protein GAP-43 is increased in the hippocampus and in the gyrus cinguli in schizophrenia. *Journal of Molecular Neuroscience*, 13, 101–109.

Boonstra, A. M., Oosterlaan, J., Sergeant, J. A. & Buitelaar, J. K. (2005). Executive functioning in adult ADHD: a meta-analytic review. *Psychological Medicine*, 35, 1097–1108.

Brewer, W. J., Pantelis, C., Anderson, V. *et al.* (2001). Stability of olfactory identification deficits in neuroleptic-naive patients with first-episode psychosis. *American Journal of Psychiatry*, 158, 107–115.

Brewer, W. J., Wood, S. J., McGorry, P. D. *et al.* (2003). Impairment of olfactory identification ability in individuals at ultra-high risk for psychosis who later develop schizophrenia. *American Journal of Psychiatry*, 160, 1790–1794.

Brewer, W. J., Wood, S. J., Pantelis, C. *et al.* (2007). Olfactory sensitivity through the course of psychosis: relationships to olfactory identification, symptomatology and the schizophrenia odour. *Psychiatry Research*, 149, 97–104.

Butler, P. V. (1999a). Diagnostic line-drawing, professional boundaries, and the rhetoric of scientific justification: a critical appraisal of the American Psychiatric Association's DSM project. *Australian Psychologist*, 34, 20–29.

Butler, P. V. (1999b). Psychiatry, naiveté, and the politics of dissimulation: a response to Parker (1999). *Australian Psychologist*, 34, 35–37.

Condren, R. M., O'Neill, A., Ryan, M. C. M., Barrett, P. & Thakore, J. H. (2002). HPA axis response to a psychological stressor in generalised social phobia. *Psychoneuroendocrinology*, 27, 693–703.

Dolan, M. & Park, I. (2002). The neuropsychology of antisocial personality disorder. *Psychological Medicine*, 32, 417–427.

Doyle, A. E., Wilens, T. E., Kwon, A. *et al.* (2005). Neuropsychological functioning in youth with bipolar disorder. *Biological Psychiatry*, 58, 540–548.

Eaton, W. W., Badawi, M. & Melton, B. (1995). Prodrome and precursors: epidemiologic data for primary prevention of disorders with slow onset. *American Journal of Psychiatry*, 152, 967–972.

Farmer, C. M., O'Donnell, B. F., Niznikiewicz, M. A. *et al.* (2000). Visual perception and working memory in schizotypal personality disorder. *American Journal of Psychiatry*, 157, 781–786.

Fava, G. A. & Kellner, R. (1993). Staging: a neglected dimension in psychiatric classification. *Acta Psychiatrica Scandinavica*, 87, 225–230.

Francey, S. M., Jackson, H. J., Phillips, L. J. *et al.* (2005). Sustained attention in young people at high risk of psychosis does not predict transition to psychosis. *Schizophrenia Research*, 79, 127–136.

Frazier, J. A., Chiu, S. F., Breeze, J. L. *et al.* (2005). Structural brain magnetic resonance imaging of limbic and thalamic volumes in pediatric bipolar disorder. *American Journal of Psychiatry*, 162, 1256–1265.

Garner, B., Pariante, C. M., Wood, S. J. *et al.* (2005). Pituitary volume predicts future transition to psychosis in individuals at ultra-high risk of developing psychosis. *Biological Psychiatry*, 58, 417–423.

Gottfries, C. G., Balldin, J., Blennow, K. *et al.* (1994). Hypothalamic dysfunction in dementia. *Journal of Neural Transmission-Supplement*, 43, 203–209.

Gould, T. D. & Gottesman, I. I. (2006). Psychiatric endophenotypes and the development of valid animal models. *Genes Brain and Behavior*, 5, 113–119.

Green, M. F. (1996). What are the functional consequences of neurocognitive deficits in schizophrenia? *American Journal of Psychiatry*, 153, 321–330.

Gross, M. J., Kahn, J. P., Laxenaire, M., Nicolas, J. P. & Burlet, C. (1994). Corticotropin-releasing-factor and anorexia-nervosa – hypothalamo-pituitary-adrenal axis response to neurotropic stress. *Annales D Endocrinologie*, 55, 221–228.

Hajek, T., Carrey, N. & Alda, M. (2005). Neuroanatomical abnormalities as risk factors for bipolar disorder. *Bipolar Disorders*, 7, 393–403.

Hirsch, A. R. & Trannel, T. J. (1996). Chemosensory disorders and psychiatric diagnoses. *Journal of*

Neurological and Orthopaedic Medicine and Surgery, **17**, 25–30.

Hughes, C., Kumari, V., Soni, W. *et al.* (2003). Longitudinal study of symptoms and cognitive function in chronic schizophrenia. *Schizophrenia Research*, **59**, 137–146.

Jorm, A. F. (2000). Mental health literacy – public knowledge and beliefs about mental disorders. *British Journal of Psychiatry*, **177**, 396–401.

Jorm, A. F., Griffiths, K. M., Christensen, H. *et al.* (2003). Providing information about the effectiveness of treatment options to depressed people in the community: a randomized controlled trial of effects on mental health literacy, help-seeking and symptoms. *Psychological Medicine*, **33**, 1071–1079.

Kariyawasam, S. H., Zaw, F. & Handley, S. L. (2002). Reduced salivary cortisol in children with comorbid attention deficit hyperactivity disorder and oppositional defiant disorder. *Neuroendocrinology Letters*, **23**, 45–48.

Katsanis, J. & Iacono, W. G. (1994). Electrodermal activity and clinical status in chronic schizophrenia. *Journal of Abnormal Psychology*, **103**, 222–283.

Kaviani, H., Rahimi-Darabad, P. & Naghavi, H. R. (2005). Autobiographical memory retrieval and problem-solving deficits of Iranian depressed patients attempting suicide. *Journal of Psychopathology and Behavioral Assessment*, **27**, 39–44.

Kendell, R. E. (1975). *The Role of Psychiatric Diagnosis in Psychiatry*. Oxford: Blackwell Scientific Publications.

Keshavan, M. S., Haas, G., Miewald, J. *et al.* (2003). Prolonged untreated illness duration from prodromal onset predicts outcome in first episode psychoses. *Schizophrenia Bulletin*, **29**, 757–769.

Kilcher, H., Schmid-Kitsikis, E., Aapro, N., Ratcliff, B. & Andreoli, A. (2000). Metacognition in borderline patients: a controlled evaluation. *Annales Medico-Psychologiques*, **158**, 558–570.

Kraemer, H. C., Stice, E., Kazdin, A. E., Offord, D. & Kupfer, D. (2001). How do risk factors work together? Mediators, moderators, and independent, overlapping, and proxy risk factors. *American Journal of Psychiatry*, **158**, 848–856.

Landro, N. I., Stiles, T. C. & Sletvold, H. (2001). Neuropsychological function in nonpsychotic unipolar major depression. *Neuropsychiatry, Neuropsychology and Behavioral Neurology*, **14**, 233–240.

Lenox, R. H., Gould, T. D. & Manji, H. K. (2002). Endophenotypes in bipolar disorder. *American Journal of Medical Genetics*, **114**, 391–406.

Lovallo, W. R., Dickensheets, S. L., Myers, D. A., Thomas, T. L. & Nixon, S. J. (2000). Blunted stress cortisol response in abstinent alcoholic and polysubstance-abusing men. *Alcoholism – Clinical and Experimental Research*, **24**, 651–658.

Mathes, B., Wood, S. J., Proffitt, T. M. *et al.* (2005). Early processing deficits in object working memory in first-episode schizophreniform psychosis and established schizophrenia. *Psychological Medicine*, **35**, 1053–1062.

McGorry, P. D., Copolov, D. L. & Singh, B. S. (1989). The validity of the assessment of psychopathology in the psychoses. *Australian and New Zealand Journal of Psychiatry*, **23**, 469–482.

McGorry, P. D., Hickie, I. B., Yung, A. R., Pantelis, C. & Jackson, H. J. (2006). Clinical staging of psychiatric disorders: a heuristic framework for choosing earlier, safer and more effective interventions. *Australian and New Zealand Journal of Psychiatry*, **40**, 616–622.

McGorry, P. D., Mihalopoulos, C., Henry, L. *et al.* (1995). Spurious precision: procedural validity of diagnostic assessment in psychotic disorders. *American Journal of Psychiatry*, **152**, 222–223.

McGorry, P. D., Yung, A. R. & Phillips, L. J. (2003). The "close-in" or ultra high-risk model: a safe and effective strategy for research and clinical intervention in prepsychotic mental disorder. *Schizophrenia Bulletin*, **29**, 771–790.

McGorry, P. D., Yung, A. R., Phillips, L. J. *et al.* (2002). Randomized controlled trial of interventions designed to reduce the risk of progression to first-episode psychosis in a clinical sample with subthreshold symptoms. *Archives of General Psychiatry*, **59**, 921–928.

Millon, T. (2005). *Masters of the Mind. Exploring the Story of Mental Illness from Ancient Times to the New Millennium*. Hoboken, NJ: Wiley.

Miquel, M. Fuentes, I., Garcia-Merita, M. & Rojo, L. (1999). Habituation and sensitization processes in depressive disorders. *Psychopathology*, **32**, 35–42.

Montoya, A., Lepage, M. & Malla, A. (2005). Temporal lobe dysfunction in patients with first-episode schizophrenia. *Salud Mental*, **28**, 33–39.

Murphy, K. R., Barkley, R. A. & Bush, T. (2001). Executive functioning and olfactory identification in young adults with attention deficit-hyperactivity disorder. *Neuropsychology*, **15**, 211–220.

O'Brien, J. T., Lloyd, A., McKeith, I., Gholkar, A. & Ferrier, N. (2004). A longitudinal study of hippocampal volume, cortisol levels, and cognition in older depressed subjects. *American Journal of Psychiatry*, **161**, 2081–2090.

Palmer, K. J. & Benfield, P. (1994). Fluvoxamine – an overview of its pharmacological properties and review of its therapeutic potential in non-depressive disorders. *CNS Drugs*, **1**, 57–87.

Pantelis, C., Barnes, T. R. E., Nelson, H. E. *et al.* (1997). Frontal-striatal cognitive deficits in patients with chronic schizophrenia. *Brain*, **120**, 1823–1843.

Pantelis, C., Velakoulis, D., McGorry, P. D. *et al.* (2003). Neuroanatomical abnormalities before and after onset of psychosis: a cross sectional and longitudinal MRI comparison. *Lancet*, **361**, 281–288.

Park, S. & Holzman, P. S. (1992). Schizophrenics show spatial working memory deficits. *Archives of General Psychiatry*, **49**, 975–982.

Parker, G. (1999). Diagnostic line-drawing: how to pick an eagle from a turkey. *Australian Psychologist*, **34**, 30–34.

Purcell, R., Maruff, P., Kyrios, M. & Pantelis, C. (1997). Neuropsychological function in young patients with unipolar major depression. *Psychological Medicine*, **27**, 1277–1285.

Purcell, R., Maruff, P., Kyrios, M. & Pantelis, C. (1998a). Cognitive deficits in obsessive-compulsive disorder on tests of frontal-striatal function. *Biological Psychiatry*, **43**, 348–357.

Purcell, R., Maruff, P., Kyrios, M. & Pantelis, C. (1998b). Neuropsychological deficits in obsessive-compulsive disorder – a comparison with unipolar depression, panic disorder, and normal controls. *Archives of General Psychiatry*, **55**, 415–423.

Raine, A., Benishay, D., Lencz, T. & Scarpa, A. (1997). Abnormal orienting in schizotypal personality disorder. *Schizophrenia Bulletin*, **23**, 75–82.

Rund, B. R. (1998). A review of longitudinal studies of cognitive functions in schizophrenia patients. *Schizophrenia Bulletin*, **24**, 425–435.

Rupp, C. I., Fleischhacker, W. W., Kemmler, G. *et al.* (2005). Olfactory functions and volumetric measures of orbitofrontal and limbic regions in schizophrenia. *Schizophrenia Research*, **74**, 149–161.

Sierra, M., Senior, C., Dalton, J. *et al.* (2002). Autonomic responses in depersonalization disorder. *Archives of General Psychiatry*, **59**, 833–838.

Simeon, D., Guralnik, O., Knutelska, M., Hollander, E. & Schmeidler, J. (2001). Hypothalamic-pituitary-adrenal axis dysregulation in depersonalization disorder. *Neuropsychopharmacology*, **25**, 793–795.

Spada, R. S., Cento, R. M., Proto, C. *et al.* (2001). Twenty-four-hour urinary free cortisol levels in vascular dementia and in Alzheimer's disease. *Archives of Gerontology and Geriatrics*, **33** (Suppl. 1), 363–367.

Stevens, A., Burkhardt, M., Hautzinger, M., Schwarz, J. & Unckel, C. (2004). Borderline personality disorder: impaired visual perception and working memory. *Psychiatry Research*, **125**, 257–267.

Stordal, K. I., Lundervold, A. J., Egeland, J. *et al.* (2004). Impairment across executive functions in recurrent major depression. *Nordic Journal of Psychiatry*, **58**, 41–47.

Suzuki, Y., Critchley, H. D., Rowe, A. *et al.* (2003). Impaired olfactory identification in Asperger's syndrome. *Journal of Neuropsychiatry and Clinical Neurosciences*, **15**, 105–107.

Turetsky, B. I., Moberg, P. J., Roalf, D. R., Arnold, S. E. & Gur, R. E. (2003). Decrements in volume of anterior ventromedial temporal lobe and olfactory dysfunction in schizophrenia. *Archives of General Psychiatry*, **60**, 1193–1200.

Tyson, P. J., Laws, K. R., Roberts, K. H. & Mortimer, A. M. (2004). Stability of set-shifting and planning abilities in patients with schizophrenia. *Psychiatry Research*, **129**, 229–239.

van Elst, L. T., Hesslinger, B., Thiel, T. *et al.* (2003). Frontolimbic brain abnormalities in patients with borderline personality disorder: a volumetric magnetic resonance imaging study. *Biological Psychiatry*, **54**, 163–171.

Velakoulis, D., Pantelis, C., McGorry, P. D. *et al.* (1999). Hippocampal volume in first-episode psychoses and chronic schizophrenia – a high-resolution magnetic resonance imaging study. *Archives of General Psychiatry*, **56**, 133–141.

Velakoulis, D., Wood, S. J., Wong, M. T. H. *et al.* (2006). Hippocampal and amygdala volumes according to psychosis stage and diagnosis – a magnetic resonance imaging study of chronic schizophrenia, first-episode psychosis, and ultra-high-risk individuals. *Archives of General Psychiatry*, **63**, 139–149.

Voglmaier, M. M., Seidman, L. J., Salisbury, D. *et al.* (1997). Verbal skill deficits in schizotypal personality disorder. *Biological Psychiatry*, **41**, 351 (Suppl.).

Westerberg, H., Hirvikoski, T., Forssberg, H. & Klingberg, T. (2004). Visuo-spatial working memory span: a sensitive measure of cognitive deficits in children with ADHD. *Child Neuropsychology*, **10**, 155–161.

World Health Organization (1992). *International Statistical Classification of Diseases and Related Health Problems* (10th Revision). Geneva: WHO.

Chapter 13

Neuropsychological methods in mental disorders research: illustrations from methamphetamine dependence

Steven Paul Woods, Jennifer E. Iudicello, J. Cobb Scott and Igor Grant

Introduction

The aim of this chapter is to provide an overview and critical examination of neuropsychological assessment methods intended for applied clinical research in mental disorders. In the first section, we will address issues of study design and test selection in studying the epidemiology, mechanisms and functional impact of cognitive impairment in mental disorders. Next, we will discuss how demographic factors, test-taking effort, disease characteristics, and data-analytic strategies can influence the interpretation of neuropsychological research in these populations. Finally, the utility of neuropsychological assessment in developing targeted remedial strategies for mental disorders, as well as in predicting and documenting treatment outcomes is considered.

Throughout the chapter, key issues will be illustrated by highlighting research on the adverse neuropsychological effects of methamphetamine (MA), which is an increasingly prevalent drug of abuse in the USA (Yacoubian & Peters, 2004). Methamphetamine is a synthetic psychostimulant with a half-life of approximately 10 hours (Harris *et al.*, 2003) that may be administered in a variety of different ways (e.g. by injection, snorting or smoking) (U.S. Department of Health and Human Services, 2002). Acute effects of MA can include euphoria, akathisia, increased respiration, vasoconstriction, appetite suppression, enhanced energy, insomnia, heightened attention, irritability and even paranoid psychosis (U.S. Department of Health and Human Services, 2002). Chronic MA use is associated with a host of adverse psychosocial (e.g. interpersonal, financial), psychological (e.g. cognitive), and physical sequelae, including marked effects on central nervous system (CNS) functioning. Long-term MA use may promote neuronal

injury via increased oxidative stress, vascular injury and/or hyperthermia (Davidson *et al.*, 2001). The neurotoxicity associated with MA use is evident in several neurotransmitter systems, but is perhaps most notable on nigrostriatal dopaminergic projections, thus altering the function of the dopamine-rich fronto-striato-thalamo-cortical loops (Nordahl *et al.*, 2003). For example, neuroimaging studies demonstrate structural, cerebral blood flow and metabolic abnormalities in the prefrontal cortex and striatum of MA-dependent persons (Chang *et al.*, 2002; Scott *et al.*, 2007). Chronic MA use is also linked to deficits in neuropsychological functioning; the nature, mechanisms, daily impact and reversibility of which will be a focus of this chapter.

Methods and approaches
Study design and test selection

A notable strength of neuropsychology is its dependence on a scientific assessment methodology that is solidly grounded in psychometric theory. As such, neuropsychology is in a unique position to guide and advance basic and clinical neuroscience research on the etiology, diagnosis and clinical features of mental disorders. A formal, standardized neuropsychological assessment is an essential tool for defining the prevalence, incidence and pattern of global and domain-specific cognitive impairments. The specific components and length of a neuropsychological battery will vary across research settings and mental disorders of interest and may include: (1) a semi-structured interview to document medical, psychiatric and psychosocial variables that might affect cognition; (2) examiner ratings of participants' behavior, effort, sensory-perception, cognition and affect; (3) objective neuropsychological tests of effort, current and pre-morbid intelligence, and a diverse range of cognitive domains, such as attention, executive functions, language, information processing speed, learning and memory, spatial abilities, praxis, motor skills, and sensory-perception; (4) standardized self- and other-report questionnaires of mood, health-related quality of life, personality characteristics, and activities of daily living; and (5) corroborating medical, neurological, psychiatric and neuroimaging examinations, as indicated (Tröster & Woods, 2003).

With regard to the selection of objective neuropsychological tests, investigators are encouraged to include at least two standardized tests of each cognitive domain being assessed to minimize the risk of diagnostic misclassification errors. Neuropsychological tests are generally considered to be useful probes of various cognitive constructs (e.g. memory); however, most are multifactorial and thus do not correspond precisely with a putative ability area (Woods & Grant, 2005). Accordingly, tests selected to assess a particular construct should provide maximal, overlapping coverage of the theorized components of that domain. In addition, most epidemiological studies of neuropsychology in mental disorders will need to cover a sufficient range of cognitive domains to allow for consistency with the diagnostic nomenclature on cognitive disorders (e.g. DSM–IV; American Psychiatric Association, 1994). For example, determining that an individual is broadly neurocognitively "impaired" will often require below normative expectations in two or more distinct cognitive domains (see Woods et al., 2004). Preference should be given to neuropsychological tests with documented administration and scoring procedures and published reliability, validity and demographically adjusted normative data. Of note, although behavioral observations and self-reported cognitive complaints are valuable interpretive tools, such measures are subject to considerable bias and are therefore not adequate substitutes for objective, performance-based neuropsychological testing in this regard (Rourke et al., 1999).

In designing a neuropsychological battery for use in mentally disordered populations, test selection will also depend on the aims of the research project and other logistical considerations. If an investigator's primary aim is to explore the cognitive sequelae of a particular mental disorder about which little is known (e.g. MA dependence), then a comprehensive neuropsychological battery assessing a broad range of domains is recommended in order to determine the nature, extent and prevalence of cognitive deficits. However, if one aims to examine the CNS impact of a newly identified comorbid condition on a disorder for which there is a large knowledge base (e.g. schizophrenia), then a much briefer battery focused on a few highly relevant measures may be indicated. Such focused neuropsychological batteries are potentially more cost-effective and may help minimize Type I error risk due to multiple statistical comparisons.

Several brief cognitive screening techniques are available in the event that a comprehensive battery is not feasible. Although they vary in length and complexity, most cognitive screenings can easily be completed in less than 1 hour, even at bedside if needed. Common approaches to screening include brief mental status tests (e.g. Mini-Mental State Examination (MMSE); Folstein et al., 1975), abbreviated screening batteries (e.g. Repeatable Battery for the Assessment of Neuropsychological Status (RBANS); Randolph, 1998), and individually selected standardized neuropsychological tests (e.g. Carey et al., 2004b). Although limited by their brevity and generally poor sensitivity, screening instruments are nevertheless highly specific and can provide valuable information for staging gross cognitive impairment or triaging participants in need of more comprehensive neuropsychological examinations.

Neuropsychological assessment in MA dependence

Given that the cognitive effects of chronic MA use are a recent area of research focus, most studies on this topic have employed relatively comprehensive neuropsychological batteries comprising well-validated tests. For example, Table 13.1 lists the battery of measures we administer in our National Institute on Drug Abuse (NIDA) sponsored Program Project on the combined CNS effects of MA, HIV, and hepatitis C (HCV). It is currently estimated that approximately 40% of persons with MA dependence demonstrate global neuropsychological impairment (i.e. deficits in at least two cognitive domains; Rippeth et al., 2004). More specifically, a recent meta-analysis on the cognitive effects of MA demonstrated moderate deficits in the domains of episodic memory, executive functions (e.g. decision-making and novel problem-solving; e.g. Simon et al., 2000), information processing speed, motor skills, language (e.g. verbal fluency), and visuoconstructional skills (Scott et al., 2007), which is generally commensurate with hypothesized MA-associated frontostriatal circuit neurotoxicity. The highest rates of impairment are evident in

Table 13.1. Neuropsychological battery for the UCSD Program project on the CNS effects of MA, HIV and hepatitis C.

Domain	Test
Psychiatric evaluation	Beck Depression Inventory-II (BDI-II)
	Semi-structured substance use history
	Composite International Diagnostic Interview (CIDI)
Test-taking effort	Hiscock Digit Memory Test (HDMT)
Premorbid IQ	WRAT-3 Reading (also Language)
Language	Action (verb) Fluency
	Animal fluency
	Letter fluency (FAS)
Executive functions	D-KEFS Color-Word Test
	Executive Control Battery
	Frontal Systems Behavior Scale (FrSBe)
	Iowa Gambling Task
	Trail Making Test, Part B
	Wisconsin Card Sorting Test (WCST-64)
Information processing speed	Trail Making Test, Part A
	WAIS-III Digit Symbol
	WAIS-III Symbol Search
Working memory	Paced Auditory Serial Addition Test (PASAT)
	WMS-III Spatial Span
Learning and memory	Brief Visuospatial Memory Test – Revised (BVMT-R)
	Hopkins Verbal Learning Test – Revised (HVLT-R)
Visuospatial	Judgment of Line Orientation (JLO)
	Hooper Visual Organization Test (HVOT)
Motor	Contraction Time
	Forced Steadiness
	Grooved Pegboard
	Velocity Scaling
Daily Functioning	Activities of Daily Living Questionnaire
	Employment Questionnaire
	Patient's Assessment of Own Functioning

Note: D-KEFS, Delis-Kaplan Executive Function Scale; UCSD, University of California, San Diego; WRAT-3, Wide Range Achievement Test, revision 3; WAIS-III, Wechsler Adult Intelligence Scale, 3rd edn.; SVT, symptom validity test.

episodic memory (Rippeth *et al.*, 2004), which may be particularly susceptible to the effects of MA relapse (Simon *et al.*, 2004). Future studies will need to expand on existing work by including a broader array of cognitive domains (e.g. spatial cognition, language). Moreover, given the observed clinical features of MA dependence, further investigation into such constructs as impulsivity and decision-making may inform conceptual models of the nosology of MA dependence.

Cognitive neuropsychology

Cognitive neuropsychology is an interdisciplinary science that utilizes conceptual models and a hypothesis-driven approach to delineate the mechanisms of cognitive impairment in clinical populations. A notable strength of the cognitive neuropsychology approach is its incorporation of theory-driven experimental tasks that dissect broader cognitive constructs into component processes. Additionally, novel assessment techniques and alternative data interpretation approaches that are rooted in cognitive neuroscience and the ever-growing understanding of neural networks (e.g. fronto-striatal loops) have proven useful in developing and validating theoretical models of mental disorders. The cognitive neuropsychology approach also helps to bridge the gap between experimental and clinical pursuits by seeking to enhance the differential diagnosis of cognitive disorders and inform remediation planning (Poreh, 2000).

The potential limitations of cognitive neuropsychology in the study of mental disorders also deserve mention. Given the multifaceted nature of most cognitive constructs, numerous component process indices (e.g. ratios, error types) are often examined that, without a well-defined hypothesis-driven analytic plan, may increase the risk for Type I error due to multiple comparisons. Also of note, component process measures often produce highly skewed distributions that may restrict test-retest reliability, especially in healthy controls (Poreh, 2000). This approach is also limited by the lack of published, demographically adjusted normative standards, which ultimately restricts its clinical utility. Clear operationalization of newly developed component process measures and ongoing critical evaluation of their psychometric properties (e.g. reliability and demographic effects) are therefore recommended (Poreh, 2000). Finally, continued evaluation of the construct validity of the cognitive neuropsychology approach in mental disorders research will be an important area for further study, such as investigation of its predictive, ecological and incremental validity relative to standard clinical tasks.

Cognitive neuropsychology of MA dependence

With few exceptions, the cognitive neuropsychology approach has been sparingly applied to the study of MA dependence, and thus little is known about the underlying cognitive mechanisms driving MA-associated neuropsychological impairments. For instance, verbal fluency deficits are common in MA dependence (Kalechstein et al., 2003), but it is not yet known whether such deficits reflect degraded semantic memory stores, executive dyscontrol of search and retrieval strategies, and/or slowed information processing. Moreover, given the hypothesized fronto-striatal neuropathogenesis of MA-related cognitive impairment, several cognitive constructs appear well suited for application in research on MA dependence, including decision-making, problem-solving, impulsivity and response inhibition, prospective memory (i.e. memory for future intentions), non-declarative memory (e.g. motor learning), and executive control of motor functions. Consistent with this notion, preliminary evidence has demonstrated significantly poorer decision-making skills (Gonzalez et al., 2007), impairments in prospective memory (Iudicello et al., in press, a) and a greater incidence of delay discounting (Monterosso et al., 2007) in MA-using individuals. Further investigation into these constructs will ostensibly advance the science and practice of the neuropsychology of MA dependence.

By way of illustration, data from standard clinical tasks indicate that MA dependence is associated with deficits in verbal learning and memory (Simon et al., 2004); however, the cognitive mechanisms driving such deficits are not well established. Accordingly, we evaluated Moscovitch's (1992) component process model of episodic verbal memory in 87 persons with MA dependence and 71 demographically comparable comparison subjects on the Hopkins Verbal Learning Test-Revised (Woods et al., 2005). Methamphetamine users were impaired in overall learning, free recall, utilization of semantic clustering strategies, repetitions, and non-semantically related intrusion errors, but not in memory consolidation (i.e. normal retention and recognition discrimination). In the context of the Moscovitch model, findings support the hypothesis that MA dependence is associated with deficient strategic (i.e. executive) control of verbal encoding and retrieval, which is consistent with the neurotoxic effects of MA on prefronto-striatal circuits. Thus, persons with MA dependence may benefit from the use of concrete behavioral strategies (e.g. reinforcement contingencies), highly structured treatment materials, and explicit reminders to enhance therapeutic interventions and maximize treatment outcomes.

Daily functioning

In recent years, recognition of the independent (and combined) effect of cognitive deficits on everyday, "real world" functioning has been a significant development in neuropsychological research in mental disorders. For example, the cognitive deficits associated with schizophrenia have been linked to impairment in treatment adherence, employment, financial management and driving (Green, 1996). There is currently no consensus regarding the optimal assessment techniques for measuring the ecological relevance of cognitive deficits. Self- and other-report measures of daily functioning, while quick and easy to administer, are subject to response bias and influence from comorbid conditions such as depression. Traditional neuropsychological instruments, which are commonly utilized in functional assessments, demonstrate variable and often limited ecological validity as measures of daily functioning (Chaytor & Schmitter-Edgecombe, 2003). With this in mind, investigators have recently developed more direct (i.e. face valid) objective methods of examining the impact of neuropsychological impairment on real-world functioning (Heaton et al., 2004). For example, laboratory measures of work performance may help rule out other factors that lead to unemployment, such as physical decline or depression. However, these direct measures also have their shortcomings. Most are relatively new and therefore have limited empirical evidence of their reliability and construct validity. These assessments can also be expensive and time-consuming, especially when given concurrently with a battery of standard neurocognitive tests. In addition, there is no clear agreement as to whether verisimilitude (i.e. how much the demands of the functional test mirror the demands of the everyday environment) or veridicality (i.e. how much the functional test is empirically related to existing cognitive tests) is more important in test construction (Chaytor & Schmitter-Edgecombe, 2003). Nonetheless, complementing traditional cognitive tests with direct tests of functional status may help in assessing severity of impairment, as well as progress in treatment and recovery in individuals with mental disorders.

When evaluating the functional impact of cognitive impairment in mental disorders, one should be aware of a number of psychiatric factors that could also adversely influence daily functioning. Psychosis can be a common occurrence in mental disorders, especially with sustained substance use, and thus orientation and reality testing should be considered as possible confounds. Although some controversy still exists regarding whether mood disorders, such as major depression and anxiety, interact with neurocognitive impairment, these factors have been shown to have a significant influence on everyday functioning in the context of mental illness (Jin et al., 2001). Patient complaints of cognitive impairments, however, are more consistently associated with depression and other affective symptoms than significant decrement in cognitive function, especially in substance-abusing populations (Errico et al., 1990). Therefore, caution is warranted in interpreting self-report of everyday functioning, and it is important to gather data from significant others, caregivers and objective testing when cognitive and functional complaints are reported.

Neuropsychology and daily functioning in MA dependence

Focused research on the impact of MA on daily functioning has been sparse, despite evidence of MA-associated cognitive impairment in ability areas (e.g. executive functions and episodic memory) with direct relevance to the successful performance of instrumental activities of daily living (IADL). The only study specifically examining MA and everyday functioning to date showed that individuals with a history of MA use displayed higher rates of cognitive complaints and impairments in IADL (e.g. preparing meals, managing money). However, IADL impairments were associated with depressive symptoms, while cognitive complaints were related to both depressive symptoms and objective neuropsychological impairment (Sadek et al., 2004). Importantly, research in populations with similar levels of cognitive impairment (e.g. HIV infection) has shown that even mild levels of neuropsychological impairment can have significant effects on everyday functioning, in such domains as employment, medication adherence and driving safety (e.g. Heaton et al., 2004). Furthermore, abusers of MA display impaired decision-making abilities (e.g. Rogers et al., 1999), which could potentially affect treatment and relapse prevention efforts, as well as money management, risky behavior and driving performance (Logan, 1996). Additional research is needed to better understand the individual and combined effects of depression and cognitive impairment on self-reported and objectively assessed functional declines in MA users, as well as the particular functional areas most susceptible to decline in this cohort.

Interpretation of neuropsychological data

A host of different environmental, psychosocial, psychiatric and psychometric factors can impact neuropsychological test performance in mental disorders. This section reviews the effects of demographic, test-taking effort, disease-related and methodological factors on the interpretation of neuropsychological research in mental disorders.

Demographic variables

It is widely accepted that demographic factors such as age, education, sex and ethnicity can exert considerable influence on certain neuropsychological tests (Heaton, 2004). For instance, older age and lower educational attainment are reliably associated with poorer performance on measures of information processing speed and executive functions. In addition, research suggests that Caucasians may perform better than certain racial/ethnic minority groups (e.g. African-Americans) on standardized tests of intelligence, verbal memory, executive functions, and information processing speed. While the magnitude of the racial/ethnic effect on cognition is generally small and may be explained by a variety of factors, including socioeconomic status, educational quality, cultural differences, test characteristics and/or reading level (Manly *et al.*, 2002), it is nonetheless an important consideration when interpreting test results. Indeed, researchers should consider the possibility that demographic factors may be interacting with disease characteristics to reveal (or mask) cognitive impairment.

Accordingly, study groups (and subgroups) should be matched on age, sex, education and ethnicity in order to minimize the potential confounding influence of demographics on study results. In addition, tests selected for the neuropsychological battery should have published, demographically adjusted normative standards available, particularly if the test results will be applied toward clinical diagnoses (Woods & Grant, 2005). A word of caution, however, is that although early research on race/ethnicity-adjusted normative standards represents a significant advance for the field, the construct validity of such

methods has yet to be fully demonstrated, particularly concerning increased risk of Type II error (i.e. false negative classifications). For instance, some authors question the incremental validity of demographically adjusted normative standards in classifying CNS disease (Reitan & Wolfson, 2005). In addition, ethnicity-based normative corrections may be a surrogate for other important factors underlying ethnic differences on cognitive tests (e.g. socioeconomic status). Finally, test selection must consider possible floor and ceiling effects related to demographics; that is, relatively "easy" tests (e.g. MMSE) may be insensitive to CNS disease in highly educated samples due to ceiling effects, whereas "difficult" tests (e.g. Paced Auditory Serial Addition Test; Gronwall, 1977) may be insensitive in samples with limited educational backgrounds due to floor effects.

Suboptimal effort

Accurate interpretation of neuropsychological data requires that the examinee has provided adequate effort in completing the examination. Individuals with mental disorders may be at high risk for suboptimal test-taking effort due to poor rapport and motivation, possible secondary gain (e.g. malingering for the purpose of disability), fatigue and/or disease-related symptoms (e.g. disorientation). Thus it is essential to ensure that observed cognitive deficits are not simply attributable to poor effort. For example, investigators may wish to exclude participants who are actively engaged in litigation, disability, or compensation claims related to their mental disorder. In addition, symptom validity testing (SVT) is increasingly common in neuropsychological research protocols involving populations at risk for suboptimal effort. As a complement to thorough behavioral observations and data screening procedures (e.g. outlier analyses), SVTs provide a relatively quick, objective, and useful means of detecting potentially invalid neuropsychological test performances due to suboptimal effort rather than genuine cognitive impairment (Bianchini *et al.*, 2001). A variety of different forced-choice SVT procedures are available and easily integrated into existing research batteries, including the Hiscock Digit Memory Test (HDMT; Hiscock & Hiscock, 1989) and the Test of Memory Malingering (Tombaugh, 1997). Researchers may also use "embedded" effort measures, which are akin to SVTs, but demand less participant time as they are readily derived from commonly used cognitive tasks (e.g. reliable digits; Greiffenstein *et al.*, 1994).

Suboptimal effort in MA dependence

Suboptimal effort may be of particular concern in research involving individuals with active MA dependence (and other substance-related disorders). For example, involvement in research investigations may be partly motivated by financial compensation (i.e. to possibly fund drug-seeking behaviors) that may diminish test-taking effort, and thus confound the validity of the cognitive data. In addition, it is possible that the acute and/or withdrawal effects of MA use (e.g. MA-induced depression) may affect test-taking effort. To address this concern, we examined the base rate of suboptimal effort in 59 MA-dependent participants in our above-described NIDA Program Project. All participants were given the HDMT, an 18-item visual forced-choice SVT whose construct validity is well supported in the neuropsychological literature (Vickery *et al.*, 2001). Results indicated that no participant fell below the established 90% performance cutoff for suboptimal effort on the HDMT; in fact, only three participants (5%) did not obtain a perfect score. This suggests that cognitive deficits evident in this MA-dependent cohort are unlikely to be a consequence of suboptimal effort.

Disease characteristics

An accurate characterization of key disease features is also important in interpreting neuropsychological research findings in mental disorders. Primary and secondary diagnoses of the mental disorders of interest, as well as any relevant diagnostic subtypes, are needed and should be based on reliable and validated diagnostic methods. Measures of symptom presence, severity and history, as well as relevant treatment characteristics (e.g. current psychotropic medications) also warrant consideration. The potential independent, additive, and/or synergistic impact of comorbid conditions on cognitive functioning also deserve statistical and methodological consideration. The use of a priori determined, detailed exclusionary and inclusionary criteria related to common comorbidities is strongly encouraged. The specific criteria used will, of course, depend on the particular mental disorders and research questions being evaluated. As a general rule, researchers should be careful to ensure the internal validity of their study (i.e. ability

to determine the effect of the independent variable on the dependent variables of interest), without sacrificing external validity (e.g. generalizability). A compromise might be to exclude confounding conditions that are not commonly associated with the mental disorder of interest and include common disease comorbidities, given that they are carefully measured and considered as potential confounds in statistical modeling and interpretation.

Methamphetamine dependence characteristics

With regard to research on the cognitive effects of MA use, investigators are well advised to provide structured diagnoses of current and prior MA abuse and dependence, as well as MA-induced disorders (e.g. MA-induced psychosis or depression). Semi-structured interviews detailing participants' lifetime histories of MA (and other substance) use should also be obtained, including onset, quantity and frequency data. Although a recent meta-analysis on MA-associated cognitive impairment found no association between length of abstinence (or other MA-use parameters) and neuropsychological impairment in chronic MA-users (Scott *et al.*, 2008), researchers should give careful consideration to the potential differential effects that may result if a participant is intoxicated, acutely withdrawn, intermediately withdrawn or abstinent. Given the lack of reliability that is inherent to self-report substance use data, urine toxicology screens for MA and other substances are useful in corroborating current abstinence. A variety of CNS-related comorbidities (e.g. alcohol dependence) are common among persons with MA dependence and may affect neuropsychological test performance. To control for such comorbidities without sacrificing generalizability, individuals with histories of HCV, HIV, depression, ADHD or remote non-MA substance-related disorders may be included in a research protocol provided that these factors are carefully documented, stratified across study cells and considered in the data analysis and interpretation. On the other hand, conditions that are less common in MA dependence or cause gross CNS impairment should be excluded, for example schizophrenia-spectrum disorders, mental retardation, seizure disorders and traumatic brain injuries.

Statistical methodologies

Statistical methods can also influence the conclusions drawn from a neuropsychological study. The mean group difference approach using null hypothesis significance testing (NHST) is commonly employed in neuropsychological research in mental disorders. However, this approach potentially increases the likelihood that abnormal performances (i.e. significantly above average) in a minority of participants will obfuscate any evidence of neuropsychological impairment at the group level. In fact, this approach may be insensitive in detecting subtle neuropsychological deficits, particularly if the base rates of impairment are low (Heaton et al., 1994). Moreover, the mean group difference approach carries with it the potential to increase the risk of Type I errors (i.e. false positives) due to multiple statistical comparisons (Ingraham & Aiken, 1996). Data reduction techniques to produce domain and global summary scores and dichotomous classifications of impairment based on statistical (Millis, 2003), actuarial (e.g. Global Deficit Scores; Carey et al., 2004a) or algorithmic clinical ratings (Heaton et al., 1994; Woods et al., 2004) may be helpful in this regard; however, such techniques have been criticized for their lack of specificity and propensity to increase Type II error risk (Zhao & Kolonel, 1992). A priori statistical power analyses are thus critical for investigators, particularly given the prevalence of NHST in mental disorders research. Power will depend on the proposed study sample size, critical alpha level (0.05 by convention), observed (or anticipated) effect size, and the specific statistical procedure being used; by convention, power values above 0.80 (range = 0, 1) are considered acceptable (Cohen, 1992). Investigators are also encouraged to consider the applicability of effect sizes (e.g. Cohen's d) and classification accuracy statistics as a complement to NHST in order to evaluate the magnitude and potential clinical relevance of neuropsychological research findings, as these statistics, most notably predictive values and risk ratios, are often underused in neuropsychological research (Woods et al., 2003).

Treatment outcomes

Neuropsychological assessment is not only integral to the identification and characterization of mental disorders, it also has important implications for planning, optimizing and assessing the effectiveness of treatment efforts. As described above, cognitive abilities are a clinically relevant predictor of an individual's functioning capacity, and therefore improvement in cognition may have important real-life

implications in the successful treatment of mental disorders. There are distinct advantages to using neuropsychological assessments for this purpose. First, neuropsychology inherently relies upon an objective, evaluative approach rooted in psychometric theory, and is thus well suited to the rigors of longitudinal study designs (Mendez et al., 1995). Second, neuropsychological data provide important information regarding the profile of relative (and absolute) cognitive strengths and weaknesses that may influence the prescription, maintenance and efficacy of treatment protocols. Third, neuropsychology can play a critical role in the evaluation of treatment outcomes and their cost-effectiveness in mental disorders (Prigatano et al., 2003).

Neuropsychological evaluations may be particularly useful in predicting which individuals with mental disorders will seek treatment, as well as those likely to succeed in treatment. For instance, Katz et al. (2005) examined the association between cognitive ability and factors related to treatment such as motivation for change and expectations for the future in 416 substance-abuse patients. Results indicated that higher cognitive abilities were associated with greater motivation for treatment as indexed by expressed desire for help and treatment readiness. In addition, subjects with higher cognitive abilities reported less hopelessness for the future, which may be associated with more positive treatment outcomes (Brown et al., 2004). Research has also shown that cognitively impaired individuals are more likely to violate substance-abuse treatment program rules, experience difficulty acquiring cognitive skills, drop out of treatment prematurely, be non-adherent to complex medication regimens and achieve overall poorer treatment outcomes (Fals-Stewart, 1993).

If cognitive deficits are a central feature of mental disorders, then measures of neuropsychological functioning will serve as important disease markers of treatment effectiveness and efficacy. Baseline and post-intervention neuropsychological evaluations can help identify the cognitive safety and benefits associated with treatment. Neuropsychological assessment also allows for the development of a focused treatment plan by informed providers who can develop interventions based on an individual's cognitive abilities and functional status, thus potentially minimizing the costs of treatment (Prigatano et al., 2003). Despite limited empirical evidence to this effect, neuropsychological assessment may minimize long-term treatment costs through proper diagnosis and knowledge of cognitive strengths and weaknesses (Welsh-Bohmer et al., 2003). By targeting known comorbid conditions or known cognitive deficits, as well as the functional impairments that they subsequently ensue, treatment may be tailored to minimize the chances of inappropriate or unsuccessful treatments and the additional costs they entail. For example, an individual with impairments in executive functioning may not benefit from treatment strategies that require planning, organizing and goal formation (Diller, 1987). Importantly, this informed adaptation of treatment may also alleviate the functional impact of such impairments on everyday skills (e.g. financial management) and facilitate independent living.

From a methodological perspective, assessing change in neuropsychological performance related to treatment is a complex undertaking. Several factors unrelated to brain functioning might explain variations in neuropsychological test performance over time, including practice effects, test-retest reliability, floor and ceiling effects, and/or individual variability (e.g. effort) (Temkin et al., 1999). As mentioned above, the use of well-standardized tests with available normative data and documented reliability and practice effects is therefore recommended. Normative standards for repeated test administration are available for many standardized neuropsychological tests (Basso et al., 2002) and represent a significant advance in interpreting cognitive changes. Moreover, alternate test forms and/or a dual (i.e. repeated) baseline approach should be used whenever possible, particularly if memory functions are being assessed (Duff et al., 2001). A variety of statistical methods are also available to assess the significance of changes in cognition, including reliable change indices and regression procedures (Temkin et al., 1999).

Neuropsychology and the treatment of MA dependence

Current treatments for MA are similar to strategies employed for stimulant dependency and include behavioral, cognitive and psychological techniques directed at increasing motivation for abstinence, developing strategies for avoiding use and preventing relapse (Schuckit, 1994). In addition, targeted pharmacological interventions are being developed to improve MA-associated cognitive impairments (Meredith et al., 2005). It nevertheless remains to be determined whether the impairments in episodic memory, processing speed and executive functions evident in MA users (Simon et al., 2000, 2002) are remediable and/or adversely impact treatment success. Future research should also investigate the extent to which neuropsychological assessments augment the strategies of treatment, predict the desire for initiation and maintenance of treatment, and effectively assess treatment outcomes in MA users. This is important and relevant because emergent data indicate that dopamine terminals in the basal ganglia may recover with abstinence from MA (Volkow et al., 2001). Consistent with this notion, recent evidence has also demonstrated partial recovery of cognitive functioning in neuropsychologically impaired MA-dependent individuals following an average year-long period of abstinence from MA, particularly in the speed of information processing and motor skills domains (Iudicello et al., in press, b). Future research examining the potential additional recovery of cognitive functioning following longer periods of abstinence (i.e. greater than a year) and the possible benefits of MA-abstinence on other factors such as instrumental activities of daily living may have important implications concerning treatment of MA-use disorders and may enhance the cost-effectiveness of treatment efforts.

Conclusion

With appropriate consideration of demographic, situational, conceptual and methodological issues, neuropsychological techniques can greatly enhance research on the epidemiology, mechanisms, functional impact and treatment of mental disorders. Multidisciplinary collaborations between neuropsychological science and neuroimaging, neurophysiology, neurobiology and neurogenetics will provide a powerful means of expanding the scientific and clinical relevance of the nosology, nature, mechanisms and social impact of psychiatric diseases.

Acknowledgments

This chapter was supported in part by grants P30 MH62512 and P01 DA12065 from the National Institutes of Health.

References

American Psychiatric Association. (1994). *Diagnostic and Statistical Manual of Mental Disorders* (4th edn.)

(DSM IV). Washington, DC: American Psychiatric Association.

Basso, M. R., Carona, F. D., Lowery, N. & Axelrod, B. N. (2002). Practice effects on the WAIS-III across 3- and 6-month intervals. *Clinical Neuropsychology*, **16**, 57–63.

Bianchini, K. J., Mathias, C. W. & Greve, K. W. (2001). Symptom validity testing: a critical review. *Clinical Neuropsychology*, **15**, 19–45.

Brown, B. S., O'Grady, K., Robert, J. & Farrell, E. V. (2004). Factors associated with treatment outcomes in an aftercare population. *American Journal of Addiction*, **13**, 447–460.

Carey, C. L., Woods, S. P., Gonzalez, R. *et al.* (2004a). Predictive validity of global deficit scores in detecting neuropsychological impairment in HIV infection. *Journal of Clinical and Experimental Neuropsychology*, **26**, 307–319.

Carey, C. L., Woods, S. P., Rippeth, J. *et al.* (2004b). Initial validation of a screening battery for the detection of HIV-associated cognitive impairment. *Clinical Neuropsychology*, **18**, 234–248.

Chang, L., Ernst, T., Speck, O. *et al.* (2002). Perfusion MRI and computerized cognitive test abnormalities in abstinent methamphetamine users. *Psychiatry Research*, **114**, 65–79.

Chaytor, N. & Schmitter-Edgecombe, M. (2003). The ecological validity of neuropsychological tests: a review of the literature on everyday cognitive skills. *Neuropsychology Review*, **13**, 181–197.

Cohen, J. (1992). A power primer. *Psychological Bulletin*, **112**, 155–159.

Davidson, C., Gow, A. J., Lee, T. H. & Ellinwood, E. H. (2001). Methamphetamine neurotoxicity: necrotic and apoptotic mechanisms and relevance to human abuse and treatment. *Brain Research Brain Research Review*, **36**, 1–22.

Diller, L. (1987). Neuropsychological rehabilitation. In M. J. Meier, A. L. Benton & L. Diller (Eds.), *Neuropsychological Rehabilitation* (p. 475). New York, NY: Guilford Press.

Duff, K., Westervelt, H. J., McCaffrey, R. J. & Haase, R. F. (2001). Practice effects, test-retest stability, and dual baseline assessments with the California Verbal Learning Test in an HIV sample. *Archives of Clinical Neuropsychology*, **16**, 461–476.

Errico, A. L., Nixon, S. J., Parsons, O. A. & Tassey, J. (1990). Screening for neuropsychological impairments in alcoholics. *Psychological Assessment*, **2**, 45–50.

Fals-Stewart, W. (1993). Neurocognitive defects and their impact on substance abuse treatment. *Journal of Addictions and Offender Counseling*, **13**, 46–57.

Folstein, M. F., Folstein, S. E. & McHugh, P. R. (1975). "Mini-mental state". A practical method for grading the cognitive state of patients for the clinician. *Journal of Psychiatric Research*, **12**, 189–198.

Gonzalez, R., Bechara, A. & Martin, E. M. (2007). Executive functions among individuals with methamphetamine or alcohol as drugs of choice: preliminary observations. *Journal of Clinical and Experimental Neuropsychology*, **29**, 155–159.

Green, M. F. (1996). What are the functional consequences of neurocognitive deficits in schizophrenia? *American Journal of Psychiatry*, **153**, 321–330.

Greiffenstein, M., Baker, W., Gola, T. *et al.* (1994). Validity of malingered amnesia measures in a large clinical sample. *Psychological Assessment*, **6**, 218–224.

Gronwall, D. M. A. (1977). Paced Auditory Serial Addition Task: a measure of recovery from concussion. *Perceptual and Motor Skills*, **44**, 367–373.

Harris, D. S., Boxenbaum, H., Everhart, E. T. *et al.* (2003). The bioavailability of intranasal and smoked methamphetamine. *Clinical Pharmacology and Therapeutics*, **74**, 475–486.

Heaton, R. K. (2004). *Revised Comprehensive Norms for an Expanded Halstead-Reitan Battery: Demographically Adjusted Neuropsychological Norms for African American and Caucasian Adults*. Lutz, FL: Psychological Assessment Resources, Inc.

Heaton, R. K., Kirson, D., Velin, R. A. & Grant, I. (1994). The utility of clinical ratings for detecting cognitive change in HIV infection. In I. Grant & A. Martin (Eds.), *Neuropsychology of HIV Infection* (pp. 188–206). New York, NY: Oxford University Press.

Heaton, R. K., Marcotte, T. D., Mindt, M. R. *et al.* (2004). The impact of HIV-associated neuropsychological impairment on everyday functioning. *Journal of the International Neuropsychological Society*, **10**, 317–331.

Hiscock, M. & Hiscock, C. K. (1989). Refining the forced-choice method for the detection of malingering. *Journal of Clinical and Experimental Neuropsychology*, **11**, 967–974.

Ingraham, L. J. & Aiken, C. B. (1996). An empirical approach to determining criteria for abnormality in test batteries with multiple measures. *Neuropsychology*, **10**, 120–124.

Iudicello, J. E., Weber, E., Dawson, M. S. *et al.* (in press, a). Prospective memory deficits in methamphetamine dependence. [abstract]. *Clinical Neuropsychologist*.

Iudicello, J. E., Woods, S. P., Vigil, O. *et al.* (in press, b). Effects of methamphetamine abstinence on neuropsychological functioning. [abstract]. *Clinical Neuropsychologist*.

Jin, H., Zisook, S., Palmer, B. W. *et al.* (2001). Association of depressive symptoms with worse functioning in schizophrenia: a study in older outpatients. *Journal of Clinical Psychiatry*, **62**, 797–803.

203

Kalechstein, A. D., Newton, T. F. & Green, M. (2003). Methamphetamine dependence is associated with neurocognitive impairment in the initial phases of abstinence. *Journal of Neuropsychiatry and Clinical Neuroscience*, **15**, 215–220.

Katz, E. C., King, S. D., Schwartz, R. P. *et al.* (2005). Cognitive ability as a factor in engagement in drug abuse treatment. *American Journal of Drug and Alcohol Abuse*, **31**, 359–369.

Logan, B. K. (1996). Methamphetamine and driving impairment. *Journal of Forensic Science*, **41**, 457–464.

Manly, J. J., Jacobs, D. M., Touradji, P., Small, S. A. & Stern, Y. (2002). Reading level attenuates differences in neuropsychological test performance between African American and White elders. *Journal of the International Neuropsychological Society*, **8**, 341–348.

Mendez, M. F., van Gorp, W. & Cummings, J. L. (1995). Neuropsychiatry, neuropsychology, and behavioral neurology – a critical comparison. *Neuropsychiatry Neuropsychology and Behavioral Neurology*, **8**, 297–302.

Meredith, C. W., Jaffe, C., Ang-Lee, K. & Saxon, A. J. (2005). Implications of chronic methamphetamine use: a literature review. *Harvard Review of Psychiatry*, **13**, 141–154.

Millis, S. R. (2003). Statistical practices: the seven deadly sins. *Neuropsychol Dev Cogn C Child Neuropsychol*, **9**, 221–233.

Monterosso, J. R., Ainslie, G., Xu, J. *et al.* (2007). Frontoparietal cortical activity of methamphetamine-dependent and comparison subjects performing a delay discounting task. *Human Brain Mapping*, **28**, 383–393.

Moscovitch, M. (1992). Memory and working-with-memory: a component process model based on modules and central systems. *Journal of Cognition and Neuroscience*, **4**, 257–267.

Nordahl, T. E., Salo, R. & Leamon, M. (2003). Neuropsychological effects of chronic methamphetamine use on neurotransmitters and cognition: a review. *Journal of Neuropsychiatry and Clinical Neuroscience*, **15**, 317–325.

Poreh, A. M. (2000). The quantified process approach: an emerging methodology to neuropsychological assessment. *Clinical Neuropsychology*, **14**, 212–222.

Prigatano, G. P., Zigler, L. D. & Rosenstein, L. (2003). The clinical neuropsychological examination: scope, cost, and health-care value. Part 1. In G. P. Prigatano & N. P. Pliskin (Eds.), *Clinical Neuropsychology and Cost Outcome Research* (pp. 15–38). New York, NY: Psychology Press.

Randolph, C. (1998). *RBANS manual: Repeatable Battery for the Assessment of Neuropsychological Status*. San Antonio, TX: The Psychological Coorporation.

Reitan, R. M. & Wolfson, D. (2005). The effect of age and education transformations on neuropsychological test scores of persons with diffuse or bilateral brain damage. *Applied Neuropsychology*, **12**, 181–189.

Rippeth, J. D., Heaton, R. K., Carey, C. K. *et al.* (2004). Methamphetamine dependence increases risk of neuropsychological impairment in HIV infected persons. *Journal of the International Neuropsychology Society*, **10**, 1–14.

Rogers, R. D., Everitt, B. J., Baldacchino, A. *et al.* (1999). Dissociable deficits in the decision-making cognition of chronic amphetamine abusers, opiate abusers, patients with focal damage to prefrontal cortex, and tryptophan-depleted normal volunteers: evidence for monoaminergic mechanisms. *Neuropsychopharmacology*, **20**, 322–339.

Rourke, S. B., Halman, M. H. & Bassel, C. (1999). Neurocognitive complaints in HIV-infection and their relationship to depressive symptoms and neuropsychological functioning. *Journal of Clinical and Experimental Neuropsychology*, **21**, 737–756.

Sadek, J. R., Vigil, O., Woods, S. P. *et al.* (2004). Impact of depression on self-reported impairment in HIV and methamphetamine use. *Journal of the International Neuropsychological Society*, **10**, 197.

Schuckit, M. A. (1994). The treatment of stimulant dependence. *Addiction*, **89**, 1559–1563.

Scott, J. C., Woods, S. P., Matt, G. E. *et al.* (2007). Neurocognitive effects of methamphetamine: a critical review and meta-analysis. *Neuropsychology Review*, **17**, 275–297.

Simon, S. L., Dacey, J., Glynn, S., Rawson, R. & Ling, W. (2004). The effect of relapse on cognition in abstinent methamphetamine abusers. *Journal of Substance Abuse Treatment*, **27**, 59–66.

Simon, S. L., Domier, C., Carnell, J. *et al.* (2000). Cognitive impairment in individuals currently using methamphetamine. *American Journal of Addiction*, **9**, 222–231.

Simon, S. L., Domier, C. P., Sim, T. *et al.* (2002). Cognitive performance of current methamphetamine and cocaine abusers. *Journal of Addictive Diseases*, **21**, 61–74.

Temkin, N. R., Heaton, R. K., Grant, I. & Dikmen, S. S. (1999). Detecting significant change in neuropsychological test performance: a comparison of four models. *Journal of the International Neuropsychology Society*, **5**, 357–369.

Tombaugh, T. N. (1997). *TOMM: Test of Memory Malingering*. Toronto: Multi-Health Systems.

Tröster, A. I. & Woods, S. P. (2003). Neuropsychological aspects of Parkinson's disease and parkinsonian syndromes. In R. Pahwa, K. Lyons & W. C. Koller (Eds.), *Handbook of Parkinson's Disease* (3rd edn.), (pp. 127–157). New York, NY: Marcel Dekker.

U.S. Department of Health and Human Services. (2002). *Methamphetamine Abuse and Addiction*. NIH Publication No. 02–4210.

Vickery, C. D., Berry, D. T., Inman, T. H., Harris, M. J. & Orey, S. A. (2001). Detection of inadequate effort on neuropsychological testing: a meta-analytic review of selected procedures. *Archives of Clinical Neuropsychology*, **16**, 45–73.

Volkow, N. D., Chang, L., Wang, G. J. *et al.* (2001). Loss of dopamine transporters in methamphetamine abusers recovers with protracted abstinence. *Journal of Neuroscience*, **21**, 9414–9418.

Welsh-Bohmer, K. A., Attix, D. K. & Mason, D. J. (2003). The clinical utility of neuropsychological evaluation of patients with known or suspected dementia. In G. P. Prigatano & N. P. Pliskin (Eds.), *Clinical Neuropsychology and Cost Outcome Research* (pp. 177–200). New York, NY: Psychology Press.

Woods, S. P. & Grant, I. (2005). Neuropsychology of HIV. In H. E. Gendelman, I. Grant, I. Everall, S. A. Lipton & S. Swindells (Eds.), *The Neurology of AIDS* (2nd edn), (pp. 607–616). Oxford: Oxford University Press.

Woods, S. P., Rippeth, J. D., Conover, E. *et al.* (2005). Deficient strategic control of verbal encoding and retrieval in individuals with methamphetamine dependence. *Neuropsychology*, **19**, 35–43.

Woods, S. P., Rippeth, J. D., Frol, A. B. *et al.* (2004). Interrater reliability of clinical ratings and neurocognitive diagnoses in HIV. *Journal of Clinical and Experimental Neuropsychology*, **26**, 759–778.

Woods, S. P., Weinborn, M. & Lovejoy, D. W. (2003). Are classification accuracy statistics underused in neuropsychological research? *Journal of Clinical and Experimental Neuropsychology*, **25**, 431–439.

Yacoubian, G. S., Jr. & Peters, R. J. (2004). Exploring the prevalence and correlates of methamphetamine use: findings from Sacramento's ADAM program. *Journal of Drug Education*, **34**, 281–294.

Zhao, L. P. & Kolonel, L. N. (1992). Efficiency loss from categorizing quantitative exposures into qualitative exposures in case-control studies. *American Journal of Epidemiology*, **136**, 464–474.

The study of emotion and the interaction between emotion and cognition: methodological perspectives

Kimberley R. Savage, Nathan A. Gates, Aleksey Dumer, Stephanie Assuras, Michelle M. Halfacre and Joan C. Borod

Introduction

In the 1950s, when behaviorism held sway over psychology, emotion was deemed to be too "subjective" for empirical study. However, the study of emotion has seen something of a renaissance over the past 25 years. The door has opened to a more objective study of emotion, largely due to technological advances and innovative methodologies that have enabled researchers to study human emotions in the laboratory (LeDoux, 2000). These new methods have helped us gain a deeper understanding of emotional processes, including how emotion interacts with cognition. Research on the interaction between emotion and cognition is particularly relevant to neurological and psychiatric disorders, given that impairments are often seen in both domains. Not only can such research increase our understanding of the relationship between thoughts and feelings to help improve our understanding of the etiology of specific clinical disorders, it can also help generate novel and effective treatment strategies.

The goal of this chapter is to provide information about some of the approaches taken to study emotion and the interaction between emotion and cognition.[1] Included in the chapter will be discussions of behavioral methodologies, focusing on those used to evaluate emotion; the interaction between emotion and memory, learning and attention; and emotion regulation. In addition, both functional and spatiotemporal imaging techniques used to assess the emotion-cognition interaction will be described. Particular emphasis will be placed on those methodologies commonly used to conduct research in cognition and emotion with psychiatric populations.

This chapter is intended to be an introduction to the methodology used to assess the interaction between emotion and cognition in humans. Given that a considerable amount of research has been conducted in this area, only a limited number of methodologies have been selected for discussion as it is impossible to review all methodologies.

Measuring emotion

Many experimental paradigms have been used to examine emotional processing, including laterality techniques (e.g. dichotic listening, tachistoscopic viewing, free-field viewing and facial expression asymmetry), studies of individuals with brain damage, functional brain imaging and neuropsychological assessment (for reviews, see Borod *et al.*, 2001; Demaree *et al.*, 2005; Heilman *et al.*, 2000). Although each method offers certain advantages, neuropsychological assessment best enables researchers and clinicians to assess different components of emotion simultaneously. In this section, we will therefore focus on commonly used neuropsychological procedures, including a description of widely used test batteries, as well as information about eliciting and evaluating emotional expression.

Test batteries

In order to develop a framework for simplifying and organizing our discussion of the neuropsychological assessment of emotion, we have taken an approach that conceptualizes emotion as having multiple components that are each mediated by different neural substrates (Borod, 1993a; Borod *et al.*, 2000a). The components include both processing modes and communication channels. In general, primary processing modes include perception, expression and experience, and communication channels include the face, prosody and verbal content (Borod, 2000). Based on this theoretical perspective, we have chosen to highlight four batteries that assess multiple components of emotional processing. Although other batteries exist, a complete review is beyond the scope of this chapter (for a review, see Borod et al., 2000b).

The Victoria Emotion Perception Test (VERT) evaluates the perception of emotion via prosodic and facial channels (Mountain, 1993). Emotionally intoned strings of nonsense words and pictures of facial emotional expressions are paired, and the subject is asked to identify and discriminate the specific emotion category and intensity level. The categories of emotions used include anger, sadness, happiness and fear, and are presented at mild, moderate and extreme levels.

Like the VERT, the Florida Affective Battery (FAB; Bowers et al., 1991) uses a single processing mode to measure multiple communication channels. As described in Bowers et al. (1991), the FAB assesses emotional perception across facial and prosodic channels, and examines happiness, sadness, anger, fear and neutrality. The FAB includes 10 subtests (5 facial, 3 prosodic and 2 cross-modal) and is designed to investigate disturbances in the perception and understanding of non-verbal emotional signals.

The Aprosodia Battery (Ross, 1985; Ross et al., 1997) is designed to assess production (spontaneous production and repetition) and comprehension (identification and discrimination) of affective prosody through a range of listening/responding exercises. Six expression categories are examined: happy, sad, angry, surprised, disinterested/bored and neutral. The posed repetition tasks involve 12 stimuli (words, monosyllables [e.g. "ba"], and asyllables [e.g. "aaaahhhhhhh"]). For the comprehension tasks, participants are asked to identify 24 stimuli across three conditions (words, monosyllables and asyllables) and to discriminate across one condition (filtered words). For the identification tasks, participants are asked to determine which line drawing of a face goes with a verbal label. Finally, participants are asked to produce posed voice recordings, which are later rated for emotional content by trained judges.

Whereas batteries that examine affective processing via one mode or channel offer valuable information

regarding the recognition and discrimination of emotion, the New York Emotion Battery (NYEB; Borod et al., 1992) examines three processing modes (emotional expression, experience and perception [identification and discrimination]) across three channels of communication (facial, prosodic and lexical [or verbal content]); (Borod et al., 1998; Canino et al., 1999; Montreys & Borod, 1998). The NYEB divides emotion types into positive (happiness, interest and pleasant surprise) and negative (anger, disgust, fear, sadness and unpleasant surprise). Non-emotional stimuli and tasks are also included for control purposes for each emotion task. For both spontaneous and posed (to command and to imitation) emotional expression across the three channels, trained raters analyze participants' expressions for category accuracy and emotional intensity.

Emotional expression

Eliciting and evaluating the accuracy and quality of emotional expressions provides important information about emotional processing, which may not be revealed through standardized testing batteries. In this section, we describe and evaluate common procedures used to conduct such investigations.

Induction procedures

Perhaps the most popular method for eliciting emotional expressions in both normal and clinical populations is the controlled induction of mood states (for a review, see Martin, 1990). Typically, mood induction involves the auditory and/or visual presentation of emotionally evocative stimuli; Federspiel et al. (2005), for example, induced a negative mood in their study by showing participants film segments featuring sad scenes from the Krakow ghetto, followed by mood-congruent music. Another common mood-induction procedure involves the presentation of emotional slides or pictures, such as the International Affective Picture System (IAPS), which is a catalogue of pictures with well-developed normative ratings across three dimensions: valence (pleasantness/unpleasantness), arousal (calm/arousing) and dominance (or control; Lang et al., 2005). Other frequently used stimuli are slides created by Buck (1978), which consist of 32 photographs from five separate emotive categories, including scenic/neutral (e.g. a sunset over a lake), pleasant (e.g. a young child touching flowers), sexual (e.g. an embracing couple), unusual (e.g. multiple exposures of an airport) and unpleasant (e.g. a starving child).

Although mood-induction techniques are commonly used in research that examines interactions between emotion and cognition, some concerns and criticisms have been raised. First, many studies using mood induction have found that sizeable percentages of participants (ranging anywhere between 15 and 75%) fail to respond to the mood induction (Martin, 1990). Furthermore, when mood induction is successfully achieved, the intensity level of the mood produced is often low and may not be specific to the desired emotion (Martin, 1990). For these reasons, it is essential to evaluate the efficacy of the induction procedure with methods such as visual analog scaling or self-report measures (e.g. the Brief Mood Introspection Scale; Mayer & Gaschke, 1988).

Evaluation procedures

Once emotional expressions are elicited and recorded, they can be rated by trained judges in terms of measures such as accuracy (or appropriateness), expressivity, frequency and emotional intensity (for reviews, see Borod, 1993b; Borod & Koff, 1990). Judges should be carefully trained to ensure a high degree of inter-rater reliability. In addition, judges should be naïve to the characteristics (e.g. diagnosis) of the participants whom they are rating.

Other methods for evaluating the expression of emotions include the Facial Action Coding System (Ekman et al., 2002) and the Maximally Discriminative Facial Movement Coding System (Izard, 1983). Both methods systematically categorize the expression of emotions based on facial muscle movement using muscle action units. More recently, automated systems for evaluating facial action have been developed (Cohn, 2005).

The interaction between emotion and cognition

Historically, the study of cognition has excluded emotion, focusing instead on non-emotional processes, such as memory, attention and perception. However, in the past 25 years, the study of the interaction between emotion and cognition has thrived, sparked, in part, by a lively debate in the literature between Lazarus and Zajonc in the 1980s (Lazarus, 1984; Zajonc, 1984). As interest in this area grows,

methodologies for understanding the interaction between cognition and emotion are being developed and refined. This section will provide a description of some of the approaches commonly used to study emotion as it relates to cognition, including behavioral methodologies and neuroimaging techniques.

Behavioral methodologies
Emotion and attention

There are an inestimable number of stimuli in the environment. Given, however, that our attentional capacity is limited, some stimuli must be selectively processed at the expense of others. Research in this area suggests that the allocation of attention may be particularly biased towards processing emotional stimuli, and in particular, fearful or threatening stimuli, which often require quick behavioral responses (Mogg et al., 2000; Pratto & John, 1991). It has also been suggested that the bias towards negative stimuli may play a role in the etiology and maintenance of mood-related disorders (Beck, 1976; for review, see Mogg & Bradley, 1998).

In line with this theory are investigative findings using modifications of traditional attention paradigms, such as the emotional Stroop paradigm, which was modeled after Stroop's (1935) original color-interference task (Pratto & John, 1991; for review, see Williams et al., 1996). In this task, participants are asked to name the color of emotionally valenced and neutral words. The words may be presented individually on a computer or tachistoscope or presented as a list on a single card. Modifications of the paradigm have also been generated for use in the functional imaging environment (Whalen et al., 1998; see description below). Results from these studies typically reveal longer color-naming latencies for negative words, as compared with positive or neutral words. This paradigm has been used to investigate attentional processes in a variety of clinical syndromes, such as post-traumatic stress disorder (PTSD) (McNally et al., 1990), phobias (Watts et al., 1986), depression (Segal et al., 1995) and panic disorder (Lim & Kim, 2005). Findings suggest that the bias towards negative stimuli may be disorder-specific; for example, McNally et al. (1990) found that Vietnam combat veterans diagnosed with PTSD had slower color-naming latencies for negative words associated with their war experience (e.g. bodybags and firefight) as compared with negative words associated with obsessive-compulsive disorders (e.g. germs and filthy) or positive words (e.g. love and friendship).

These findings suggest an attentional bias towards stimuli that are judged by an individual to be either threatening or fearful. Specifically, negative stimuli may automatically capture the attention of participants, thereby interfering with processing the stimuli's other characteristics and causing increased reaction time. Alternatively, slower color-naming latencies for negative stimuli may reflect an inability to disengage from threatening stimuli rather than a bias to orient toward them (Fox et al., 2001). Fox and colleagues provide initial support for this argument in a study using an exogenous cue paradigm. In this paradigm, a cue (such as a word or picture) appears on a screen, automatically drawing the participant's attention to the location where a target is most likely to appear. If the cue is validly placed (i.e. it correctly indicates the location of the target), then the cue facilitates detection of the target stimulus. On the other hand, if the cue is invalid (i.e. it does not correctly indicate the location of the target), then it will delay the detection of the stimulus, as attention must be disengaged from the cue and re-oriented to the target. Most notably, Fox et al. (2001) modified the paradigm to incorporate emotional cues (positive, neutral and threat-related words). Participants took longer to localize a target after seeing threatening cue words than after seeing either positive or neutral cue words. The authors interpreted the results as an indication that the threatening cue impeded the detachment process, thus delaying the detection of the target.

Findings from a recent study using the dot probe paradigm (Koster et al., 2004) also corroborate this interpretation. The dot probe paradigm is a visual detection task in which a pair of stimuli (one threatening in nature and the other neutral) is shown for a brief period of time at various locations on a screen. Immediately following presentation of the stimuli, a dot appears on the screen, either at the location of the neutral stimulus (incongruent presentation) or the threatening stimulus (congruent presentation). The participant indicates when the dot appears as quickly as possible, with response latency to detect the stimulus used as an index of attention allocation (MacLeod et al., 1986). Results typically indicate that participants respond faster to congruent than to incongruent trials (for review, see Mogg & Bradley, 1998), suggesting enhanced vigilance for

threat. However, Koster et al. (2004) compared response latency on neutral trials (two neutral stimuli) with response time on trials with one threatening stimulus and found no significant difference between the two times. The authors concluded that their results might reflect a difficulty in disengaging attention from threat rather than a heightened vigilance towards negative stimuli.

Emotion and memory

It has been well established that emotions generally enhance memory and that memories of emotional events tend to be more persistent and vivid than other memories. Emotions appear to bring salience to memories, helping memory processes determine which information is important and, therefore, what should and should not be remembered. Understanding emotional memory formation, including its underlying neural mechanisms, may have important implications for psychiatry. Such knowledge may clarify the etiology of disorders such as PTSD and depression, which have significant emotionally based symptoms, as well as deficits in memory and attention (Cahill, 1997; Dolan, 2002).

A variety of different methodologies have been developed for investigating the effect of emotion on memory, including both laboratory experiments and more naturalistic field studies. Laboratory experiments offer the advantage of increased control over potential confounds, enabling more direct interpretation. In these studies, subjects are typically asked to remember specific stimuli that vary in their emotional valence. Memory for the stimuli is later tested and compared with memory for non-emotional (i.e. neutral) stimuli. Affective word lists, such as the Auditory Affective Learning Test (Snyder & Harrison, 1997), are commonly used in these designs (Berrin-Wasserman et al., 2003; Demaree, et al. 2004). Additionally, studies have used emotional narratives (Kensinger et al., 2004; Nitschke et al., 2004), short films with emotional content (Cahill et al., 1996), or pictures from the IAPS (see description above; Lang et al., 2005) to study the relationship between emotion and memory.

Regardless of the methodology used, it is important that the emotional stimuli be matched as closely as possible to the "neutral" or "control" stimuli in order to ensure that it is the emotional valence, and not another characteristic of the stimuli, that is accounting for any between-group differences

(Cahill & McGaugh, 1995). For example, if emotionally arousing words are used, they should be closely matched with the neutral words in terms of their frequency of occurrence in the English language (Kucera & Francis, 1967; Thorndike & Lorge, 1944) and their difficulty level (e.g. Chapman & Chapman, 1973). Or, in the case of emotional narratives, the grammatical and syntactical structure of text should be carefully constructed to ensure equivalence. Cahill & McGaugh (1995) avoided this potential confound by using identical pictures for both the emotional and neutral conditions and varying only the emotional valence of the narratives accompanying the pictures. Results from this study showed that participants who heard the arousing story remembered significantly more information than did participants who heard the neutral story. As the visual stimuli used in both conditions were identical, the enhanced memory could not have been due to the content of the slides themselves, but rather the emotional meaning attributed to them.

Although laboratory experiments offer more controlled investigations, some researchers have chosen to take a more naturalistic approach to the study of emotion in order to maximize generalizability. One method commonly used is the examination of "flashbulb" memories, which are the vivid, long-lasting memories of the circumstances under which an individual learns of emotionally arousing or shocking news (Brown & Kulik, 1977). For example, researchers have evaluated the accuracy of memories surrounding unexpected events such as the assassinations of John F. Kennedy and Martin Luther King, Jr. (Brown & Kulik, 1977), the Challenger explosion (Neisser & Harsch, 1992), the death of Princess Diana (Hornstein et al., 2003) and the terrorist attacks of September 11 (Luminet et al., 2004). These studies compare successive recollections of the event (e.g. "Where were you when you heard the news?") by measuring the consistency between the participants' memories shortly after the event and their memories several months later. In general, flashbulb memories have been found to be more stable than other autobiographical memories (Brown & Kulik, 1977), although there are conflicting reports in the literature (Neisser & Harsch, 1992). Researchers have examined numerous attributes of flashbulb memories in an attempt to determine the factors responsible for the formation and consolidation of these memories. For example, research has demonstrated a relationship between recall and the personal (or national) importance of an event (Conway et al., 1994). The amount of rehearsal (i.e. talking about the event or media exposure to it) also appears to impact the consolidation of flashbulb memories. Nonetheless, it remains unclear whether rehearsal has an enhancing effect or whether it causes distortion of the memories due to the potential interjection of inaccurate information each time the memory is rehearsed (Bohannon, 1988; Conway et al., 1994). Of particular relevance is the finding that an affective response is central to the creation of flashbulb memories (Bohannon & Symons, 1992; Otani et al., 2005). In their study of the disaster involving the space shuttle *Challenger*, Bohannon & Symons noted that the participants who reported being "upset" by the event were more likely to have consistent memories of the disaster. In contrast, the participants who remained "calm" were equally likely to have either consistent or inconsistent memories. Given these results, it is clearly important for investigations of flashbulb memories to include a measure of the participant's emotional reaction(s) to the target event.

Emotion and learning

Every day we learn to associate neutral stimuli with a particular emotional valence. For example, if eating ice cream brings you pleasure, then eventually just thinking about ice cream may be enough to make you happy. The study of emotional learning focuses on how associations between neutral stimuli and emotional valence are formed (Phelps, 2006).

A common method for studying emotional learning is the fear conditioning paradigm, which is based upon classical Pavlovian conditioning. Specifically, a neutral stimulus, such as a tone, is paired with an aversive stimulus, typically a shock. After repeated pairings of the stimuli, the animal learns that the neutral stimulus is associated with the aversive event and therefore begins to display fear responses even when the neutral stimulus is presented alone. Researchers studying animals have used the fear conditioning paradigm to elucidate emotional circuits in the brain (for review, see LeDoux, 2000). The paradigm has also been applied to humans, particularly in studies using functional neuroimaging (e.g. Buchel et al., 1998; LaBar & Phelps, 2005).

Although many studies about emotional learning have focused on negative stimuli, studies using the conditioned preference paradigm have also examined how associations are formed between stimuli and positive emotions or reward. In the conditioned preference paradigm, which is based upon stimulus-reward learning, previously neutral stimuli elicit approach responses after being paired with a reward. For example, Johnsrude et al. (2000) presented three monochrome patterns to healthy adults and to patients with unilateral surgical lesions that included the amygdaloid nuclear complex. One of the patterns was consistently paired with a food reward. When pattern preferences were assessed at the end of the study, the healthy participants preferred the pattern paired with the reward more often than the other patterns. The patients with brain damage did not show a conditioned preference. The participants in the study were not explicitly aware of the conditioning procedures. When asked why they showed the preferences they did, all participants attributed their preference to characteristics of the pattern.

Functional imaging

Similarly to other areas of neuropsychology, the neuropsychology of emotion has benefited from functional neuroimaging techniques in at least two ways. First, such techniques have enabled the localization of emotional processes in the brain with a degree of precision that could only be achieved previously in animal studies. Second, this new opportunity for a precise study of the neural bases of emotion in normal volunteers (for reviews, see Borod et al., 2001; Phan et al., 2004) has lessened the need for inferences about emotion in an intact brain from studies with patients. Below, we provide a few examples of what neuroimaging is teaching brain researchers about the neuropsychology of cognitive–emotional interactions in normal and clinical populations.

Hemodynamic–metabolic approaches

Several neuroimaging techniques are based on the fact that a rise in the neural activity of a brain region is followed by a change in blood flow and oxygenation in that region (Logothetis & Pfeuffer, 2004; Raichle, 1987; see Chapter 16, this volume). Some of the most common techniques in this category are functional magnetic resonance imaging (fMRI), positron emission tomography (PET) and single photon emission computerized tomography (SPECT). These techniques are used to map the brain regions that are most active during specific tasks.

Due to differences in several parameters (e.g. paradigm design and methods of data analysis), both fMRI and PET studies of emotion have often produced inconsistent results regarding the neural substrates of various emotions. Nevertheless, consistent patterns emerge when results across many studies are examined in a meta-analysis. An analysis by Phan et al. (2002) identified a considerable degree of dissociation among neural circuits underlying different emotions; although the activations corresponding to the processing of several emotions overlap in the medial prefrontal cortex, they also include other brain regions that seem to be activated preferentially by one emotion only. Thus, stimuli conveying fear preferentially activate the amygdala, whereas stimuli conveying sadness preferentially activate the subcallosal cingulate (Phan et al., 2002). Moreover, processing of happiness or disgust tends to activate the basal ganglia (Phan et al., 2002). As demonstrated by Calder et al. (2001), these dissociations challenge dimensional models of emotion (e.g. Russell, 1980) that view a given emotion as a manifestation of two underlying factors (e.g. arousal and valence), such that various emotions differ from one another only in the degree to which they express these factors. Thus, fear may be viewed as a state of negative valence that is high in arousal, whereas sadness is represented as a state of negative valence that is low in arousal. In their two-dimensional space, these models place disgust close to fear and distant from happiness. Yet, neuroimaging studies indicate the opposite pattern of results (Phan et al., 2002) and provide evidence that emotions, at their most basic level, may be discrete states that do not necessarily lie along a continuous dimension.

Neuroimaging data have also illuminated the neural mechanisms subserving the interplay of emotion and cognition during various tasks. Such research often makes clever use of behavioral paradigms by modifying them for the scanning environment. For instance, a variation of the emotional Stroop has been developed for use with fMRI. As described above, the emotional Stroop measures a participant's color-naming latency for emotional words. This method is not feasible in the fMRI environment, as head movement caused by speech could result in image distortion. To address this problem, Whalen et al. (1998) altered the original paradigm to create the emotional counting Stroop (ecStroop). In this task, word stimuli are presented in sets of one to four identical words. Participants are asked to report the number of words appearing on the screen by pressing a button. The words are presented in blocks of either neutral (e.g. cushion) or negative (e.g. murder) words. Delays in the negative condition as compared to the neutral condition are used as a measure of emotional interference. Performance on the ecStroop has been associated with activation of the rostral anterior cingulate cortex (ACC) in normal controls (Whalen *et al.*, 1998). By using another Stroop variant, Wagner *et al.* (2006) extended the study of emotional interference in cognitive processing to clinical populations, showing that relative to control participants, there was an increased activation of the rostral ACC and the dorsolateral prefrontal cortex (DLPFC) during the Stroop task in unmedicated and performance-matched patients with a major depressive disorder.

Transcranial magnetic stimulation

Another exciting technique in the field of neuroimaging, transcranial magnetic stimulation (TMS), will likely have an impact on the study of the interplay between cognition and emotion. During TMS, an alternating current is produced in the stimulating coil of a TMS device and as a result *pulsed* magnetic fields are created around the coil. Since the coil is placed over a region of interest on a participant's brain, a pulsed magnetic field passes through the skull and into the brain of the participant, inducing focal neuronal depolarization in that region. Two basic modes of TMS administration exist. In one mode, TMS is administered one pulse at a time, whereas in the other mode (termed repetitive TMS [rTMS]), trains of TMS pulses are delivered. Depending on the mode of TMS administration and the frequency of TMS pulses in a train, TMS results in a temporary focal excitation or inhibition of neuronal activity (Maeda *et al.*, 2000; Robertson *et al.*, 2003), thereby allowing for non-invasive, real-time investigations of neuronal circuitry (for reviews, see Lisanby & Sackeim, 2000; Robertson *et al.*, 2003). Because TMS involves manipulation of neuronal activity, it allows causal inferences regarding the role of a particular brain region and its role in task performance. Such inferences are often not possible with the imaging methods discussed earlier which, without corroborating evidence, are unable to distinguish activity that is necessary for the performance of a given task from activity that is merely epiphenomenal to it. At the present time, however, this advantage of TMS is somewhat attenuated by our limited knowledge of information processing in neural networks. Namely, it is often not clear whether a disruption of neuronal activity in a brain region causes changes in task performance directly or through its connections with other brain regions. The solution to this fundamental problem may lie in manipulating neuronal activity with TMS and visualizing TMS-affected brain regions with fMRI or PET at the same time. A number of studies (e.g. Bohning *et al.*, 1998) have successfully combined these methods, and research aimed at overcoming major challenges that face this field is rapidly developing (for review, see Paus, 2005).

Transcranial magnetic stimulation investigations into the neuropsychology of emotion are faced with another limitation of this technique – its inability to directly affect neuronal activity in structures that lie deeper than roughly 2.5 cm from the skull surface (Cowey, 2005), including many subcortical regions involved in emotional processing (e.g. the amygdala). Despite this limitation, a number of successful attempts to affect the interplay of cognition and emotion have been reported in the TMS literature, with two basic types of experimental design utilized. In one type, rTMS is applied for an extended period of time (e.g. 10 minutes) to induce a long-lasting effect, and experimental measures are administered after the TMS application has ended. This approach was adopted by Bermpohl *et al.* (2006), who found that rTMS administered over the right DLPFC led to improved performance on an affective go/no-go task relative to the control condition in a group of depressed participants, whereas it tended to impair performance in a group of participants who had remitted from depression. The latter effect failed to reach statistical significance. Additionally, rTMS over the left DLPFC impaired performance in the remitted group. Because 1 Hz rTMS was used, which has been shown to inhibit neuronal activity (Maeda *et al.*, 2000), these findings support the "imbalance" hypothesis of depression which states that a hyperactivity of the right, relative to the left, prefrontal region underlies this disorder (Sackeim *et al.*, 1982). The lack of an rTMS effect when the left DLPFC was stimulated in the depressed group could possibly have reflected a floor effect stemming from the putative hypoactivity in this area during depression.

In the second type of design, TMS is administered during the performance of a cognitive task. Since each TMS pulse is usually accompanied by unpleasant sensations (e.g. contraction of head muscles) that may have a confounding effect on task performance, the single-pulse mode of TMS administration is usually used in this design. Compared with rTMS, the advantage of the single-pulse approach is its excellent temporal resolution (on the order of tens of milliseconds; Walsh & Rushworth, 1999). Thus, single-pulse TMS may not only reveal whether a certain brain region is involved in a task, but also provide information regarding *when* in the task it becomes involved. Processes that can be empirically monitored in real time (e.g. movement) are particularly amenable to this technique. Unfortunately, because the disruption in neural processing caused by a single pulse is very transient (as opposed to rTMS), many cognitive processes (e.g. memory) which cannot be monitored in real time are consequently not appropriate for study with single-pulse TMS (Wassermann, 1998). A related problem is that single TMS pulses may "miss" the time during which the stimulated brain region is involved in a cognitive task unless, based on previous findings, a researcher has some knowledge of when in a task trial the involvement may occur. Studies using single-pulse TMS to study the involvement of a brain region in the processing of emotional information have only recently started appearing in the literature (Pourtois *et al.*, 2004). It is likely that as this area of research develops, TMS studies of cognitive–emotional interplay will be able to investigate interactions among several brain regions, in addition to the function of a single region, as has been previously done. As discussed earlier, combining TMS with fMRI or PET is a promising approach toward this aim.

It is undeniable that functional imaging techniques have revolutionized cognitive, affective and social neuroscience. However, certain aspects of neuroimaging make it inherently problematic for use with clinical populations. First, many scanning protocols require the patient to lie still in a tunnel-like magnetic coil, sometimes for long periods of time, as excessive movement can cause distortion in the image being captured. Though this may be relatively simple for healthy adult individuals, certain psychiatric and neurological patients may find it particularly difficult to remain motionless for the required amount of time or may be unable to monitor their body movements. Therefore, functional neuroimaging may not be appropriate for every clinical population (cf. Breiter & Rauch, 1996; Raz *et al.*, 2005).

Another potential problem is that many of the functional imaging procedures are inherently stressful and can evoke feelings of fear or anxiety in the patient. According to a comprehensive review by Melendez & McCrank (1993), up to 30% of patients in functional neuroimaging studies experience anxiety-related reactions that are severe enough to warrant interruption of the scanning procedure. And 4.3% experience full-blown panic attacks. Besides the obvious concern for the welfare and comfort of the patient, these findings have particular implications for researchers investigating the neural underpinnings of emotion, as anxiety experienced by the patient (either reported or not) is likely to seriously confound the outcome of a study. For example, Tabert *et al.* (2001) found that state anxiety levels do increase as a result of the scanning procedure, and that under certain conditions, the increase in participant state anxiety as evaluated by a self-report questionnaire was correlated with amygdala activation. One potential remedy for this problem is to have patients "practice" the scanning procedure using a mock scanner. A mock scanner is designed to provide a realistic simulation of the scanning environment so that participants can be desensitized, resulting in relatively less anxiety during the actual scanning session. The use of mock scanners has proven successful in acclimating participants to the scanning environment (e.g. Slifer *et al.*, 1993).

A final concern for researchers is that some patients may find that lying supine and motionless in a scanner, combined with the rhythmic thumping of the magnet can induce fatigue and drowsiness. Clearly, the success of an imaging study depends on the participants' ability to focus on the presented stimuli. Therefore, researchers must be careful to ensure that participants are awake and alert throughout each session (Raz *et al.*, 2005).

Event-related potentials

Event-related potentials (ERPs) offer much to the investigation of cognitive and emotional processes, as they provide a measure of the brain's electrical activity in response to external stimuli and of its subsequent cognitive and/or emotional processing. Event-related potentials record electrical activity from populations of neurons underlying electrodes that are applied to standard positions on the scalp. There are two features of ERPs that are particularly useful: (1) temporal characteristics of electrical activity are measured in near to real-time (i.e. milliseconds) and (2) the amplitude of electrical activity provides a good measure of the extent to which cognitive operations are engaged (Duncan-Johnson & Donchin, 1982). Temporal and spatial changes in ERP amplitude are helpful in determining which cortical regions are involved in a specific mental process, as well as the sequence in which these regions are recruited.

There are several methodological advantages to applying ERPs in the study of emotion and cognition. For one, like other functional imaging techniques, ERPs offer researchers the ability to study cognitive and emotional processes independent of conventional, overt behavioral measures (e.g. response time and accuracy). Measures like reaction time and response accuracy are limited in terms of explaining the underlying neuropsychological processes involved in a given experimental task (e.g. the relative amount of attention and evaluation allocated to an experimental stimulus). However, ERPs can directly address some of the inadequacies of simple behavioral measures by directly examining cortical activity related to early sensory or attentional processes (e.g. as reflected by P1 or N1), as well as later stages of information processing (e.g. as reflected by the N2-P3 complex). Thus, phasic measures of perception, classification and discrimination can be investigated in regard to task-related processing.

Event-related potentials are generally analyzed by averaging the sum of an individual's waveforms across a particular experimental condition; therefore, repeated-measures are inherent to ERP methods. This characteristic is advantageous as it enables studies to achieve statistically reliable effects even with small samples, since statistical power is gained by exposing each subject to each experimental condition (e.g. Sprinthall, 2003). In doing so, each participant serves as his/her own control, which eliminates the between-subjects variance caused by extraneous factors (i.e. individual differences). This is especially useful when sufficient numbers of a certain clinical population are difficult to obtain.

Various procedures have been used to examine the relationship between emotion and cognition in research utilizing ERPs. One such procedure involves having participants categorize stimuli according to emotional content. Analysis of the resulting stimulus-locked ERP waveforms can help elucidate differences in early selective attention for stimuli characterized by different emotional content (e.g. Schupp et al., 2003, 2004, 2006). Further, an analysis of components related to later stages of stimulus processing (e.g. P3/P300) can assess the extent to which increases in early attentional allocation paid to emotional stimuli (seen as augmented early components) result in augmentation of later components. Augmentation of the P3/P300 component resulting from emotionally laden stimuli would further indicate an interaction of emotion and cognition, as the P3/P300 has been interpreted as an index of the level of stimulus evaluation (Duncan-Johnson & Donchin, 1982).

Based on this concept, paradigms have been developed that attempt to control for the degree to which emotional or cognitive processes are involved, thereby enabling researchers to examine the interrelatedness or independence of emotion and cognition. For instance, Kayser et al. (1997) argue that the use of paradigms requiring some behavioral output or decision on the part of the research participant make it difficult to distinguish emotional processes from overlapping cognitive operations. Therefore, they constructed a paradigm to decrease the impact of cognitive and motor-related processes by having participants view highly emotional visual stimuli (pictures of facial areas directly before or after surgery) and neutral stimuli (same facial regions years after surgery) without requiring overt responses. Further, they incorporated a visual-half field paradigm (i.e. lateralized exposures in order to directly stimulate one hemisphere) in order to study the role that each hemisphere plays in the regulation of affect. Findings from this study revealed augmentation of the N2-P3 complex for emotional stimuli compared with neutral stimuli over right parietal regions. Because no overt response was required, thus suggesting little cognitive involvement, the authors could conclude that their findings indicated "a basic lateralized neuronal mechanism... responsible for an involuntary classification (N2) and evaluation (P3) of the affective significance of the stimulus" (Kayser et al., 1997, p. 425; see Endnote 1).

It is also important to consider subtle aspects of the experimental paradigm, such as whether or not participants are instructed to attend to the emotional content of stimuli, as this can affect early perceptual processes. For example, if a participant is instructed to attend to the emotional content of a stimulus, early ERP components (e.g. P1 and N1) related to attentional allocation mediated by extrastriate cortex

(Gomez *et al.*, 1994) will be enhanced, compared with when the subject is not explicitly instructed to attend to emotional content (cf. Kayser *et al.*, 1997, 2000; Smith *et al.*, 2003, 2006).

The oddball paradigm has also been shown to be a robust tool to investigate the nature of stimulus evaluation. Stimulus evaluation and categorization is best represented by the P3/P300 component (for reviews, see Johnson, 1988; Picton, 1992). In this paradigm, an occasional or infrequent target stimulus must be detected within blocks of frequently presented standard stimuli. The amplitude of the P3/P300 component is inversely correlated with the frequency to which targets are presented and positively correlated with the amount of attention allocated to the task (i.e. detecting target stimuli; Spencer *et al.*, 2001).

Variations of the oddball paradigm have been developed to investigate the modulation of stimulus evaluation via emotional content. For instance, Ito *et al.* (1998) examined whether infrequent target stimuli characterized by negative valence influence evaluative processes preferentially more than positive valence, when couched in the "context" of neutral stimuli (i.e. frequent neutral stimuli). Blocks of emotionally positive pictures or blocks of negative pictures were presented as target stimuli while emotionally neutral pictures served as the standard frequent stimuli in both conditions. Participants were asked to indicate the emotional content of the picture by pressing one of two labeled buttons: one key indicated emotional content (either positive or negative, depending on which block was being presented), and the other indicated neutral content. This study replicated similar findings of traditional oddball studies in that the rare targets (i.e. emotional pictures) yielded larger P3 amplitudes compared with the standard neutral stimuli. However, their findings also revealed larger P3 amplitudes to negative rare targets compared with positive rare targets. The authors concluded that these findings suggest negative stimuli are evaluated and categorized to a greater extent than emotionally neutral or positive stimuli.

Another variation of the oddball paradigm is the use of dichotic listening tasks in which syllables (e.g. ba, ta, ga) are presented binaurally and differ in emotional prosody (e.g. Erhan *et al.*, 1998). This procedure offers the ability to study not only the effect of emotional prosody on auditory discrimination, but also to examine differential effects between the cerebral hemispheres. This procedure is also amenable for use in clinical populations. Comparisons on the dichotic listening task (without the use of emotional prosody) have been made between healthy and depressed samples (Bruder *et al.*, 1998); healthy individuals and individuals with anxiety disorders with and without comorbid depression (Bruder *et al.*, 2002, 2004); and healthy individuals to those with post-traumatic stress disorder (Kimble *et al.*, 2000).

Advances in methods for conducting ERP analyses, such as the use of principal component analysis (PCA; e.g. Dien *et al.*, 2005; Kayser & Tenke, 2003, 2006a, 2006b) have facilitated the identification of distinct ERP components related to cognitive and/or emotional processes. These advances in ERP methodology provide further aid in disentangling the interaction between emotion and cognition in the human brain.

Summary

The study of emotion has a long history in the field of psychology, beginning with William James at the turn of the century. With the cognitive revolution in the 1960s, the exploration of the interaction between emotion and cognition was inevitable and has become an important area of research.

As has been outlined in this chapter, the effect of emotion on cognition is pervasive, influencing what we pay attention to, how we process information, what we remember and even how we learn. As interest in the area is growing, the number of innovative methodologies to assess the interaction between emotion and cognition is increasing. Much of this progress can be attributed to technological advances in both functional and spatial imaging, which are now enabling us to study the interaction between emotion and cognition at a neural level. Activation studies using fMRI, PET and SPECT have begun to elucidate the neurobiology of emotion generation and processing. In addition, modifications of behavioral paradigms, such as the ecStroop, are enabling researchers to investigate the neural underpinnings of the interaction between emotion and cognition. To complement the advances in neuroimaging, creative behavioral paradigms are also being developed to assess the interaction between emotion and various cognitive domains, including attention, learning and memory.

This area of research is particularly relevant to clinical populations, as these populations frequently demonstrate impairment in both emotion and cognition. Further understanding of how these two domains relate to each other could help to elucidate the etiology of both mood and thought disorders and lead to the development of more targeted treatments.

Acknowledgments

This work was supported, in part, by Professional Staff Congress–City University of New York Research Awards nos. 68150-00-37 & 69683–0038 and by NIH R01 DC01150 subcontract to Queens College.

Endnote

1. We would like to note that although the work reviewed in this chapter is heavily weighted towards the study of the influence of emotion on cognition, researchers are also exploring the impact that cognition has on emotion. The goal of this other line of research is to identify the higher cognitive control processes responsible for the control and regulation of emotions and to understand interactions among the underlying neural systems (for a review, see Ochsner & Gross, 2005). Unfortunately, a discussion of this literature was beyond the scope of the current chapter.

References

Beck, A. T. (1976). *Cognitive Therapy and the Emotional Disorders*. New York, NY: International Universities Press.

Bermpohl, F., Fregni, F., Boggio, P. S. *et al.* (2006). Effect of low-frequency transcranial magnetic stimulation on an affective go/no-go task in patients with major depression: role of stimulation site and depression severity. *Psychiatry Research*, **30**, 1–13.

Berrin-Wasserman, S., Winnick, W. A. & Borod, J. C. (2003). Effects of stimulus emotionality and sentence generation on memory for words in adults with unilateral brain damage. *Neuropsychology*, **17**, 429–438.

Bohannon, J. N. (1988). Flashbulb memories for the Space Shuttle disaster: a tale of two theories. *Cognition*, **29**, 179–196.

Bohannon, J. N. & Symons, V. L. (1992). Flashbulb memories: confidence, consistency, and quantity. In E. Winograd & U. Neisser (Eds.), *Affect and Accuracy in Recall: Studies of "Flashbulb Memories"* (pp. 65–94). Cambridge: Cambridge University Press.

Bohning, D. E., Shastri, A., Nahas, Z. *et al.* (1998). Echoplanar BOLD fMRI of brain activation induced by concurrent transcranial magnetic stimulation. *Investigative Radiology*, **33**, 336–340.

Borod, J. C. (1993a). Emotion and the brain – anatomy and theory: an introduction to the Special Section. *Neuropsychology*, 7, 427–432.

Borod, J. C. (1993b). Cerebral mechanisms underlying facial, prosodic, and lexical emotional expression: a review of neuropsychological studies and methodological issues. *Neuropsychology*, 7, 445–463.

Borod, J. C. (Ed.). (2000). *The Neuropsychology of Emotion*. New York, NY: Oxford University Press.

Borod, J. C. & Koff, E. (1990). Lateralization for facial emotional behavior: a methodological perspective. *International Journal of Psychology*, **25**, 157–177.

Borod, J. C., Cicero, B., Obler, L. *et al.* (1998). Right hemisphere emotional perception: evidence across multiple channels. *Neuropsychology*, **12**, 446–458.

Borod, J. C., Pick, L. H., Hall, S. *et al.* (2000a). Relationships among facial, prosodic, and lexical channels of emotional perceptual processing. *Cognition and Emotion*, **14**, 193–211.

Borod, J. C., Tabert, M. H., Santschi, C. & Strauss, E. H. (2000b). Neuropsychological assessment of emotional processing in brain-damaged patients. In J. C. Borod (Ed.), *The Neuropsychology of Emotion* (pp. 80–105). New York, NY: Oxford University Press.

Borod, J. C., Welkowitz, J. & Obler, L. K. (1992). *The New York Emotion Battery*. Unpublished materials, Department of Neurology, Mount Sinai Medical Center, New York, NY.

Borod, J. C., Zgaljardic, D., Tabert, M. & Koff, E. (2001). Asymmetries of emotional perception and expression in normal adults. In F. Boller & J. Grafman (Series Eds.) and G. Gainotti (Vol. Ed.), *Handbook of Neuropsychology: Emotional Behavior and its Disorders* (pp. 181–205). Oxford: Elsevier Science.

Bowers, D., Blonder, L. X. & Heilman, K. M. (1991). *The Florida Affect Battery*. Gainesville, FL: University of Florida.

Breiter, H. C. & Rauch, S. L. (1996). Functional MRI and the study of OCD: from symptom provocation to cognitive-behavioral probes of cortico-striatal systems and the amygdala. *Neuroimage*, **4**, S127–S138.

Brown, R. & Kulik, J. (1977). Flashbulb memories. *Cognition*, **5**, 73–99.

Bruder, G. E., Kayser, J., Tenke, C. E. *et al.* (2002). Cognitive ERPs in depressive and anxiety disorders during tonal and phonetic oddball tasks. *Clinical Electroencephalography*, **33**, 119–124.

Bruder, G. E., Schneier, F. R., Stewart, J. W., McGrath, P. J. & Quitkin, F. (2004). Left hemisphere dysfunction during verbal dichotic listening tests in patients who have social phobia with or without comorbid depressive disorder. *American Journal of Psychiatry*, **161**, 72–78.

Bruder, G. E., Tenke, C. E., Towey, J. P. *et al.* (1998). Brain ERPs of depressed patients to complex tones in an oddball task: relation of reduced P3 asymmetry to physical anhedonia. *Psychophysiology*, **35**, 54–63.

Buchel, C., Morris, J., Dolan, R. J. & Friston, K. J. (1998). Brain systems mediating aversive conditioning: an event-related fMRI study. *Neuron*, **20**, 947–957.

Buck, R. (1978). The slide-viewing technique for measuring nonverbal sending accuracy: a guide for replication. *Catalog of Selected Documents in Psychology*, **8**, 63.

Cahill, L. (1997). The neurobiology of emotionally influenced memory. Implications for understanding traumatic memory. *Annals of the New York Academy of Sciences*, **21**, 238–246.

Cahill, L. & McGaugh, J. L. (1995). A novel demonstration of enhanced memory associated with emotional arousal. *Consciousness and Cognition*, **4**, 410–421.

Cahill, L., Haier, R. J., Fallon, J. *et al.* (1996). Amygdala activity at encoding correlated with long-term free recall of emotional information. *Proceedings of the National Academy of Sciences*, **93**, 8016–8021.

Calder, A. J., Lawrence, A. D. & Young, A. W. (2001). Neuropsychology of fear and loathing. *National Review of Neuroscience*, **2**, 352–363.

Canino, E., Borod, J. C., Madigan, N., Tabert, M. & Schmidt, J. M. (1999). The development of procedures for rating posed emotional expressions across facial, prosodic, and lexical channels. *Perceptual and Motor Skills*, **89**, 57–71.

Chapman, L. J. & Chapman, J. P. (1973). Problems in the measurement of cognitive deficits. *Psychological Bulletin*, **79**, 380–385.

Cohn, J. F. (2005). Automated analysis of the configuration and timing of facial expression. In P. Ekman & E. L. Rosenberg (Eds.), *What the face reveals: Basic and applied studies of spontaneous expression using the Facial Action Coding System (FACS)* (2nd edn.), (pp. 388–392). New York: Oxford University Press.

Conway, M. A., Anderson, S. J., Larsen, S. F. *et al.* (1994). The formation of flashbulb memories. *Memory and Cognition*, **22**, 326–342.

Cowey, A. (2005). The Ferrier Lecture 2004: What can transcranial magnetic stimulation tell us about how the brain works? *Philosophical Transactions of the Royal Society of London. Series B: Biological Sciences*, **360**, 1185–1205.

Delplanque, S., Silvert, L., Hot, P. & Sequeira, H. (2005). Event-related P3a and P3b in response to unpredictable emotional stimuli. *Biological Psychology*, **68**, 107–120.

Demaree, H. A., Everhart, D. E., Youngstrom, E. A. & Harrison, D. W. (2005). Brain lateralization of emotional processing: Historical roots and a future incorporating

"dominance". *Behavioral and Cognitive Neuroscience Reviews*, **4**, 3–20.

Demaree, H. A., Shenal, B. V., Everhart, D. E. & Robinson, J. L. (2004). Primacy and recency effects found using affective word lists. *Cognitive and Behavioral Neurology*, **17**, 102–108.

Dien, J., Beal, D. J. & Berg, P. (2005). Optimizing principal components analysis of event-related potentials: matrix type, factor loading weighting, extraction, and rotations. *Clinical Neurophysiology*, **116**, 1808–1825.

Dolan, R. J. (2002). Emotion, cognition, and behavior. *Science*, **8**, 1191–1194.

Duncan-Johnson, C. C. & Donchin, E. (1982). The P300 component of the event-related brain potential as an index of information processing. *Biological Psychology*, **14**, 1–52.

Ekman, P., Friesen, W. V. & Hager, J. C. (2002). *The Facial Action Coding System* (2nd edn.). London: Weisdenfeld & Nicolson.

Erhan, H., Borod, J. C., Tenke, C. E. & Bruder, G. E. (1998). Identification of emotion in a dichotic listening task: event-related brain potential and behavioral findings. *Brain and Cognition*, **37**, 286–307.

Federspiel, E., Imfeld, A., Keller, M. & Zimprich, D. (2005). Effects of sad mood on time-based prospective memory. *Cognition and Emotion*, **19**, 1199–1213.

Fox, E., Russo, R., Bowles, R. & Dutton, K. (2001). Do threatening stimuli draw and hold visual attention in subclinical anxiety? *Journal of Experimental Psychology: General*, **130**, 681–700.

Gomez Gonzalez, C. M., Clark, V. P., Fan, S., Luck, S. J. & Hillyard, S. A. (1994). Sources of attention-sensitive visual event-related potentials. *Brain Topography*, **7**, 41–51.

Heilman, K. M., Blonder, L. X., Bowers, D. & Crucian, G. P. (2000). Neurological disorders and emotional dysfunction. In J. C. Borod (Ed.), *The Neuropsychology of Emotion* (pp. 367–412). New York, NY: Oxford University Press.

Hornstein, S. L., Brown, A. S. & Mulligan, N. W. (2003). Long-term flashbulb memory for learning of Princess Diana's death. *Memory*, **11**, 293–306.

Ito, T. A., Larsen, J. T., Smith, N. K. & Cacioppo, J. T. (1998). Negative information weighs more heavily on the brain: the negativity bias in evaluative categorizations. *Journal of Personality and Social Psychology*, **75**, 887–900.

Izard, C. E. (1983). *The Maximally Discriminative Facial Movement Coding System (Revised)*. Newark: University of Delaware, Instructional Resources Center.

Johnson, R. (1988). The amplitude of the P300 component of the event-related potential: Review and synthesis. In P. K. Ackles, J. R. Jennings & M. G. H. Coles (Eds.),

Advances in Psychophysiology (Vol. 3, pp. 69–137). Greenwich, CT: JAI Press.

Johnsrude, I. S., Owen, A. M., White, N. M., Zhao, W. V. & Bohbot, V. (2000). Impaired preference conditioning after anterior temporal lobe resection in humans. *Journal of Neuroscience*, **20**, 2649–2656.

Kayser, J., Bruder, G. E., Tenke, C. E., Stewart, J. E. & Quitkin, F. M. (2000). Event-related potentials (ERPs) to hemifield presentations of emotional stimuli: differences between depressed patients and healthy adults in P3 amplitude and asymmetry. *International Journal of Psychophysiology*, **36**, 211–236.

Kayser, J., Tenke, C., Nordby, H. *et al.* (1997). Event-related potential (ERP) asymmetries to emotional stimuli in a visual half-field paradigm. *Psychophysiology*, **34**, 414–426.

Kayser, J. & Tenke, C. E. (2003). Optimizing PCA methodology for ERP component identification and measurement: theoretical rationale and empirical evaluation. *Clinical Neurophysiology*, **114**, 2307–2325.

Kayser, J. & Tenke, C. E. (2006a). Principal components analysis of Laplacian waveforms as a generic method for identifying ERP generator patterns: I. Evaluation with auditory oddball tasks. *Clinical Neurophysiology*, **117**, 348–368.

Kayser, J. & Tenke, C. E. (2006b). Principal components analysis of Laplacian waveforms as a generic method for identifying ERP generator patterns: II. Adequacy of low-density estimates. *Clinical Neurophysiology*, **117**, 369–380.

Kensinger, E. A., Anderson, A., Growdon, J. H. & Corkin, S. (2004). Effects of Alzheimer disease on memory for verbal emotional information. *Neuropsychologia*, **42**, 791–800.

Kimble, M., Kaloupek, D., Kaufman, M. & Deldin, P. (2000). Stimulus novelty differentially affects attentional allocation in PTSD. *Biological Psychiatry*, **47**, 880–890.

Koster, E. H. W., Crombez, G., Verschuere, B. & De Houwer, J. (2004). Selective attention to threat in the dot probe paradigm: differentiating vigilance and difficulty to disengage. *Behaviour Research and Therapy*, **42**, 1183–1192.

Kucera, H. & Francis, W. N. (1967). *Computational Analysis of Present-day American English*. Providence, RI: Brown University Press.

LaBar, K. S. & Phelps, E. A. (2005). Reinstatement of conditioned fear in humans is context dependent and impaired in amnesia. *Behavioral Neuroscience*, **119**, 677–686.

Lang, P. J., Bradley, M. M. & Cuthbert, B. N. (2005). *The International Affective Picture System (IAPS): Affective Ratings of Pictures and Instruction Manual*. Technical Report A-6, University of Florida, Gainesville, FL.

Lazarus, R. S. (1984). On the primacy of cognition. *American Psychologist*, **39**, 124–129.

LeDoux, J. E. (2000). Emotion circuits in the brain. *Annual Review of Neuroscience*, **23**, 155–184.

Lim, S. & Kim, J. (2005). Cognitive processing of emotional information in depression, panic, and somatoform disorder. *Journal of Abnormal Psychology*, **114**, 50–61.

Lisanby, S. H. & Sackeim, H. A. (2000). Therapeutic brain interventions in mood disorders and the nature of emotion. In J. C. Borod (Ed.), *The Neuropsychology of Emotion* (pp. 456–492). New York, NY: Oxford University Press.

Logothetis, N. K. & Pfeuffer, J. (2004). On the nature of the BOLD fMRI contrast mechanism. *Magnetic Resonance Imaging*, **22**, 1517–1531.

Luminet, O., Curci, A., Marsh, E. J. *et al.* (2004). The cognitive, emotional, and social impacts of the September 11 attacks: group differences in memory for the reception context and the determinants of flashbulb memory. *Journal of General Psychology*, **131**, 197–224.

MacLeod, C., Mathews, A. & Tata, P. (1986). Attentional bias in emotional disorders. *Journal of Abnormal Psychology*, **95**, 15–20.

Maeda, F., Keenan, J. P., Tormos, J. M., Topka, H. & Pascual-Leone, A. (2000). Modulation of corticospinal excitability by repetitive transcranial magnetic stimulation. *Clinical Neurophysiology*, **111**, 800–815.

Martin, M. (1990). On the induction of mood. *Clinical Psychology Review*, **10**, 669–697.

Mayer, J. D. & Gaschke, Y. N. (1988). The experience and meta-experience of mood. *Journal of Personality and Social Psychology*, **55**, 102–111.

McNally, R. J., Kaspi, S. P., Riemann, B. C. & Zeitlin, S. B. (1990). Selective processing of threat cues in posttraumatic stress disorder. *Journal of Abnormal Psychology*, **99**, 398–402.

Melendez, J. C. & McCrank, E. (1993). Anxiety-related reactions associated with magnetic resonance imaging examinations. *Journal of the American Medical Association*, **270**, 745–747.

Mogg, K. & Bradley, B. P. (1998). A cognitive-motivational analysis of anxiety. *Behaviour Research and Therapy*, **36**, 809–848.

Mogg, K., Millar, N. & Bradley, B. P. (2000). Biases in eye movements to threatening facial expressions in generalized anxiety disorder and depressive disorder. *Journal of Abnormal Psychology*, **109**, 695–704.

Montreys, C. & Borod, J. C. (1998). A preliminary evaluation of emotional experience and expression following unilateral brain damage. *International Journal of Neuroscience*, **96**, 269–283.

Mountain, M. A. (1993). *The Victoria Emotion Recognition Test*. Unpublished doctoral Dissertation, University of Victoria, British Columbia, Canada.

Neisser, U. & Harsch, N. (1992). Phantom flashbulbs: false recollections of hearing the news about *Challenger*. In E. Winograd & U. Neisser (Eds.), *Affect and Accuracy of Recall: Studies of "Flashbulb Memories"* (pp. 65–91). Cambridge: Cambridge University Press.

Nitschke, J. B., Heller, W., Etienne, M. A. & Miller, G. A. (2004). Prefrontal cortex activity differentiates processes affecting memory in depression. *Biological Psychology*, **67**, 125–143.

Ochsner, K. N. & Gross, J. J. (2005). The cognitive control of emotion. *Trends in Cognitive Sciences*, **9**, 242–249.

Otani, H., Kusumi, T., Kato, K. *et al.* (2005). Remembering a nuclear accident in Japan: did it trigger flashbulb memories? *Memory*, **13**, 6–20.

Paus, T. (2005). Inferring causality in brain images: A perturbation approach. *Philosophical Transactions of the Royal Society of London. Series B: Biological Sciences*, **360**, 1109–1114.

Phan K. L., Wager, T. D., Taylor, S. F. & Liberzon, I. (2002). Functional neuroanatomy of emotion: a meta-analysis of emotion activation studies in PET and fMRI. *Neuroimage*, **16**, 331–348.

Phan, K. L., Wager, T. D., Taylor, S. F. & Liberzon, I. (2004). Functional neuroimaging studies of human emotions. *CNS Spectrums*, **9**, 258–266.

Phelps, E. (2006). Emotion and cognition: insights from studies of the human amygdala. *Annual Review of Psychology*, **57**, 27–53.

Picton, T. W. (1992). The P300 wave of the human event-related potential. *Journal of Clinical Electrophysiology*, **9**, 456–479.

Pourtois, G., Sander, D., Andres, M. *et al.* (2004). Dissociable roles of the human somatosensory and superior temporal cortices for processing social face signals. *European Journal of Neuroscience*, **20**, 3507–3515.

Pratto, F. & John, O. P. (1991). Automatic vigilance: the attention-grabbing power of negative social information. *Journal of Personality and Social Psychology*, **61**, 380–391.

Raichle, M. E. (1987). Circulatory and metabolic correlates of brain function in normal humans. In V. B. Mountcastle, F. F. Plum & S. R. Geiger (Eds.), *Handbook of Physiology. The Nervous System* (Vol. V, Pt. 2, pp. 643–674). Baltimore, MD: Williams & Wilkins.

Raz, A., Lieber, B., Soliman, F. *et al.* (2005). Ecological nuances in functional magnetic resonance imaging (fMRI): psychological stressors, posture, and hydrostatics. *Neuroimage*, **25**, 1–7.

Robertson, E. M., Theoret, H. & Pascual-Leone, A. (2003). Studies in cognition: the problems solved and created by transcranial magnetic stimulation. *Journal of Cognitive Neuroscience*, **15**, 948–960.

Ross, E. D. (1985). Modulation of affect and nonverbal communication by the right hemisphere. In M.-M. Mesulam (Ed.), *Principles of Behavioral Neurology* (pp. 239–257). Philadelphia, PA: F. A. Davis.

Ross, E. D., Thompson, R. D. & Yenkosky, J. (1997). Lateralization of affective prosody in brain and the colossal integration of hemispheric language functions. *Brain and Language*, **56**, 27–54.

Russell, J. A. (1980). A circumplex model of affect. *Journal of Personality and Social Psychology*, **39**, 1161–1178.

Sackeim, H. A., Greenberg, M. S., Weiman, A. L. *et al.* (1982). Hemispheric asymmetry in the expression of positive and negative emotions. Neurologic evidence. *Archives of Neurology*, **39**, 210–218.

Schupp, H. T., Junghofer, M., Weike, A. I. & Hamm, A. O. (2003). Attention and emotion: an ERP analysis of facilitated emotional stimulus processing. *Neuroreport*, **14**, 1107–1110.

Schupp, H. T., Junghofer, M., Weike, A. I. & Hamm, A. O. (2004). The selective processing of briefly presented affective pictures: an ERP analysis. *Psychophysiology*, **41**, 441–449.

Schupp, H. T., Stockburger, J., Codispoti, M. *et al.* (2006). Stimulus novelty and emotion perception: the near absence of habituation in the visual cortex. *Neuroreport*, **17**, 365–369.

Segal, Z. V., Gemar, M., Truchon, C., Guirguis, M. & Horowitz, L. M. (1995). A priming methodology for studying self-representation in major depressive disorder. *Journal of Abnormal Psychology*, **104**, 205–213.

Slifer, K. J., Cataldo, M. F., Cataldo, M. D., Llorente, A. M. & Gerson, A. C. (1993). Behavior analysis of motion control for pediatric neuroimaging. *Journal of Applied Behavior Analysis*, **26**, 469–470.

Smith, N. K., Cacioppo, J. T., Larsen, J. T. & Chartrand, T. L. (2003). May I have your attention, please: electrocortical responses to positive and negative stimuli. *Neuropsychologia*, **41**, 171–183.

Smith, N. K., Larsen, J. T., Chartrand, T. L. *et al.* (2006). Being bad isn't always good: affective context moderates the attention bias toward negative information. *Journal of Personality and Social Psychology*, **90**, 210–220.

219

Snyder, K. A. & Harrison, D. W. (1997). The affective auditory verbal learning test. *Archives of Clinical Neuropsychology*, **12**, 477–482.

Spencer, K. M., Dien, J. & Donchin, E. (2001). Spatiotemporal analysis of the late ERP responses to deviant stimuli. *Psychophysiology*, **38**, 343–358.

Sprinthall, R. C. (2003). *Basic Statistical Analysis* (7th edn). Boston: Allyn & Bacon, Inc.

Stroop, J. R. (1935). Studies of interference in serial verbal reactions. *Journal of Experimental Psychology*, **18**, 643–662.

Tabert, M., Borod, J. C., Tang, C. *et al.* (2001). Differential amygdala activation during emotional decision and recognition memory tasks using unpleasant words: an fMRI study. *Neuropsychologia*, **39**, 556–573.

Thorndike, E. & Lorge, I. (1944). *The Teacher's Workbook of 30,000 words*. New York, NY: Bureau of Publications, Teacher's College, Columbia University.

Wagner, G., Sinsel, E., Sobanski, T. *et al.* (2006). Cortical inefficiency in patients with unipolar depression: an event-related fMRI study with the Stroop task. *Biological Psychiatry*, **59**, 958–965.

Walsh, V. & Rushworth, M. (1999). A primer of magnetic stimulation as a tool for neuropsychology. *Neuropsychologia*, **37**, 125–135.

Wassermann, E. M. (1998). Risk and safety of repetitive transcranial magnetic stimulation: report and suggested guidelines from the International Workshop on the Safety of Repetitive Transcranial Magnetic Stimulation, June 5–7, 1996. *Electroencephalography and Clinical Neurophysiology*, **108**, 1–16.

Watts, F. N., McKenna, F. P., Sharrock, R. & Trezise, L. (1986). Colour-naming of phobia-related words. *British Journal of Psychology*, **77**, 97–108.

Whalen, P. J., Bush, G., McNally, R. J. *et al.* (1998). The emotional counting Stroop paradigm: a functional magnetic resonance imaging probe of the anterior cingulate affective division. *Biological Psychiatry*, **44**, 1219–1228.

Williams, J. M. G., Mathews, A. & MacLeod, C. (1996). The emotional Stroop task and psychopathology. *Psychological Bulletin*, **120**, 3–24.

Zajonc, R. B. (1984). On the primacy of affect. *American Psychologist*, **39**, 117–123.

Chapter 15

Using neurophysiological techniques to study auditory hallucinations in schizophrenia

Judith M. Ford and Daniel H. Mathalon

Introduction

This chapter will explore the utility of using the neurophysiological techniques of event-related potentials (ERPs) and functional magnetic resonance imaging (fMRI) to understand the pathophysiology of mental illness, by using our own work with auditory hallucinations as an example. We will also explore the benefits and limitations of both techniques, while briefly discussing some of the other neurophysiological methodologies being used by others, such as magnetoencephalography (MEG) and positron emission tomography (PET).

Approaches to studying mental illness

Syndrome vs symptom approach

Although the use of categorical psychiatric disorders, such as those provided by the DSM–IV, can facilitate patient care and research into the etiology of clinical disorders, there is considerable heterogeneity, and many patients don't "fit" neatly into defined disorders. This seems to be especially true of schizophrenia and makes it a difficult disorder to study. Instead of a diagnosis-oriented approach, a symptom-oriented one enables investigations of specific mechanisms that may underlie the symptom and lead to targeted, biologically based treatment strategies.

Choosing a symptom to study – auditory hallucinations

In trying to elucidate the pathophysiology of schizophrenia, the symptom of auditory hallucinations is a good place to start, as it is both a cardinal symptom of schizophrenia and few other illnesses are characterized by auditory hallucinations. Although estimates

vary, as many as 75% of schizophrenic patients have experienced auditory hallucinations (Nayani & David, 1996). Auditory hallucinations are experienced as voices even though no one is speaking. Voices can be commenting, conversing or commanding. They can be menacing or comforting, male or female, coming from inside or outside the head.

Choosing a method to study auditory hallucinations

A variety of brain imaging methods can be used to study the pathophysiology of auditory hallucinations. However, unless the phenomenology of the hallucinatory experience is understood, the utility of neurophysiology methods is limited. For example, knowing that most patients distinguish between "voices" and their own thoughts has forced us to abandon our earlier conceptualization that "voices" are simply incorrectly tagged inner speech.

Once we understand the phenomenon we are trying to study, there are several neurophysiological methods to chose from, varying in their ability to resolve information spatially and temporally. Hemodynamic methods, such as fMRI and PET, provide excellent spatial resolution but very poor temporal resolution. Electrophysiological methods such as electroencephalography (EEG) and MEG provide excellent temporal resolution but poor spatial resolution. If a patient signaled every time he heard a "voice," with hemodynamic imaging we would not know if the brain activation happened seconds before or seconds after the signal. We would know, however, whether primary or secondary auditory cortex was involved. With EEG, we would know whether there was distinct activity within milliseconds of the signal and how

The Neuropsychology of Mental Illness, ed. Stephen J. Wood, Nicholas B. Allen and Christos Pantelis. Published by Cambridge University Press. © Cambridge University Press 2009.

long the "voice" lasted, but would not know if primary or secondary auditory cortex was involved. With MEG we would be able to make that distinction, as it has superior spatial resolution. However, MEG is not as accessible as EEG, due to cost and technical difficulties. While EEG and MEG have the same temporal resolution as the neural activity they measure, EEG is sensitive to activity parallel to the electrode in cortical gyri, while MEG is sensitive to activity tangential to the sensor in cortical sulci (see Roth *et al.*, 1995). Both are most sensitive to activity in the cortex, as the signal falls off with the square of the distance from the sensor or electrode. To get the best cortical coverage, both would be used simultaneously.

Although both hemodynamic and EEG methods are believed to reflect the underlying global field potentials (Logothetis *et al.*, 2001), they resolve on very different temporal scales. Nevertheless, they can be combined successfully to address specific questions. We have adopted an individual-differences approach where we are able to see which brain regions are most active in people who have the largest amplitude ERP component. For example, we reported that healthy controls with larger No-Go P300s had greater activation in brain regions typically considered to be involved in detecting conflict (ACC), withholding responses (right IPL), and stopping a response in-action (caudate). This neural system was not correlated with No-Go P300 amplitude in the patients. Instead, patients with the largest No-Go P300s had greater activation only in ACC. This is interesting for two reasons. First, it appears that patients approached the task differently, and because prepotent response tendencies were not established, they did not need to inhibit or stop in-action incorrect responses. Second, P300 generation may not depend on the same structures across normal and clinical groups, or situations.

For our studies of auditory hallucinations, we chose to use both EEG-based and hemodynamically based methods.

Approaches to studying auditory hallucinations
Symptom capture
With hemodynamic and electrophysiological brain imaging, we have the opportunity to understand the neural mechanisms underlying this perplexing symptom. With these tools some investigators attempt "symptom capture;" this is a naturalist approach

where neurobiological data are collected as patients experience a hallucination. While this approach is conceptually simple, it is extremely difficult in practice because it relies not only on the timely occurrence of an illusive subjective experience, but also on the ability of the patient to reliably report its initiation and completion. Symptom capture requires patience from the research team and cooperation and insight from the patient. Nevertheless, a number of investigators have used it successfully, variously reporting that auditory hallucinations are associated with activation of speech production areas (Dierks *et al.*, 1999), primary (Dierks *et al.*, 1999) and secondary auditory cortices, and various polymodal association cortices (Dierks *et al.*, 1999; Shergill *et al.*, 2000a; Silbersweig & Stern, 1996).

Fundamental deficits underlying auditory hallucinations
A more mechanistic approach that does not rely on timing, patience, cooperation and endurance is the "fundamental deficit" approach (see Silbersweig & Stern, 1996). The first step in this approach is to identify a fundamental psychological mechanism that could cause auditory hallucinations when malfunctioning. The second step is to identify the neurobiological process underlying this psychological mechanism, and the third step is to assess the integrity of this neurobiological process. Following a suggestion by Frith and colleagues (Frith, 1987), we hypothesized that a self-monitoring deficit is the fundamental dysfunctional psychological mechanism responsible for auditory hallucinations. The underlying assumption is that if voices that come from "inside the head" (i.e. old memories, preoccupations) are not identified as self-generated through a failure of self-monitoring, they will be experienced as coming from an external source (i.e. hallucinations). Next, we adopted the proposal of Feinberg (1978) who suggested that self-monitoring deficits in schizophrenia reflect dysfunction of the efference copy/corollary discharge mechanism. Then we sought a neurobiological assay of this efference copy/corollary discharge mechanism. And finally, we attempted to relate abnormalities in this assay to auditory hallucinations.

Efference copy/corollary discharge mechanism
Communication between frontal and temporal lobes during talking and inner speech may involve

an efference copy/corollary mechanism. For example, as you begin to speak, an efference copy of the motor command is sent to auditory cortex, resulting in a corollary discharge that represents the anticipated speech sounds. Presumably, via some kind of computational process involving subtraction of the corollary discharge signal from the signal generated by incoming speech sounds ("sensory reafference"), there is a net cancellation or suppression of the auditory cortical response to self-produced speech. Von Holst & Mittelstaedt (1950) and Sperry (1950) were the first to describe the operation of corollary discharge mechanisms in the visual systems of horseflies and fish, respectively. Based on their seminal experiments, they independently suggested that a motor action is accompanied by an "efference copy" of the action that produces a "corollary discharge" in sensory cortex. In the visual system, the operation of an efference copy/corollary discharge mechanism may serve to stabilize the visual image during eye movements, maintaining visuospatial constancy (Sperry, 1950; Von Holst & Mittelstaedt, 1950). In the somatosensory system, the operation of such a mechanism may account for why we cannot tickle ourselves (Blakemore *et al.*, 1998). In its simplest form, the efference copy/corollary discharge mechanism works to dampen or suppress perception of sensory events that result from self-generated actions. Thus, in addition to serving as a mechanism for learning and fine-tuning our actions, it may allow an automatic distinction between internally and externally generated percepts.

Efference copy/corollary discharge mechanism in the auditory system

In the auditory system, efference copies from speech production and vocalization regions in the frontal lobes may prepare the auditory cortex for imminent self-generated speech sounds, minimizing the auditory cortical response to these sounds and providing a mechanism for recognizing these sounds as self-generated.

Support for this mechanism comes from studies in which recordings were made during a pre-surgical planning procedure from the exposed surface of the right and left temporal cortices while patients talked and listened to others talking. Several important findings were highlighted by Creutzfeldt *et al.* (1989). First, they noted no significant differences between the right and left hemisphere. Second, during listening,

all neurons in STG responded to various aspects of spoken language within 200 ms following speech onset. Neurons in MTG were relatively less responsive to listening to speech than were those in STG. Third, during overt talking, they observed suppression of ongoing activity in ~1/3 of the MTG neurons. This suppression preceded vocalization by up to a few hundred milliseconds, and could outlast it up to 1 second.

This is similar, in some ways, to the findings of Eliades & Wang (2003, 2005) who recorded from primary auditory cortex single units in marmoset monkeys during vocalization. Like Creutzfeldt and colleagues, they reported vocalization-induced suppression beginning before vocalization, with excitation of units beginning after vocal onset (Eliades & Wang, 2003). They suggested that the origin of the suppression was from the speech production areas and also from excitation from sensory responses to the re-afferent of the self-produced vocalization. Like Creutzfeldt and colleagues, they also noted that most neurons inhibited during vocalization were not excited by external sounds, and vice versa, although some units were both suppressed and excited. They also described a laminar organization to this inhibition and excitation, with 75–80% of the units in the upper cortical layers favoring suppression, and units in the deeper cortical layers exhibiting more equal proportions of suppression and excitation. They also commented that neurons in the upper layers of cortex receive both long and short projections from frontal cortex, the likely source of inhibitory input.

These findings of auditory cortical suppression during vocalization in monkeys and humans, using direct recordings of neuronal activity, are consistent with non-invasive, human electrophysiological studies employing EEG or MEG potentials synchronized to the onset of vocalization (Curio *et al.*, 2000; Ford *et al.*, 2001a; Heinks-Maldonado *et al.*, 2005; Houde *et al.*, 2002). This occurs even when the speech sound does not result from speaking, but from a self-initiated button press (Martikainen *et al.*, 2005). In these studies, the N1 of the EEG-based ERP, or the M100 of the MEG-based response, reveals that there is increased activity in the auditory areas during speaking, but that the level of activity is lower than that observed when the same speech sound is recorded and played back to the speaker. To reconcile this with the marmoset data, Eliades & Wang (2005) approximated the global activity in the auditory cortex by averaging together large, small and

223

multi-unit activity. In spite of their finding of more suppressed than excited units, they found a net excitatory pattern of response. They suggested that this might be due to the fact that excitation is unbounded in amplitude, while inhibition is bounded by zero (no firing). This asymmetry allows a small number of excitatory neurons to mask a larger number of inhibited neurons when summed together as a group. Because of this, they suggested that finding suppression in multi-unit recordings and human imaging studies may be difficult. However, perhaps because EEG and MEG methods are more sensitive to activity in the upper than deeper layers of cortex, we and others have had success in showing dampened cortical activity during talking, although the methods do not allow precise localization to specific cortical regions or layers.

Because the only intra-cortical human study of suppression during talking found greater suppression in MTG than STG (Creutzfeldt *et al.*, 1989), MTG is an excellent focus of study. While STG is largely involved in auditory processing, MTG is traditionally considered more integrative and multi-modal (Mesulam, 1998). In fact, MTG is not essential for language comprehension or speaking, even in the language-dominant hemisphere (Creutzfeldt *et al.*, 1989). Instead, it seems to have a modulatory role in language production and comprehension. Its on-going activity is dampened during talking, perhaps allowing you to hear what others say as you talk over them, or signaling the source of the sound. It is activated when subjects observe lips mouthing numbers (Calvert *et al.*, 1997), a crutch we use to improve speech perception.

Importantly, MTG also has a role in auditory hallucinations. During auditory verbal imagery, control subjects show reduced activation of left MTG, while patients who experience hallucinations showed less suppression (McGuire *et al.*, 1995). Both left and right MTG are activated during symptom capture studies (Dierks *et al.*, 1999; Lennox *et al.*, 2000; Shergill *et al.*, 2000b; Woodruff *et al.*, 1995). Finally, a careful structural MRI study revealed reduced (13%) left MTG gray matter volumes in patients with schizophrenia, and 10% reduction of bilateral inferior temporal gyrus gray matter volumes (Onitsuka *et al.*, 2004).

Efference copy/corollary discharge dysfunction in schizophrenia

It has been suggested that failures of corollary discharge may contribute to the positive symptoms of schizophrenia (Feinberg, 1978; Feinberg & Guazzelli, 1999). If an efference copy of an intended action (or thought) does not produce a corollary discharge of the expected experience in relevant sensory areas, patients may fail to distinguish their own inner experiences from external stimuli, resulting in passivity experiences, delusions of alien control or hallucinations. Although corollary discharge is typically associated with sensorimotor systems, it is plausible to apply it to thinking, considered by some to be "our most complex motor act" (Jackson, 1958). Indeed, it has been postulated (Jackson, 1958) that thinking "might conserve and utilize the computational and integrative mechanisms evolved for physical movement."

We have reported that the auditory N1, emanating from auditory cortex, is not suppressed during talking in patients with schizophrenia (Ford *et al.*, 2001a). While our efforts to relate corollary discharge dysfunction during talking to auditory hallucinations has met with some modest success using EEG measures of spatial coherence (Ford & Mathalon, 2005; Ford *et al.*, 2002), correlations between lack of N1 amplitude suppression during talking and hallucination severity have been difficult to obtain (Ford *et al.*, 2001a, 2001b).

Functional MRI to study corollary discharge dysfunction in schizophrenia
Predictions

In spite of the warnings issued by Eliades and colleagues (Eliades & Wang, 2005), we attempted to use fMRI to study the corollary discharge and its dysfunction in schizophrenia. Like Eliades and colleagues, we compared activity during vocalizing to that of activity during relative silence, looking for relative suppression in auditory processing areas. First, we predicted that successful action of a corollary discharge mechanism during Talking would suppress MTG activity relative to a Resting baseline. That is, we predicted that healthy controls would show some MTG de-activation during Talk compared with Rest. Second, we predicted that this de-activation would be less evident in patients with schizophrenia. Third, we predicted that patients with more severe auditory hallucinations would show less MTG de-activation during Talk, consistent with compromise of an underlying corollary discharge mechanism.

Methods

We acquired fMRI data from 21 patients (17 schizophrenia; 4 schizoaffective) and 20 healthy comparison subjects. Subjects said "ah" for 1.66 s every time they saw a yellow X (5 times per blocklet), and rested every time they saw a black X (5 times per blocklet). Using a clustered acquisition sequence, fMRI data were collected for 1.66 s after each 1.66 s of talking (TR = 3.3 s). Each talk/rest block was repeated six times. Instructions were presented on the screen, and at the end of the six repeats, the word "END" appeared on the screen. During the ERP session, pre-recorded MR noise was played for 1.66 s between utterances to duplicate the fMRI environment. Each subject practiced the task before entering the MR suite. After entering the scanner but before data acquisition, subjects uttered "ah" several times to facilitate sound system calibration and acclimation to the environment.

Images were acquired on a GE 3 Tesla MRI scanner using a clustered acquisition sequence allowing for whole brain coverage (1.667 s acquisition + 1.667 s silence = 3.334 s inter-trial interval). Subjects' heads were stabilized by a bite-bar coated with dental impression material.

SPM2 was used for analysis, much as we have done in the past (Ford & Mathalon 2005). A random-effects model was applied to individual subject contrast images derived from the first-level fixed-effects analyses of single subject data. Details of acquisition and analysis appear in our earlier papers (Ford et al., 2004a, 2004b).

As in the Eliades studies, we looked for areas that were "excited" and "inhibited" by talking. Thus, Talk–Rest (activation) and Rest–Talk (de-activation) contrasts were estimated for patients and healthy subjects, separately, and were tested for significance using one-sample t-tests. Group comparisons of these contrasts were also performed using independent sample t-tests. Grand mean scaling adjusted images for global differences in image intensity across scan runs and across subjects.

As in the Eliades studies, we focused on MTG. Thus, we constructed masks of left and right BA21 and BA37 using WFU PickAtlas from Wake Forrest University (Maldjian et al. 2003, 2004) with their automated anatomic labeling atlas (Tzourio-Mazoyer et al., 2002). We correlated Talk–Rest activation heights with the Brief Psychiatric Rating Scale (BPRS) auditory hallucinations scores using the simple regression option in SPM2.

This produced SPMs showing voxels whose activation height during Talking was significantly correlated with hallucination severity (or de-activation height during Rest was negatively correlated with hallucination severity). This was done for the whole brain and for the MTG regions of interest (ROIs).

Results

Like Eliades and colleagues (Eliades & Wang, 2005), we were able to find modest evidence of "inhibition" or de-activation during talking, especially in controls. In Figure 15.1, we show the group comparison, where healthy controls have significantly greater de-activations ($P < 0.05$, uncorrected). An arrow indicates a voxel that exceeds $P < 0.05$, FDR corrected. None exceeded this threshold for patients.

Figure 15.2 displays the MTG masked correlation maps showing areas of the temporal lobes where de-activation is associated with more severe hallucinations, $P < 0.05$, uncorrected. The voxels surviving the $P < 0.05$ correction for FDR are shown with arrows. The correlation between hallucination severity and Talk–Rest mean activation height for left BA21 was $R = 0.74$, $P < 0.0001$. This relationship is plotted on the right of Figure 15.2. There was no area where patients with more severe hallucinations had significantly more de-activation during Talking corrected for FDR.

Like Eliades, we also saw areas of "excitation" during talking. Talking activated large areas of the brain in both groups, even when FDR corrected. These areas included primary and secondary auditory areas of the temporal lobe (BA41, 42, 22, 21), insula (BA13), inferior frontal gyrus (BA44, 45), anterior cingulate gyrus (BA24, 32), dorsolateral prefrontal cortex (BA9, 46) motor and supplementary motor areas (BA4, 6), somatosensory areas (BA1, 2, 3), parietal lobe (BA40), cerebellum, thalamus and basal ganglia (putamen, caudate, globus pallidus). At this threshold, there was no area that was more active in healthy comparison subjects than in patients; however, five voxels in left parietal lobe (BA7) were more active in patients than comparison subjects.

Using ERPs to study corollary discharge dysfunction in schizophrenia

Using the identical paradigm that we used for the fMRI study described above, we recorded EEG from

De-activation during talking

Healthy controls > Schizophrenics   Schizophrenics > Healthy controls

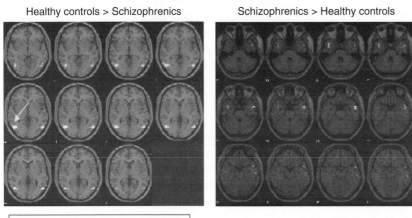

BA37: −52, −64, 4 → P = 0.041 FDR

Figure 15.1. This figure is also reproduced in the color plate section. Group contrast for Rest–Talk, showing activations exceeding $P < 0.05$, uncorrected levels with MTG mask. On the left are shown voxels where healthy controls have greater de-activation than patients during talking, and on the right, where patients have greater de-activation than controls. Voxels exceeding the $P < 0.05$ FDR are indicated by arrows, and the location is given as a Brodmann area and an x, y, z coordinate.

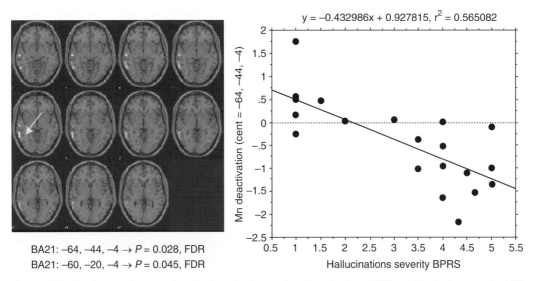

BA21: −64, −44, −4 → P = 0.028, FDR
BA21: −60, −20, −4 → P = 0.045, FDR

Figure 15.2. This figure is also reproduced in the color plate section. De-activation of MTG vs. Hallucinations severity. MTG masked correlation maps showing areas of MTG where de-activation is associated with more severe hallucinations, $P < 0.05$, uncorrected. The voxels surviving the $P < 0.05$ correction for FDR are shown with an arrow and their location is given as a Brodmann area and as x, y, z coordinates. The correlation between hallucination severity and Talk–Rest mean activation height for left BA21 was $R = 0.74$, $P < 0.0001$. This relationship is plotted on the right. Patients with less left MTG de-activation during talking had significantly more severe auditory hallucinations.

a subsample of subjects participating in the fMRI experiment (controls = 19, patients = 18). Previously, we showed that the N1 to the self-produced sound during talking was dampened compared with listening, and that this dampening was greater in controls than in patients (Ford *et al.*, 2001). Because we initially showed

this in a small sample of patients (n = 7) and controls (n = 7), we wanted to replicate it in a larger sample under better-controlled conditions and from a larger array of electrodes. In order to provide maximal comparability with the fMRI experiment, we played pre-recorded scanner noise during the 1.33 s

Chapter 15: Techniques to study auditory hallucinations in schizophrenia

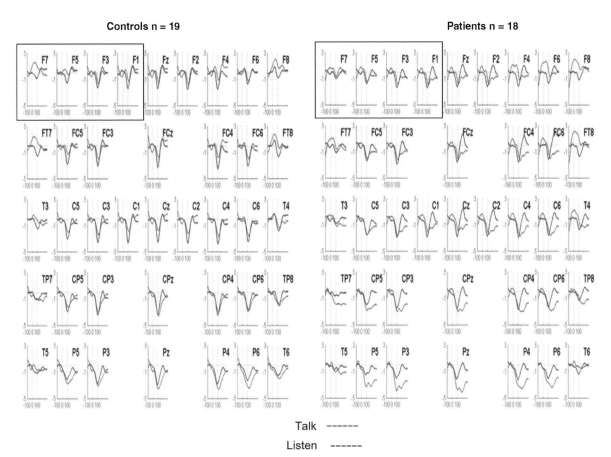

Controls n = 19   **Patients n = 18**

Talk ------
Listen ------

Figure 15.3. This figure is also reproduced in the color plate section. Event-related potentials to speech onset are shown for controls (left) and patients (right) during Talking (red) and Listening (blue). Single trials were corrected for eye movements and blinks. Negativity is plotted down. Even numbered electrode sites are over right hemisphere, odd numbered sites are over left hemisphere; F = frontal, T = temporal, C = central, P = parietal, Z = midline. Sites are positioned on figure as they appear on the head.

no-talking interval. For an optimal comparison with the fMRI experiment and the data from Eliades and colleagues, responses during talking should be compared with a period of relative quiet. This is a problem for *event*-related potentials, as quiet, or rest, is not an event. While a pre-stimulus baseline of an ERP is typically considered an adequate contrast for post-stimulus activity, our 100 ms pre-stimulus baseline was compromised because of pre-speech activity. Instead, we compared N1s during talking to those recorded to the same sounds played back during listening. In Figure 15.3, we show ERPs from a large array of electrodes to the onset of the spoken sound ("ah" during talking and listening). Earlier, we only recorded from the midline sites and reported this effect for frontal-central midline electrodes. With this new study, we were able to show greater suppression over left hemisphere sites in the controls than in the patients (Talk/Listen × Group: $F(1, 35) = 4.18$, $P < 0.05$). We did not see significant suppression over left MTG (sites TP7, etc.), the area in which modest de-activation in the fMRI study was identified.

With this more extensive recording montage and larger sample, we also noticed that N1 was considerably slower during talking than listening, especially over the left frontal region; but only in controls. The N1 to self-produced speech sounds was significantly ($P = 0.045$) later in controls (124 ms) than in patients (109 ms). This relative speeding of the response to self-initiated speech in the patients may be due to faster transmission of the neural signals from speech production to speech perception areas. In fact, the left arcuate fasciculus has greater "integrity" in patients who hallucinate than those who do not (Hubl *et al.*, 2004),

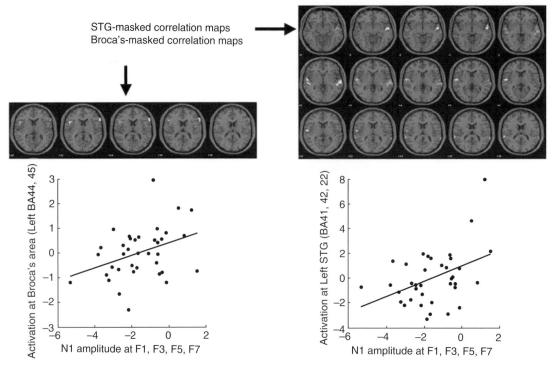

Figure 15.4. This figure is also reproduced in the color plate section. (Upper left) Broca's area-masked correlation maps showing areas of Broca's area where activation was associated with N1 suppression during talking recorded from F1, 3, 5, 7 ($P < 0.05$, uncorrected). This relationship is plotted in the lower left for left Broca's area. Subjects with more N1 suppression had greater Broca's activation during talking. (Upper right) STG-masked correlation maps showing areas of STG where activation was associated with N1 suppression ($P < 0.05$, uncorrected). This relationship is plotted in the lower right for left STG.

suggesting that speedy transmission may account for hallucinations. However, we were not able to find correlations between hallucination severity and N1 latency during talking except at TP7, over left MTG ($r = -0.51$, $P = 0.03$).

Combining EEG-based measures with fMRI

We attempted to understand the dynamics of the corollary discharge system by combining ERP and fMRI data. In spite of the inherent problems of relating signals with drastically different temporal resolutions (milliseconds vs seconds), we have had some success using an "individual differences" approach that we used for relating hallucinations to de-activation of the blood oxygen level dependent (BOLD) signal described above (Ford *et al.*, 2004a, 2004c; Mathalon *et al.*, 2003).

We calculated the mean N1 amplitude during talking from the left frontal sites boxed in Figure 15.3. We correlated this mean value with the BOLD signal

from each voxel in the brain across groups. This individual-differences analysis allowed us to interpret activations in terms of individual subjects' N1 amplitudes. To test our hypothesis about the origin and destination of the corollary discharge activity during talking, we focused this analysis on Broca's area and temporal lobe structures. Specifically, we asked whether subjects who showed the most suppression of N1 (more positive N1 values) during talking showed the greatest activation in Broca's area, reflecting a stronger corollary discharge signal (more positive BOLD signal) and the least activation in MTG reflecting suppression of responsiveness (more negative BOLD signal). While our primary interest was in left hemisphere activation, uttering non-semantic repetitive sounds would also involve right hemisphere structures.

Using a Broca's area mask (BA44, 45), we found that N1 suppression during talking was positively correlated with activity in seven voxels on the left ($P < 0.02$, uncorrected) and 10 voxels on the right ($P < 0.01$, uncorrected). In Figure 15.4, we show that subjects who had more suppression of N1 during talking had more activation in Broca's area. While this is not a statistically strong finding, it supports our notions of a corollary discharge from speech production areas dampening auditory cortex, where N1 is likely generated. That is, the stronger the signal from Broca's area, the more suppression of cortical responsiveness. To determine if there were group differences in this relationship, we did a multiple regression analysis to compare the slopes of relationships in the two groups. The slope relating Broca's area activation to N1 suppression was not different in the two groups.

We found no support for our hypothesis that N1 suppression (relatively positive value) would be related to MTG suppression (relatively negative value). Because inhibition is itself an energetic process, we also asked whether an increase in the BOLD signal (relatively positive value) would be associated with N1 suppression (relatively positive value). We found that people with greater activity in the STG had more N1 suppression during talking, although it did not reach corrected levels of significance. Specifically, we found that 48 voxels in right STG and 36 voxels in left STG (Ps ranging from 0.005 to 0.02, uncorrected) were more active when N1 was more suppressed (see Figure 15.4). This raises the possibility that the activity needed to suppress responsiveness of the N1 generators may come from STG, as suggested by Guenther (2002). To determine if there were group differences in this relationship, we did a multiple regression analysis to compare the slopes of relationships in the two groups. The slope relating STG activation to N1 suppression was not different in the two groups. It is important to note that N1 can be both generated in STG and suppressed by activity in STG, as excitation and inhibition occur within the same cortical column.

Discussion

Our decision to adopt the symptom approach to understand the pathophysiology of schizophrenia led us to explore auditory hallucinations, a cardinal symptom of the illness. Unlike cognitive dysfunctions, which are also characteristic of the illness, auditory hallucinations are difficult to study. They are phenomenologically varied, and there is no external manifestation of their occurrence. Our next decision was to test the hypothesis that auditory hallucinations are due to a dysfunctional corollary discharge (Feinberg, 1978; Feinberg & Guazzelli, 1999) resulting in a misperception of the source of inner thoughts and memories. To study the corollary discharge in action, we decided to observe it in the act of speaking, as speaking is the most easily observed motor act related to thinking (Jackson, 1958). Because of our experience with ERPs, we initiated a series of studies in which we recorded ERPs to the spoken sound *as it was being uttered*. These studies yielded ERP evidence of corollary discharge function in controls (Ford et al., 2001a; Heinks-Maldonado et al., 2005), and its dysfunction in patients (Ford et al., 2001). As we showed above (Figure 15.3), N1, emanating from auditory cortex, is dampened about 100 ms after the onset of speech. A spatial coherence analysis of EEG data during talking (Ford et al., 2002) suggested that this suppression comes from frontal lobe areas. Although we suggested that the corollary discharge signal was coming from Broca's area in the frontal lobes, and that its target was temporal lobe structures, our ERP and EEG methods were not able to address this level of neuroanatomical precision. Thus, we decided to combine data from ERP and fMRI brain imaging modalities to try to understand the neuroanatomical origins and destinations of the corollary discharge in healthy controls, their dysfunction in patients, and their relationship to auditory hallucinations.

Thus, our first step in this effort was to document BOLD signal de-activation during talking in healthy controls using fMRI. We found only modest evidence for MTG de-activation during talking, consistent with the warning of Eliades and Wang that it would be difficult to find multi-unit evidence of speech-related inhibition (Eliades & Wang, 2003, 2005). Perhaps contributing to our disappointing level of de-activation is the fact that suppression and excitation both occur within a single cortical column, a level of distinction not possible with our voxel size. Furthermore, Eliades & Wang (2005) found that activity in adjacent columns was not necessarily correlated, further challenging the coarse spatial resolution of fMRI. Nevertheless, some significant suppression was seen, but only when ROI analyses (BA21 and BA37) within MTG were done. Functional MRI has proven to be a very disappointing tool in the search for evidence of suppression of activity in auditory cortex. Single-unit studies, if possible, would have been better. Instead, we may have to wait for animal models of schizophrenia.

Our second step was to find evidence of corollary discharge dysfunction in patients. We predicted that the pattern of MTG suppression during speech production would be less prominent in patients with schizophrenia. Indeed, at the thresholds used, patients showed less suppression than controls.

Our third step was to find an association between corollary discharge dysfunction and auditory hallucinations. As predicted, we found that patients who had the most severe auditory hallucinations showed the least de-activation (the most activation) during Talking. The correlation with auditory hallucinations was significant at corrected levels of significance for left MTG (BA21) de-activations. The left hemisphere pattern was consistent with a failure of the corollary discharge mechanism to suppress responses to inner speech and inner verbal experiences (Jackson, 1958). Correlations with right MTG activity did not meet the corrected level of significance.

Finally, we attempted to understand the dynamics of the corollary discharge system by combining ERP and fMRI data. To the extent that the N1 component of the auditory ERP emanates from secondary auditory cortical regions, the de-activation of MTG in healthy controls was consistent with N1 data showing reduced responsiveness to the spoken sound during talking (Curio *et al.*, 2000; Ford *et al.*, 2001a; Heinks-Maldonado *et al.*, 2005; Houde *et al.*, 2002). However, we found no direct support for a relationship between suppression of N1 and BOLD signal de-activation. Our failure to relate N1 suppression to temporal lobe de-activation might be due to inherent limitations of the BOLD response to strongly reflect inhibition. Indeed, as Eliades & Wang pointed out, neural excitation is unbounded in amplitude, while inhibition is bounded by zero. Our failure might also be due to the fact that inhibition requires energy and might produce more of a BOLD signal increase than decrease. Indeed, our efforts to relate data from the two imaging modalities suggest that *excitation* in Broca's area and superior temporal gyrus during talking contributes to suppression of N1. At this point in our understanding of the concepts and the methods, it appears that fMRI can tell us where suppression *is coming from* and is less able to tell us where it *is happening*. Activity before an intention is actuated may be easier to study and provide better insight into the mechanisms underlying corollary discharge failures and, ultimately, their relationship to symptoms. In light of this, we have begun time-frequency analyses of pre-speech (Ford *et al.*, 2007) and pre-movement (Ford *et al.*, 2008) neural phase synchrony. About 100 ms before an action is taken, there is a significant increase in synchrony across a wide range of EEG frequencies. This is not seen in patients. We consider this to be a neural reflection of the corollary discharge, but it awaits confirmation with additional studies. We feel that these methods of analysis are more closely akin to those used by bench neuroscientists with in vivo and in vitro preparations, and have greater translational potential. Furthermore, neural synchrony measures may be more sensitive to intra-cerebral communication than voltage-based ones (Pinto *et al.*, 2003).

References

Blakemore, S., Rees, G. & Frith, C. (1998). How do we predict the consequences of our actions? A functional imaging study. *Neuropsychologia*, **36**, 521–529.

Calvert, G. A., Bullmore, E. T., Brammer, M. J. *et al.* (1997). Activation of auditory cortex during silent lipreading. *Science*, **276**, 593–596.

Creutzfeldt, O., Ojeman, G. & Lettich, E. (1989). Neuronal activity in the human lateral temporal lobe. II Responses to the subject's own voice. *Experimental Brain Research*, 77, 476–489.

Curio, G., Neuloh, G., Numminen, J., Jousmaki, V. & Hari, R. (2000). Speaking modifies voice-evoked activity in the human auditory cortex. *Human Brain Mapping*, **9**, 183–191.

Dierks, T., Linden, D., Jandl, M. *et al.* (1999). Activation of Heschl's Gyrus during auditory hallucinations. *Neuron*, **22**, 615–621.

Eliades, S. J. & Wang, X. (2003). Sensory-motor interaction in the primate auditory cortex during self-initiated vocalizations. *Journal of Neurophysiology*, **89**, 2194–2207.

Eliades, S. J. & Wang, X. (2005). Dynamics of auditory-vocal interaction in monkey auditory cortex. *Cerebral Cortex*, **15**(10), 1510–1523.

Feinberg, I. (1978). Efference copy and corollary discharge: implications for thinking and its disorders. *Schizophrenia Bulletin*, **4**, 636–640.

Feinberg, I. & Guazzelli, M. (1999). Schizophrenia – a disorder of the corollary discharge systems that integrate the motor systems of thought with the sensory systems of consciousness. *British Journal of Psychiatry*, **174**, 196–204.

Ford, J. M. & Mathalon, D. H. (2005). Corollary discharge dysfunction in schizophrenia: can it explain auditory hallucinations? *International Journal of Psychophysiology*, **58**, 179–189.

Ford, J. M., Gray, E. M., Whitfield, S. L. *et al.* (2004a). Acquiring and inhibiting pre-potent responses in schizophrenia: event related potentials and functional magnetic resonance imaging. *Archives of General Psychiatry*, **61**, 119–129.

Ford, J. M., Johnson, M. B., Whitfield, S. L. & Mathalon, D. H. (2004b). Schizophrenic patients have slow neural and hemodynamic responses: ERP and fMRI evidence (abstract). In *Schizophrenia Research. 12th Biennial Winter Workshop on Schizophrenia* (p. 128). Davos, Switzerland, February 7–13.

Ford, J. M., Mathalon, D. H., Heinks, T., Kalba, S. & Roth, W. T. (2001a). Neurophysiological evidence of corollary discharge dysfunction in schizophrenia. *American Journal of Psychiatry*, **158**, 2069–2071.

Ford, J. M., Mathalon, D. H., Kalba, S. *et al.* (2001b). Cortical responsiveness during talking and listening in schizophrenia: an event-related brain potential study. *Biological Psychiatry*, **50**, 540–549.

Ford, J. M., Mathalon, D. H., Whitfield, S., Faustman, W. O. & Roth, W. T. (2002). Reduced communication between frontal and temporal lobes during talking in schizophrenia. *Biological Psychiatry*, **21**, 485–492.

Ford, J. M., Roach, B. J., Faustman, W. O. & Mathalon, D. H. (2007). Synch before you speak: auditory hallucinations in schizophrenia. *American Journal of Psychiatry*, **164**, 456–466.

Ford, J. M., Roach, B. J., Faustman, W. O. & Mathalon, D. H. (2008). Out-of-synch and out of sorts: dysfunction of motor-sensory communication in schizophrenia. *Biological Psychiatry*, **63**(8), 736–743.

Ford, J. M., Whitfield, S. L. & Mathalon, D. H. (2004c). The neuroanatomy of conflict and error: ERP and fMRI. In M. Ullsperger & M. Falkenstein (Eds.), *Errors, Conflicts and the Brain. Current Opinions on Performance Monitoring* (pp. 42–48). Leipzig: MPI of Cognitive Neuroscience.

Frith, C. D. (1987). The positive and negative symptoms of schizophrenia reflect impairments in the perception and initiation of action. *Psychological Medicine*, **17**, 631–648.

Guenther, F. H. (2002). Neural control of speech movement. In A. Meyer & N. Schiller (Eds.), *Phonetics and Phonology in Language Comprehension and Production: Differences and Similarities*. Berlin: Mouton de Gruyter.

Heinks-Maldonado, T. H., Mathalon, D. H., Gray, M. & Ford, J. M. (2005). Fine-tuning of auditory cortex during speech production. *Psychophysiology*, **42**, 180–190.

Houde, J. F., Nagarajan, S. S., Sekihara, K. & Merzenich, M. M. (2002). Modulation of the auditory cortex during speech: an MEG study. *Journal of Cognitive Neuroscience*, **14**, 1125–1138.

Hubl, D., Koenig, T., Strik, W. *et al.* (2004). Pathways that make voices: white matter changes in auditory hallucinations. *Archives of General Psychiatry*, **61**, 658–668.

Jackson, J. H. (1958). *Selected Writings of John Hughlings Jackson*. New York: Basic Books.

Lennox, B. R., Park, S. B., Medley, I., Morris, P. G. & Jones, P. B. (2000). The functional anatomy of auditory hallucinations in schizophrenia. *Psychiatry Research*, **100**, 13–20.

Logothetis, N., Pauls, J., Augath, M., Trinath, T. & Oeltermann, A. (2001). Neurophysiological investigation of the basis of the fMRI signal. *Nature*, **412**, 150–157.

Maldjian, J. A., Laurienti, P. J. & Burdette, J. H. (2004). Precentral gyrus discrepancy in electronic versions of the Talairach atlas. *Neuroimage*, **21**, 450–455.

Maldjian, J. A., Laurienti, P. J., Kraft, R. A. & Burdette, J. H. (2003). An automated method for neuroanatomic and cytoarchitectonic atlas-based interrogation of fMRI data sets. *Neuroimage*, **19**, 1233–1239.

Martikainen, M. H., Kaneko, K. & Hari, R. (2005). Suppressed responses to self-triggered sounds in the human auditory cortex. *Cerebral Cortex*, **15**, 299–302.

Mathalon, D. H., Whitfield, S. L. & Ford, J. M. (2003). Anatomy of an error: ERP and fMRI. *Biological Psychology*, **64**, 119–141.

McGuire, P. K., Silbersweig, D. A., Wright, I. *et al.* (1995). Abnormal monitoring of inner speech: a physiological basis for auditory hallucinations. *Lancet*, **346**, 596–600.

Mesulam, M. M. (1998). From sensation to cognition. *Brain*, **121**, 1013–1052.

Nayani, T. H. & David, A. S. (1996). The auditory hallucination: a phenomenological survey. *Psychological Medicine*, **26**, 177–189.

Onitsuka, T., Shenton, M. E., Salisbury, D. F. (2004). Middle and inferior temporal gyrus gray matter volume abnormalities in chronic schizophrenia: an MRI study. *American Journal of Psychiatry*, **161**, 1603–1611.

Pinto, D. J., Hartings, J. A., Brumberg, J. C. & Simons, D. J. (2003). Cortical damping: analysis of thalamocortical response transformations in rodent barrel cortex. *Cerebral Cortex*, **13**, 33–44.

Roth, W. T., Ford, J. M., Pfefferbaum, A. & Elbert, T. (1995). Methodological issues in event-related brain potential and magnetic field studies. In F. E. Bloom (Eds.), *Psychopharmacology: The Fourth Generation of Progress* (pp. 895–910). New York, NY: Raven Press.

Shergill, S., Brammer, M., Williams, S., Murray, R. & McGuire, P. (2000a). Mapping auditory hallucinations in schizophrenia using functional magnetic resonance imaging. *Archives of General Psychiatry*, **57**, 1033–1038.

231

Shergill, S. S., Bullmore, E., Simmons, A., Murray, R. & McGuire, P. (2000b). Functional anatomy of auditory verbal imagery in schizophrenic patients with auditory hallucinations. *American Journal of Psychiatry*, **157**, 1691–1693.

Silbersweig, D. & Stern, E. (1996). Functional neuroimaging of hallucinations in schizophrenia: toward an integration of bottom-up and top-down approaches. *Molecular Psychiatry*, **1**, 367–375.

Sperry, R. W. (1950). Neural basis of the spontaneous optokinetic response produced by visual inversion. *Journal of Comparative and Physiological Psychology*, **43**, 482–489.

Tzourio-Mazoyer, N., Landeau, B., Papathanassiou, D. *et al.* (2002). Automated anatomical labeling of activations in SPM using a macroscopic anatomical parcellation of the MNI MRI single-subject brain. *Neuroimage*, **15**, 273–289.

Von Holst, E. & Mittelstaedt, H. (1950). Das Reafferenzprinzip. *Naturwissenschaften*, **37**, 464–476.

Woodruff, P., Brammer, M., Mellers, J. *et al.* (1995). Auditory hallucinations and perception of external speech. *Lancet*, **346**, 1035.

Chapter 16

Neuroimaging

Paolo Fusar-Poli and Philip McGuire

Introduction

In this chapter, we will consider the role of neuroimaging techniques in neuropsychological research on psychiatric illness. Neuroimaging has rapidly developed into a powerful tool in cognitive neuroscience and in recent years has seen widespread application in psychiatry. Although imaging methods provide an unprecedented opportunity for investigation of physiological function of the human brain, there are fundamental methodological questions that remain to be addressed. We will first outline the basic principles of structural magnetic resonance imaging (sMRI), positron emission tomography (PET), single photon emission computed tomography (SPECT), functional magnetic resonance imaging (fMRI), magnetic resonance spectroscopy (MRS) and diffusion tensor imaging (DTI), and highlight their potential uses and limitations. We will also discuss the integration of neuroimaging data across modalities and with data from electrophysiological and magnetoencephalography (MEG) studies. These issues will be explored using studies on psychosis as an example. However, the issues generalize to neuroimaging studies in all psychiatric disorders.

Structural magnetic resonance imaging (sMRI)

The term "structural" MRI (sMRI) refers to the use of MRI to examine the anatomy (as opposed to the activity or function) of the brain. Magnetic resonance imaging provides good contrasts between the three principal compartments of the brain (gray and white matter and cerebrospinal fluid (CSF)); consequently these compartments are usually easier to distinguish in MR images than in data collected using computerized tomography (CT) (Diwadkar & Keshavan, 2002; McCarley et al., 1999). In most studies, the volume of these compartments in a given brain region or the whole brain is estimated, hence the term "volumetric." Magnetic resonance imaging is based on the ability of tissues to absorb energy from radio waves and to re-emit those waves proportional to the concentration of mobile hydrogen ions in that tissue. The technique exploits the magnetic properties of hydrogen ions in water, which is abundant in brain tissue. Normally, the magnetic moments of the hydrogen protons in a subject's brain are aligned randomly in space. However, when the subject's head is placed in a powerful magnetic field, a proportion of the mobile hydrogen ions become aligned with the direction of that field. The longitudinally aligned protons are temporarily displaced out of equilibrium by the application of a radio-frequency (RF) pulse. Then the RF pulse is turned off and the rate of realignment of the protons with the external magnetic field is measured. Two simultaneous processes principally characterize this realignment: "T1-relaxation" and "T2-decay." T1 and T2 relaxation times are different in each tissue. By changing the interval between the application of the RF pulse and when the MR signal is read, either the T1 or the T2 component can be differently weighted leading to different types of tissue contrast. A T1-weighted image will provide very good contrast between white matter (which has a short T1-time), gray matter (which has an intermediate T1-time) and CSF (which has a relatively long T1-time). In T1-weighted scans, white matter appears relatively bright and CSF appears relatively dark. The ordering of intensities is the opposite in the case of T2-weighted scans (Gibby, 2005). Magnetic

The Neuropsychology of Mental Illness, ed. Stephen J. Wood, Nicholas B. Allen and Christos Pantelis. Published by Cambridge University Press. © Cambridge University Press 2009.

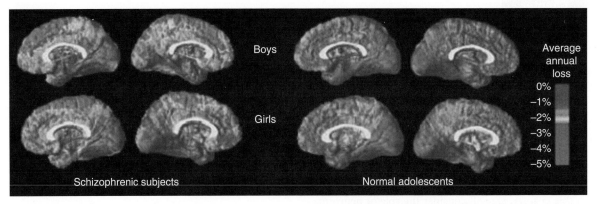

Figure 16.1. This figure is also reproduced in the color plate section. Dynamic changes of gray matter loss in boys and girls in both groups of schizophrenic subjects and normal adolescents. These maps show similar patterns of deficits for both sexes in both groups of subjects (from Vidal *et al.*, 2006, with permission).

resonance imaging is marked by excellent overall spatial resolution, the ability to image most of the brain volume (as opposed to a focal region), and by not requiring ionizing radiation.

Potentials of sMRI

In the last 20 years, MRI has been used extensively to identify structural brain abnormalities in schizophrenia. Meta-analyses of MRI studies indicate that patients with schizophrenia, compared with healthy controls, show reduced total brain volume (Ward *et al.*, 1996; Woods *et al.*, 2005; Wright *et al.*, 2000), enlarged lateral and third ventricles (Lawrie & Abukmeil, 1998; Wright *et al.*, 2000) and reduced volume in the frontal lobes (Wright *et al.*, 2000), temporo-limbic structures (Honea *et al.*, 2005; Nelson *et al.*, 1998; Ward *et al.*, 1996; Wright *et al.*, 2000), thalamus (Konick & Friedman, 2001) and corpus callosum (Woodruff *et al.*, 1995). Structural MRI has also been used to investigate how these abnormalities emerge over the course of the disorder (for a review see Toga *et al.*, 2006). Some of the brain abnormalities observed in chronic patients (such as enlargement of the ventricular system and reduction of hippocampal and total brain volume) are also evident in first-episode psychosis (Vita *et al.*, 2006), suggesting that these findings are not due to illness chronicity or treatment. Structural MRI studies in the early phase of psychosis have the potential to address the stage of development that structural abnormalities first appear (Borgwardt *et al.*, 2006; Pantelis *et al.*, 2003; Velakoulis *et al.*, 2006); the extent to which

these are related to vulnerability to psychosis (Garner *et al.*, 2005) or to psychotic symptoms (Sumich *et al.*, 2005; Whitford *et al.*, 2005); the effects of early treatment (Girgis *et al.*, 2006; Lappin *et al.*, 2006; Lieberman *et al.*, 2005); and the dynamic course over time (Vidal *et al.*, 2006) (Figure 16.1).

Limits of sMRI in schizophrenia research

There are several difficulties in interpreting this literature. First, sample sizes have often been small, and because the magnitudes of brain differences in psychiatric disorders are usually small, the results of individual studies may be unduly influenced by sampling variation. Second, the results of the studies are generally reported with an emphasis on tests of significance rather than confidence intervals, and this may give a misleading impression of a large number of inconsistent positive or negative findings. Third, many early studies used MRI acquisitions with "gaps" in between slices, with interpolation used to estimate the volume in the "gap," which limits precision of measurement. Studies with thinner slices, smaller units of volume analysis (called voxels, for volume element), and no gaps between slices are likely to yield more precise results. Fourth, in the imaging literature, the most prominent method used to investigate structural abnormalities is a region of interest analysis (ROI) (McCarley *et al.*, 1999). This approach relies on a priori defined regions of interest and the outlining of these regions to obtain volumetric measurements. As these are often dependent on the subjective judgment of the investigator, it could contribute a bias to the results (Kubicki *et al.*, 2002). In addition it may lead to a focus on a small number of regions at the expense of other areas that may also be relevant (Goldstein *et al.*, 1999). An alternative approach is voxel-based morphometry (VBM) (Ashburner & Friston, 2000; Wright *et al.*, 1995), an automated method that permits examination of the entire brain volume in a relatively user-independent way. Many recent studies have employed this approach (for a review see Giuliani *et al.*, 2005), although it is also associated with methodological concerns, particularly the effects of warping of individual brains into a standard stereotactic space (Bookstein, 2001).

PET–SPECT

The ability of single photon emission computed tomography (SPECT) and positron emission tomography (PET) to image specific biomolecules in the living brain provides a unique tool for neuropsychological researchers (for reviews of PET/SPECT in psychiatry see Smith *et al.*, 2003; Warwick, 2004). The instruments traditionally used include gamma cameras capable of detecting standard single-photon emitting radionuclides (i.e. technetium-99m, iodine-123, thallium-201) for SPECT, and scanners capable of detecting positron-emitting radionuclides (fluorine-18, oxygen-15, carbon-11), usually produced by cyclotrons, for PET (Costa *et al.*, 1999). SPECT is the nuclear medicine equivalent of computed tomography (CT) similarly combining a series of two-dimensional images obtained by moving a gamma camera on a gantry in a circular or elliptical orbit around the patient. The nature of the functional information obtained from a brain SPECT scan is determined by the biochemical interactions occurring between brain tissue and the injected substance used. These chemical substances on their own are invisible to the gamma camera, and are therefore labeled with a radioactive marker such as 99mTc or 123I to enable it to be imaged. The labeled compound is referred to as a radiopharmaceutical. Although PET can provide superior spatial resolution, SPECT has the advantage that it is much more widely available both in the developing and the developed world, while still being able to provide much of the same information (Warwick, 2004). PET, like a standard nuclear medicine gamma camera, images the distribution of radioactivity in the region being examined but, unlike SPECT, can provide both quantitative information and a higher spatial and contrast

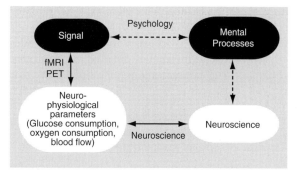

Figure 16.2. Relation of the signal obtained from fMRI or PET to mental processes. In the usual experimental plan and interpretation, on the basis of psychology, a direct relationship between the signal and mental processes is assumed, as represented by the upper pathway. The definition of mental processes comes from psychology, while the imaging experiment serves to localize and quantify the brain activity identified with the process. The lower pathway assumes that mental processes have a molecular and cellular basis, which is broken into three steps leading to the signal. The signal in fMRI or PET experiments is primarily a measure of the neurophysiological parameters of the cerebral metabolic rate of glucose consumption, the cerebral metabolic rate of oxygen consumption, or cerebral blood flow (CBF). PET methods have been developed for measuring each of these three parameters separately, while fMRI signals respond to differences in the changes in CBF and the cerebral metabolic rate of oxygen consumption, whose quantitative relationships are being investigated. The cerebral metabolic rate of glucose consumption and the cerebral metabolic rate of oxygen consumption measure cerebral energy consumption, while the change in each measures its increment. The unsolved "hard" problem of neuroscience: what is the relationship between mental processes and neuronal activity? (From Shulman, 2001 with permission).

resolution (Turkington, 2001). While these performance characteristics of the PET scanner are important, the PET scanner's main advantage over gamma cameras is its unique ability to quantitatively image in vivo the only radioactive forms of common atoms in living systems that can be detected externally: the positron-emitting forms of oxygen, carbon, nitrogen and fluorine. Since an organic molecule labeled with a positron emitting atom will behave exactly like the naturally occurring molecule, it allows the investigator to obtain a quantitative image of the bio-distribution of the molecules so labeled at a given point in time (Moresco *et al.*, 2001).

The accurate relationship of the signal obtained from PET or SPECT to mental processes involves model-based methodology (Frankle *et al.*, 2005) (Figure 16.2). These tools are currently being used in schizophrenia research to: (i) investigate the pre-, post- and intra-synaptic abnormalities of dopaminergic and serotonergic systems, (ii) compare the dopaminergic, serotonergic, glutamatergic receptor binding between patients and controls, and (iii) assess the magnitude of occupancy of the target sites of action of antipsychotics relative to treatment response, drug concentrations and side-effects (for reviews see Kasper *et al.*, 1999; Soares & Innis, 1999; Verhoeff, 1999).

Studies of neurotransmitters

Neurochemical brain imaging of schizophrenia largely began in the early 1980s and focused on SPECT and PET measurements of post-synaptic dopamine receptors, using radiolabeled ligands for dopamine D1 and D2 receptors. Early work suggested that there was an increase in the density of post-synaptic D2 receptors in the striatum (Wong *et al.*, 1986), although this finding was not replicated in later studies (Nordstrom *et al.*, 1995; Pilowsky *et al.*, 1994). However a meta-analysis of the literature suggests that there is a modest but significant increase in D2 receptor density in schizophrenia (Laruelle, 1998). Extensions of these initial SPECT and PET receptor imaging studies have examined pre-synaptic targets (e.g. dopamine synthesis) and the "intra-synaptic" levels of the transmitter itself, assessed with stimulant-induced release (for review see Volkow *et al.*, 1996). The pre-synaptic site can be labeled with probes for the dopamine transporter (DAT) or the synthetic enzyme aromatic L-amino acid decarboxylase ("dopa decarboxylase"). PET studies indicate that striatal dopamine transporter (DAT) binding in vivo is unaltered in neuroleptic-naïve first-episode schizophrenic patients (Laakso *et al.*, 2000) but decreased in chronic schizophrenia (Laakso *et al.*, 2001), suggesting a relative loss of striatal dopaminergic nerve terminals and/or decreased expression of DAT in a subset of chronic schizophrenic patients. Studies with fluorodopa have consistently found that both first-episode and chronic schizophrenia is associated with increased pre-synaptic dopamine activity (McGowan *et al.*, 2004). The "synaptic" measurements are made indirectly by measurements of the interaction/displacement of receptor tracers by endogenous dopamine (DA). Agents are used which either release (e.g. amphetamine) or deplete (e.g. alpha-methyl-paratyrosine (AMPT) an inhibitor of tyrosine hydroxylase) tissue stores of DA (Verhoeff, 1999). Studies of transmitter release suggest that schizophrenia is associated with increased amphetamine-induced DA release in the striatum, most pronounced during episodes of illness exacerbation (Abi-Dargham *et al.*, 2004).

Receptor binding

PET and SPECT techniques have been used to compare binding to the receptors of transmitters implicated in psychosis in schizophrenic patients and controls (e.g. DR1-4, 5HT2, NMDA). While the D2 receptor has been examined in several studies (Corripio *et al.*, 2006) (Figure 16.3), more recently PET/SPECT research addressed the role of D1 (Karlsson *et al.*, 2002) and D3 (Yang *et al.*, 2004) receptor binding in the pathophysiology of schizophrenia. Central serotonergic function has been assessed

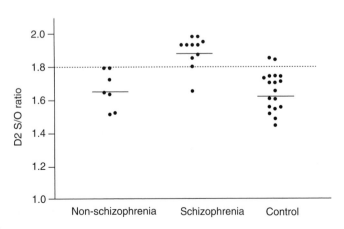

Figure 16.3. D2 receptor binding (measured as D2 striatum/occipital ratio, D2 S/0) at diagnosis in schizophrenia, non-schizophrenia and control groups. Dotted line shows the threshold ratio (D2 S/O > 1.8) (From Corripio *et al.*, 2006 with permission. Copyright © 2005 Elsevier Inc. All rights reserved.)

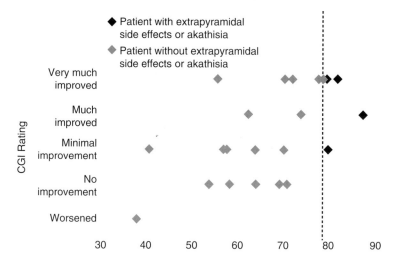

Figure 16.4. Relation of dopamine D2 occupancy to the Clinical Global Impression scale (CGI) among patients with first-episode schizophrenia receiving haloperidol. Dotted line indicates 78% D2 occupancy, which was associated with a significantly greater likelihood of extrapyramidal side effects or akathisia (From Kapur *et al.*, 2000 with permission.)

in PET studies investigating 5-HT2A and 5-HT1A binding potentials (Lewis *et al.*, 1999). Finally, reductions in NMDA receptor binding in the left hippocampus have recently been described in medication-free, but not antipsychotic-treated schizophrenic patients, implicating modulation of glutamate dysfunction at NMDA receptors by antipsychotic drugs (Pilowsky *et al.*, 2006).

Studies of medication occupancy

Using PET and SPET techniques, pharmacokinetic behavior may be detailed and pharmacodynamic relationships defined. The models derived from these techniques complement, and in some instances may supersede animal behavior models. SPET and PET measurements of striatal D2 receptor occupancy have informed the use of antipsychotic drugs, as they have revealed that the 70% level of occupancy associated with a therapeutic response could be achieved with what was initially regarded as relatively low doses of medication (for a review see Grunder *et al.*, 2003). Moreover, once this level has been reached, further increases in dose have little additional therapeutic effect, and only serve to increase the risk of motor side-effects (Farde *et al.*, 1992; Kapur *et al.*, 2000) (Figure 16.4).

PET and SPECT can also be used to measure blood flow and metabolism, and thus assess neural activity (McGuire *et al.*, 1993). However, while these techniques can still be very usefully employed in this

way, most current neuroimaging studies aimed at assessing regional neural activity use functional MRI.

Functional magnetic resonance imaging

Principles of blood oxygenation level dependent (BOLD) fMRI

A functional imaging study involves the collection of images, which show signal changes that reflect neural activity. Its superior temporal and spatial resolution compared with SPECT and PET has established fMRI as the major tool for the study of regional activity in relation to neuropsychology in mental disorders (for reviews see Honey *et al.*, 2002a; McGuire & Matsumoto, 2004). In particular, this technique has been recently used to address the pathophysiology of schizophrenia from its early stages (Fusar-Poli *et al.*, 2007b). Functional MRI generally involves the acquisition of a large series of images in each subject, and to compensate for subject head movement it is usual to realign the images to one of the images in the series. In most studies the statistical analysis is conducted after the images from each subject in a group are transformed into a standard stereotactic space, such as that described by Talairach & Tournoux (1988). This is designed to facilitate comparison of the same region in brain images from different subjects that may have different sizes and shapes. Following this spatial normalization, statistical analysis may involve a number of methods, most of which result in some index at each voxel of how the brain has responded to the experimental manipulation of interest. In the final step of the analysis, voxels where there is a significant difference in signal are displayed, producing a statistical map of activation in the brain (Figure 16.5).

Block design studies

Block design fMRI generally involves "epochs" of different conditions (Friston *et al.*, 1998), often alternated during the scanning session. Commonly, the comparison of two or more conditions that are intended to differ in the demands on the aspects of cognitive or emotional processing of interest is conducted. For example, in a verbal fluency task subjects may be required to articulate words beginning with a presented letter in one condition, and to simply articulate the presented letter (without generating a word) in the other (Holt *et al.*, 2005). The basic theoretical principle behind this design is cognitive subtraction (Friston *et al.*, 1996). This assumes that differences in activation between the conditions are related to the differences in the demands of the two conditions. However, the conditions employed may differ in several ways, making interpretation difficult. This potential confound can be minimized by making the two conditions as similar as possible, with the exception of the specific cognitive/emotional component of interest.

Event-related design studies

A limitation of block design techniques is the lack of information regarding the time-course of an individual response within a block. In an event-related design, images are acquired serially after discrete stimuli or responses. The importance of event-related fMRI is that it allows the response to a single event to be examined in a context independent fashion (Friston *et al.*, 1998). By averaging data acquired after many such discrete events, the time course of the hemodynamic response can be thus defined. The major drawback of this approach is sensitivity: an fMRI study that attempts to measure individual events (event-related fMRI) may demonstrate less robust results than one in which several events are averaged in a blocked design (Rosen & Gur 2002).

Psychopharmacological fMRI studies

Recently, there has been growing interest in using fMRI for the evaluation of psychopharmacological agents. These are often compounds known to act on central transmitter systems, such as amphetamine (influencing dopamine release), tryptophan depletion (affecting serotonin function) and ketamine (acting at NMDA receptors). This approach provides a means of examining the interaction between a given transmitter system and the cognitive or emotional processes engaged by the fMRI paradigm. Although this approach can be combined with resting state studies, using a cognitive task increases the likelihood that the mental activity being modulated by the drug is similar across subjects. fMRI studies of this kind in schizophrenia have also included investigations of the acute (Fusar-Poli *et al.*, 2007a) and long-term effects of antipsychotic medication (Davis *et al.*, 2005). For example, substitution of risperidone for typical antipsychotic drugs in the treatment of schizophrenia has been associated with enhanced functional activation of frontal cortex, indicating the potential value of fMRI as a tool for longitudinal assessment of psychopharmacological effects on cerebral physiology (Honey *et al.*, 1999).

Neural correlates of specific symptoms

The ultimate validity of a case-control methodology, in which a diagnostic category (such as schizophrenia) is a necessary and sufficient inclusion criterion, hinges upon the validity of the taxonomy used. However, psychiatric conditions are not discrete and homogeneous entities, and this could explain some (although by no means uniquely) inconclusive aspects of the functional imaging research of schizophrenia. To avoid the problems highlighted with disease level categories, neuroimaging research has alternatively focused on the major symptoms of psychosis. In accordance with such arguments, some functional imaging studies have adopted the symptom approach to schizophrenia research, focusing on auditory hallucinations (McGuire *et al.*, 1995; Woodruff *et al.*, 1997) and formal thought disorder (Kircher *et al.*, 2001). For example, the severity of positive formal thought disorder has been inversely correlated with the level of activity in the left superior temporal cortex, a region implicated in the production of coherent speech, suggesting that reduced activity in

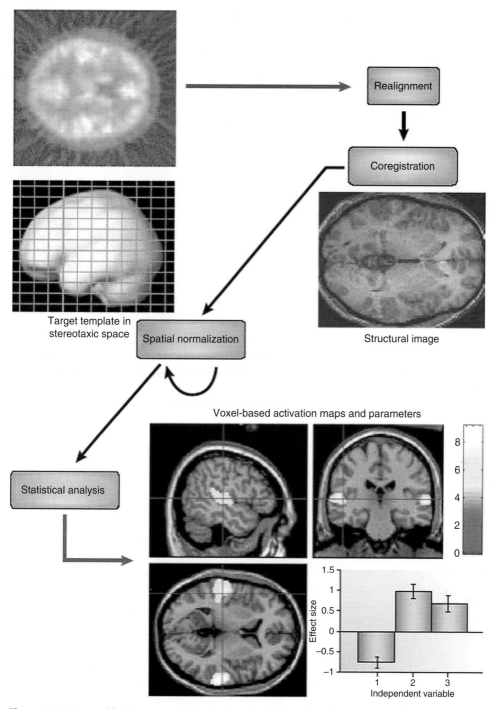

Target template in
stereotaxic space

Structural image

Voxel-based activation maps and parameters

Independent variable

Figure 16.5. Stages of fMRI image processing. The functional images for each subject are realigned to correct for subject movement, and then coregistered with a structural image. If required, the images are spatially normalized to align brains across subjects. Statistical analysis attempts to detect areas that have been activated by the experimental manipulation. The results can be displayed on individual or average structural images (From Brett *et al.*, 2002 with permission. Copyright © 2002, Nature Publishing Group.)

this area might contribute to the articulation of incoherent speech (Kircher *et al.*, 2001).

Parametric design studies

Parametric studies are useful for determining whether neural responses are linear, non-linear, whether they vary in different regions of the brain, and whether they have any specific relevance to any cognitive function (Buchel *et al.*, 1998). They are based on the assumption that the magnitude of the hemodynamic response changes as a function of cognitive load, or of another continuous variable such as symptom severity or dose of medication. This approach raises concerns about the interpretation of subtractive designs and the validity of rest/baseline conditions. In psychiatric research, these studies are often used to explore how regional activity varies with parametrically increasing task demand, and provide a means of clarifying whether activation during cognitive tasks reflects the operation of general processes associated with task difficulty and mental effort, or even specific components of the tasks themselves.

Functional connectivity studies

Although schizophrenia has been associated with regional functional deficits, it has not been possible to explain the complex features of the disorder on the basis of discrete focal abnormalities. This has led to the suggestion that the core pathology of schizophrenia could be based within abnormal interactions or disconnectivity between a distributed network of brain regions (Friston, 1998; McGuire & Frith 1996). In neuroimaging, this can be assessed in terms of functional connectivity, defined as *the temporal correlations between spatially remote neurophysiological events* (Friston *et al.*, 1993). Functional connectivity is simply a statement about correlations and does not necessarily infer that the correlations are based on anatomical connections. A related concept is effective connectivity, *the influence one neuronal system exerts over another* (Friston *et al.*, 1993). Effective connectivity is closer to the notion of a connection and is estimated using a mathematical model that describes how activity in two areas is related, and a neuroanatomical model based on knowledge of the projections between them. A range of methods can be used to assess effective connectivity, such as multiple linear regression, covariance structural equation modeling and variable parametric

regression. Early connectivity studies examined correlations between spontaneously active regions in normal subjects during the resting state, learning (McIntosh & Gonzalez-Lima 1998), auditory (McIntosh *et al.*, 1998) and mnemonic processes (McIntosh, 1999). Schizophrenic subjects have been investigated with both resting-state fMRI and conventional task activation methods. The first approach showed a decreased functional connectivity during rest, providing quantitative support for the hypothesis that schizophrenia may arise from the disrupted functional integration of widespread brain areas (Liang *et al.*, 2006). The latter strategy has been applied to investigate the cortico-cerebellar-thalamo-cortical disconnectivity associated with cognitive dysmetria (Honey *et al.*, 2005); the prefrontal functional disconnectivity characterizing the schizophrenic phenotype (Frith *et al.*, 1995; Spence *et al.*, 2000); and the neural basis of hallucinations and delusions (Frith 2005). For example, it has been demonstrated that defective communication between frontal and temporal areas leads to the misidentification of internally generated verbal material as "alien" speech, and is likely a critical factor underlying auditory hallucinations in schizophrenia (Shergill *et al.*, 2002). Key areas for future connectivity research in schizophrenia concern the mechanisms underlying specific signs and symptoms associated with illness (Frith, 1997), the effects of antipsychotics on cerebral functional connectivity (Stephan *et al.*, 2001), and the evaluation of genetically mediated functional disconnectivity in subjects at high genetic risk of schizophrenia (Whalley *et al.*, 2005).

Limits

One of the main limitations of this technique is the issue of task-related co-activity. If two regions are both activated by a task, they will inevitably be seen to be co-active and hence viewed as functionally connected (Xiong *et al.*, 1999). Therefore, examining connectivity that is not modulated by transient activity associated with task-related activation may be more related to underlying anatomical connectivity (Koch *et al.*, 2002). Several approaches have been undertaken to overcome this problem: (i) via the exclusion of rest or baseline conditions, and examining correlations during 'active' periods only (Just *et al.*, 2004), or in a cognitive-load dependent fashion (Fu *et al.*, 2006; Honey *et al.*, 2002b); (ii) by the implementation of statistical methods to remove effects of task activation from the data (Arfanakis *et al.*, 2000). Furthermore, time resolution is limited by the rate of the hemodynamic response, which occurs over a time-course that is orders of magnitude slower than the primary neural response. This technique has intrinsically low signal-to-noise and contrast-to-noise, which leads to the need for repetition of stimuli in order to decrease variance in results. Finally, even though functional brain connectivity is an influential concept in modern cognitive neuroscience, it remains a very controversial notion (for a critical review on functional connectivity see Fingelkurts & Kahkonen, 2005).

Diffusion tensor imaging (DTI)

Diffusion tensor imaging (DTI) is a relatively new neuroimaging technique that can be used to examine the microstructure of white matter in vivo (for a review on DTI principles see Le Bihan *et al.*, 2001). Diffusion tensor imaging uses a conventional MRI scanner; however, by imposing additional magnetic field gradients, the scanned images are sensitized to the diffusion of water in the direction of those gradients. Fractional anisotropy (FA) roughly represents the degree to which diffusion is directionally hindered (anisotropic). It is high in areas of high structural coherence, such as white matter (WM), lower in gray matter (GM), and close to zero in cerebrospinal fluid (CSF), where diffusion is expected to be equal in all directions (isotropic) (Kanaan *et al.*, 2005) (Figure 16.6). A reduction in WM FA is therefore usually interpreted as reflecting a reduction in WM integrity. As with volumetric MRI, there are two principal methods employed in the analysis of FA: region of interest (ROI) and whole-brain and voxel-based analysis. The majority of studies to date have adopted the former, manually defining ROIs on the unregistered images. This allows a powerful examination of regions selected on the basis of existing information. However, because the placement of ROIs is subjective, this should be guided by unambiguous criteria and with demonstrated inter-rater/intra-rater reliability (Kanaan *et al.*, 2005) (for review on DTI in mental disorders see Taylor *et al.*, 2004).

In the case of schizophrenia, in which the regions of white matter abnormality are still being determined and the alterations may be distributed rather than focal, a voxel-based approach may be a more useful alternative. However, there are particular difficulties in the stereotactic normalization of DTI data and this approach has yet to be well established. Interest in disconnectivity models of schizophrenia (Liang *et al.*, 2006; Whalley *et al.*, 2005) has led to an increasing focus on white matter. Most DTI studies in schizophrenia found significant FA differences between patients and controls in different brain areas, although others found only negative results (for reviews on DTI in schizophrenia see Kanaan *et al.*, 2005; Kubicki *et al.*, 2005). Results of these studies are frequently inconsistent as there are no accepted gold standards for data acquisition, processing and analysis. In addition, several different factors could affect the results including small sample size (Type II errors), different ROI definitions, low signal-to-noise ratio, different number of acquisition angles and different scanner gradient performance and field strength, as well as partial volume effects due to the low image resolution. Diffusion tensor imaging findings in schizophrenia should therefore be interpreted within the context of the acquisition parameters used, as well as in the context of the different methodological strategies adopted by different investigators (Kanaan *et al.*, 2005; Kubicki *et al.*, 2005). Diffusion tensor imaging is still a relatively immature research

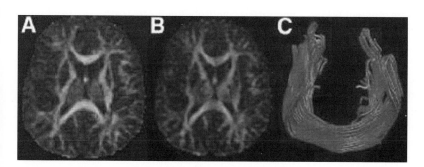

Figure 16.6. This figure is also reproduced in the color plate section. Representations of diffusion tensor imaging datasets. (A) A fractional anisotropy (FA) axial slice from a single subject. (B) FA slice, colored to represent directions: red, left-right; green, anterior-posterior; blue, superior-inferior. (C) Tractography performed on the genu of the same subject (From Kanaan *et al.*, 2005 with permission. Copyright © 2005 Society of Biological Psychiatry.)

technique and the methods of image acquisition and analysis are still evolving. Some of the inconsistency of the findings across DTI studies in schizophrenia to date may therefore be related to differences in methodology (Basser & Jones 2002). Studies involving larger, more homogeneous patient groups, such as those defined by a common phase of illness and treatment (Kumra *et al.*, 2004) or by symptom profile (Hubl *et al.*, 2004) may improve its potential as a means of examining anatomical connectivity. Combining DTI with data from other imaging modalities may shed light on the nature of FA deficits detected and allow the correlation of structure and function (Toosy *et al.*, 2004), although there have been few such studies to date. Finally, the promise of DTI in schizophrenia research may be more fully realized through fiber tractography (Kanaan *et al.*, 2006). Tractography usually takes an initial ROI and traces the fiber tracts using the diffusion tensor. The validity of these putative "tracts" is difficult to ascertain due to a lack of neuroanatomical standards, however (Catani *et al.*, 2002). With tractography, researchers may be able to define WM tracts and examine measures of WM integrity (such as FA) on a tract-by-tract basis (Kanaan *et al.*, 2006). For example, recent measurements of mean diffusivity in early-onset schizophrenia were performed within fronto-temporal fasciculi by forming 3D reconstructions of the cingulum, uncinate, superior longitudinal and inferior fronto-occipital fasciculi using diffusion tensor tractography (Jones *et al.*, 2006).

Magnetic resonance spectroscopy (MRS)

Magnetic resonance spectroscopy is a complex and sophisticated neuroimaging technique that allows reliable and reproducible quantification of brain neurochemistry, provided its limitations are acknowledged. Magnetic resonance spectroscopy imaging (MRSI) can be used to provide information on the relative concentration and distribution of compounds of ions with nuclei that have a magnetic moment (1H, 13C, 31P, 23Na). There are large differences between resonance frequencies for different nuclei in an applied magnetic field. Even the same nuclei will resonate at slightly different frequencies in different molecules or at different positions in a molecule (Malhi *et al.*, 2002). Furthermore, the use of MR imaging plus MR spectroscopy provides a unique advantage, because information on cerebral structure and physiology can be gleaned in vivo in a non-invasive fashion in the same session on the same patients (Stanley, 2002). In some branches of medicine, this technique is already used clinically, for instance, to diagnose tumors. In psychiatry, MRS applications are extending beyond research. It allows direct in vivo measurement of medication levels within the brain (lithium), endogenous cerebral metabolites (glutamate, GABA), and macromolecules such as synaptic proteins (Keshavan *et al.*, 2000; Stanley *et al.*, 2000) (for reviews on MRs in psychiatry see Lyoo & Renshaw, 2002; Malhi *et al.*, 2002; Stanley, 2002; for reviews on MRS applications in schizophrenia see Keshavan *et al.*, 1997; Stanley *et al.*, 2000). Two MRS-visible nuclei have been widely used in MRS studies in psychiatry: phosphorus-31 (31P) and hydrogen-1 (1H).

In vivo phosphorus magnetic resonance spectroscopy (31P MRS) is a non-invasive technique that can assess the membrane phospholipid and high-energy phosphate metabolism in localized brain regions (Stanley, 2002), revealing important information about the integrity of neuronal cell membranes. Specifically, the phosphomonoester (PME) resonance in 31P MRS includes the freely mobile precursors of membrane phospholipids such as phosphocholine, phosphoethanolamine; the phosphodiester (PDE) resonance comprises breakdown products such as glycerophosphocholine and glycerophosphoethanolamine (Pettegrew *et al.*, 1987). Observations that schizophrenia is associated with reduced prefrontal function and membrane phospholipid alterations in peripheral cells (Horrobin *et al.*, 1994) stimulated early 31P MRS studies. Overall, there appear to be alterations in membrane phospholipids in the fronto-temporal regions in schizophrenia, especially in first-episode patients (Jensen *et al.*, 2006). The pathophysiological basis of 31P MRS alterations in schizophrenia has been much debated. Decreased PMEs and increased PDEs have been thought to reflect decreased synthesis and increased breakdown of membrane phospholipids in early schizophrenia (Klemm *et al.*, 2001). The possibility that these alterations may represent "trait" markers underscores the importance of MRS studies in genetically at-risk subjects for schizophrenia (Fukuzako *et al.*, 1999). Consistently, young offspring at risk for schizophrenia are found to have a decreased synthesis of membrane phospholipids, as well as an altered content or molecular environment of synaptic vesicles in the prefrontal cortex (Keshavan *et al.*, 2003).

Hydrogen-1 MRS can be used to measure the second most abundant amino acid, *N*-Acetyl aspartate (NAA), which can be localized to neurons and is thought to reflect overall neuronal functional integrity (Maier *et al.*, 1995) (for a review on 1H MRS in schizophrenia see Steen *et al.*, 2005). Evidence has accumulated to suggest that there are NAA reductions among schizophrenic patients in the frontal lobe and the hippocampus, although these differences may be rather subtle (Steen *et al.*, 2005). Though the pathophysiological significance of NAA reduction in schizophrenia remains unclear, reduced NAA may reflect the volume loss observed in the temporal and frontal cortex (McCarley *et al.*, 1999) and may be related to reductions in synaptic neuropil or to changes in energy metabolism. Another intriguing question is whether neuronal damage, potentially detectable via lower NAA, may characterize individuals at risk for schizophrenia. Consistently, significant NAA reductions in hippocampal area and ventral prefrontal cortex were observed respectively in unaffected siblings of patients with schizophrenia (Callicott *et al.*, 1998) and in offspring at risk for schizophrenia (Keshavan *et al.*, 1997). In a later work, however, Wood and colleagues failed to find reduced levels of hippocampal NAA in individuals at ultra-high risk of psychosis (Wood *et al.*, 2003) but different methodological issues may have played a significant role in generating these contrasting findings.

Levels of glutamate, glutamine, total creatine, choline-containing compounds, taurine, *scyllo*-inositol and *myo*-inositol can be measured simultaneously by using in vivo short-echo-time 1H MRS. Given the putative role of NMDA receptors in the pathophysiology of psychosis (Farber, 2003), measures of glutamate might be particularly instructive. A higher level of glutamine has been observed using such methods in the anterior cingulate and thalamus of never-treated first-episode psychosis, consistent with the glutamatergic models of schizophrenia (Theberge *et al.*, 2002). Similarly, glutamate/glutamine has been shown to be significantly higher in subjects at increased genetic risk for schizophrenia as compared with healthy subjects (Tibbo *et al.*, 2004).

Finally, both proton and phosphorus MR have been used to study the pathophysiology of other psychiatric conditions such as major depression, bipolar disorders, panic disorders, obsessive-compulsive disorders, post-traumatic stress disorders and substance abuse, and to address the pharmacokinetic and pharmacodynamic properties of a number of psychotropic medications in the human brain (Lyoo & Renshaw, 2002).

Integration of imaging data across modalities

The complementary strengths and weaknesses of available neuroimaging techniques have driven efforts by a number of investigators to combine data from multiple imaging modalities. The integration of imaging data across modalities, such as fMRI-sMRI co-registration, magnetoencephalography and a combination of fMRI and electrophysiological techniques is of great interest, given that it would be very useful to know the relationship between abnormalities of structure, function and neurochemistry. To date, however, this has rarely been done. This is because most neuroimaging studies do not collect multiple types of imaging data from the same subjects, partly because it is both logistically difficult and financially expensive to examine the same individual with several methods. In addition, techniques for directly integrating data of different types are not well established.

Volumetric MRI and fMRI co-registration

While co-registration of changes in blood oxygenation levels or blood flow rates onto structural MRI scans of individual brains can be achieved with high levels of accuracy, grouping these data for quantitative comparisons (e.g. between diagnostic groups) poses a major methodological challenge due to the inter-individual variability of regional brain morphology (Brett *et al.*, 2002). Joint independent component analysis (jICA) is a novel methodology useful to perform independent component analysis across image modalities; specifically, gray matter images and fMRI activation images, as well as a joint histogram visualization techniques (James & Hesse, 2005). For example, using this approach, schizophrenic patients showed an association between low gray matter concentration and low hemodynamic activity in bilateral anterior temporal regions while performing a target detection in an auditory oddball fMRI task (Calhoun *et al.*, 2006).

An alternative strategy to overcome such difficulty is the application of cortical pattern-matching methodologies that permit aggregation of imaging datasets in the same anatomical reference locations across subjects, explicitly modeling and adjusting for

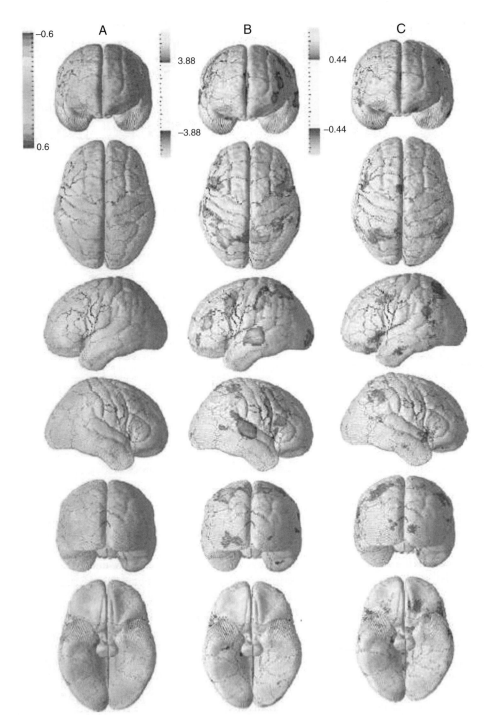

Figure 16.7. This figure is also reproduced in the color plate section. Combined structural and functional magnetic resonance imaging data of first-episode schizophrenia patients and matched healthy control subjects. Views from top to bottom: frontal, superior, left lateral, right lateral, posterior and inferior. Brodmann areas are warped into the probabilistic model of the brain surface. (A) Unthresholded correlation maps of cortical gray matter thickness by group. Positive values indicate increased gray matter while negative values indicate reduced gray matter in patients, particularly in the right anterior temporal lobe, prefrontal, frontal and parietal cortex and hippocampus. (B) Combined group BOLD response as a function of task difficulty when performing the Tower of London task showing increasing activation in the prefrontal and parietal cortex and a negative BOLD response predominantly in the superior and middle temporal gyrus. (C) Correlation maps of cortical gray matter thickness by BOLD response suggest reduced BOLD response with decreased cortical gray matter thickness in the left prefrontal, right orbitofrontal, right superior temporal and bilateral parietal cortices across groups (From Rasser *et al.*, 2005 with permission. Copyright © 2005 Published by Elsevier Inc.)

individual differences in the cortical folding pattern as well as in overall brain size (Thompson *et al.*, 2001, 2003). Cortical pattern matching has been applied in a recent study to compare the spatial properties of brain activation of first-episode schizophrenia patients with those of matched healthy control subjects when performing the Tower of London (TOL) task. Reduced regional gray-matter thickness correlated with reduced left-hemispheric prefrontal/frontal and bilateral parietal BOLD activation in first-episode patients (Figure 16.7). This study demonstrated that reduction of regional gray matter in first-episode schizophrenia patients was associated with impaired brain function when performing executive attention and working memory (Rasser *et al.*, 2005).

Magnetoencephalography

Magnetoencephalography (MEG) measures the extracranial magnetic fields produced by intraneuronal ionic current flow within appropriately oriented cortical pyramidal cells. Magnetoencephalography offers excellent temporal and spatial resolution for selected sources, and can complement information obtained from electroencephalograms and other functional imaging strategies. Magnetoencephalographic studies of schizophrenia have shown disturbances in cerebral lateralization (Reite *et al.*, 1989), short-term auditory memory (Reite *et al.*, 1996), somatosensory processing, cortical reorganization (Rojas *et al.*, 1997) and P50 response (Clementz *et al.*, 1997) (for a review see Reite *et al.*, 1999). One limitation of this technique is that it can only measure surface activity and not activity in subcortical structures.

Combination of functional neuroimaging and electrophysiological techniques

With the improvement of whole-head sensor arrays and improved analytical strategies, neural electromagnetic techniques (MEG, EEG and related methods) are becoming increasingly important tools for human brain mapping (Hamalainen, 1992). In fact, one limitation of fMRI/PET is their relatively low temporal resolution. Electroencephalography (EEG)/MEG signals have a higher temporal resolution but poorer spatial resolution. One of the most promising perspectives in neuropsychological research of mental disorder is the combination of electrophysiological (EEG/MEG) measures with fMRI/PET; this combines the high temporal resolution of the former with the

high spatial resolution of the latter (Ashburner & Friston 1997; Gallinat & Heinz 2006). There are now several classes of computational techniques that allow the integration of data from MEG and MRI to improve the accuracy and reliability of fMRI by MEG (George *et al.*, 1995), although collecting both types of data in the scanner is technically difficult, particularly in the case of fMRI, as the magnetic field can interfere with the electrophysiological signal. Nevertheless such studies are beginning to be applied in basic neurosciences (Laufs *et al.*, 2006) and in schizophrenia research (Kircher *et al.*, 2004).

Conclusions

In the past ten years, rapid improvements in imaging technology and methodology have had an enormous impact on our understanding of the neurocognitive basis of psychiatric disorders. Detailed images of the anatomy of gray and white matter can be obtained using sMRI and DTI, while fMRI is a key tool to address the neurofunctional abnormalities underlying mental diseases. The main transmitter systems implicated in psychiatric disorders can be examined in vivo using SPECT and PET, while the biochemistry of the brain can be investigated using MRS. While further advances are likely with technological improvements, neuroimaging may prove particularly useful when it is applied to larger samples than have been examined hitherto: this may entail the pooling of data from different centers, and reliable methods for this are under development (Poline *et al.*, 1996; Schnack *et al.*, 2004; Stocker *et al.*, 2005). The potential of neuroimaging may also be realized when data are integrated across imaging modalities and with other forms of data, such as electrophysiological, neuropsychological and genetic information.

References

Abi-Dargham, A., Kegeles, L. S., Zea-Ponce, Y. *et al.* (2004). Striatal amphetamine-induced dopamine release in patients with schizotypal personality disorder studied with single photon emission computed tomography and [123I]iodobenzamide. *Biological Psychiatry*, **55**, 1001–1006.

Arfanakis, K., Cordes, D., Haughton, V. M. *et al.* (2000). Combining independent component analysis and correlation analysis to probe interregional connectivity in fMRI task activation datasets. *Magnetic Resonance Imaging*, **18**, 921–930.

Ashburner, J. & Friston, K. (1997). Multimodal image coregistration and partitioning – a unified framework. *Neuroimage*, **6**, 209–217.

Ashburner, J. & Friston, K. J. (2000). Voxel-based morphometry – the methods. *Neuroimage*, **11**, 805–821.

Basser, P. J. & Jones, D. K. (2002). Diffusion-tensor MRI: theory, experimental design and data analysis – a technical review. *NMR Biomedicine*, **15**, 456–467.

Bookstein, F. L. (2001). "Voxel-based morphometry" should not be used with imperfectly registered images. *Neuroimage*, **14**, 1454–1462.

Borgwardt, S. J., Radue, E. W., Gotz, K. *et al.* (2006). Radiological findings in individuals at high risk of psychosis. *Journal of Neurology, Neurosurgery and Psychiatry*, 77, 229–233.

Brett, M., Johnsrude, I. S. & Owen, A. M. (2002). The problem of functional localization in the human brain. *Nature Reviews Neuroscience*, 3, 243–249.

Buchel, C., Holmes, A. P., Rees, G. & Friston, K. J. (1998). Characterizing stimulus-response functions using nonlinear regressors in parametric fMRI experiments. *Neuroimage*, **8**, 140–148.

Calhoun, V. D., Adali, T., Giuliani, N. R. *et al.* (2006). Method for multimodal analysis of independent source differences in schizophrenia: combining gray matter structural and auditory oddball functional data. *Human Brain Mapping*, **27**, 47–62.

Callicott, J. H., Egan, M. F., Bertolino, A. *et al.* (1998). Hippocampal N-acetyl aspartate in unaffected siblings of patients with schizophrenia: a possible intermediate neurobiological phenotype. *Biological Psychiatry*, **44**, 941–950.

Catani, M., Howard, R. J., Pajevic, S. & Jones, D. K. (2002). Virtual in vivo interactive dissection of white matter fasciculi in the human brain. *Neuroimage*, **17**, 77–94.

Clementz, B. A., Blumenfeld, L. D. & Cobb, S. (1997). The gamma band response may account for poor P50 suppression in schizophrenia. *Neuroreport*, **8**, 3889–3893.

Corripio, I., Perez, V., Catafau, A. M. *et al.* (2006). Striatal D2 receptor binding as a marker of prognosis and outcome in untreated first-episode psychosis. *Neuroimage*, **29**, 662–666.

Costa, D. C., Pilowsky, L. S. & Ell, P. J. (1999). Nuclear medicine in neurology and psychiatry. *Lancet*, **354**, 1107–1111.

Davis, C. E., Jeste, D. V. & Eyler, L. T. (2005). Review of longitudinal functional neuroimaging studies of drug treatments in patients with schizophrenia. *Schizophrenia Research*, **78**, 45–60.

Diwadkar, V. A. & Keshavan, M. S. (2002). Newer techniques in magnetic resonance imaging and their potential for neuropsychiatric research. *Journal of Psychosomatic Research*, **53**, 677–685.

Farber, N. B. (2003). The NMDA receptor hypofunction model of psychosis. *Annals of the New York Academy of Sciences*, **1003**, 119–130.

Farde, L., Nordstrom, A. L., Wiesel, F. A. *et al.* (1992). Positron emission tomographic analysis of central D1 and D2 dopamine receptor occupancy in patients treated with classical neuroleptics and clozapine. Relation to extrapyramidal side effects. *Archives of General Psychiatry*, **49**, 538–544.

Fingelkurts, A. A. & Kahkonen, S. (2005). Functional connectivity in the brain – is it an elusive concept? *Neuroscience and Biobehavior Review*, **28**, 827–836.

Frankle, W. G., Slifstein, M., Talbot, P. S. & Laruelle, M. (2005). Neuroreceptor imaging in psychiatry: theory and applications. *International Review of Neurobiology*, **67**, 385–440.

Friston, K. J. (1998). The disconnection hypothesis. *Schizophrenia Research*, **30**, 115–125.

Friston, K. J., Fletcher, P., Josephs, O. *et al.* (1998). Event-related fMRI: characterizing differential responses. *Neuroimage*, **7**, 30–40.

Friston, K. J., Frith, C. D., Liddle, P. F. & Frackowiak, R. S. (1993). Functional connectivity: the principal-component analysis of large (PET) data sets. *Journal of Cerebral Blood Flow and Metabolism*, **13**, 5–14.

Friston, K. J., Price, C. J., Fletcher, P. *et al.* (1996). The trouble with cognitive subtraction. *Neuroimage*, **4**, 97–104.

Frith, C. (2005). The neural basis of hallucinations and delusions. *C R Biol*, **328**, 169–175.

Frith, C. D. (1997). Functional brain imaging and the neuropathology of schizophrenia. *Schizophrenia Bulletin*, **23**, 525–527.

Frith, C. D., Friston, K. J., Herold, S. *et al.* (1995). Regional brain activity in chronic schizophrenic patients during the performance of a verbal fluency task. *British Journal of Psychiatry*, **167**, 343–349.

Fu, C. H., McIntosh, A. R., Kim, J. *et al.* (2006). Modulation of effective connectivity by cognitive demand in phonological verbal fluency. *Neuroimage*, **30**, 266–271.

Fukuzako, H., Fukuzako, T., Hashiguchi, T. *et al.* (1999). Changes in levels of phosphorus metabolites in temporal lobes of drug-naive schizophrenic patients. *American Journal of Psychiatry*, **156**, 1205–1208.

Fusar-Poli, P., Broome, M., Matthiasson, P. *et al.* (2007a). Effects of acute antipsychotic treatment on brain activation in first episode psychosis: an fMRI study. *European Neuropsychopharmacology*, **17**, 492–500.

Fusar-Poli, P., Perez, J., Broome, M. *et al.* (2007b). Neurofunctional correlates of vulnerability to psychosis: a systematic review and meta-analysis. *Neuroscience and Biobehavior Review*, **31**, 465–484.

Gallinat, J. & Heinz, A. (2006). Combination of multimodal imaging and molecular genetic information to investigate complex psychiatric disorders. *Pharmacopsychiatry*, **39**, 76–79.

Garner, B., Pariante, C. M., Wood, S. J. *et al.* (2005). Pituitary volume predicts future transition to psychosis in individuals at ultra-high risk of developing psychosis. *Biological Psychiatry*, **58**, 417–423.

George, J. S., Aine, C. J., Mosher, J. C. *et al.* (1995). Mapping function in the human brain with magnetoencephalography, anatomical magnetic resonance imaging, and functional magnetic resonance imaging. *Journal of Clinical Neurophysiology*, **12**, 406–431.

Gibby, W. A. (2005). Basic principles of magnetic resonance imaging. *Neurosurgery Clinics of North America*, **16**, 1–64.

Girgis, R. R., Diwadkar, V. A., Nutche, J. J. *et al.* (2006). Risperidone in first-episode psychosis: a longitudinal, exploratory voxel-based morphometric study. *Schizophrenia Research*, **82**, 89–94.

Giuliani, N. R., Calhoun, V. D., Pearlson, G. D., Francis, A. & Buchanan, R. W. (2005). Voxel-based morphometry versus region of interest: a comparison of two methods for analyzing gray matter differences in schizophrenia. *Schizophrenia Research*, **74**, 135–147.

Goldstein, J. M., Goodman, J. M., Seidman, L. J. *et al.* (1999). Cortical abnormalities in schizophrenia identified by structural magnetic resonance imaging. *Archives of General Psychiatry*, **56**, 537–547.

Grunder, G., Carlsson, A. & Wong, D. F. (2003). Mechanism of new antipsychotic medications: occupancy is not just antagonism. *Archives of General Psychiatry*, **60**, 974–977.

Hamalainen, M. S. (1992). Magnetoencephalography: a tool for functional brain imaging. *Brain Topography*, **5**, 95–102.

Holt, D. J., Kunkel, L., Weiss, A. P. *et al.* (2005). Increased medial temporal lobe activation during the passive viewing of emotional and neutral facial expressions in schizophrenia. *Schizophrenia Research*, **82**, 153–162.

Honea, R., Crow, T. J., Passingham, D. & Mackay, C. E. (2005). Regional deficits in brain volume in schizophrenia: a meta-analysis of voxel-based morphometry studies. *American Journal of Psychiatry*, **162**, 2233–2245.

Honey, G. D., Bullmore, E. T., Soni, W. *et al.* (1999). Differences in frontal cortical activation by a working memory task after substitution of risperidone for typical antipsychotic drugs in patients with schizophrenia. *Proceedings of the National Academy of Sciences USA*, **96**, 13432–13437.

Honey, G. D., Fletcher, P. C. & Bullmore, E. T. (2002a). Functional brain mapping of psychopathology. *Journal of Neurology, Neurosurgery and Psychiatry*, **72**, 432–439.

Honey, G. D., Fu, C. H., Kim, J. *et al.* (2002b). Effects of verbal working memory load on corticocortical connectivity modeled by path analysis of functional magnetic resonance imaging data. *Neuroimage*, **17**, 573–582.

Honey, G. D., Pomarol-Clotet, E., Corlett, P. R. *et al.* (2005). Functional dysconnectivity in schizophrenia associated with attentional modulation of motor function. *Brain*, **128**, 2597–2611.

Horrobin, D. F., Glen, A. I. & Vaddadi, K. (1994). The membrane hypothesis of schizophrenia. *Schizophrenia Research*, **13**, 195–207.

Hubl, D., Koenig, T., Strik, W. *et al.* (2004). Pathways that make voices: white matter changes in auditory hallucinations. *Archives of General Psychiatry*, **61**, 658–668.

James, C. J. & Hesse, C. W. (2005). Independent component analysis for biomedical signals. *Physiological Measurement*, **26**, R15–R39.

Jensen, J. E., Miller, J., Williamson, P. C. *et al.* (2006). Grey and white matter differences in brain energy metabolism in first episode schizophrenia: (31)P-MRS chemical shift imaging at 4 Tesla. *Psychiatry Research*, **146**, 127–135.

Jones, D. K., Catani, M., Pierpaoli, C. *et al.* (2006). Age effects on diffusion tensor magnetic resonance imaging tractography measures of frontal cortex connections in schizophrenia. *Human Brain Mapping*, **27**, 230–238.

Just, M. A., Cherkassky, V. L., Keller, T. A. & Minshew, N. J. (2004). Cortical activation and synchronization during sentence comprehension in high-functioning autism: evidence of underconnectivity. *Brain*, **127**, 1811–1821.

Kanaan, R. A., Kim, J. S., Kaufmann, W. E. *et al.* (2005). Diffusion tensor imaging in schizophrenia. *Biological Psychiatry*, **58**, 921–929.

Kanaan, R. A., Shergill, S. S., Barker, G. J. *et al.* (2006). Tract-specific anisotropy measurements in diffusion tensor imaging. *Psychiatry Research*, **146**, 73–82.

Kapur, S., Zipursky, R., Jones, C., Remington, G. & Houle, S. (2000). Relationship between dopamine D(2) occupancy, clinical response, and side effects: a double-blind PET study of first-episode schizophrenia. *American Journal of Psychiatry*, **157**, 514–520.

Karlsson, P., Farde, L., Halldin, C. & Sedvall, G. (2002). PET study of D(1) dopamine receptor binding in neuroleptic-naive patients with schizophrenia. *American Journal of Psychiatry*, **159**, 761–767.

Kasper, S., Tauscher, J., Kufferle, B. *et al.* (1999). Dopamine- and serotonin-receptors in schizophrenia: results of imaging-studies and implications for pharmacotherapy in schizophrenia. *European Archives of Psychiatry and Clinical Neuroscience*, **249**, 83–89.

Keshavan, M. S., Montrose, D. M., Pierri, J. N. *et al.* (1997). Magnetic resonance imaging and spectroscopy in offspring at risk for schizophrenia: preliminary studies. *Progress in Neuropsychopharmacology and Biological Psychiatry*, **21**, 1285–1295.

Keshavan, M. S., Stanley, J. A., Montrose, D. M., Minshew, N. J. & Pettegrew, J. W. (2003). Prefrontal membrane phospholipid metabolism of child and adolescent offspring at risk for schizophrenia or schizoaffective disorder: an in vivo 31P MRS study. *Molecular Psychiatry*, **8**, 316–323, 251.

Keshavan, M. S., Stanley, J. A. & Pettegrew, J. W. (2000). Magnetic resonance spectroscopy in schizophrenia: methodological issues and findings – part II. *Biological Psychiatry*, **48**, 369–380.

Kircher, T. T., Liddle, P. F., Brammer, M. J. *et al.* (2001). Neural correlates of formal thought disorder in schizophrenia: preliminary findings from a functional magnetic resonance imaging study. *Archives of General Psychiatry*, **58**, 769–774.

Kircher, T. T., Rapp, A., Grodd, W. *et al.* (2004). Mismatch negativity responses in schizophrenia: a combined fMRI and whole-head MEG study. *American Journal of Psychiatry*, **161**, 294–304.

Klemm, S., Rzanny, R., Riehemann, S. *et al.* (2001). Cerebral phosphate metabolism in first-degree relatives of patients with schizophrenia. *American Journal of Psychiatry*, **158**, 958–960.

Koch, M. A., Norris, D. G. & Hund-Georgiadis, M. (2002). An investigation of functional and anatomical connectivity using magnetic resonance imaging. *Neuroimage*, **16**, 241–250.

Konick, L. C. & Friedman, L. (2001). Meta-analysis of thalamic size in schizophrenia. *Biological Psychiatry*, **49**, 28–38.

Kubicki, M., Shenton, M. E., Salisbury, D. F. *et al.* (2002). Voxel-based morphometric analysis of gray matter in first episode schizophrenia. *Neuroimage*, **17**, 1711–1719.

Kubicki, M., Westin, C. F., McCarley, R. W. & Shenton, M. E. (2005). The application of DTI to investigate white matter abnormalities in schizophrenia. *Annals of the New York Academy of Sciences*, **1064**, 134–148.

Kumra, S., Ashtari, M., McMeniman, M. *et al.* (2004). Reduced frontal white matter integrity in early-onset schizophrenia: a preliminary study. *Biological Psychiatry*, **55**, 1138–1145.

Laakso, A., Bergman, J., Haaparanta, M. *et al.* (2001). Decreased striatal dopamine transporter binding in vivo in chronic schizophrenia. *Schizophr Research*, **52**, 115–120.

Laakso, A., Vilkman, H., Alakare, B. *et al.* (2000). Striatal dopamine transporter binding in neuroleptic-naive patients with schizophrenia studied with positron emission tomography. *American Journal of Psychiatry*, **157**, 269–271.

Lappin, J. M., Morgan, K., Morgan, C. *et al.* (2006). Gray matter abnormalities associated with duration of untreated psychosis. *Schizophrenia Research*, **82**, 145–153.

Laruelle, M. (1998). Imaging dopamine transmission in schizophrenia. A review and meta-analysis. *Quarterly Journal of Nuclear Medicine*, **42**, 211–221.

Laufs, H., Lengler, U., Hamandi, K., Kleinschmidt, A. & Krakow, K. (2006). Linking generalized spike-and-wave discharges and resting state brain activity by using EEG/fMRI in a patient with absence seizures. *Epilepsia*, **47**, 444–448.

Lawrie, S. M. & Abukmeil, S. S. (1998). Brain abnormality in schizophrenia. A systematic and quantitative review of volumetric magnetic resonance imaging studies. *British Journal of Psychiatry*, **172**, 110–120.

Le Bihan, D., Mangin, J. F., Poupon, C. *et al.* (2001). Diffusion tensor imaging: concepts and applications. *Journal of Magnetic Resonance Imaging*, **13**, 534–546.

Lewis, R., Kapur, S., Jones, C. *et al.* (1999). Serotonin 5-HT2 receptors in schizophrenia: a PET study using [18F] setoperone in neuroleptic-naive patients and normal subjects. *American Journal of Psychiatry*, **156**, 72–78.

Liang, M., Zhou, Y., Jiang, T. *et al.* (2006). Widespread functional disconnectivity in schizophrenia with resting-state functional magnetic resonance imaging. *Neuroreport*, **17**, 209–213.

Lieberman, J. A., Tollefson, G. D., Charles, C. *et al.* (2005). Antipsychotic drug effects on brain morphology in first-episode psychosis. *Archives of General Psychiatry*, **62**, 361–370.

Lyoo, I. K. & Renshaw, P. F. (2002). Magnetic resonance spectroscopy: current and future applications in psychiatric research. *Biological Psychiatry*, **51**, 195–207.

Maier, M., Ron, M. A., Barker, G. J. & Tofts, P. S. (1995). Proton magnetic resonance spectroscopy: an in vivo method of estimating hippocampal neuronal depletion in schizophrenia. *Psychological Medicine*, **25**, 1201–1209.

Malhi, G. S., Valenzuela, M., Wen, W. & Sachdev, P. (2002). Magnetic resonance spectroscopy and its applications in psychiatry. *Australian and New Zealand Journal of Psychiatry*, **36**, 31–43.

McCarley, R. W., Wible, C. G., Frumin M. *et al.* (1999). MRI anatomy of schizophrenia. *Biological Psychiatry*, **45**, 1099–1119.

McGowan, S., Lawrence, A. D., Sales, T., Quested, D. & Grasby, P. (2004). Presynaptic dopaminergic dysfunction in schizophrenia: a positron emission tomographic [18F]fluorodopa study. *Archives of General Psychiatry*, **61**, 134–142.

McGuire, P. & Matsumoto, K. (2004). Functional neuroimaging in mental disorders. *World Psychology*, **3**, 6–11.

McGuire, P. K. & Frith, C. D. (1996). Disordered functional connectivity in schizophrenia. *Psychological Medicine*, **26**, 663–667.

McGuire, P. K., Shah, G. M. & Murray, R. M. (1993). Increased blood flow in Broca's area during auditory hallucinations in schizophrenia. *Lancet*, **342**, 703–706.

McGuire, P. K., Silbersweig, D. A., Wright, I. *et al.* (1995). Abnormal monitoring of inner speech: a physiological basis for auditory hallucinations. *Lancet*, **346**, 596–600.

McIntosh, A. R. (1999). Mapping cognition to the brain through neural interactions. *Memory*, **7**, 523–548.

McIntosh, A. R. & Gonzalez-Lima, F. (1998). Large-scale functional connectivity in associative learning: interrelations of the rat auditory, visual, and limbic systems. *Journal of Neurophysiology*, **80**, 3148–3162.

McIntosh, A. R., Cabeza, R. E. & Lobaugh, N. J. (1998). Analysis of neural interactions explains the activation of occipital cortex by an auditory stimulus. *Journal of Neurophysiology*, **80**, 2790–2796.

Moresco, R., Messa, C., Lucignani, G. *et al.* (2001). PET in psychopharmacology. *Pharmacological Research*, **44**, 151–159.

Nelson, M. D., Saykin, A. J., Flashman, L. A. & Riordan, H. J. (1998). Hippocampal volume reduction in schizophrenia as assessed by magnetic resonance imaging: a meta-analytic study. *Archives of General Psychiatry*, **55**, 433–440.

Nordstrom, A. L., Farde, L., Eriksson, L. & Halldin, C. (1995). No elevated D2 dopamine receptors in neuroleptic-naive schizophrenic patients revealed by positron emission tomography and [11C]N-methylspiperone. *Psychiatry Research*, **61**, 67–83.

Pantelis, C., Velakoulis, D., McGorry, P. D. *et al.* (2003). Neuroanatomical abnormalities before and after onset of psychosis: a cross-sectional and longitudinal MRI comparison. *Lancet*, **361**, 281–288.

Pettegrew, J. W., Kopp, S. J., Minshew, N. J. *et al.* (1987). 31P nuclear magnetic resonance studies of phosphoglyceride metabolism in developing and degenerating brain: preliminary observations. *Journal of Neuropathology and Experimental Neurology*, **46**, 419–430.

Pilowsky, L. S., Bressan, R. A., Stone, J. M. *et al.* (2006). First in vivo evidence of an NMDA receptor deficit in medication-free schizophrenic patients. *Molecular Psychiatry*, **11**, 118–119.

Pilowsky, L. S., Costa, D. C., Ell, P. J. *et al.* (1994). D2 dopamine receptor binding in the basal ganglia of antipsychotic-free schizophrenic patients. An 123I-IBZM single photon emission computerised tomography study. *British Journal of Psychiatry*, **164**, 16–26.

Poline, J. B., Vandenberghe, R., Holmes, A. P., Friston, K. J. & Frackowiak, R. S. (1996). Reproducibility of PET activation studies: lessons from a multi-center European experiment. EU concerted action on functional imaging. *Neuroimage*, **4**, 34–54.

Rasser, P. E., Johnston, P., Lagopoulos, J. *et al.* (2005). Functional MRI BOLD response to Tower of London performance of first-episode schizophrenia patients using cortical pattern matching. *Neuroimage*, **26**, 941–951.

Reite, M., Teale, P., Goldstein, L., Whalen, J. & Linnville, S. (1989). Late auditory magnetic sources may differ in the left hemisphere of schizophrenic patients. A preliminary report. *Archives of General Psychiatry*, **46**, 565–572.

Reite, M., Teale, P. & Rojas, D. C. (1999). Magnetoencephalography: applications in psychiatry. *Biological Psychiatry*, **45**, 1553–1563.

Reite, M., Teale, P., Sheeder, J., Rojas, D. C. & Schneider, E. E. (1996). Magnetoencephalographic evidence of abnormal early auditory memory function in schizophrenia. *Biological Psychiatry*, **40**, 299–301.

Rojas, D. C., Teale, P., Sheeder, J., Simon, J. & Reite, M. (1997). Sex-specific expression of Heschl's gyrus functional and structural abnormalities in paranoid schizophrenia. *American Journal of Psychiatry*, **154**, 1655–1662.

Rosen, A. C. & Gur, R. C. (2002). Ethical considerations for neuropsychologists as functional magnetic imagers. *Brain and Cognition*, **50**, 469–481.

Schnack, H. G., van Haren, N. E., Hulshoff Pol, H. E. *et al.* (2004). Reliability of brain volumes from multicenter MRI acquisition: a calibration study. *Human Brain Mapping*, **22**, 312–320.

Shergill, S. S., Brammer, M. J., Fukuda, R. *et al.* (2002). Modulation of activity in temporal cortex during generation of inner speech. *Human Brain Mapping*, **16**, 219–227.

Shulman, R. G. (2001). Functional imaging studies: linking mind and basic neuroscience. *American Journal of Psychiatry*, **158**, 11–20.

Smith, G. S., Koppel, J. & Goldberg, S. (2003). Applications of neuroreceptor imaging to psychiatry research. *Psychopharmacology Bulletin*, **37**, 26–65.

Soares, J. C. & Innis, R. B. (1999). Neurochemical brain imaging investigations of schizophrenia. *Biological Psychiatry*, **46**, 600–615.

Spence, S. A., Liddle, P. F., Stefan, M. D. *et al.* (2000). Functional anatomy of verbal fluency in people with schizophrenia and those at genetic risk. Focal dysfunction and distributed disconnectivity reappraised. *British Journal of Psychiatry*, **176**, 52–60.

Stanley, J. A. (2002). In vivo magnetic resonance spectroscopy and its application to neuropsychiatric disorders. *Canadian Journal of Psychiatry*, **47**, 315–326.

Stanley, J. A., Pettegrew, J. W. & Keshavan, M. S. (2000). Magnetic resonance spectroscopy in schizophrenia: methodological issues and findings – part I. *Biological Psychiatry*, **48**, 357–368.

Steen, R. G., Hamer, R. M. & Lieberman, J. A. (2005). Measurement of brain metabolites by 1H magnetic resonance spectroscopy in patients with schizophrenia: a systematic review and meta-analysis. *Neuropsychopharmacology*, **30**, 1949–1962.

Stephan, K. E., Magnotta, V. A., White, T. *et al.* (2001). Effects of olanzapine on cerebellar functional connectivity in schizophrenia measured by fMRI during a simple motor task. *Psychological Medicine*, **31**, 1065–1078.

Stocker, T., Schneider, F., Klein, M. *et al.* (2005). Automated quality assurance routines for fMRI data applied to a multicenter study. *Human Brain Mapping*, **25**, 237–246.

Sumich, A., Chitnis, X. A., Fannon, D. G. *et al.* (2005). Unreality symptoms and volumetric measures of Heschl's gyrus and planum temporal in first-episode psychosis. *Biological Psychiatry*, **57**, 947–950.

Talairach, J. & Tournoux, P. (1988). *A Co-planar Stereotactic Atlas of the Human Brain*. New York, NY: Thieme Medical Publishers.

Taylor, W. D., Hsu, E., Krishnan, K. R. & MacFall, J. R. (2004). Diffusion tensor imaging: background, potential, and utility in psychiatric research. *Biological Psychiatry*, **55**, 201–207.

Theberge, J., Bartha, R., Drost, D. J. *et al.* (2002). Glutamate and glutamine measured with 4.0 T proton MRS in never-treated patients with schizophrenia and healthy volunteers. *American Journal of Psychiatry*, **159**, 1944–1946.

Thompson, P. M., Hayashi, K. M. & de Zubicaray, G. (2003). Dynamics of gray matter loss in Alzheimer's disease. *Journal of Neuroscience*, **23**, 994.

Thompson, P. M., Vidal, C. N. & Giedd, J. N. (2001). Mapping adolescent brain changes reveals dynamic wave of accelerated gray matter loss in very early onset schizophrenia. *Proceedings of the National Academy of Sciences USA*, **98**, 11650–11655.

Tibbo, P., Hanstock, C., Valiakalayil, A. & Allen, P. (2004). 3-T proton MRS investigation of glutamate and glutamine in adolescents at high genetic risk for schizophrenia. *American Journal of Psychiatry*, **161**, 1116–1118.

Toga, A. W., Thompson, P. M. & Sowell, E. R. (2006). Mapping brain maturation. *Trends in Neuroscience*, **29**, 148–159.

Toosy, A. T., Ciccarelli, O., Parker, G. J. *et al.* (2004). Characterizing function-structure relationships in the human visual system with functional MRI and diffusion tensor imaging. *Neuroimage*, **21**, 1452–1463.

Turkington, T. G. (2001). Introduction to PET instrumentation. *Journal of Nuclear Medicine Technology*, **29**, 4–11.

Velakoulis, D., Wood, S. J., Wong, M. T. *et al.* (2006). Hippocampal and amygdala volumes according to psychosis stage and diagnosis: a magnetic resonance imaging study of chronic schizophrenia, first-episode psychosis, and ultra-high-risk individuals. *Archives of General Psychiatry*, **63**, 139–149.

Verhoeff, N. P. (1999). Radiotracer imaging of dopaminergic transmission in neuropsychiatric disorders. *Psychopharmacology (Berlin)*, **147**, 217–249.

Vidal, C. N., Rapoport, J. L., Hayashi, K. M. *et al.* (2006). Dynamically spreading frontal and cingulate deficits mapped in adolescents with schizophrenia. *Archives of General Psychiatry*, **63**, 25–34.

Vita, A., De Peri, L., Silenzi, C. & Dieci, M. (2006). Brain morphology in first-episode schizophrenia: a meta-analysis of quantitative magnetic resonance imaging studies. *Schizophrenia Research*, **82**, 75–88.

Volkow, N. D., Fowler, J. S., Gatley, S. J. *et al.* (1996). PET evaluation of the dopamine system of the human brain. *Journal of Nuclear Medicine*, **37**, 1242–1256.

Ward, K. E., Friedman, L., Wise, A. & Schulz, S. C. (1996). Meta-analysis of brain and cranial size in schizophrenia. *Schizophrenia Research*, **22**, 197–213.

Warwick, J. M. (2004). Imaging of brain function using SPECT. *Metabolic Brain Disease*, **19**, 113–123.

Whalley, H. C., Simonotto, E., Marshall, I. *et al.* (2005). Functional disconnectivity in subjects at high genetic risk of schizophrenia. *Brain*, **128**, 2097–2108.

Whitford, T. J., Farrow, T. F., Gomes, L. *et al.* (2005). Grey matter deficits and symptom profile in first episode schizophrenia. *Psychiatry Research*, **139**, 229–238.

Wong, D. F., Wagner, H. N., Jr., Tune, L. E. *et al.* (1986). Positron emission tomography reveals elevated D2 dopamine receptors in drug-naive schizophrenics. *Science*, **234**, 1558–1563.

Wood, S. J., Berger, G., Velakoulis, D. *et al.* (2003). Proton magnetic resonance spectroscopy in first episode psychosis and ultra high-risk individuals. *Schizophrenia Bulletin*, **29**, 831–843.

Woodruff, P. W., McManus, I. C. & David, A. S. (1995). Meta-analysis of corpus callosum size in schizophrenia. *Journal of Neurology, Neurosurgery and Psychiatry*, **58**, 457–461.

Woodruff, P. W., Wright, I. C., Bullmore, E. T. *et al.* (1997). Auditory hallucinations and the temporal cortical response to speech in schizophrenia: a functional magnetic resonance imaging study. *American Journal of Psychiatry*, **154**, 1676–1682.

Woods, B. T., Ward, K. E. & Johnson, E. H. (2005). Meta-analysis of the time-course of brain volume reduction in schizophrenia: implications for pathogenesis and early treatment. *Schizophrenia Research*, **73**, 221–228.

Wright, I. C., McGuire, P. K., Poline, J. B. *et al.* (1995). A voxel-based method for the statistical analysis of gray and white matter density applied to schizophrenia. *Neuroimage*, **2**, 244–252.

Wright, I. C., Rabe-Hesketh, S., Woodruff, P. W. *et al.* (2000). Meta-analysis of regional brain volumes in schizophrenia. *American Journal of Psychiatry*, **157**, 16–25.

Xiong, J., Parsons, L. M., Gao, J. H. & Fox, P. T. (1999). Interregional connectivity to primary motor cortex revealed using MRI resting state images. *Human Brain Mapping*, **8**, 151–156.

Yang, Y. K., Yu, L., Yeh, T. L. *et al.* (2004). Associated alterations of striatal dopamine D2/D3 receptor and transporter binding in drug-naive patients with schizophrenia: a dual-isotope SPECT study. *American Journal of Psychiatry*, **161**, 1496–1498.

Psychopharmacological modeling of psychiatric illness

Garry D. Honey

Introduction

The success with which preclinical models of mental illness can appropriately represent the complexities of disorders of higher cognitive function is limited. There are also confounds which often limit the insights which can be gained from directly studying patients with these disorders, such as the effects of the chronicity of disease and treatment, for example. Human psychopharmacological models of psychiatric illness, involving drug manipulations resulting in the reproduction of key features of the syndrome, therefore provide an important contribution in understanding the pathophysiology underlying neuro-psychological impairments in psychiatry. However, as with any model, the fundamental aspects in which the model departs from the real-world situation one attempts to approximate must be acknowledged and appreciated, in order to evaluate the ways in which this impacts on the interpretation of important findings which can be gained from this approach.

Modeling cognitive impairment

Human pharmacological models of disease involve the administration of psychoactive compounds to healthy individuals in order to reproduce symptoms which are qualitatively similar to those experienced by people with mental illness. The assumption is that if symptoms of a disease process are convincingly replicated by the drug model, then the mechanisms mediating the effects of both drug and disease may share important commonalities. The drug model can thus be manipulated in a controlled environment, in order to provide insights into disease processes, often providing information which would be otherwise inaccessible. In this chapter, specific instances where

drug models have provided such information will be highlighted.

On what criteria should a drug model of a psychiatric illness be considered a useful model? Clearly, one should expect that key symptoms of the illness should be descriptively similar under the drug condition and in patients. Thus the phenomenology experienced by healthy subjects receiving the drug, in comparison with placebo, should be quantifiable and qualitatively comparable with patients, ideally using psychiatric ratings used routinely in clinical settings. This will be considered in the next section, in which we examine the overlap in symptoms produced by drug and disease.

One might also hope to identify physiological changes associated with clinical symptomatology which are similarly observed following drug administration. These might include, for example, autonomic responses (e.g. skin conductance), biochemical changes (e.g. metabolites in cerebrospinal fluid) or central measures (e.g. resting state electroencephalography (EEG) or functional neuroimaging data acquired during cognitive stimulation). Given increasing evidence that cognitive deficits are a core feature of psychiatric illnesses, a third measure by which drug models may be assessed is the extent to which the cognitive deficits are common across drug and disease states. Indeed, modeling cognitive impairment might be seen as central for two reasons. First, the importance of cognitive dysfunction is increasingly recognized as a primary factor of mental illness, and not simply attributable to the distraction and disorientation of pervasive psychopathology. Indeed, there is evidence that cognitive dysfunction may precede the emergence of psychopathology, and is of practical importance in terms of correlating with incapacity and predicting outcome (Green, 1996; Green & Nuechterlein, 1999). Second,

The Neuropsychology of Mental Illness, ed. Stephen J. Wood, Nicholas B. Allen and Christos Pantelis. Published by Cambridge University Press. © Cambridge University Press 2009.

cognitive function may provide the conceptual link between the other two levels of description: psychiatric symptomatology and physiological alterations. For example, one might hypothesize that thought disorder is a reflection of disturbed working-memory processes, and that working-memory impairment is mediated by aberrant dopaminergic innervation of prefrontal cortex. Pharmacological models of disease allow us to test whether the consequences of perturbations of the dopaminergic system include these predicted effects in humans. Modeling cognitive impairment is therefore of practical significance, in that insights may facilitate improvements in early diagnosis, intervention and treatment; and it is of theoretical importance in conceptualizing disease mechanisms comprehensively, providing the central link in the association between brain, cognition and psychopathology.

However, the evolution of psychiatric illness in an individual is a complex and gradual process, possibly involving biological predispositions initiated at or during birth, revealing themselves over subsequent years, into early adulthood. Limitations in the extent to which the administration of a single acute dose of a drug given in a laboratory to an otherwise healthy subject can reproduce the myriad experiences associated with the insidious onset of a mental disorder must be acknowledged. Some of these shortcomings will be considered in this chapter. Despite these limitations, given appropriately focused questions within these constraints, it is likely that human psychopharmacological models will lead to important developments in neuropsychiatry.

The issues outlined above will be discussed in this chapter, largely in reference to the most intensively investigated model, ketamine. The disproportionate emphasis on this model reflects the imbalance evident in the current scientific literature. In an attempt to draw conclusions across psychopharmacological models of disease, other compounds will also be briefly considered where evidence is available.

Psychopathology of drug models of schizophrenia
Assumptions and expectations of a model of schizophrenia

The heterogeneity of psychotic phenomena and the variability of outcomes in schizophrenia, and its

precursor, dementia praecox, can be traced to Kraepelin, who stated "The course of the illness can take the most varied forms" (Kraepelin, 1896). Indeed, Bentall (Bentall, 1993; Bentall et al., 1988) argues that this is an inevitable and insurmountable problem inherent in its conceptualization. Bentall argues that over 100 years of schizophrenia research has been misconceived, as the concept of schizophrenia has fallen short of the requirements of validity and reliability necessary to justify its existence. None of the symptoms of the illness are pathognomonic, thus it is conceivable that two patients with the same diagnosis of schizophrenia could have no overlapping symptoms.

How then are we to expect a model of the illness to be useful, if it is not at all clear whether the illness is itself a meaningful entity? There are at least two observations which arise from this taxonomic confusion in clinical psychiatry in relation to attempts to conceptualize and develop a model. First, it will be unreasonable to expect any model to reproduce all of the symptoms which comprise the concept of schizophrenia; since this is not a clinical requirement for diagnostic purposes, it would be unrealistic to expect the model to perform beyond this. Second, it should be expected that the effect of the drug would be variable across individuals, with some individuals more susceptible to some symptoms than others. Indeed, it is likely that this variability in disease-related psychopathology represents a predisposition to a specific pattern of symptoms, or sub-syndrome of the illness. Similarly, these factors may predispose some individuals towards particular symptoms induced by the drug, and this may provide a rich area of research to determine the basis for such vulnerability. This point will be revisited later, in considering further the advantages of the drug modeling approach. Below, the extent to which two drugs, ketamine and delta-9-tetrahydrocannabinol (THC) reproduce the symptoms of schizophrenia will be considered, with these caveats in mind.

Ketamine
Historical background
The association between glutamate, the principal excitatory neurotransmitter in the brain, and schizophrenia was suggested by Kim et al. (1980) on the basis of their observation of reduced glutamate concentration in cerebrospinal fluid (CSF) of schizophrenic patients. The involvement of the glutamatergic system in the

pathophysiology of schizophrenia was further supported by post-mortem evidence of increased NMDA receptor densities in schizophrenia (Deakin *et al.*, 1989; Ishimaru *et al.*, 1994; Kornhuber *et al.*, 1989; Nishikawa *et al.*, 1983; Simpson *et al.*, 1991), though non-replications have also been reported. The discovery that phencyclidine (PCP), known to induce both positive and negative symptoms of psychosis in healthy volunteers (Luby *et al.*, 1962), non-competitively blocks the ion channel of the NMDA receptor complex (Lodge & Anis, 1982) formed the mainstay for the NMDA hypofunction model. Such findings reinvigorated debate concerning the role of glutamatergic systems in schizophrenia (Carlsson & Carlsson, 1990; Deutsch *et al.*, 1989; Hirsch *et al.*, 1997; Javitt & Zukin, 1991; Jentsch & Roth, 1999; Olney & Farber, 1995). While PCP is unsuitable as a psychopharmacological tool in humans due to its neurotoxicity, ketamine, with approximately one-tenth the potency of PCP, provides a safe alternative, with no discernible long-term effects in healthy volunteers (Carpenter, 1999; Malhotra *et al.*, 1996). Ketamine non-competitively blocks the NMDA receptor with affinity several times greater than its action at other sites, including the σ receptor, the μ opiate receptor, acetylcholinesterate and monoamine transporter sites. Furthermore, it is the blockade of the NMDA receptor that is thought to mediate its psychotomimetic properties, since blockade of other effects of ketamine does not block its psychotomimetic effects (Byrd *et al.*, 1987).

Safety

Ketamine has been used clinically as a general anesthetic for many years. Interestingly, it is not typically used as a first-line option due to adverse side-effects, known as "emergence phenomena," in which patients experience bizarre perceptual changes during recovery. Indeed, it is these very phenomena which are exploited in its use as a pharmacological model of schizophrenia. It is also interesting to note that these experiences are generally not observed in children, which is thought to relate to the maturation of the NMDA system occurring in late adolescence. This provides a parallel to the clinical course of schizophrenia, and gives further support that ketamine may impact the same systems as the disease process.

Ketamine is well-suited to an acute dosing regime in the laboratory as an experimental tool. It may be administered intravenously and has a rapid onset and short half-life, which conveys specific advantages for experimental investigation, as discussed later. Plasma assays are routinely used to confirm target drug levels.

Psychotomimetic effects

The most frequent effects of ketamine administration are distortions of visual perception and increased intensity of colors, lights and sounds (Duncan *et al.*, 2001; Newcomer *et al.*, 1999). Subjectively, participants report feeling detached from their surroundings and amotivational, having difficulty initiating action or sustaining attention (Krystal *et al.*, 1994). They also report alterations in body perception, feelings of unreality and depersonalization (Duncan *et al.*, 2001; Krystal *et al.*, 1994). With respect to the psychopathology associated with ketamine administration, the Brief Psychiatric Rating Scale (BPRS) is the most commonly used measure. On this measure, participants who have received 100–250 ng/ml of ketamine show an increase in overall BPRS score (Duncan *et al.*, 2001; Malhotra *et al.*, 1997; Umbricht *et al.*, 2000). More specifically, they experience visual and conceptual distortion, suspiciousness and unusual thought content, including ideas of references and paranoid delusions (Duncan *et al.*, 2001; Krystal *et al.*, 1994; Malhotra *et al.*, 1997; Newcomer *et al.*, 1999). These studies also show that this level of ketamine leads to an increase in negative symptoms rated on the BPRS such as emotional withdrawal, motor retardation and affective flattening.

There is some evidence of formal thought disorder associated with ketamine administration at levels between 50 and 250 ng/ml, including negative and positive symptoms of thought disorder (Malhotra *et al.*, 1996). Negative thought disorder symptoms include blocking, poverty of speech, poverty of content and increased latency of response (Newcomer *et al.*, 1999). Positive thought disorder symptoms include concreteness, loose associations, derailment and stilted speech (Duncan *et al.*, 2001; Krystal *et al.*, 1994). The symptoms of formal thought disorder associated with ketamine administration appear similar to those displayed by patients with schizophrenia (Adler *et al.*, 1999).

The administration of ketamine to patients with schizophrenia appears to induce or exacerbate psychotic symptoms that typify schizophrenia. Generally, there is an increase in BPRS scores following acute administration of ketamine to patients with schizophrenia, including increases on the thought disturbance and withdrawal-retardation subscales (Lahti *et al.*, 1995a, 1995b, 2001: Malhotra *et al.*, 1997). These studies suggest that ketamine induces symptoms that are qualitatively similar to those experienced by patients during a psychotic episode. For example, patients with a history of auditory hallucinations will also experience this phenomenon under ketamine administration. This consistency also holds for formal thought disorder, delusions, paranoia and negative symptoms.

Delta-9-tetrahydrocannabinol (THC)

Whilst the ketamine model is undoubtedly the most intensively investigated, other drug models of schizophrenia are also available. This is important since it relates to a further advantage of the drug-modeling approach, namely the comparison of different manipulations of transmitter systems, which allow further refinement of the association between cognitive and molecular processes, and also the exclusion of nonspecific effects. Commonalities between these drug models and the disease itself are therefore important to elucidate, as they may represent a final common pathway mediating specific symptoms, as elaborated later.

The cannabinoid hypothesis of schizophrenia (Emrich *et al.*, 1997) is based on several observations. Like ketamine, acute administration of the psychoactive component of cannabis, delta-9-tetrahydrocannabinol (THC), produces symptoms characteristic of schizophrenia, including delusions of control, grandiosity, persecution, thought insertion, auditory hallucinations, altered perception and emotional blunting in healthy volunteers (Iversen, 2003). As will be considered later in this chapter, cognitive dysfunction (including memory, attention and executive processing impairments) is also evident following exposure to THC. Patients with schizophrenia show enhanced sensitivity to these effects of THC (D'Souza *et al.*, 2005). There is also strong evidence that chronic recreational use of cannabis significantly increases vulnerability to schizophrenia, particularly in high-risk individuals, and in sub-clinical populations is associated with schizotypal personality (Johns, 2001). The psychotropic effects of THC are primarily mediated via modulation of transmitter release via activation of pre-synaptic CB1 receptors. These are distributed with high density in regions implicated in psychosis, particularly in the limbic system. These observations support the hypothesis that schizophrenia is associated with hyperactivity of endocannabinoid mechanisms.

Other models

Both ketamine and THC produce a range of symptoms which are similar to those of schizophrenia, and the co-occurrence of these effects, as occurs in the disease itself, is an important factor in assessing the validity of drug models. However, it should be noted that other drugs, whilst not providing the range of schizophrenia-like symptoms associated with ketamine and THC, specifically produce hallucinatory effects. These include, amongst others, lysergic acid, psilocybin and N,N-dimethyltryptamine (DMT). Hallucinations are notably absent from the array of psychotic effects associated with these drugs, therefore these hallucinogens provide a useful alternative for research into this aspect of psychosis.

Cognitive impairments associated with drug models

Working memory

The concept of "working memory" is a hypothetical construct that refers to a limited capacity system that facilitates the simultaneous storage and processing of information, which can then be utilized to guide subsequent behavior (Baddeley, 1986, 1992, 1998; Baddeley & Hitch, 1974). It is proposed that working memory comprises a central executive that organizes the allocation and coordination of processing resources to utilize stored representations, and modality-specific short-term "slave stores" (i.e. a speech-based, "phonological loop" verbal storage system and a "visuospatial scratchpad" for storage of non-verbal information). Working-memory deficits have consistently been demonstrated in patients with schizophrenia, incorporating both verbal (Bell *et al.*, 2001; Condray *et al.*, 1996; Conklin *et al.*, 2000; Fleming *et al.*, 1995, 1997; Granholm *et al.*, 1997; Honey *et al.*, 2002) and non-verbal memoranda (Keefe *et al.*, 1995; Okada, 2002; Pantelis *et al.*, 2001; Park & Holzman, 1992, 1993; Park *et al.*, 1999). Working-memory dysfunction is thought to have important implications for the expression of disparate cognitive deficits, and the physiological basis of working memory is therefore considered to be fundamental to pathophysiological mechanisms of schizophrenia (Cohen &

Servan-Schreiber, 1992; Goldman-Rakic, 1990, 1994, 1999; Weinberger, 1993). A greater understanding of the mechanisms by which working memory is disrupted in schizophrenia is therefore likely to be useful in characterizing the syndrome more fully.

An important distinction in the way information is processed in working memory is that between maintenance and manipulation. Maintenance refers to the simple process of storing the information in the limited capacity system over a period of time. An everyday example might include remembering an unfamiliar phone number from a telephone directory and maintaining the information for the delay during which you walked across the room to the telephone to dial the number. The information simply sits in storage until it is required. This may be facilitated by subvocally rehearsing the information, but no further processing of the information is required in order to perform the task. Alternatively, one might have to remember three telephone numbers, but dial the numbers in the alphabetical order of the surnames to which the numbers were associated. This would require reordering of the information, by way of manipulating the contents of working memory in order to achieve a desired goal.

This distinction between maintenance and manipulation of information is relevant to the dysfunction of working memory observed in schizophrenia. While patients show impairment of both functions, the deficit appears greater for manipulation (Fleming et al., 1995; Glahn et al., 2000; Kim et al., 2004; Morice & Delahunty, 1996; Perry et al., 2001; Rushe et al., 1999) and is not due to the increased maintenance requirements associated with manipulation tasks (Kim et al., 2004). An indication that the requirement to manipulate information may be central to working-memory deficits in schizophrenia comes from evidence of selective deficits observed in non-psychotic relatives of patients with schizophrenia. Using a series of working-memory tasks graded with respect to manipulation demands, Conklin et al. (2005) recently reported that first-degree relatives of patients with schizophrenia showed increasing impairment as the requirement to manipulate information in working memory increased. The distinction between maintenance and manipulation is further supported on the basis of functional neuroimaging studies, indicating a ventrodorsal dissociation respectively within the prefrontal cortex. Accordingly, Conklin et al. (2005) interpret the difficulties with manipulation as

indicative of a functional deficit within the dorsolateral prefrontal cortex, in line with similar findings in patients with schizophrenia (Perlstein et al., 2001).

The disruptive effects of ketamine on verbal working memory in healthy volunteers support its validity as a model detailing disrupted processes in schizophrenia (Adler et al., 1998; Ahn et al., 2003; Honey et al., 2003; Malhotra et al., 1996; Morgan et al., 2004; Umbricht et al., 2000). Discrepant findings reported in two studies may relate to doses and/or sample sizes (Ghoneim et al., 1985; Rowland et al., 2005). Furthermore, there is evidence suggesting that the effect of ketamine may be due to a disruption of the ability to manipulate information in working memory. Honey et al. (2003) found that subjects' performance was impaired by ketamine on tasks engaging working-memory manipulation but not on those requiring maintenance only. This effect, which is consistent with the study reported by Conklin et al. (2005) in non-psychotic relatives, is unlikely to be due to simple considerations of difficulty, since no effect was observed in other more difficult tasks, including a spatial working-memory maintenance and manipulation task. Whilst the differential effect of ketamine on spatial and verbal working memory in this study is intriguing, it should be interpreted cautiously; however, it is consistent with the only previous study to examine the effects of ketamine on spatial working memory (Newcomer et al., 1999). The effects of ketamine on working memory were subsequently shown to augment fronto-parietal responses to a working memory-manipulation condition, relative to a maintenance-only condition (Honey et al., 2004). This effect was observed specifically at a low cognitive load (maintaining/manipulating two items in working memory), but not at a higher load (five items), indicating that as load increases, fronto-parietal activation is increased under both placebo and ketamine treatments, but also that a similarly high level of activation is required for manipulation under ketamine even at low cognitive load. This parallels similar observations from studies in patients with schizophrenia, in which patients exhibit exaggerated frontal activation ("hyperfrontality") in response to working-memory tasks, until the physiological capacity of the prefrontal cortex to respond to task-related requirements is exceeded by the cognitive load (Callicott et al., 2000; Manoach et al., 1999, 2000; Perlstein et al., 2001; Walter et al., 2003). Similar findings were also observed in two cohorts of non-schizophrenic siblings of patients with schizophrenia (Callicott *et al.*, 2003).

The neuropharmacological mechanism underlying the disruption of working memory following ketamine exposure is unclear at present. However, there may be some insight gained from research involving THC. Several studies have examined the effects of THC on verbal working memory. Comparable to the effects of ketamine, there is evidence that working memory manipulation may be preferentially disrupted. McDonald *et al.* (2003) administered the forward and backward digit span tests to subjects exposed to 7.5 or 15 mg THC. Consistent with a primary effect on the requirement to manipulate information in working memory, both doses significantly impaired backward but not forward span. This may reconcile discrepant findings from other studies of the effects of THC on working memory, which have involved tests of simple maintenance of verbal material, and have failed to find an effect of the drug (Fant *et al.*, 1998; Heishman *et al.*, 1997; Nicholson *et al.*, 2004).

The observation that both ketamine and THC induce psychopathology and lead to specific working-memory impairments that overlap with those seen in schizophrenia is an important insight. Further research into the shared mechanisms that underlie these effects across drug and disease is likely to be of considerable value in advancing theoretical neurobiological models of schizophrenia.

Working-memory dysfunction in schizophrenia is likely to be related to abnormalities in the dopaminergic innervation of the frontal cortex (Goldman-Rakic, 1987). Egan *et al.* (2001) link cognitive performance and DLPFC response to polymorphisms in the catechol-*O*-methyltransferase (COMT) gene, important for metabolism of synaptically released dopamine in the prefrontal cortex. A potential mechanism for the effects of both disease and drug on working memory may be the dysregulation of dopaminergic innervation of the prefrontal cortex via the mesocortical dopaminergic system (Jentsch *et al.*, 1997; Verma & Moghaddam, 1996). Animal models may also provide important evidence in understanding these effects.

Dopamine transmission in prefrontal cortex is increased by administration of both THC and phencyclidine (PCP) in animal models (Bowers & Morton, 1994). Furthermore, administration of a selective NMDA agonist prevents the increase associated with THC, and ameliorates its disruption of working memory (Jentsch *et al.*, 1997). Similarly, clonidine (an α2 noradrenergic agonist) has been shown to potently block the increase in prefrontal dopamine following both THC and PCP (Jentsch *et al.*, 1998), and to prevent working-memory deficits associated with PCP (Jentsch & Anzivino, 2004). Interestingly, clonidine also improves memory function in schizophrenia (Fields *et al.*, 1988). An intriguing alternative explanation emerges from a recent study which suggests that both drugs may act via the cannabinoid CB1 receptor. Haller *et al.* (2005) have recently shown that the behavioral effect of PCP on social interaction in mice, thought to mimic the psychotomimetic properties of the drug, was absent in CB1-knockout mice.

Episodic memory

Impairment of episodic memory has been widely reported following ketamine administration (Curran & Morgan, 2000; Ghoneim *et al.*, 1985; Harris *et al.*, 1975; Hetem *et al.*, 2000; Krystal *et al.*, 1994, 1998b, 2000; Malhotra *et al.*, 1996, 1997; Murman *et al.*, 1997; Newcomer *et al.*, 1999; Pfenninger *et al.*, 2002; Radant *et al.*, 1998). Disruption of memory has been elicited using a range of cognitive tasks, including word-list recall and recognition, picture recognition and paragraph recall. However, a small number of studies have failed to observe effects on memory. Ghoneim *et al.* (1985) reported intact word recognition, despite impaired word recall; Krystal *et al.* (1994) found that delayed but not immediate paragraph recall was disrupted, whilst Murman *et al.* (1997) found the opposite pattern for word-list recall, and preserved immediate and delayed picture recognition. Most studies have generally focused on verbal memory, whilst relatively fewer studies have examined non-verbal memory processes; however a consistent finding of disrupted visuospatial memory is also beginning to emerge (Oye *et al.*, 1992; Pandit *et al.*, 1980; Pfenninger *et al.*, 2002), suggesting that episodic memory disruption following ketamine may be insensitive to the content of the memoranda. This is consistent with the large number of studies in rodents and non-human primates which have described impaired performance on both verbal (Danysz *et al.*, 1988; Morris *et al.*, 1986, 1989; Spangler *et al.*, 1991) and non-verbal tasks (Jones *et al.*, 1990; Parada-Turska & Turski, 1990; Tonkiss & Rawlins, 1991;

Tonkiss *et al.*, 1988) following treatment with competitive and non-competitive NMDA antagonists.

Similarly, this parallels the impairment noted in patients with schizophrenia, whereby memory deficits for both verbal (Bell *et al.*, 2001; Calev *et al.*, 1983; Cannon *et al.*, 1994; Clare *et al.*, 1993; Conklin *et al.*, 2000; Fleming *et al.*, 1995; Landro *et al.*, 1993; Lyons *et al.*, 1995; Manschreck *et al.*, 2000; Nopoulos *et al.*, 1994; Paulsen *et al.*, 1995; Saykin *et al.*, 1994; Stirling *et al.*, 1997; Wexler *et al.*, 1998) and non-verbal material (Carter *et al.*, 1996; Fleming *et al.*, 1997; Gooding & Tallent, 2002; Keefe *et al.*, 1995; Okada, 2002; Pantelis *et al.*, 2001; Park & Holzman, 1992; Park *et al.*, 1999; Spindler *et al.*, 1997; Tek *et al.*, 2002) have been reported.

The cognitive mechanism by which ketamine disrupts long-term memory remains unknown at present: impaired performance could plausibly relate to anomalous acquisition of information, a failure of storage, an inability to retrieve successfully stored information, or some combination of these. The possibility that ketamine affects encoding or retrieval processes has been addressed indirectly by several studies based on the assumption that encoding deficits would be expected to impair both recall and recognition mnemonic performance. Alternatively, a disproportionate deficit on recall compared with recognition performance would implicate retrieval processes, given the reduced engagement of retrieval in recognition tasks (as the target stimulus is presented to the subject, and not self-generated as required in free-recall tasks). However, contradictory findings based on this approach have been reported. Malhotra *et al.* (1996) found similar impairment of both recall and recognition performance, which they suggested was compatible with a preferential impairment of encoding processes, perhaps secondary to inhibition of long-term potentiation in the hippocampus (Zhang & Levy, 1992). Equivalent impairment of recognition and recall has also been reported by Radant *et al.* (1998) and Hetem *et al.* (2000). However, Ghoneim *et al.* (1985) found relative sparing of recognition memory, despite dose-related impairment of recall, perhaps suggestive of disrupted retrieval of information successfully encoded and stored. A potential complication with the assumptions employed in some of these studies is that impairment of both recall and recognition performance may not necessarily imply a specific encoding deficit. It is possible that a failure to retain information in temporary/permanent storage

that has been successfully encoded would equally lead to similar performance deficits across recall and recognition tasks. In addition, a disproportionate effect on free recall would not preclude an effect of ketamine on retrieval processes. Impairment of retrieval could primarily underlie recall deficits, and to a lesser extent, impair recognition, with recognition performance compounded by additional effects of ketamine on encoding or storage processes. The pattern of impairment on recall and recognition tasks does not, therefore, specifically isolate the cognitive mechanism by which ketamine impairs episodic memory tasks.

An alternative approach that avoids this assumption and capitalizes on a central advantage of the pharmacological approach is to present stimuli pre- and post-drug treatment: impairment of memory selectively for items presented post-infusion indicates a failure of encoding, whereas failure to recall/recognize both item sets presented before and after ketamine treatment would suggest disrupted retrieval mechanisms. Using this method, several studies have identified a primary disruption of encoding under ketamine. Oye *et al.* (1992) and Hetem *et al.* (2000) reported selective deficits for items presented subsequent to drug administration, indicating that the effect of ketamine on episodic memory is to selectively disrupt encoding processes. A potential complication to this approach, however, is that memory for items encoded both pre- and post-drug treatment was tested during drug exposure. The possibility of an interactive effect of ketamine on both encoding and retrieval processes cannot therefore be refuted, which would require encoding and retrieval to be performed both in the presence and in the absence of the drug. This design was reported by Honey *et al.* (2005b), involving encoding and recognition of two word lists: the first was presented before the drug was administered and recognition was tested during drug administration. Impairment of recognition on this list could only be due to an effect on retrieval, since the words were encoded prior to receiving the drug. A second list was then presented for encoding whilst subjects were still receiving ketamine, following which the drug was terminated, and plasma levels allowed to return to near baseline. Recognition was then tested for these items, with any impairment attributable to encoding, since the items were retrieved in the relative absence of the drug. Using this design, deficits were observed for the second list, indicating that ketamine disrupts episodic memory via an effect on encoding.

In this study, a depth-of-processing manipulation was also included. Subjects encoded the words according to a deep (pleasant/unpleasant judgment), intermediate (active/passive judgment) or shallow (syllable counting) strategy. Deeper encoding was robustly associated with improved recognition. Memory disruption produced by ketamine was specifically related to the intermediate level of processing, suggesting that ketamine disrupts memory by a disturbance of encoding processes that leads to recollective processing, compared with recognition based on familiarity. The preservation of the deepest encoded items suggests that if information is sufficiently deeply encoded, this may be protective against the effects of the drug, at least at low dose. Disruption of encoding processes suggests that ketamine may impact on the fronto-hippocampal system, critical for the encoding of episodic information. This was confirmed in a subsequent study (Honey *et al.*, 2005a). However, interestingly, this study also showed that despite the lack of evidence of a behavioral effect of ketamine on retrieval processes, attenuation of frontal activation was observed at retrieval, suggesting that functional imaging may provide a more sensitive marker of the effects of drug manipulations, and that compensatory behavioral responses may mask these effects from performance measures.

It was also noted that subjects were more likely to guess the source of the item, that is, when having recognized a word, subjects were more likely to guess which of the the encoding tasks were used to remember the word (Honey *et al.*, 2005b). This is interesting, because source memory deficits are thought to underlie a range of psychotic symptoms. Hallucinations for example, are suggested to occur when subjects fail to recognize the source of their own thoughts/actions, and thus erroneously attribute these to an external source (Frith, 1992). Honey *et al.* (2006) examined the effect of ketamine on reality monitoring: recognition of the source of information that was internally or externally generated, that is, whether a presented word had been generated by the subject themselves or by the experimenter. In accordance with previous studies in patients (Brebion *et al.*, 2000, 2002; Keefe *et al.*, 1999, 2002) it was predicted that under ketamine, subjects would be more likely to attribute the source externally. In fact, the opposite was observed: subjects were less likely under ketamine to externalize source guessing. Given the psychopathological profile of ketamine, this pattern of results is intriguing.

Subjects do not experience hallucinations, associated with abnormal externalization of information, but do show referential delusions, which could be seen as an abnormal internalization of information, consistent with the source memory bias observed under ketamine.

The effects of THC on episodic memory have not been as extensively investigated as for ketamine, however a consistent pattern is beginning to emerge. Most studies have reported a disruption of recall and recognition (Curran *et al.*, 2002; D'Souza *et al.*, 2004; Heishman *et al.*, 1997; Ilan *et al.*, 2004; Nicholson *et al.*, 2004) though others have found no effect (Hart *et al.*, 2001; McDonald *et al.*, 2003). In these studies, it is important to control for subjects' level of prior exposure to cannabis, since the effect of THC is likely to be attenuated in subjects who are not drug-naïve. The much longer half-life of THC would preclude the pre/post dosing strategy used with ketamine to dissociate effects on encoding and retrieval. To date, further exploration of specific encoding processes impacted by THC have not been reported.

Attention

Patients with schizophrenia show impairments in attention, both in terms of their ability to sustain attention over a period of time, and also to selectively attend to a specific stimulus. The continuous performance test (CPT) (Roswold *et al.*, 1956) is perhaps the most widely used assessment of sustained attention, and impaired performance in schizophrenic patients has been reported using this task (Binder *et al.*, 1998). However, studies using ketamine have in general failed to find a disruption of sustained attentional processes as measured by the CPT and similar tasks (Adler *et al.*, 1998; Morgan *et al.*, 2004; Newcomer *et al.*, 1999; Oranje *et al.*, 2000) or selective attention, as measured using the Stroop test (Krystal *et al.*, 2005b; Newcomer *et al.*, 1999; Rowland *et al.*, 2005). Ketamine does impair performance using a modified version of the CPT, however, this version is likely to engage working-memory processes (Krystal *et al.*, 1998a, 1999, 2005b), and was not replicated in a subsequent study by the same group (Krystal *et al.*, 2000). Ketamine does appear to increase distractability (Krystal *et al.*, 1998a, 1999, 2000, 2005b). Therefore, whilst relatively few studies have employed tasks to isolate attentional deficits, the impairments reported in patients with schizophrenia are not reproduced by ketamine. This may represent a departure from the neuropsychological profile of schizophrenia. Alternatively, at the doses used, it may be possible for subjects to engage compensatory processes, and thereby maintain performance. This hypothesis could be tested using functional imaging, which may more sensitively index drug effects on attentional systems, and also implicate brain regions which may be involved in a compensatory response. From a methodological point of view, the failure to demonstrate attentional deficits under ketamine suggests that other cognitive effects of the drug are unlikely to be due to non-specific factors, such as fatigue, sedation or impaired attention.

A similar pattern emerges from studies examining the effects of THC on attention, which appears to be intact under drug administration (Curran *et al.*, 2002; D'Souza *et al.*, 2004; Hart *et al.*, 2001; Heishman *et al.*, 1997; Nicholson *et al.*, 2004). Interestingly, D'Souza *et al.* (2004) showed that THC does impair distractibility. The pattern of findings therefore appears to be remarkably similar across both drug conditions. The significance of the increase in distractibility under these drugs is not clear, and may simply represent a secondary consequence of the other experiences to which subjects are exposed under drugs.

Executive function

Executive functioning is a rather vague concept which is generally used to refer to a range of 'higher' cognitive functions, often used synonymously with functions involving the prefrontal cortex (see Chapter 9, this volume for discussion). The most widely reported test of executive function under ketamine is the verbal fluency test, involving both the phonological and semantic variants (subject produces as many words as possible of a given letter or category, respectively). Whilst there is evidence of impaired performance on this task in schizophrenia, it is a complex multifaceted task and it is not clear precisely what processes are engaged or which may be disrupted in patients. The findings from this task under ketamine are accordingly equivocal, with impaired (Adler *et al.*, 1998; Krupitsky *et al.*, 2001; Krystal *et al.*, 1998b) and intact (Krystal *et al.*, 1999; LaPorte *et al.*, 1996; Morgan *et al.*, 2004; Newcomer *et al.*, 1999; Rowland *et al.*, 2005) performance reported. A single study which has investigated the effects of THC on verbal fluency found no effect of the drug (Curran *et al.*, 2002). The inconsistency of the effects of ketamine reported on tasks involving executive function may reflect the range and complexity of processes engaged by such tasks, and also the potential for subjects to adopt alternative strategies to maintain performance. This could potentially obscure psychopharmacological effects and contribute to the inconsistent findings across studies. Another test of executive function widely in use is the Wisconsin Card Sort test. Ketamine has been shown to impair performance (Krystal *et al.*, 1998a, 1999, 2000), however, given the working-memory component of this task, it is unclear to what extent impairment on this task reflects disruption of working memory, or indicates further deficits, for example in strategy formation and set shifting. Cognitive tasks which refine process specificity will be needed to address these issues.

Advantages of psychopharmacological modeling

The administration of ketamine is a safe and routine procedure, however, the advantages of administering any psychotropic drug for experimental purposes must be carefully considered and justified. One might reasonably ask, what are the benefits of this approach compared with more direct investigations involving patients with the disorder? Here we consider some of the advantages of the drug-modeling technique in more detail, and specifically highlight where the drug model offers insights where similar observations from patient studies would be unfeasible.

Exploring neurochemical mechanisms of psychiatric disease

The neurochemical basis of schizophrenia likely involves a complex interaction of multiple neurotransmitter effects. However, dysfunction of a single transmitter may be central, resulting in complex downstream effects on other systems and reciprocal feedback mechanisms. The identification of this putative fundamental pathology is clearly difficult in patients. Post-mortem studies have failed to reveal any consistent neuropathological insult that would be consistent with a transmitter dysfunction, such as altered regulation of receptor densities, or structural abnormalities to receptors affecting transmitter affinity. The pathophysiological mechanism is therefore likely to be functional in origin, i.e. dynamic changes in transmitter availability, uptake, etc. The measurement of metabolites in CSF in patients is an extremely indirect approximation of the functional integrity of the nervous system, often compared to the diagnosis of mechanical failure in a car engine on the basis of the chemical constituents of the exhaust fumes. In vivo chemical imaging is possible in patients, using magnetic resonance spectroscopy, but the technique is presently limited to the analysis of small regions of interest. Pharmacological models therefore provide some insight into the neurochemical basis of psychotic symptoms, which is difficult to obtain from other methods.

Ketamine primarily affects the NMDA system, however it is not selective, and has a range of other effects at other sites. As a result, the effects of ketamine administration cannot be simply attributed to glutamatergic mechanisms, but a pre-treatment strategy in which one aims to block the effects of the drug using more selective compounds can be used to facilitate interpretation of the mechanisms associated with its specific effects. Using this approach, Krystal and colleagues have demonstrated that the psychotic effects of ketamine are not ameliorated by benzodiazepine blockade (Krystal *et al.*, 1998b) or dopamine D2 blockade (Krystal *et al.*, 1999). However, haloperidol was found to reduce the associated deficits in executive function, suggesting an interaction of these drugs in frontal cortex in mediating cognitive function (Krystal *et al.*, 1999). Similarly, disruption of working memory following ketamine is prevented by pre-treatment with a group II metabotropic receptor agonist (Krystal *et al.*, 2005b). Both cognitive and psychotic effects were attenuated following blockade of voltage-sensitive calcium channels, using nimodipine, suggesting that this may also be an important mechanism in the pathophysiology of ketamine-related psychosis (Krystal *et al.*, 1996). These studies are important in suggesting novel mechanisms by which the cognitive deficits in schizophrenia may be targeted for treatment. A similar approach has also been reported in which one aims to potentiate the effects of ketamine using a second compound. Krystal *et al.* (2005a) found that amphetamine and ketamine did not have additive effects on psychosis, thought disorder and euphoria, suggesting a dissociability of the effects of dopaminergic and glutamatergic mechanisms. However, amphetamine attenuated the disruption of working memory associated with ketamine, again supporting the role of prefrontal dopaminergic transmission in the cognitive effects of ketamine.

A related strategy which has the potential to identify fundamental neurobiological mechanisms of psychosis is the combination of drug models. Both THC and ketamine induce psychopathology in healthy subjects. However, these drugs ostensibly act via distinct mechanisms: the cannabinoid CB1 receptor is believed to mediate the psychotropic effects of THC, whereas ketamine is believed to exert its psychopathological effects via the NMDA receptor. Both the endocannabinoid and glutamatergic systems are intricately connected to the dopaminergic system, suggesting this may be a common mechanism of action. A testable prediction for the central involvement of dopamine in the generation of specific psychotic symptoms would be that symptoms following administration of both ketamine and THC should be prevented by blocking dopaminergic transmission. Observing commonalities between these drug models may indicate a final common pathway mediating specific symptoms. Similarly, differences between drug models may prove equally informative: drug-specific effects of ketamine and THC might reasonably be related to distinctive mechanisms associated with these compounds.

Individual differences as measures of symptom vulnerability

The heterogeneity of schizophrenia indicates that vulnerability to specific patterns of symptoms varies considerably between patients, and over the course of the illness. The biological factors which predispose patients to such vulnerability is unknown, but would be extremely valuable information in early treatment of high-risk subjects, and in pre-empting relapse. Healthy volunteers also show a wide variability in the subjective and cognitive response to ketamine. An intriguing possibility is that parallel mechanisms which confer vulnerability to specific psychotic symptoms under ketamine may also confer vulnerability to disease-related psychopathology. Ketamine induces delusional ideation, similar to that observed in patients with schizophrenia. An increasingly prominent theory is that delusions develop as a result of abnormal perceptual associations, in response to which the patient engages in delusional reasoning to impose a causal structure (Kapur, 2003). In a recent study, it was shown that the level of lateral prefrontal response to a causal learning task under placebo strongly predicted the degree of referential delusions subjects subsequently experienced under ketamine

(Corlett *et al.*, 2006). This suggests that physiological variability present within the normal population may represent a predisposition to specific symptoms under ketamine. It remains to be determined whether this physiological marker in the prefrontal cortex is also predictive of psychosis in patients. The advantage of this design is that subjects can be studied before and after the psychotic episode. Equivalent studies in patient populations are extremely difficult and time-consuming, requiring the identification and assessment of subjects before the onset of illness, followed by longitudinal assessments over the period in which the disease emerges. Whilst findings are beginning to emerge from such studies (Whalley *et al.*, 2006; see also Chapter 26, this volume, on schizophrenia), this naturalistic design relies on disease occurring in a subgroup of the identified individuals, which may take several months or years to emerge. The drug model approach offers the flexibility to relate vulnerability to outcome in a short period of time, and to test specific hypotheses in a controlled experimental context.

Fractionating cognitive processes

The flexibility of the drug-model approach also allows the effects of the drug to be specified with greater precision in terms of the specific processes which are disrupted. This is illustrated in the example cited earlier in which assessment of episodic memory pre- and post-drug administration facilitates dissociation of drug effects on encoding from retrieval processes (Honey *et al.*, 2005b). When the drug is given subsequent to encoding and items are retrieved in the presence of the drug, detrimental mnemonic effects can be attributed to the disruption of retrieval. Similarly, when the drug is administered prior to the subject encoding the information, but is terminated and levels allowed to return to baseline prior to retrieval of the items, the effect of the drug can be attributed to a disruption of encoding. Clearly, this design would be untenable in patient studies, since one cannot experimentally manipulate psychosis in this way in patients. Such designs may therefore prove useful in interpreting cognitive deficits in patients, where one must make assumptions about whether information has been appropriately encoded/retrieved, and rely on indirect methods.

Separating cognitive and psychotic effects

Finally, careful manipulation of the dosage enables the separation of cognitive effects at low, sub-psychotic doses, from the psychotomimetic effects of the drug. This has been reported in a number of studies in which the observed psychotic effects of ketamine at between 50–100 ng/ml plasma concentrations are minimal, but in which deficits in both working memory (Honey *et al.* 2003, 2004) and episodic memory (Honey *et al.*, 2005a, 2005b, 2006) have been reported. The non-specific distracting effects of psychosis can be effectively eliminated in interpreting precise effects of drug on cognitive function. This is an important advantage, since the mechanisms which mediate the cognitive and psychotic symptoms in schizophrenia are often thought to be relatively independent, as evidenced by the limited efficacy of antipsychotics to improve cognitive and negative symptoms, whilst effectively treating positive symptoms.

Limitations of the approach
Validity

Pharmacological models of schizophrenia differ in important respects with regard to the illness itself, and it is important to acknowledge and understand these issues, in order to appropriately interpret findings obtained using this approach. Perhaps the most important consideration is the clinical validity of these models: are the symptoms experienced under psychotomimetic drugs truly similar in nature to those experienced as a consequence of disease? Certainly, the symptoms typically reported following exposure to ketamine are evident as quantified using standard psychiatric rating scales. Further, the exacerbation of existing symptoms when patients with schizophrenia are exposed to ketamine is supportive of the idea that drug-related symptoms are qualitatively related. Two cardinal symptoms in particular highlight important differences between an acute dose model and the insidious onset of psychotic symptoms.

Auditory hallucinations are not generally observed following administration of ketamine, perhaps suggesting that ketamine is not a valid model of this aspect of psychosis. However, subjects do report auditory illusory experiences: difficulty in locating sounds, changes in the acoustic nature of sounds, and difficulty in filtering background sounds. Reports of patients' descriptions of the early prodromal symptoms of schizophrenia include a heightening of sensory vividness in auditory and visual fields (McGhie & Chapman, 1961). Such perceptual changes, if experienced chronically and in the absence of a clear precipitating factor (such as an experimental drug infusion) could conceivably contribute to the perception that sounds (even those generated internally) are alien in nature and of external origin; therefore, forming the basis for an auditory hallucination. The central distinction between the experience associated with drugs, and that with disease, is that the evaluative process that occurs in response to the perceptual changes in disease may occur over weeks and months in order to rationalize the experience. In the acute drug setting, it is possible that the drug provides a valid model of the same perceptual changes that occur during the illness and may be central to the genesis of the symptom, but by definition, it cannot model the protracted evaluative response to this experience. Furthermore, the setting of the clinical experiment provides a context which the subject is able to use to attribute abnormal experiences and thereby retain insight; whereby, they remain aware that the drug is causing the perceptual changes. Under these experimental conditions, subjects are less likely to engage in the more bizarre rationalizations of their experience that patients adopt when they may experience similar changes, but do not have similar causal information. It is possible that there is overlap in the central pathophysiological mechanism which supports symptoms in both drug and disease states, but the phenomenological outcome may differ as a result of the context in which they occur.

A second example is that of referential delusions. A prominent theory of the formation of delusions asserts that dysregulated dopaminergic firing increases the salience of randomly occurring events, thereby biasing the subject to form inappropriate associations between these events (Kapur, 2003). According to this view, the delusion forms and crystallizes as a rationalization of the inappropriate association. Again, it is possible that an acute drug model may impact upon the same perceptual changes which lead to the formation of inappropriate associations, however, it is clearly beyond the setting of this approach to capture the subsequent process of evaluation which leads to the delusional belief.

Reliability

The cognitive effects of drug models of psychosis reviewed earlier show some consistent findings, however, it is clear that this literature is not without discrepancies. Furthermore, some of the findings,

particularly so with respect to THC effects, have yet to be replicated and must therefore be interpreted cautiously in light of this. Methodological considerations may account to some extent for these discrepancies. In particular, the considerable variation in choices of subjects (drug-naïve subjects versus regular drug users) and different doses, routes of administration, dosing regimes and the inconsistent use of drug plasma level monitoring during experimental procedures should be considered carefully in interpreting findings across studies. The dosing regime in studies involving steady-state plasma concentrations is typically based on a three-compartment model of ketamine pharmacokinetics, combining a bolus dose, a constant rate infusion to compensate for drug elimination, and an exponentially decreasing infusion to compensate for drug distribution (Kruger-Theimer, (1968). Based on this pharmacokinetic model, Radant et al. (1998) reported a mean variation of measured to target concentration of $<30\%$; they also noted greater variability with higher dose ranges (150 and 200 ng/ml), with actual levels tending to exceed predicted levels at these higher doses. Other studies in which plasma levels have not been monitored complicate interpretation of discrepant findings across studies.

Specificity

To what extent are the effects of ketamine and other similar drugs seen in, and only in, schizophrenia? This is a difficult question, since the blurred taxonomic boundaries of schizophrenia mean that there are no symptoms which are specific to the illness, and some patients will have symptoms not seen in other patients. With this caveat in mind, there are some experiences reported under ketamine which differ from the typical clinical profile of schizophrenia. Euphoria, for example, is not characteristic of the illness, but is frequently observed following ketamine. Ketamine, of course, has actions at other non-NMDA sites, and these effects presumably relate to other aspects of ketamine's pharmacological profile. Other effects of ketamine such as sedation and fatigue are similarly not representative of the illness, and it is important to bear in mind the extent to which these non-specific effects interact or confound interpretation of the symptoms of schizophrenia one is attempting to model. A related point regarding specificity is that some of the symptoms which are common to both drug and disease state, are unique to neither. Memory impairments, for example, are characteristic of a broad range of other illnesses, and it is therefore difficult to interpret the implications of deficits seen using behaviorally complex and multifaceted tasks which may also appear in numerous other conditions. It is important therefore to establish the extent to which memory deficits under ketamine represent more precise process deficits seen in, and (ideally) only in, schizophrenia. Ultimately, we must attempt to relate these cognitive deficits to the psychotic symptoms of the illness.

Conclusions

Psychopharmacological models of psychosis provide important insights into the cognitive and neurobiological mechanisms which may be impaired in patients. The flexibility of this approach means that central questions can be addressed efficiently and iteratively, where similar investigations in patients would be intractable. The findings from such studies are beginning to yield important observations, and may inform our understanding of key issues in clinical psychiatry, such as individual differences which predispose to vulnerability to specific symptoms. The identification of such markers will require an appreciation of the experimental medicine context in which the data are acquired.

References

Adler, C. M., Goldberg, T. E., Malhotra, A. K., Pickar, D. & Breier, A. (1998). Effects of ketamine on thought disorder, working memory, and semantic memory in healthy volunteers. *Biological Psychiatry*, **43**, 811–816.

Adler, C. M., Malhotra, A. K., Elman, I. *et al.* (1999). Comparison of ketamine-induced thought disorder in healthy volunteers and thought disorder in schizophrenia. *American Journal of Psychiatry*, **156**, 1646–1649.

Ahn, K. H., Youn, T., Cho, S. S. *et al.* (2003). N-methyl-D-aspartate receptor in working memory impairments in schizophrenia: event-related potential study of late stage of working memory process. *Progress in Neuropsychopharmacology and Biological Psychiatry*, **27**, 993–999.

Baddeley, A. (1986). *Working Memory*. Oxford: Clarendon Press.

Baddeley, A. (1992). Working memory. *Science*, **256**, 556–559.

Baddeley, A. (1998). Recent developments in working memory. *Current Opinion in Neurobiology*, **8**, 234–238.

Baddeley, A. & Hitch, G. (1974). Working memory. In G. Bower (Ed.), *The Psychology of Learning and Motivation* (pp. 47–90). New York, NY: Academic Press.

Bell, M. D., Bryson, G. & Wexler, B. (2001). Verbal working memory impairment in schizophrenia. *American Journal of Psychiatry*, **158**, 660–661.

Bentall, R. (1993). Deconstructing the concept of schizophrenia. *Journal of Mental Health*, **2**, 223–238.

Bentall, R. P., Jackson, H. F. & Pilgrim, D. (1988). The concept of schizophrenia is dead: long live the concept of schizophrenia? *British Journal of Clinical Psychology*, **27**, 329–331.

Binder, J., Albus, M., Hubmann, W. *et al.* (1998). Neuropsychological impairment and psychopathology in first-episode schizophrenic patients related to the early course of illness. *European Archives of Psychiatry and Clinical Neuroscience*, **248**, 70–77.

Bowers, M. B., Jr. & Morton, J. B. (1994). Regional brain catecholamines and metabolites following THC, PCP and MK-801. *Progress in Neuropsychopharmacology and Biological Psychiatry*, **18**, 961–964.

Brebion, G., Amador, X., David, A. *et al.* (2000). Positive symptomatology and source-monitoring failure in schizophrenia – an analysis of symptom-specific effects. *Psychiatry Research*, **95**, 119–131.

Brebion, G., Gorman, J. M., Amador, X., Malaspina, D. & Sharif, Z. (2002). Source monitoring impairments in schizophrenia: characterisation and associations with positive and negative symptomatology. *Psychiatry Research*, **112**, 27–39.

Byrd, L. D., Standish, L. J. & Howell, L. L. (1987). Behavioral effects of phencyclidine and ketamine alone and in combination with other drugs. *European Journal of Pharmacology*, **144**, 331–341.

Calev, A., Venables, P. H. & Monk, A. F. (1983). Evidence for distinct verbal memory pathologies in severely and mildly disturbed schizophrenics. *Schizophrenia Bulletin*, **9**, 247–264.

Callicott, J. H., Egan, M. F., Mattay, V. S. *et al.* (2003). Abnormal fMRI response of the dorsolateral prefrontal cortex in cognitively intact siblings of patients with schizophrenia. *American Journal of Psychiatry*, **160**, 709–719.

Callicott, J. H., Bertolino, A., Mattay, V. S. *et al.* (2000). Physiological dysfunction of the dorsolateral prefrontal cortex in schizophrenia revisited. *Cerebral Cortex*, **10**, 1078–1092.

Cannon, T. D., Zorrilla, L. E., Shtasel, D. *et al.* (1994). Neuropsychological functioning in siblings discordant for schizophrenia and healthy volunteers. *Archives of General Psychiatry*, **51**, 651–661.

Carlsson, M. & Carlsson, A. (1990). Schizophrenia: a subcortical neurotransmitter imbalance syndrome? *Schizophrenia Bulletin*, **16**, 425–432.

Carpenter, W. T., Jr. (1999). The schizophrenia ketamine challenge study debate. *Biological Psychiatry*, **46**, 1081–1091.

Carter, C., Robertson, L., Nordahl, T. *et al.* (1996). Spatial working memory deficits and their relationship to negative symptoms in unmedicated schizophrenia patients. *Biological Psychiatry*, **40**, 930–932.

Clare, L., McKenna, P. J., Mortimer, A. M. & Baddeley, A. D. (1993). Memory in schizophrenia: what is impaired and what is preserved? *Neuropsychologia*, **31**, 1225–1241.

Cohen, J. D. & Servan-Schreiber, D. (1992). Context, cortex, and dopamine: a connectionist approach to behavior and biology in schizophrenia. *Psychological Review*, **99**, 45–77.

Condray, R., Steinhauer, S., van Kammen, D. & Kasparek, A. (1996). Working memory capacity predicts language comprehension in schizophrenic patients. *Schizophrenia Research*, **20**, 1–13.

Conklin, H. M., Curtis, C. E., Calkins, M. E. & Iacono, W. G. (2005). Working memory functioning in schizophrenia patients and their first-degree relatives: cognitive functioning shedding light on etiology. *Neuropsychologia*, **43**, 930–942.

Conklin, H., Curtis, C., Katsanis, J. & Iacono, W. (2000). Verbal working memory impairment in schizophrenia patients and their first-degree relatives: evidence from the digit span task. *American Journal of Psychiatry*, **157**, 275–277.

Corlett, P. R., Honey, G. D., Aitken, M. R. F. *et al.* (2006). Frontal responses during learning predict vulnerability to the psychotogenic effects of ketamine: linking cognition, brain activity and psychosis. *Archives of General Psychiatry*, **63** (6), 611–621.

Curran, H. V. & Morgan, C. (2000). Cognitive, dissociative and psychotogenic effects of ketamine in recreational users on the night of drug use and 3 days later. *Addiction*, **95**, 575–590.

Curran, H. V., Brignell, C., Fletcher, S., Middleton, P. & Henry, J. (2002). Cognitive and subjective dose-response effects of acute oral delta 9-tetrahydrocannabinol (THC) in infrequent cannabis users. *Psychopharmacology (Berlin)*, **164**, 61–70.

Danysz, W., Wroblewski, J. T. & Costa, E. (1988). Learning impairment in rats by N-methyl-D-aspartate receptor antagonists. *Neuropharmacology*, **27**, 653–656.

Deakin, J. F., Slater, P., Simpson, M. D. *et al.* (1989). Frontal cortical and left temporal glutamatergic dysfunction in schizophrenia. *Journal of Neurochemistry*, **52**, 1781–1786.

Deutsch, S. I., Mastropaolo, J., Schwartz, B. L., Rosse, R. B. & Morihisa, J. M. (1989). A "glutamatergic hypothesis" of schizophrenia. Rationale for pharmacotherapy with glycine. *Clinical Neuropharmacology*, **12**, 1–13.

D'Souza, D. C., Abi-Saab, W. M., Madonick, S. *et al.* (2005). Delta-9-tetrahydrocannabinol effects in schizophrenia: implications for cognition, psychosis, and addiction. *Biological Psychiatry*, **57**, 594–608.

D'Souza, D. C., Perry, E., MacDougall, L. *et al.* (2004). The psychotomimetic effects of intravenous delta-9-tetrahydrocannabinol in healthy individuals: implications for psychosis. *Neuropsychopharmacology*, **29**, 1558–1572.

Duncan, E. J., Madonick, S. H., Parwani, A. *et al.* (2001). Clinical and sensorimotor gating effects of ketamine in normals. *Neuropsychopharmacology*, **25**, 72–83.

Egan, M. F., Goldberg, T. E., Kolachana, B. S. *et al.* (2001). Effect of COMT Val108/158 Met genotype on frontal lobe function and risk for schizophrenia. *Proceedings of the National Academy of Sciences USA*, **98**, 6917–6922.

Emrich, H. M., Leweke, F. M. & Schneider, U. (1997). Towards a cannabinoid hypothesis of schizophrenia: cognitive impairments due to dysregulation of the endogenous cannabinoid system. *Pharmacology, Biochemistry and Behavior*, **56**, 803–807.

Fant, R. V., Heishman, S. J., Bunker, E. B. & Pickworth, W. B. (1998). Acute and residual effects of marijuana in humans. *Pharmacology, Biochemistry and Behavior*, **60**, 777–784.

Fields, R. B., Van Kammen, D. P., Peters, J. L. *et al.* (1988). Clonidine improves memory function in schizophrenia independently from change in psychosis. Preliminary findings. *Schizophrenia Research*, **1**, 417–423.

Fleming, K., Goldberg, T. E., Binks, S. *et al.* (1997). Visuospatial working memory in patients with schizophrenia. *Biological Psychiatry*, **41**, 43–49.

Fleming, K., Goldberg, T. E., Gold, J. M. & Weinberger, D. R. (1995). Verbal working memory dysfunction in schizophrenia: use of a Brown-Peterson paradigm. *Psychiatry Research*, **56**, 155–161.

Frith, C. (1992). *The Cognitive Neuropsychology of Schizophrenia*. Hove, UK: Lawrence Erlbaum Associates.

Ghoneim, M. M., Hinrichs, J. V., Mewaldt, S. P. & Petersen, R. C. (1985). Ketamine: behavioral effects of subanesthetic doses. *Journal of Clinical Psychopharmacology*, **5**, 70–77.

Glahn, D. C., Cannon, T. D., Gur, R. E., Ragland, J. D. & Gur, R. C. (2000). Working memory constrains abstraction in schizophrenia. *Biological Psychiatry*, **47**, 34–42.

Goldman-Rakic, P. (1987). Circuitry of primate prefrontal cortex and regulation of behaviour by representational memory. In F. Plum (Ed.), *Handbook of Physiology: The Nervous System* (pp. 373–417). Bethesda, MD: American Physiological Society.

Goldman-Rakic, P. (1990). Prefrontal cortical dysfunction in schizophrenia: the relevance of working memory. In B. Carroll & J. Bartrett (Eds.), *Psychopathology and the Brain* (pp. 1–23). New York, NY: Raven Press.

Goldman-Rakic, P. S. (1994). Working memory dysfunction in schizophrenia. *Journal of Neuropsychiatry and Clinical Neuroscience*, **6**, 348–357.

Goldman-Rakic, P. S. (1999). The physiological approach: functional architecture of working memory and disordered cognition in schizophrenia. *Biological Psychiatry*, **46**, 650–661.

Gooding, D. C. & Tallent, K. A. (2002). Spatial working memory performance in patients with schizoaffective psychosis versus schizophrenia: a tale of two disorders? *Schizophrenia Research*, **53**, 209–218.

Granholm, E., Morris, S. K., Sarkin, A. J., Asarnow, R. F. & Jeste, D. V. (1997). Pupillary responses index overload of working memory resources in schizophrenia. *Journal of Abnormal Psychology*, **106**, 458–467.

Green, M. F. (1996). What are the functional consequences of neurocognitive deficits in schizophrenia? *American Journal of Psychiatry*, **153**, 321–330.

Green, M. F. & Nuechterlein, K. H. (1999). Should schizophrenia be treated as a neurocognitive disorder? *Schizophrenia Bulletin*, **25**, 309–319.

Haller, J., Szirmai, M., Varga, B., Ledent, C. & Freund, T. F. (2005). Cannabinoid CB1 receptor dependent effects of the NMDA antagonist phencyclidine in the social withdrawal model of schizophrenia. *Behavioral Pharmacology*, **16**, 415–422.

Harris, J. A., Biersner, R. J., Edwards, D. & Bailey, L. W. (1975). Attention, learning, and personality during ketamine emergence: a pilot study. *Anesthesia and Analgesia*, **54**, 169–172.

Hart, C. L., van Gorp, W., Haney, M., Foltin, R. W. & Fischman, M. W. (2001). Effects of acute smoked marijuana on complex cognitive performance. *Neuropsychopharmacology*, **25**, 757–765.

Heishman, S. J., Arasteh, K. & Stitzer, M. L. (1997). Comparative effects of alcohol and marijuana on mood, memory, and performance. *Pharmacology, Biochemistry and Behavior*, **58**, 93–101.

Hetem, L. A., Danion, J. M., Diemunsch, P. & Brandt, C. (2000). Effect of a subanesthetic dose of ketamine on memory and conscious awareness in healthy volunteers. *Psychopharmacology (Berlin)*, **152**, 283–288.

Hirsch, S. R., Das, I., Garey, L. J. & de Belleroche, J. (1997). A pivotal role for glutamate in the pathogenesis of schizophrenia, and its cognitive dysfunction. *Pharmacology, Biochemistry and Behavior*, **56**, 797–802.

Honey, G. D., Bullmore, E. T. & Sharma, T. (2002). De-coupling of cognitive performance and cerebral functional response during working memory in schizophrenia. *Schizophrenia Research*, **53**, 45–56.

Honey, G. D., Honey, R. A., O'Loughlin, C. *et al.* (2005a). Ketamine disrupts frontal and hippocampal contribution to encoding and retrieval of episodic memory: an FMRI study. *Cerebral Cortex*, **15**, 749–759.

Honey, G. D., O'Loughlin, C., Turner, D. C. *et al.* (2006). The effects of a subpsychotic dose of ketamine on recognition and source memory for agency: implications for pharmacological modelling of core symptoms of schizophrenia. *Neuropsychopharmacology*, **31**, 413–423.

Honey, G. D., Honey, R. A., Sharar, S. R. *et al.* (2005b). Impairment of specific episodic memory processes by sub-psychotic doses of ketamine: the effects of levels of processing at encoding and of the subsequent retrieval task. *Psychopharmacology (Berlin)*, **181**, 445–457.

Honey, R. A., Turner, D. C., Honey, G. D. *et al.* (2003). Subdissociative dose ketamine produces a deficit in manipulation but not maintenance of the contents of working memory. *Neuropsychopharmacology*, **30**, 30.

Honey, R. A., Honey, G. D., O'Loughlin, C. *et al.* (2004). Acute ketamine administration alters the brain responses to executive demands in a verbal working memory task: an FMRI study. *Neuropsychopharmacology*, **29**, 1203–1214.

Ilan, A. B., Smith, M. E. & Gevins, A. (2004). Effects of marijuana on neurophysiological signals of working and episodic memory. *Psychopharmacology (Berlin)*, **176**, 214–222.

Ishimaru, M., Kurumaji, A. & Toru, M. (1994). Increases in strychnine-insensitive glycine binding sites in cerebral cortex of chronic schizophrenics: evidence for glutamate hypothesis. *Biological Psychiatry*, **35**, 84–95.

Iversen, L. (2003). Cannabis and the brain. *Brain*, **126**, 1252–1270.

Javitt, D. C. & Zukin, S. R. (1991). Recent advances in the phencyclidine model of schizophrenia. *American Journal of Psychiatry*, **148**, 1301–1308.

Jentsch, J. D. & Anzivino, L. A. (2004). A low dose of the alpha2 agonist clonidine ameliorates the visual attention and spatial working memory deficits produced by phencyclidine administration to rats. *Psychopharmacology (Berlin)*, **175**, 76–83.

Jentsch, J. D. & Roth, R. H. (1999). The neuropsychopharmacology of phencyclidine: from NMDA receptor hypofunction to the dopamine hypothesis of schizophrenia. *Neuropsychopharmacology*, **20**, 201–225.

Jentsch, J. D., Andrusiak, E., Tran, A., Bowers, M. B., Jr. & Roth, R. H. (1997). Delta 9-tetrahydrocannabinol increases prefrontal cortical catecholaminergic utilization and impairs spatial working memory in the rat: blockade of dopaminergic effects with HA966. *Neuropsychopharmacology*, **16**, 426–432.

Jentsch, J. D., Wise, A., Katz, Z. & Roth, R. H. (1998). Alpha-noradrenergic receptor modulation of the phencyclidine- and delta9-tetrahydrocannabinol-induced increases in dopamine utilization in rat prefrontal cortex. *Synapse*, **28**, 21–26.

Johns, A. (2001). Psychiatric effects of cannabis. *British Journal of Psychiatry*, **178**, 116–122.

Jones, K. W., Bauerle, L. M. & DeNoble, V. J. (1990). Differential effects of sigma and phencyclidine receptor ligands on learning. *European Journal of Pharmacology*, **179**, 97–102.

Kapur, S. (2003). Psychosis as a state of aberrant salience: a framework linking biology, phenomenology, and pharmacology in schizophrenia. *American Journal of Psychiatry*, **160**, 13–23.

Keefe, R. S. E., Arnold, M. C., Bayen, U. J. & Harvey, P. D. (1999). Source monitoring deficits in patients with schizophrenia; a multinomial modelling analysis. *Psychological Medicine*, **29**, 903–914.

Keefe, R. S. E., Arnold, M. C., Bayen, U. J., McEvoy, J. P. & Wilson, W. H. (2002). Source-monitoring deficits for self-generated stimuli in schizophrenia: multinomial modeling of data from three sources. *Schizophrenia Research*, **57**, 51–67.

Keefe, R. S., Roitman, S. E., Harvey, P. D. (1995). A pen-and-paper human analogue of a monkey prefrontal cortex activation task: spatial working memory in patients with schizophrenia. *Schizophrenia Research*, **17**, 25–33.

Kim, J., Glahn, D. C., Nuechterlein, K. H. & Cannon, T. D. (2004). Maintenance and manipulation of information in schizophrenia: further evidence for impairment in the central executive component of working memory. *Schizophrenia Research*, **68**, 173–187.

Kim, J. S., Kornhuber, H. H., Schmid-Burgk, W. & Holzmuller, B. (1980). Low cerebrospinal fluid glutamate in schizophrenic patients and a new hypothesis on schizophrenia. *Neuroscience Letters*, **20**, 379–382.

Kornhuber, J., Mack-Burkhardt, F., Riederer, P. et al. (1989). [3H]MK-801 binding sites in postmortem brain regions of schizophrenic patients. *Journal of Neural Transmission*, **77**, 231–236.

Kraepelin, E. (1896). *Psychiatrie*. Leipzig: Barth.

Kruger-Theimer, E. (1968). Continuous intravenous infusion and multicompartment accumulation. *European Journal of Pharmacology*, **4**, 317–324.

Krystal, J. H., Abi-Saab, W., Perry, E. et al. (2005b). Preliminary evidence of attenuation of the disruptive effects of the NMDA glutamate receptor antagonist, ketamine, on working memory by pretreatment with the group II metabotropic glutamate receptor agonist, LY354740, in healthy human subjects. *Psychopharmacology (Berlin)*, **179**, 303–309.

Krystal, J. H., Bennett, A., Abi-Saab, D. et al. (2000). Dissociation of ketamine effects on rule acquisition and rule implementation: possible relevance to NMDA receptor contributions to executive cognitive functions. *Biological Psychiatry*, **47**, 137–143.

Krupitsky, E. M., Burakov, A. M., Romanova, T. N. et al. (2001). Attenuation of ketamine effects by nimodipine pretreatment in recovering ethanol dependent men: psychopharmacologic implications of the interaction of NMDA and L-type calcium channel antagonists. *Neuropsychopharmacology*, **25**, 936–947.

Krystal, J. H., Compere, S., Nestler, E. J. & Rasmussen, K. (1996). Nimodipine reduction of naltrexone-precipitated locus coeruleus activation and abstinence behavior in morphine-dependent rats. *Physiology and Behavior*, **59**, 863–866.

Krystal, J. H., D'Souza, D. C., Karper, L. P. et al. (1999). Interactive effects of subanesthetic ketamine and haloperidol in healthy humans. *Psychopharmacology (Berlin)*, **145**, 193–204.

Krystal, J. H., Karper, L. P., Bennett, A. et al. (1998b). Interactive effects of subanesthetic ketamine and subhypnotic lorazepam in humans. *Psychopharmacology (Berlin)*, **135**, 213–229.

Krystal, J. H., Karper, L. P., Seibyl, J. P. (1994). Subanesthetic effects of the noncompetitive NMDA antagonist, ketamine, in humans. Psychotomimetic, perceptual, cognitive, and neuroendocrine responses. *Archives of General Psychiatry*, **51**, 199–214.

Krystal, J. H., Perry, E. B., Jr., Gueorguieva, R. et al. (2005a). Comparative and interactive human psychopharmacologic effects of ketamine and amphetamine: implications for glutamatergic and dopaminergic model psychoses and cognitive function. *Archives of General Psychiatry*, **62**, 985–994.

Krystal, J. H., Petrakis, I. L., Webb, E. et al. (1998a). Dose-related ethanol-like effects of the NMDA antagonist, ketamine, in recently detoxified alcoholics. *Archives of General Psychiatry*, **55**, 354–360.

Lahti, A. C., Holcomb, H. H., Medoff, D. R. & Tamminga, C. A. (1995a). Ketamine activates psychosis and alters limbic blood flow in schizophrenia. *Neuroreport*, **6**, 869–872.

Lahti, A. C., Koffel, B., LaPorte, D. & Tamminga, C. A. (1995b). Subanesthetic doses of ketamine stimulate psychosis in schizophrenia. *Neuropsychopharmacology*, **13**, 9–19.

Lahti, A. C., Weiler, M. A., Tamara Michaelidis, B. A., Parwani, A. & Tamminga, C. A. (2001). Effects of ketamine in normal and schizophrenic volunteers. *Neuropsychopharmacology*, **25**, 455–467.

Landro, N. I., Orbeck, A. L. & Rund, B. R. (1993). Memory functioning in chronic and non-chronic schizophrenics, affectively disturbed patients and normal controls. *Schizophrenia Research*, **10**, 85–92.

LaPorte, D. J., Lahti, A. C., Koffel, B. & Tamminga, C. A. (1996). Absence of ketamine effects on memory and other cognitive functions in schizophrenia patients. *Journal of Psychiatric Research*, **30**, 321–330.

Lodge, D. & Anis, N. A. (1982). Effects of phencyclidine on excitatory amino acid activation of spinal interneurones in the cat. *European Journal of Pharmacology*, **77**, 203–204.

Luby, E. D., Gottlieb, J. S., Cohen, B. D., Rosenbaum, G. & Domino, E. F. (1962). Model psychoses and schizophrenia. *American Journal of Psychiatry*, **119**, 61–67.

Lyons, M. J., Toomey, R., Seidman, L. J. *et al.* (1995). Verbal learning and memory in relatives of schizophrenics: preliminary findings. *Biological Psychiatry*, **37**, 750–753.

Malhotra, A. K., Pinals, D. A., Adler, C. M. *et al.* (1997). Ketamine-induced exacerbation of psychotic symptoms and cognitive impairment in neuroleptic-free schizophrenics. *Neuropsychopharmacology*, **17**, 141–150.

Malhotra, A. K., Pinals, D. A., Weingartner, H. *et al.* (1996). NMDA receptor function and human cognition: the effects of ketamine in healthy volunteers. *Neuropsychopharmacology*, **14**, 301–307.

Manoach, D. S., Gollub, R. L., Benson, E. S. *et al.* (2000). Schizophrenic subjects show aberrant fMRI activation of dorsolateral prefrontal cortex and basal ganglia during working memory performance. *Biological Psychiatry*, **48**, 99–109.

Manoach, D.-S., Press, D.-Z., Thangaraj, V. *et al.* (1999). Schizophrenic subjects activate dorsolateral prefrontal cortex during a working memory task, as measured by fMRI. *Biological Psychiatry*, **45**, 1128–1137.

Manschreck, T. C., Maher, B. A., Candela, S. F. *et al.* (2000). Impaired verbal memory is associated with impaired motor performance in schizophrenia: relationship to brain structure. *Schizophrenia Research*, **43**, 21–32.

McDonald, J., Schleifer, L., Richards, J. B. & de Wit, H. (2003). Effects of THC on behavioral measures of impulsivity in humans. *Neuropsychopharmacology*, **28**, 1356–1365.

McGhie, A. & Chapman, J. (1961). Disorders of attention and perception in early schizophrenia. *British Journal of Medical Psychology*, **34**, 103–116.

Morgan, C. J., Mofeez, A., Brandner, B., Bromley, L. & Curran, H. V. (2004). Acute effects of ketamine on memory systems and psychotic symptoms in healthy volunteers. *Neuropsychopharmacology*, **29**, 208–218.

Morice, R. & Delahunty, A. (1996). Frontal/executive impairments in schizophrenia. *Schizophrenia Bulletin*, **22**, 125–137.

Morris, R. G., Anderson, E., Lynch, G. S. & Baudry, M. (1986). Selective impairment of learning and blockade of long-term potentiation by an N-methyl-D-aspartate receptor antagonist, AP5. *Nature*, **319**, 774–776.

Morris, R. G., Halliwell, R. F. & Bowery, N. (1989). Synaptic plasticity and learning. II: Do different kinds of plasticity underlie different kinds of learning? *Neuropsychologia*, **27**, 41–59.

Murman, D. L., Giordani, B., Mellow, A. M. *et al.* (1997). Cognitive, behavioral, and motor effects of the NMDA antagonist ketamine in Huntington's disease. *Neurology*, **49**, 153–161.

Newcomer, J. W., Farber, N. B., Jevtovic-Todorovic, V. *et al.* (1999). Ketamine-induced NMDA receptor hypofunction as a model of memory impairment and psychosis. *Neuropsychopharmacology*, **20**, 106–118.

Nicholson, A. N., Turner, C., Stone, B. M. & Robson, P. J. (2004). Effect of Delta-9-tetrahydrocannabinol and cannabidiol on nocturnal sleep and early-morning behavior in young adults. *Journal of Clinical Psychopharmacology*, **24**, 305–313.

Nishikawa, T., Takashima, M. & Toru, M. (1983). Increased [3H]kainic acid binding in the prefrontal cortex in schizophrenia. *Neuroscience Letters*, **40**, 245–250.

Nopoulos, P., Flashman, L., Flaum, M., Arndt, S. & Andreasen, N. (1994). Stability of cognitive functioning early in the course of schizophrenia. *Schizophrenia Research*, **14**, 29–37.

Okada, A. (2002). Deficits of spatial working memory in chronic schizophrenia. *Schizophrenia Research*, **53**, 75–82.

Olney, J. W. & Farber, N. B. (1995). Glutamate receptor dysfunction and schizophrenia. *Archives of General Psychiatry*, **52**, 998–1007.

Oranje, B., van Berckel, B. N., Kemner, C. *et al.* (2000). The effects of a sub-anaesthetic dose of ketamine on human selective attention. *Neuropsychopharmacology*, **22**, 293–302.

Oye, I., Paulsen, O. & Maurset, A. (1992). Effects of ketamine on sensory perception: evidence for a role of N-methyl-D-aspartate receptors. *Journal of Pharmacological and Experimental Therapeutics*, **260**, 1209–1213.

Pandit, S. K., Kothary, S. P. & Kumar, S. M. (1980). Low dose intravenous infusion technique with ketamine.

Amnesic, analgesic and sedative effects in human volunteers. *Anaesthesia*, **35**, 669–675.

Pantelis, C., Stuart, G. W., Nelson, H. E., Robbins, T. W. & Barnes, T. R. (2001). Spatial working memory deficits in schizophrenia: relationship with tardive dyskinesia and negative symptoms. *American Journal of Psychiatry*, **158**, 1276–1285.

Parada-Turska, J. & Turski, W. A. (1990). Excitatory amino acid antagonists and memory: effect of drugs acting at N-methyl-D-aspartate receptors in learning and memory tasks. *Neuropharmacology*, **29**, 1111–1116.

Park, S. & Holzman, P. S. (1992). Schizophrenics show spatial working memory deficits. *Archives of General Psychiatry*, **49**, 975–982.

Park, S. & Holzman, P. S. (1993). Association of working memory deficit and eye tracking dysfunction in schizophrenia. *Schizophrenia Research*, **11**, 55–61.

Park, S., Puschel, J., Sauter, B. H., Rentsch, M. & Hell, D. (1999). Spatial working memory deficits and clinical symptoms in schizophrenia: a 4-month follow-up study. *Biological Psychiatry*, **46**, 392–400.

Paulsen, J. S., Heaton, R. K., Sadek, J. R. *et al.* (1995). The nature of learning and memory impairments in schizophrenia. *Journal of the International Neuropsychology Society*, **1**, 88–99.

Perlstein, W. M., Carter, C. S., Noll, D. C. & Cohen, J. D. (2001). Relation of prefrontal cortex dysfunction to working memory and symptoms in schizophrenia. *American Journal of Psychiatry*, **158**, 1105–1113.

Perry, W., Heaton, R. K., Potterat, E. *et al.* (2001). Working memory in schizophrenia: transient "online" storage versus executive functioning. *Schizophrenia Bulletin*, **27**, 157–176.

Pfenninger, E. G., Durieux, M. E. & Himmelseher, S. (2002). Cognitive impairment after small-dose ketamine isomers in comparison to equianalgesic racemic ketamine in human volunteers. *Anesthesiology*, **96**, 357–366.

Radant, A. D., Bowdle, T. A., Cowley, D. S., Kharasch, E. D. & Roy-Byrne, P. P. (1998). Does ketamine-mediated N-methyl-D-aspartate receptor antagonism cause schizophrenia-like oculomotor abnormalities? *Neuropsychopharmacology*, **19**, 434–444.

Roswold, H. E., Mirsky, A., Sarason, I., Bransome, E. D. & Beck, L. H. (1956). A continuous performance test of brain damage. *Journal of Consulting Psychology*, **20**, 343–350.

Rowland, L. M., Astur, R. S., Jung, R. E. *et al.* (2005). Selective cognitive impairments associated with NMDA receptor blockade in humans. *Neuropsychopharmacology*, **30**, 633–639.

Rushe, T. M., Morris, R. G., Miotto, E. C. *et al.* (1999). Problem-solving and spatial working memory in patients with schizophrenia and with focal frontal and temporal lobe lesions. *Schizophrenia Research*, **37**, 21–33.

Saykin, A. J., Shtasel, D. L., Gur, R. E. *et al.* (1994). Neuropsychological deficits in neuroleptic naive patients with first-episode schizophrenia. *Archives of General Psychiatry*, **51**, 124–131.

Simpson, M. D., Slater, P., Royston, M. C. & Deakin, J. F. (1991). Alterations in phencyclidine and sigma binding sites in schizophrenic brains. Effects of disease process and neuroleptic medication. *Schizophrenia Research*, **6**, 41–48.

Spangler, E. L., Bresnahan, E. L., Garofalo, P. *et al.* (1991). NMDA receptor channel antagonism by dizocilpine (MK-801) impairs performance of rats in aversively motivated complex maze tasks. *Pharmacology, Biochemistry and Behavior*, **40**, 949–958.

Spindler, K. A., Sullivan, E. V., Menon, V., Lim, K. O. & Pfefferbaum, A. (1997). Deficits in multiple systems of working memory in schizophrenia. *Schizophrenia Research*, **27**, 1–10.

Stirling, J. D., Hellewell, J. S. & Hewitt, J. (1997). Verbal memory impairment in schizophrenia: no sparing of short-term recall. *Schizophrenia Research*, **25**, 85–95.

Tek, C., Gold, J., Blaxton, T. *et al.* (2002). Visual perceptual and working memory impairments in schizophrenia. *Archives of General Psychiatry*, **59**, 146–153.

Tonkiss, J. & Rawlins, J. N. P. (1991). The competitive NMDA antagonist Ap5, but not the noncompetitive antagonist Mk801, induces a delay-related impairment in spatial working memory in rats. *Experimental Brain Research*, **85**, 349–358.

Tonkiss, J., Morris, R. G. & Rawlins, J. N. (1988). Intra-ventricular infusion of the NMDA antagonist AP5 impairs performance on a non-spatial operant DRL task in the rat. *Experimental Brain Research*, **73**, 181–188.

Umbricht, D., Schmid, L., Koller, R. *et al.* (2000). Ketamine-induced deficits in auditory and visual context-dependent processing in healthy volunteers: implications for models of cognitive deficits in schizophrenia. *Archives of General Psychiatry*, **57**, 1139–1147.

Verma, A. & Moghaddam, B. (1996). NMDA receptor antagonists impair prefrontal cortex function as assessed via spatial delayed alternation performance in rats: modulation by dopamine. *Journal of Neuroscience*, **16**, 373–379.

Walter, H., Wunderlich, A. P., Blankenhorn, M. *et al.* (2003). No hypofrontality, but absence of prefrontal lateralization comparing verbal and spatial working memory in schizophrenia. *Schizophrenia Research*, **61**, 175–184.

Weinberger, D. R. (1993). A connectionist approach to the prefrontal cortex. *Journal of Neuropsychiatry and Clinical Neuroscience*, **5**, 241–253.

Wexler, B. E., Stevens, A. A., Bowers, A. A., Sernyak, M. J. & Goldman-Rakic, P. S. (1998). Word and tone working memory deficits in schizophrenia. *Archives of General Psychiatry*, **55**, 1093–1096.

Whalley, H. C., Simonotto, E., Moorhead, W. *et al.* (2006). Functional imaging as a predictor of schizophrenia. *Biological Psychiatry*, **60**, 454–462.

Zhang, D. X. & Levy, W. B. (1992). Ketamine blocks the induction of LTP at the lateral entorhinal cortex-dentate gyrus synapses. *Brain Research*, **593**, 124–127.

Chapter 18

Cognitive phenomics

Robert M. Bilder, Russell A. Poldrack, D. Stott Parker, Steven Paul Reise, J. David Jentsch, Tyrone Cannon, Edythe London, Fred W. Sabb, Lara Foland-Ross, Angela Rizk-Jackson, Donald Kalar, Nik Brown, Audrey Carstensen and Nelson Freimer

Neuropsychology enjoys unprecedented opportunities for discovery in the post-genomic era, but also faces major challenges, particularly in finding genetic causes and rational treatments for mental disorders. Now that the Human Genome Project (HGP) has generated a complete draft of the genome, it has been argued that the Human Phenome Project (HPP) is the highest priority in biomedicine (Freimer & Sabatti, 2003). In comparison to the delineation of a relatively simple one-dimensional sequence of nucleotides that was the target of the HGP, the HPP poses enormous challenges – to characterize the myriad phenotypes from molecular expression through complex behavior of complete organisms. Research on mental disorders poses particularly formidable challenges because the "illness" phenotypes are so far removed from more basic biological processes. The phenotypic territory to be addressed by neuropsychology, while only a small fraction of the whole phenome, is still vast, including all the neuronal elements, neural systems, cognitive phenotypes and cognitive syndromes. Major questions confronting our discipline include:

(1) How are neuropsychological phenotypes best characterized and articulated in modern biomedical science?

(2) How can we systematically study the genetic and environmental contributions to these complex phenotypes?

(3) How can we relate information about neuropsychological phenotypes to other repositories of biological knowledge to foster discovery of causes and new treatments?

Major advances in genetics and genomics have now fostered the advent of *phenomics*, which broadly can be considered the systematic study of phenotypes as

these apply to the whole genome. Given the specific domains required to apply phenomics strategies to brain function and dysfunction, it is valuable to specify a new discipline of *cognitive phenomics*, which is dedicated to the systematic study of cognitive phenotypes. The unique conceptual space within which cognitive phenomics operates is illustrated schematically in Figure 18.1. This figure highlights the fact that formulation of a complete biological hypothesis about cognitive disorders from genome to syndrome requires traversal across multiple levels of analysis ranging over diverse disciplines. The figure further highlights domains that are shared between *cognitive phenomics* and other phenomics disciplines (i.e. all human physiological systems share a foundation at levels 1–3: from genetic, through proteomic, to cellular systems and signaling pathways) but at higher levels of analysis (at levels 4–7: from neural systems, to cognitive phenotypes, to symptoms and syndromes), there is clear divergence and specialization of phenotypes uniquely relevant to the clinical neurosciences. As will be discussed further below, the "top-down" influences of the cognitive phenomics strategy can further limit the scope of concepts that are most relevant in the lower-level domains. For example, the subsets of gene, protein and cellular systems/signaling pathways can be limited to those with known expression in the central nervous system for cognitive phenomics applications. With support from the NIH Roadmap Initiative (P20 RR020750) we assembled an interdisciplinary team at UCLA to develop a Center for Cognitive Phenomics (see http://www.phenomics.ucla.edu). This project has two overarching goals: (1) development of systematic empirical research strategies that will advance the discipline of cognitive phenomics; and (2) development of an informatics

---

The Neuropsychology of Mental Illness, ed. Stephen J. Wood, Nicholas B. Allen and Christos Pantelis. Published by Cambridge University Press. © Cambridge University Press 2009.

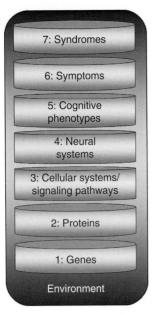

Figure 18.1. Seven-level model illustrating the types of concepts to be traversed in comprehensive hypotheses of mental disorders from genome to syndrome.

more are affected by disorders that are considered "neurological" but profoundly affect behavior (e.g. dementia, stroke, Parkinson's disease). Mental illness, neurological disorders and other behavioral disorders are thought to cost ~$500 billion annually in the USA alone, and this figure does not include the costs from behaviors that impact upon other medical conditions (e.g. cardiovascular disease, diabetes, obesity, HIV/ AIDS) (Zerhouni, 2005). Even defined narrowly, mental illness is the leading cause of disability in North America among people 15–44 years of age, accounting for ~15% of the global burden of disease from all causes (Murray & Lopez, 1996). Despite major investments by the NIH and other agencies, and concerted efforts by advocacy groups, research on mental illness lags behind other areas of biomedical research due to historical perceptions of "mental" disorders as separate from "medical" disorders, stigma associated with mental illness and the complexities of understanding behavioral and brain functions.

A major challenge for neuropsychiatry research is that basic aspects of diagnosis remain controversial and lack solid scientific foundations. Prior to the publication of the *Diagnostic and Statistical Manual of Mental Disorders* (3rd edn) (DSM–III) (American Psychiatric Association, 1980) diagnostic agreement was poor. The DSM–III introduced explicit criteria for diagnosis, enhancing *reliability* but not *validity* of diagnosis, as the criteria were divorced from etiological or pathophysiological hypotheses. The task forces for DSM–IV (American Psychiatric Association, 1994) and DSM–V (estimated publication, 2011) have strived to consider more empirical data, but with little impact so far on either the overall taxonomy or the specific criteria. A group considering plans for DSM–V noted a litany of signs marking its poor performance as a taxonomic device (Kupfer *et al.*, 2002). Specifically the diagnoses suffer from: (1) a lack of biological markers; (2) a lack of specific treatments (i.e. treatment specificity is the exception rather than the rule); (3) high "comorbidity" (i.e. individuals are difficult to classify); and (4) a lack of longitudinal stability (Kupfer *et al.*, 2002). A discipline known as *taxometrics* has demonstrated that many accepted categorical boundaries between diagnoses are invalid and that only a handful of distinctions are supported empirically (Haslam, 2003; Haslam & Kim, 2002). Future understanding of neuropsychiatric syndromes may rely more heavily on well-defined dimensions of functioning rather than

infrastructure that can support literature mining, knowledge representation and modeling of relationships among phenotypes of high relevance to cognitive phenomics, and link these to other repositories of biological knowledge. This chapter summarizes aspects of these goals that are most important for neuropsychological investigation of mental disorders.

Unique challenges for the neuropsychological investigation of mental disorders

Before turning to the empirical research and informatics strategies that are being developed to enable the new inter-discipline of cognitive phenomics, it is important to recognize the unique challenges faced by clinicians and researchers interested in the neuropsychology of mental disorders. In contrast to neuropsychological, neurological and radiological investigation of some other brain disorders where etiology and/or pathophysiology may be better understood, the investigation of mental disorders suffers from poor definition of the disorders themselves.

The lack of biologically useful definitions of mental disorders is unfortunate given their public health significance. Some 28–30% of people in the USA suffer from "mental" or "addictive" disorders (Kessler *et al.*, 1994; Regier *et al.*, 1993), and many discrete categories (Acton & Zodda, 2005), and genetic analysis may be advanced more by application of the study of quantitative traits rather than categorical diagnoses (Bearden & Freimer, 2006). Given this background, it is not surprising that gene and drug discovery for neuropsychiatric disorders has been disappointing. Improved phenotype definitions could increase the power of genetic studies and point to mechanisms that will advance rational diagnosis and treatment for neuropsychiatric syndromes.

Neuropsychiatric phenotype definitions will be advanced most effectively by research that: (1) spans conventional diagnostic boundaries and (2) examines phenotypic variation across species. First, research focused on a complex syndrome that lacks a unitary pathophysiology necessarily confounds relevant with irrelevant features. By studying multiple syndromes that share pathological features, we can enhance power to detect the shared pathology and possibly shared etiologies. Even if syndromes share a feature that reflects *different* pathological bases, studying the syndromes together will better isolate the unique mechanisms leading to final common paths. Second, while some syndromes involve "uniquely human" features (e.g. language), many if not most brain and behavioral functions overlap substantially with non-human attributes, and understanding mechanisms depends on our ability to examine this overlap in animal models. These considerations prompted our team to form *cross-disorder* and *cross-species* workgroups to identify phenotypes that would be most informative for neuropsychiatric research teams of the future.

Focusing on cognitive or neuropsychological phenotypes rather than the psychiatrically defined syndromal phenotypes may generate greater traction and foster more rapid discovery. There is considerable variability in the degree to which specific "psychiatric" phenotypes offer credible targets for gene discovery. One window on the possible likelihood of success for gene discovery is offered by epidemiological studies of inheritance. Heritability of the most widespread psychiatric disorders, such as anxiety disorders and depression, is modest to moderate but well replicated (20–40%), higher for some syndromes such as alcohol and drug dependence (40–60%), and relatively strong for certain severe syndromes such as schizophrenia or bipolar disorder (60–80%) or autism (80–100%; Kendler 2005, personal communication). While heritability statistics offer only one index of the degree to which specific traits are tractable targets

for gene discovery, there is usually greater optimism that biological mechanisms will be easier to identify for the more heritable characteristics, and phenotypes such as schizophrenia or autism appear to offer reasonable targets from this perspective.

At the same time, "gene finding" methods that focus on determining specifically the locations and identities of the responsible genes have been difficult to replicate, and the effect sizes for any specific gene have usually been quite small, even for highly heritable syndromes. For example, Kendler's summary of meta-analytic results of gene-finding studies published since 2000, found odds ratios of only 1.07–1.57 with a median of 1.30 for 10 "candidate" genes identified as significantly associated with various psychiatric disorders (Kendler, 2005). These are clearly modest effects. We note that Kendler suggested an odds ratio greater than 3.0 would be needed to refer to an effect as "moderate." For comparison, this is roughly the increased risk of Alzheimer's disease for individuals who are heterozygous for the apolipoprotein E4 allele. While there is so far little direct evidence, there is optimism that work on cognitive phenotypes, which arguably are more directly related to biological processes, can lead to stronger and more easily replicable findings. Heritability statistics for the many cognitive traits, including IQ, approximate to 50%, even using conservative estimates (Devlin *et al.*, 1997). For more specific cognitive characteristics, presumably those that are more tightly linked to the operation of specific functional systems in the brain, heritability may be even higher (Fan *et al.*, 2001; see also discussion below about catechol-*O*-methyltransferase). Although it is assumed that the genetics of cognitive traits will be complex, there is optimism that moving the phenotype closer to the functioning of neural systems will be productive. Just how much traction this will afford remains an open, empirical question.

The phenomics research strategy

Neuropsychology, traditionally established as the discipline concerned with the study of brain–behavior relations, is intrinsically interdisciplinary and has always been at the forefront of science in the definition of cognitive phenotypes in the broad sense. As noted in the introductory comments above, the phenotypes considered by our field embrace not only the behavioral manifestations of brain function, but the complex physiological operations of neural systems, and the cellular processes and molecular expressions that underlie these. The reader may therefore wonder: What is new about the "phenomics" approach that is not already science-as-usual for neuropsychology?

The shift in emphasis is principally strategic, focusing on establishing validity of phenotypes using convergent horizontal and vertical approaches. By *horizontal* we mean those approaches that are used to validate a specific phenotype construct within its own level of analysis. For most neuropsychological procedures, this focuses on establishing construct validity using psychometric approaches, including assessment of various forms of reliability, internal consistency, and the convergent and divergent validity of a given indicator with respect to other psychological test constructs. Following Figure 18.1, this would imply fleshing out the territory within "Level 5." By *vertical* we mean those approaches that validate the phenotype construct with respect to constructs at other levels. For neuropsychology, this usually means linking a specific behavioral phenotype to phenotypes at other levels such as the anatomic level, or to a genotype. Again following Figure 18.1, this would mean establishing links of a concept or construct at Level 5 with concepts or constructs at other levels.

Most current neuropsychology research proceeds with measures that have undergone prior "horizontal" reliability and validity testing, but this is highly variable. For some measures there is little information about internal consistency (coefficient alpha or similar), test–retest reliability and stability, or the degree to which the measure adequately covers the domain of interest. Each of these psychometric characteristics has unique salience in the phenomics era. Coefficient alpha or alternate measures of true score reliability are important to know how well the test measures the construct it was intended to measure. This in turn constrains heritability estimates, which are also essential for phenomics investigations, and are so far available for relatively few measures. Stability of test scores also carries a unique value for phenomics, because it is assumed (usually) that gene discovery is targeting persistent trait functions; unfortunately it is rarely known how much, and in what ways, transient state effects influence neuropsychological measures. The convergent and divergent validity data are of high importance in phenomics investigations because: (1) we rarely know the true scope of the construct

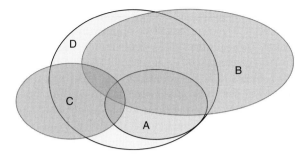

Figure 18.2. Domain assessment in neuropsychology. D = true construct domain of interest; test A is specific but not sensitive; test B is sensitive but not specific; test C is neither very sensitive nor very specific, but measures possibly important variance in domain D that is not assessed by either test A or test B.

domain that we aim to assess, so we usually need to "overmeasure" to be confident that the most relevant phenotypic variance has been assessed; (2) to link findings to a broader literature, the incorporation of "reference tests" in the validation process may help enable inclusion of findings in systematic searches and knowledge-bases that would otherwise not be possible. An example is illustrated in Figure 18.2, which shows how typical measures of a neuropsychological construct might overlap with each other and with the overall domain space. Further complicating this process of test selection for phenomic investigations is the fact that we still lack accepted methods for maximizing the *biological validity* of neuropsychological constructs. Thus we can use psychometric methods to assess quantitatively the degree to which a test or set of tests measure a specific psychological construct (for example, by estimating coefficient alpha or similar metrics we can say how much true score variance we are explaining with our tests). But it is rare to see comparable methods defining the variance explained in another construct (say, the variance in a biological process) by some set of psychological variables. These are methods that the new discipline of phenomics will be dedicated to developing (see also the discussion of "vertical validation strategies") below.

Even limiting our discussion to horizontal validation strategies, modern psychometric theory is surprisingly absent from consideration in most neuropsychological test procedures. There have been major developments in item response theory (IRT), for example, which have the potential to overcome multiple problems with traditional neuropsychological test procedures (Embretson & Reise, 2002; Reise & Henson, 2003). Item response theory involves defining, for any specific test of a construct, how individual items on that test relate to an individual's true scores on the underlying construct. One advantage of an IRT approach is its ability to help overcome "instrumentation inertia," because it is possible to use different combinations of items to estimate individual true scores, and thus new items can be included without jeopardizing the measurement of the construct. Another asset of IRT methods is that new tests can be constructed with high efficiency, and investigators can determine the minimal item set necessary to enable predetermined degrees of measurement precision. Since an individual's response to a given item allows one to compute how much incremental precision has been added to the estimation of that individual's true score, IRT also fosters the generation of *adaptive* testing, with optimized item selection based on the individual's prior response history. Now that computerized testing is increasingly being embraced by both researchers and clinicians, the incorporation of adaptive testing is markedly facilitated.

Most published neuropsychology research studies are "vertical" validation studies from the phenomics perspective. In these studies, some neuropsychological measure(s) usually serves as the dependent variable(s), while the independent variables are some alteration in anatomy, exposure to some environmental insult or treatment, or in genetics research, individual subject classification according to allelic variation in some gene or genes. Although incremental validation of this sort offers the simplest approach to hypothesis testing, there is now an increased need to examine more complex mechanistic hypotheses that traverse multiple steps simultaneously. While obviously adding to the complexity and magnitude of research projects and programs, the simultaneous convergence on multiple elements of a complex hypothesis in the same participants offers unique and powerful leverage on the inferential process. The phenomics perspective emphasizes this *multilevel vertical validation*, which can better evaluate the overall validity of a mechanistic model. For cognitive phenotypes, this means developing tests of plausibility for the relations that take us all the way from the genetic level up to the level of cognition, with specification of the proteomic, cellular systems and signaling pathways, and neural system level intermediate steps that are linked successively back to the genetic level.

To take a concrete example, there has been recent interest in the catechol-*O*-methyltransferase (COMT)

val158met polymorphism in schizophrenia research. Meta-analysis of multiple studies investigating the association of this genetic variation with the phenotype "schizophrenia" (as diagnosed by the DSM–IV) reveals that the correlation is very weak (Glatt *et al.*, 2003). Using the descriptors of Figure 18.1, we can see that this link from the "genetic" level (level 1) to the "syndromal" level (level 7) has limited validity. In contrast, there are now multiple studies showing various relations of this polymorphism with different cognitive measures (i.e. from level 1 to level 5). While for some measures, these associations are modest (e.g. the link to Wisconsin Card Sorting Test performance has an $R^2 < 5\%$), there may be stronger associations (e.g. $R^2 \sim 40\%$) with simpler cognitive phenotypes involving response reversal (Nolan *et al.*, 2004). Basic science studies confirming the functional nature of this polymorphism reveal much larger effect sizes; for example, the effect of this polymorphism on the functional activity of the COMT enzyme (i.e. the link from level 1 to level 2) is quite robust, with heritability estimates in some studies as high as 1.0 for COMT enzyme activity in the red blood cell (RBC), and with correlations of enzyme activity across tissue types suggesting strong relationships of genotype with enzyme activity phenotype (with $R^2 \sim 38\%$ to 66%). There are now several proposals regarding the ways in which the COMT *val158met* polymorphism, via expression of variations of COMT enzyme that differ in activity, may affect catabolism of dopamine in the prefrontal cortex and/or the striatum (i.e. an effect of level 1 on level 3 via level 2), and further how the cellular effects may influence activity in broader neural systems (level 4; Bilder *et al.*, 2004).

Although this kind of mechanistic hypothesis validation across multiple levels of analysis may reflect the desiderata of many research projects and programs, it is surprising how infrequently the specific links between relevant and necessary levels are explicated. We believe this is a useful goal for phenomics investigations, which will help guide the scientific research strategy. Given the complexity of these hypotheses, novel approaches to hypothesis specification and visualization are needed. We believe that the use of graphical modeling techniques may offer useful insights into complex phenomics hypotheses. Specifically, it is possible to represent the relevant constructs and their relations in terms of a probabilistic graph, with nodes representing the concepts and edges representing the hypothesized relations

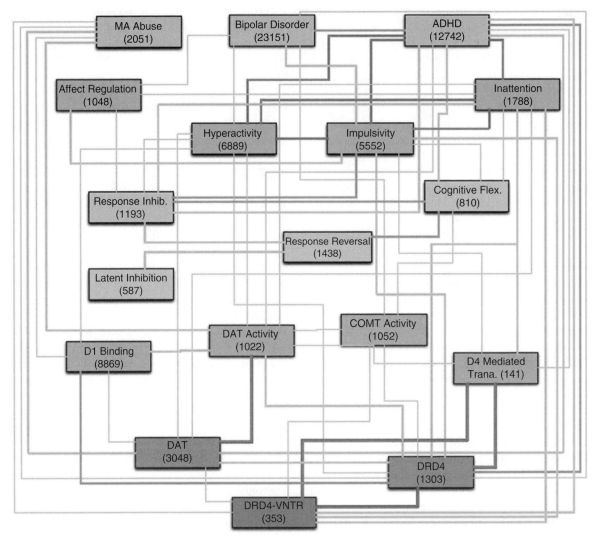

Figure 18.3. Map of concepts relating DRD4 polymorphism to phenotypes involving "response inhibition." Nodes are concepts identified in *PubMed*, while edges represent the Jaccard coefficients that indicate the co-occurrence of the relevant concepts in 14 million *PubMed* abstracts. ADHD = attention-deficit hyperactivity disorder; COMT = catechol-*O*-methyltransferase; DAT = dopamine transporter; MA = methamphetamine.

between constructs (e.g. see Figure 18.3). This approach bears some relation to widely used methods such as structural equation modeling (SEM) or covariance structure analysis (CSA), which are used primarily for hypothesis specification and estimation of fit to the data for empirical models. What remains to be developed are mixed models, whereby a given set of experimental data is used to partially specify a given set of relationships, while other aspects of the full hypothesis, including nodes and edges that are never measured, are incorporated based on prior observations in the literature. Bayesian approaches could

further facilitate identification of nodes and weighting of relationships among these.

The representation of multilevel hypotheses can thus become a tool for evaluating results of a given experiment in the context of the broader literature, and usefully involve the methods of meta-analysis and literature mining. For example, Figure 18.3 illustrates some of the primary concepts involved in a multi-level hypothesis, possibly relating a candidate gene (a variable nucleotide tandem repeat polymorphism in the dopamine D4 receptor gene or DRD4) to complex syndromes such as bipolar disorder and attention-deficit hyperactivity disorder, via intermediate effects on dopamine metabolism, response inhibition and impulsivity. This figure, however, does not involve any empirically observed effects or "indicators" with their associated error terms, but rather uses concept labels reflecting terms derived using literature mining tools, and edges reflecting literature associations between concepts. This brings us to discuss informatics approaches that comprise another major thrust of cognitive phenomics.

The informatics strategy

Much as *genomics* was formed from the interaction of multiple disciplines including genetics, molecular biology and bioinformatics, *phenomics* demands novel informatics strategies for its realization. The explosion of biological knowledge that has accompanied the human genome project, and promulgated new industries in the other "-omics," is yielding more data than any single expert can digest. The capacity to represent, visualize and analyze these data is arguably the highest priority for advancing knowledge in biomedicine. This in turn requires new strategies for information management using a combination of measurement theory, biology and bioinformatics. To focus on phenotypes relevant to neuropsychology requires a platform to connect diverse types of information, including brain images, results of cognitive

experiments, symptoms and syndromes. A valuable architecture should be designed to support exploratory analyses across many scales and multilevel modeling of phenotype constructs (endophenotypes), the relationships among them, and testing of hypotheses. Projects that follow the cognitive phenomics strategy can be conceptualized as developing a new kind of atlas following the multilevel schema shown in Figure 18.1. By an "atlas," we do not mean a conventional brain atlas, but instead an integrated collection of maps. Conceptually each element in Figure 18.1 corresponds to a type of map, ranging across genetic to syndromal levels. A related depiction is provided in Figure 18.4, which further highlights how such an "atlas" comprises maps of many different types. An atlas should also enable viewers to zoom within any given level to see finer granularity of concepts, instances and relations within that level, and enable users to perform approximate matching of concepts and instances whenever exact matching is unavailable. A multilevel atlas can help organize interdisciplinary efforts for multivariate characterization of phenotypes and statistical associations that connect genome to syndrome. Collectively, these efforts take steps towards a Neuropsychiatric Phenomics Atlas (NPA).

Among the many challenges of developing informatics resources for cognitive phenomics is that the relevant *ontologies* are so far under-developed. The concept of ontology comes from philosophy,

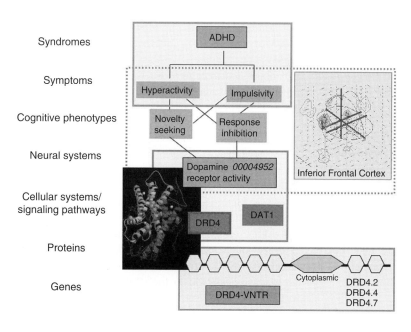

Figure 18.4. This figure is also reproduced in the color plate section. An atlas is an integrated collection of "maps" (indexed information sources). In the Neuro-psychiatric Phenomics Atlas (NPA) maps must span multiple levels and scales, and support zooming to see finer granularity of concepts and/or data within levels.

Syndromes

Symptoms

Cognitive phenotypes

Neural systems

Cellular systems/
signaling pathways

Proteins

Genes

ADHD

Hyperactivity

Impulsivity

Novelty seeking

Response inhibition

Dopamine *00004952* receptor activity

Inferior Frontal Cortex

DRD4

DAT1

Cytoplasmic DRD4.2
DRD4.4
DRD4.7

DRD4-VNTR

where it refers to the study of being or existence. However, the term has been adopted in modern biomedical informatics to refer to a formal characterization of the entities that make up a particular domain and their relations. More specifically, a "cognitive ontology" would reflect an explicit characterization of the entities (such as mental processes or representations) that are thought to make up the mind, and the relations between those entities. For example, a cognitive ontology might denote that "working memory" is an entity, that it is a kind of memory, and that it encompasses maintenance and manipulation of mental representations.

Ontologies may have different levels of specification:

(1) Specification of a controlled vocabulary – while this may seem trivial, the simple cataloging of terms and concepts, identification of synonyms, and their definitions, is a substantial undertaking even for a domain limited in scope.

(2) Specification of a simple taxonomy – following the definition of a controlled vocabulary, this level of specification implies that some simple relations between concepts are identified, and particularly that "is a" and "part of" relations are stated, to indicate that some concepts are subsets, or hierarchically related to others in a conceptual classification tree (for example, "declarative memory" may be considered a subset of "memory").

(3) Specification of more complex relations among entities – in addition to specifying the simple class hierarchy, this demands enumeration of other relations, sometimes complex relations, among concepts. For example, "scopolamine" (which may be represented in a class hierarchy itself (e.g. "is an anticholinergic drug," which in turn "is a" drug") also "affects" memory, or the relation might be more specifically coded as "impairs" memory. Any arbitrary relational term can be designed to specify causal, correlational or other probabilistic relations between entities. The greatest challenge in this effort is parsimony.

(4) Specification of formal logical rules governing the relations among entities and among relations – these specifications usually take the form of full-fledged grammars with syntactic rules, such as the rules governing computer languages and operations.

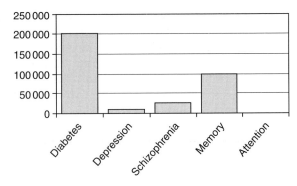

Figure 18.5. Hits by diagnostic search term in Entrez-GEO Expressions Database.

To enable the systematic study of observable phenotypes, and advance identification of more meaningful latent constructs, an ontology representing these phenotypic domains is necessary. In contrast to other areas of biomedicine where the concepts have been better defined and formalized (as is the case in genetics, and now emerging in proteomics and metabolomics), the development of ontologies for cognition and for mental disorders more broadly is still very incomplete. Phenomic descriptions of neuropsychiatric disorders are poorly represented in existing genomic and related gene-expression databases. In one such database, Entrez-GEO Expressions, a search for the term "diabetes" yields ~200 000 hits, while similar searches for psychiatric syndromes yield values less than 30 000 (see Figure 18.5). Even very broad cognitive terms such as "memory" still generate fewer than half the hits of a term like "diabetes," and for some terms arguably important to cognition and neuropsychology (e.g. "attention") there are no database entries.

There is a clear need for increased representation of psychiatric and cognitive phenotypes in public data repositories, so that these can be linked to other growing biological databases; this requires elaboration of cognitive ontologies. Considerable development in informatics depends on existing ontologies or controlled vocabularies, most notably the Unified Medical Language System (UMLS) and related resources (i.e. Metathesaurus, the Semantic Network, NIH Specialist Lexicon and Medical Subject Headings [MeSH]), which are coordinated by the National Library of Medicine (see http://www.nlm.nih.gov/research/umls/). We have identified several interesting lacunae specific to the study of psychiatric disorders and cognition in these resources.

For psychiatric disorders broadly speaking, we have found that the ontologies in the UMLS, while acknowledging the DSM–IV–TR as a source vocabulary, do not encode the relationships that are defined in the DSM, and only some of the "top level" diagnostic terms are included. For example, the term "schizophrenia" is in the UMLS, but all of its subtypes are not listed; nor is the concept "schizophrenia" in UMLS linked explicitly to the defining symptoms of the disorder. The Center for Cognitive Phenomics has undertaken the task of constructing all the explicit relations of diagnostic concepts with the symptoms that are used to define these. In this way, searches on the term "schizophrenia" can be "expanded" to search also for links to directly related concepts including "delusions," "hallucinations," and "negative symptoms." It might be considered inefficient or even misleading to reproduce the DSM ontology, since this could reinforce and reify erroneous relationships. To avoid this, it is important to recognize explicitly the source of relationships between concepts: some are empirically determined via associations in literature or data, but others (like those in the DSM) are largely the result of expert consensus only variably supported by empirical findings. In the ultimate informatics applications, it is therefore important to be able to relax constraints that might be imposed by relationships that lack empirical validation; for example, one should have the facility to "turn off" DSM diagnostic algorithms when searching for links to symptoms or syndromes.

For the representation of cognition and neuropsychology, we have found that existing ontologies are particularly sparse. For example, the UMLS currently includes only 39 concepts to represent all *mental processes* and only six concepts under the heading *Cognition*. The categories that are included are not necessarily those that would be considered complete, or even representative of the domain of cognition as conceptualized by contemporary cognitive science (i.e. the "children" of Cognition in the UMLS are: *Awareness*; *Cognitive Dissonance*; *Consciousness*; *Imagination*; *Comprehension*; and *Intuition*). There is a slightly greater representation of other concepts that are relevant to cognition. For example, "Learning" has 23 child concepts, one of which is *Verbal Learning*, which in turn is further divided into *Paired Associate Learning* and *Serial Learning*. While these concept labels come closer to describing cognitive functions and procedures in a

manner that seem useful for literature searching, the UMLS still lacks a coherent, comprehensive and up-to-date ontology of cognitive concepts.

Other databases also have relatively sparse representation of cognitive concepts. For example, the BrainMap database (http://ric.uthscsa.edu/projects/brainmap.html) uses a simple cognitive ontology to help users identify functional neuroimaging experiments that may relate to important cognitive processes, and the fMRI data center at Dartmouth (soon to be at the University of California, Santa Barbara; see http://www.fmridc.org/f/fmridc) uses a sparse set of nine terms to label fMRI experiments. A somewhat more elaborate ontology of cognitive processes is used to label the neuroimaging experiments in the Brede Database (http://hendrix.imm.dtu.dk/services/jerne/brede/). This database includes a total of ∼565 labels to describe the experiments; many of these terms would be considered "cognitive," but others refer to neurotransmitter receptors, drugs, syndromes and other concepts useful in characterizing the studies. In the Center for Cognitive Phenomics, we identified a class hierarchy developed by the Defense Advanced Research Projects Agency (DARPA), that includes 416 cognitive terms, and used this as a starting point in the development of a cognitive ontology. With these terms to "seed" the concept space of cognitive terms, we have identified other terms that are strongly associated to expand the lexicon of cognitive terms. We also have used other methods from text mining, such as the detection of terms that are probabilistically more likely to be found in "cognitive" journals compared with other scientific journals, to enrich the lexicon of cognitive terms. We already have identified more than 2000 new terms that are likely candidates for membership in a future cognitive lexicon, and are currently curating these terms (see http://www.phenomics.ucla.edu). We would anticipate that once codified, the ontologies developed by our group and others will be adopted by the National Library of Medicine and used to expand or enhance the UMLS and MeSH terms that now are used to guide literature searches in scientific literature search engines such as *PubMed*. It is also likely that similar tools will be adopted by commercial engines such as *Google Scholar*.

In addition to enabling more effective searches in existing literature, and explicit recognition of conceptual links that are widely agreed by neuropsychologists and cognitive scientists, there are further implications of these developments for the modeling

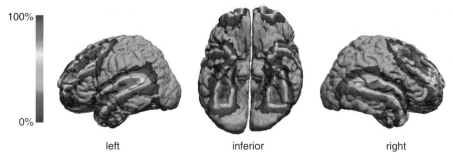

100%

0%

left   inferior   right

Figure 18.6. This figure is also reproduced in the color plate section. Probability maps for three cortical structures. Probabilistic data from the LPBA40 atlas was mapped back to the space of one of the atlas subjects. The surface model has been colored according to the probability values for middle frontal gyrus, superior temporal gyrus and fusiform gyrus to indicate the likelihood of one of those structures at a given surface point. From Shattuck *et al.*, 2008, with permission.

and visualization of relationships among cognitive concepts, and the testing of complex scientific hypotheses. Different models of the structure of cognition can be tested against various data sources such as: (1) existing term-term association statistics in *PubMed*; (2) curated effect sizes that link concepts to each other; or (3) empirically collected data on individual cases with scores on test indicators of cognitive concepts. For example, someone interested in the relationship between the concepts "working memory" and "attention" could examine: (1) the association of these concepts with each other directly, or implicitly via their shared relationships with other terms (for example, both "working memory" and "attention" might co-occur in scientific literature abstracts that also have the word "frontal lobe"), using text mining methods; (2) the association of these concepts using a model that specified the effect sizes observed in different empirical studies. This amounts to extracting the information about reported relationships and summarizing these in the same way that meta-analysis usually proceeds, but in this case possibly across many different relationships for a specific domain of interest; or (3) using the same basic structural model, test its validity directly with observations made in individual people (i.e. use structural equation modeling in its conventional sense to test model validity).

We already have begun to develop some applications that we hope will leverage improved informatics capacities pertinent to cognitive phenomics. Our informatics team has further developed several software applications. We previously described a literature- and data-mining study in which we generated a map of cognitive brain activations relevant for schizophrenia, but without studying a single patient with schizophrenia (Bilder, 2005). This stimulated

development of an application that takes any arbitrary literature search, mines *PubMed* for intersections with neuroanatomic terms, and displays this as a map on the human brain. While conceptually straightforward, a key limitation is that concepts used to define brain regions vary in precision, and anatomic variability is sufficient that overlaps of labels might be confounded with differences in individual anatomy thus creating errors. To address this we are collaborating with colleagues in the Laboratory of NeuroImaging (LONI) and the Center for Computational Biology, and have created a probabilistic atlas based on healthy people (see Figure 18.6). In parallel, we developed software (*PubBrain*, http://www.pubbrain.org, now in prototype) to take *PubMed* queries and display these on the probabilistic atlas. This probabilistic atlas may have widespread application in functional imaging as a source of templates from which researchers can select regions of interest for analysis of specific brain regions, better reflecting population variability than the single-subject atlases currently used by the field (Shattuck *et al.*, 2008 [presented at the *Human Brain Mapping* meeting, June 2006]).

We also developed *PubGraph*, a visualization tool for exploring associations between user-specified sets of terms. *PubGraph* allows entry of arbitrary term sets as *PubMed* queries, and exploration of the documents corresponding to edges and nodes in the resulting graphs. Thus it is an interface for visualizing associations between *PubMed* documents, as well as exploring or hypothesizing their multilevel structure. There are examples at http://www.pubgraph.org. These tools also generated the "concept map" (Figure 18.3), which lays out a vertical hypothesis relating the gene "DRD4" to several neuropsychiatric syndromes via a series of intervening biological constructs, and encodes literature association strengths using different edge weights. These tools are beginning to offer new ways to conceptualize links between diverse data types and data sources, that will ultimately be needed to advance the new discipline of phenomics.

Summary

With the completion of the Human Genome Project and the advent of lower-cost whole genome approaches to genotyping, there is enormous excitement that we may soon be poised to identify the genetic underpinnings of complex traits including those underlying neuropsychological functions. It is likely that cognitive traits, via presumably closer links to brain function and neurobiology, may offer more tractable phenotypic targets relative to the psychiatric syndromes as these are diagnosed by the DSM–IV. To realize this vision will demand a variety of new methods, and indeed the establishment of a new discipline, which we refer to as *cognitive phenomics*. Cognitive phenomics research will require novel vertically integrated research spanning basic and clinical sciences, and a strong focus on psychometric theory to enhance efficiency for high throughput phenotyping that will be necessary to test hypotheses. This work will need to be augmented by novel informatics strategies that enable the representation, visualization, and modeling of complex relations among measured variables and theoretical concepts. The development of these new strategies is now fostering dramatic changes in the ways we approach interdisciplinary research in general, and neuropsychology in particular.

Acknowledgments

This work was supported by a grant from the NIH Director's Roadmap Initiative (P20 RR020750; R Bilder, PI).

References

Acton, G. S. & Zodda, J. J. (2005). Classification of psychopathology – goals and methods in an empirical approach. *Theory and Psychology*, **15**, 373–399.

American Psychiatric Association (1980). *Diagnostic and Statistical Manual of Mental Disorders* (3rd edn.) (DSM–III). Washington, DC: APA.

American Psychiatric Association (1994). *Diagnostic and Statistical Manual of Mental Disorders* (4th edn.) (DSM–IV). Washington, DC: APA.

Bearden, C. & Freimer, N. (2006). Endophenotypes for psychiatric disorders: Ready for primetime? *Trends in Genetics*, **22**, 306–313.

Bilder, R. M. (2005). Cognitive phenomics for neuropsychiatric therapeutics. *Schizophrenia Bulletin*, **31**, 318–319.

Bilder, R. M., Volavka, J., Lachman, H. M. & Grace, A. A. (2004). The catechol-O-methyltransferase polymorphism: relations to the tonic-phasic dopamine hypothesis and neuropsychiatric phenotypes. *Neuropsychopharmacology*, **29**, 1943–1961.

Devlin, B., Daniels, M. & Roeder, K. (1997). The heritability of IQ. *Nature*, **388**, 468–471.

Embretson, S. E. & Reise, S. P. (2002). *Item Response Theory for Psychologists*. Mahwah, NJ: Lawrence Erlbaum Associates.

Fan, J., Wu, Y., Fossella, J. & Posner, M. (2001). Assessing the heritability of attentional networks. *BMC Neuroscience*, **2**, 14.

Freimer, N. & Sabatti, C. (2003). The human phenome project. *Nature Genetics*, **34**, 15–21.

Glatt, S. J., Faraone, S. V. & Tsuang, M. T. (2003). Association between a functional catechol-O-methyltransferase gene polymorphism and schizophrenia: meta-analysis of case-control and family-based studies. *American Journal of Psychiatry*, **160**, 469–476.

Haslam, N. (2003). The dimensional view of personality disorders: a review of the taxometric evidence. *Clinical Psychology Review*, **23**, 75–93.

Haslam, N. & Kim, H. C. (2002). Categories and continua: a review of taxometric research. *Genetic Social and General Psychology Monographs*, **128**, 271–320.

Kendler, K. S. (2005). "A gene for ...": the nature of gene action in psychiatric disorders. *American Journal of Psychiatry*, **162**, 1243–1252.

Kessler, R. C., McGonagle, K. A., Zhao, S., *et al.* (1994). Lifetime and 12-month prevalence of DSM–III–R psychiatric disorders in the United States. Results from the National Comorbidity Survey. *Archives of General Psychiatry*, **51**, 8–19.

Kupfer, D. J., First, M. B. & Regier, D. A. (2002). *A Research Agenda for DSM–V*. Washington, DC: American Psychiatric Association.

Murray, C. J. L. & Lopez, A. D. (1996). *The Global Burden of Disease and Injury Series, Vol. 1: A Comprehensive Assessment of Mortality and Disability from Diseases, Injuries, and Risk Factors in 1990 and Projected to 2020.* Cambridge, MA: Harvard University Press.

Nolan, K. A., Bilder, R. M., Lachman, H. M. & Volavka, J. (2004). Catechol-O-methyltransferase Val158Met polymorphism in schizophrenia: differential effects of

Val and Met alleles on cognitive stability and flexibility. *American Journal of Psychiatry*, **161**, 359–361.

Regier, D. A., Narrow, W. E., Rae, D. S. *et al.* (1993). The de facto US mental and addictive disorders service system. Epidemiologic catchment area prospective 1-year prevalence rates of disorders and services. *Archives of General Psychiatry*, **50**, 85–94.

Reise, S. P. & Henson, J. M. (2003). A discussion of modern versus traditional psychometrics as applied to

personality assessment scales. *Journal of Personal Assessment*, **81**, 93–103.

Shattuck, D. W., Mirza, M., Adisetiyo, V. *et al.* (2008). Construction of a 3D probabilistic atlas of human cortical structures. *Neuroimage*, **39**, 1064–1080.

Zerhouni, E. (2005). *Fiscal Year 2006 Budget Request*. House Subcommittee on Labor-HHS-Education Appropriations.

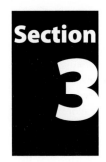

Section 3

The neuropsychology of psychiatric disorders

Why examine neuropsychological processes in specific psychiatric disorders?

Although we noted some limitations of the current nosological system in our introduction to the first section of this volume, examining the neuropsychology of specific psychiatric disorders and syndromes remains a critical task, if not *the* critical task, of the neuropsychological study of mental illness. As noted by Jackson & McGorry in this volume (Chapter 12), the major functions of diagnosis are to indicate the type of treatment that is required for the presenting patient, as well as predicting course and prognosis, and understanding etiology and factors leading to the condition. Given that so much clinical information and clinical decision making is organized around clinical diagnosis, the neuropsychological study of specific psychiatric disorders is clearly essential. If neuropsychological models are to be able to inform treatment selection, and describe the mechanisms that underlie treatment response then integrating neuropsychological models with the significant clinical database that is organised around diagnostic entities will be required. Of course, eventually neuropsychological models may improve clinical diagnosis, by identifying which processes are unique to specific disorders (and their associated treatment responses), as well as those that are common across a range of disorders.

Jackson & McGorry (Chapter 12, this volume) identify two approaches to understanding psychiatric diagnoses. The "clinical" approach posits the clinical picture (i.e. the observations of clinicians, the reports of patients and of others) as being the defining feature of psychopathology. As they note, critics of this approach point out the importance of less directly observable factors (e.g. intermediate phenotypes and endophenotypes) and propose that the findings of neuropsychological, neurological, psychophysiological, biochemical, genetic and neuroradiological investigations are likely to significantly clarify disease phenotypes in a way that will be impossible using descriptive psychiatry alone. These data may provide enhanced reliability and validity when compared with clinical observation, due to their objective nature and ease of quantification. However, as Jackson & McGorry also point out, linking disease phenotypes with neuropsychological data is not necessarily straightforward. One critical issue is which set of criteria (i.e. the neuropsychological versus descriptive/diagnostic) is treated as the "gold standard" in analyses. Proponents of the biological viewpoint argue that focusing initially on neuro-cognitive and biological biases or deficits prior to linking them to disease phenotypes will enhance progress in the area. However, as noted above, the significant research and clinical databases organized around diagnostic entities suggest that there is likely to be value in treating these phenomena as primary as well. (Indeed, Jackson & McGorry argue for a conciliation of these two approaches.)

This section begins with Valera, Brown & Seidman considering the neuropsychology of attention-deficit hyperactivity disorder (ADHD) and other disorders of childhood such as conduct disorder, oppositional defiant disorder and autism-spectrum disorders. They particularly focus on the neuropsychological heterogeneity of ADHD, and recommended that an integration of current neuropsychological models of ADHD is necessary. They also discuss the clinical evaluation of neurocognitive functioning in ADHD and provide an overview of the structural and functional neuroimaging findings. They conclude that a neuropsychological approach is a key to understanding the heterogeneous nature of these disorders (particularly ADHD), and propose that this will ultimately lead to the most effective treatment.

Depue proposes a multidimensional neuropsychological model of personality disorder. He begins with a critique of the current approach to diagnosis, and goes on to propose an alternative approach based on individual differences in the function of neurochemical systems. His work demonstrates clearly how our understanding of fundamental neuropsychological processes can be used to reorganize our diagnostic understanding of a particular domain of mental illness in a potentially more valid way.

Eating disorders are reviewed by Southgate, Tchanturia & Treasure. They note that despite the fact that the general intellectual ability of those suffering from eating disorders is usually found to be in the average to high-average range, poor cognitive function has been noted across a variety of domains. However, they conclude that this decrement in cognitive function is not purely a result of current illness, but has etiological significance as well. Indeed, they argue that abnormal processing of information and emotion is a key maintaining factor in eating disorders, and describe the treatment implications of this perspective.

Yücel, Lubman, Solowij & Brewer describe the neuropsychological factors that lay the foundation for vulnerability to addiction. They review models that suggest addictive behavior may involve deficits in inhibitory control, decision-making and affect regulation. They also particularly focus on how understanding the neurodevelopmental processes in adolescence may help understand why this is a key period of vulnerability for the initiation of substance use and abuse. They propose a model where neuropsychological impairments directly due to substance use interact with both premorbid neuro-psychological vulnerabilities and the particular developmental changes occurring during adolescence to increase risk for addictive disorders.

Obsessive-compulsive disorder (OCD) represents another psychiatric syndrome characterized by difficulties in inhibiting thoughts and behavior. Deckersbach, Savage & Rauch conclude that although neuropsychological research has consistently demonstrated cognitive impairments in OCD in the domains of visuospatial skill, memory and executive functioning, a general impairment in inhibiting ongoing cognitive processes may represent a core cognitive deficit that underlies the various forms of cognitive impairment that has been noted.

The neuropsychology of unipolar and bipolar mood disorders is addressed by Keedwell, Surguladze & Philips. They note the utility of simultaneously taking a syndromal and dimensional approach, and also note the importance of the neuropsychological evaluation and follow up of high-risk samples in order to further understand the role of neuropsychological factors of precursors versus sequelae of mood disorders. Fleck, Shear & Strakowski provide a complementary chapter that focuses on bipolar disorder, especially the manic phase. They conclude that there may be fewer stable neuropsychological vulnerabilities in bipolar disorder than previously assumed. Cognitive deficits observed during manic states are likely to reflect the need for additional resources from functional cortical regions to compen-sate for decreased attentional capacity. As such, attentional capacity is likely to be influenced not only by factors such as effort and motivation, but also neurophysiological changes and emotional factors such as manic distractibility.

In the final chapter in this section, Testa, Wood & Pantelis take a longitudinal approach to neuropsychological deficits associated with schizophrenia. They note that although cross-sectional studies do demonstrate some differences in neuropsychological performance by stage of illness, the findings from longitudinal studies are much less clear. They conclude that the current evidence indicates that cognitive impairments are likely to be present from the start of the illness and do not progress appreciably, although some decline may occur across the transition to frank disorder. They argue strongly for the examination of trajectories of change across developmentally sensitive periods, especially adolescence and early adulthood.

The chapters in this section therefore provide an excellent set of reviews of the current state of play with respect to neuropsychological processes in various psychiatric disorders. Although most of the major disorders are covered, there is a range of psychiatric (e.g. post-traumatic stress disorder, phobias) and neuropsychiatric (e.g. dementia) disorders that are not covered. Nevertheless, the issues elucidated by the chapters in this section do provide a clear picture of the current knowns and unknowns, as well as prescriptions for future research.

Neuropsychology of ADHD and other disorders of childhood

Eve M. Valera, Ariel Brown and Larry J. Seidman

Introduction

The focus of this chapter is on the neuropsychology of attention-deficit hyperactivity disorder (ADHD) through childhood.[1] We begin with a brief history of how ADHD has been conceptualized over the past 100 years and discuss a primary cognitive model of ADHD and how it may hold up to the existing neuropsychological data. We then discuss heterogeneity of neuropsychological findings across ADHD children and present some potential sources of such heterogeneity. This leads to a general summary of the literature on the most common neuropsychological deficits found in preschoolers and children 6–12 years of age with ADHD. Because of the increasing awareness that ADHD is a neurobiological disorder, we briefly summarize the structural and functional neuroimaging findings which indicate the most likely brain regions implicated in ADHD. Although limited in data, we also briefly discuss structure–function relationships. Finally, we provide a brief review of how the neuropsychological deficits found in children with conduct disorder/oppositional defiant disorder (CD/ODD) and those with autism-spectrum disorders compare with what has been found in ADHD children.

Development of the concept of neuropsychological dysfunction in ADHD

Formerly called "hyperactivity," "hyperkinesis disorder of childhood," and "minimal brain dysfunction," ADHD was first described 100 years ago as a childhood disorder found mainly in boys (Still, 1902). Revisions in the diagnostic construct have been made a number of times over the past century (Barkley, 1990). The most important shift occurred in the 1970s, when the concept of attention dysfunction was introduced as the defining feature (Douglas, 1972), and the disorder was renamed accordingly. However, the key symptoms needed for the diagnosis remain the behavioral descriptions of motor and attentional problems rather than laboratory cognitive measures of "inattention."

The diagnosis of ADHD is currently made on the basis of developmentally inappropriate symptoms of inattention, impulsivity and motor restlessness. There are three recognized subtypes: "inattentive," "hyperactive-impulsive," and "combined" (reflecting a combination of the other two types). Symptoms must be: (1) present early in life (before age seven); (2) pervasive across at least two situations; and (3) chronic. The clinical presentation has suggested that ADHD is a neuropsychological disorder, and current theories emphasize a central role for deficits in attentional and executive functions such as behavioral inhibition (Barkley, 1997).

Early investigators of ADHD noted that there were similarities between the ADHD phenotype (i.e. impulsivity, hyperactivity, inattention) and patients with frontal lobe lesions (Mattes, 1980). This observation led some researchers to believe that ADHD was a frontal lobe disorder and, consequently, they focused many of their studies on frontal brain regions. This idea was later expanded to include the potential involvement of brain regions with projections to the frontal cortex, and the term "frontal-subcortical" was used to describe the putative brain abnormalities in ADHD. Treatment studies have since provided an abundance of evidence for the involvement of dopaminergic and noradrenergic systems, which are particularly prominent in the frontal-subcortical regions (Pliszka, 2005). Evidence from neuropsychological (Frazier et al., 2004) and neuroimaging (Makris

The Neuropsychology of Mental Illness, ed. Stephen J. Wood, Nicholas B. Allen and Christos Pantelis. Published by Cambridge University Press. © Cambridge University Press 2009.

et al., 2007; Seidman *et al.*, 2005b, 2006b) studies has also supported the notion that frontal structures along with their connecting regions are implicated in ADHD. Nonetheless, it should be mentioned that recent neuroimaging studies have implicated structures across the entire brain, not just limited to the classical "frontal-subcortical" network (see the section on neuroimaging, below).

Attention and executive functions have become the dominant focus of current theories concerning the neuropsychological basis of ADHD. In contrast to early studies, when cognitive neuropsychological research in ADHD concentrated on the "attention deficit" (e.g. vigilance or distractibility), current studies commonly examine multiple executive processes that putatively control subordinate cognitive processes. Although there is a lack of consensus about the taxonomy of executive processes, there is some agreement that these processes include inhibition, working memory, set-shifting and task switching, planning and organization, and interference control (Willcutt *et al.*, 2005).

Some researchers have suggested that the core deficit in ADHD involves one particular executive process, namely inhibitory control (Barkley, 1997). Executive inhibition (as contrasted with motivational inhibition) has a role in situations that require withholding or suddenly interrupting an ongoing action or thought (suppression of a primary response, as on the Stop-Signal task; Logan *et al.*, 1997). It also occurs with the suppression of information that one wishes to ignore, such as an interfering or conflicting stimulus, as on the Stroop test (Nigg, 1999). According to this model, deficient inhibitory control impairs the ability of persons with ADHD to engage other executive control strategies to optimize behavior. Fuster (1989), in particular, has argued that the proficiency of a related executive function, working memory, is dependent on response inhibition and interference control. Deficient inhibitory control can disrupt working-memory capacity and interfere with planning and organized behavior. While neuropsychologically based theories appear to be conceptually sound, and have face validity with respect to observed behavior, it is important to carefully evaluate whether they are supported by empirical literature. Based on the published literature to date, it remains unclear whether specific components of executive functions are selectively impaired and if they can account for other deficits.

Although a core disturbance of executive functions has been the dominant model for explaining

ADHD over the past two to three decades, this model is only partially supported in the research literature (Sergeant *et al.*, 2003). There is growing consensus that the executive function "single deficit" model is insufficient to explain ADHD (Nigg *et al.*, 2005; Pennington, 2005; Sonuga-Barke, 2005), and some researchers have begun to synthesize new models to provide more comprehensive explanations. Recently published work suggests that a new neuropsychological model of ADHD is likely to encompass subtypes and multiple deficits in executive functions and in motivation and reward (Pennington, 2005). For example, Sonuga-Barke (2005) has proposed a dual pathway model of ADHD development in which one pathway involves executive deficits associated with abnormalities in fronto-dorsal striatal circuits, and the other pathway involves delay aversion associated with abnormalities in fronto-ventral striatal circuits. Castellanos and colleagues (2006), using ideas from Zelazo & Muller (2004), propose that both "cool" (cognitive) and "hot" (affective) executive-function deficits need to be considered in ADHD individuals, as different types of executive dysfunction may be related to different ADHD symptomatology. Cognitive aspects of executive function such as inhibition or maintaining representations in working memory would be considered "cool" and associated with inattentive symptoms. In contrast, affective aspects of executive function such as assessing the emotional significance of information would be considered "hot" and associated with hyperactive/impulsive symptoms. Although evidence is still limited, there has been some support showing that risky decision-making ("hot" executive function) is associated with hyperactive/impulsive symptomatology but not inattention or other "cool" executive measures (Toplak *et al.*, 2005). It is possible that the emergence of such integrated models may bring us closer to a more accurate and comprehensive etiological model of deficits in ADHD children.

Neuropsychological heterogeneity in childhood ADHD: clinical heterogeneity and methodological issues
Clinical heterogeneity
Groups of children with ADHD on average perform worse than normal controls on tests of attention and executive function. However, accumulating data

suggest that not all children with ADHD exhibit cognitive dysfunctions. Using a battery of conventional neuropsychological tests (i.e. Stroop, Wisconsin Card Sorting Test (WCST), Continuous Performance Task (CPT), etc.), Doyle *et al.* (2000) demonstrated neuropsychological impairment (defined as impairment on two or more tests, one standard deviation below the control mean) in roughly 35–40% of boys with ADHD (n = 113), compared with approximately 10% of normal boys (n = 103). Moreover, the majority of children with ADHD did not perform poorly on most tests of cognitive function. Even when ADHD individuals exhibited cognitive deficits, these varied between individuals across a range of tests of attention and executive function. These data are consistent with a number of other studies assessing the ability of neuropsychological test performances to classify children with ADHD (Grodzinsky & Barkley, 1999; Nigg *et al.*, 1998). Exactly why some individuals with ADHD exhibit cognitive deficits while others do not is unclear, but not terribly surprising, given the clinical heterogeneity of the disorder: a diagnosis of ADHD can be made based on inattentive, hyperactive/impulsive *or* a combination of inattentive and hyperactive/impulsive symptoms.

It could be hypothesized that certain cognitive deficits may be associated with a certain pattern of ADHD symptoms. There has been relatively little support for different neuropsychological profiles mapping onto particular ADHD subtypes; although this may be a result of theories being too narrowly defined, or alternatively, the definition of ADHD subtypes being too broad. Creating more integrated models may help us find potential connections between clinical and neuropsychological heterogeneity. Through structural and functional neuroimaging techniques we are becoming increasingly aware that there are widespread abnormalities across the ADHD brain. This suggests that there may be multiple networks, and consequently different cognitive functions, affected across ADHD individuals. To date, the current data suggest that the ability to use neuropsychological tests to specifically diagnose ADHD is weak, and we emphasize that while there is a general "neuropsychological profile" in ADHD, it would be unwise to try to apply it broadly across all ADHD individuals. In this next section we present some developmental and methodological issues which should be considered when interpreting data pertaining to the neuropsychology of ADHD.

Potential methodological issues contributing to heterogeneity

In addition to "true" heterogeneity across children with ADHD, there are a number of methodological issues that could contribute to apparent heterogeneity found in and across research studies. Some potential sources of heterogeneity include: (1) the age of the individuals being assessed; (2) medication status of the individuals in the ADHD sample; (3) psychiatric comorbidity of the ADHD and control groups; (4) IQ and how it is dealt with in the analyses; and (5) the potential effect that motor abnormalities may have on test performance.

Age of the ADHD sample is important because some age groups present particular methodological issues that are not as common with other ages; for example, preschoolers aged 3–5. Many of the behaviors characteristic of ADHD are behaviors that are typically observed in *normally* developing children at preschool age (American Psychiatric Association, 1994). Therefore, differentiating "normal" from "abnormal" or "problematic" behavior could require a modification of the diagnostic assessment and criteria in order to adequately diagnose ADHD preschoolers, and also to decrease the potential rate of false positive diagnoses (see Dalen *et al.*, 2004). Further, preschoolers' normal level of cognitive and motor abilities is below that of older children. Such differences may necessitate tailoring standard neuropsychological tests to fit this younger age group. It therefore becomes important to obtain convergent data among tests to help ensure that the cognitive function of interest is being assessed accurately by the modified tests. Finally, some cognitive processes may only be emerging during the preschool years and may not yet be fully developed. Therefore, finding a difference between normal and abnormal cognitive functioning may be more difficult, requiring more sensitive assessment techniques or analyses.

Another issue requiring consideration is medication status. This is important because studies have shown that while medicated children with ADHD tend to be cognitively impaired as a group, their performance may be less impaired in general or on specific tests compared with unmedicated ADHD children (Barnett *et al.*, 2001; Seidman *et al.*, 2006a). Therefore, the variety of ways in which studies deal with medication status (e.g. not reporting it, not taking it into account when analyzing data, mixing groups of medicated and unmedicated children) can contribute to heterogeneity in neuropsychological assessment results both within and across such studies.

The presence or absence of psychiatric comorbidities could also influence the heterogeneity observed in neuropsychology data in ADHD. Youth with ADHD frequently have comorbid conditions including conduct disorder, oppositional defiant disorder, substance abuse, mood or anxiety disorders. Studies of ADHD children have generally shown that neuropsychological deficits in ADHD remain robust after statistically adjusting for the presence of psychiatric comorbidities (Klorman et al., 1999; Seidman et al., 2000), providing support that neuropsychological abnormalities in ADHD can be demonstrated independent of psychiatric comorbidity. However, the degree to which comorbidities contribute to variability in neuropsychological performance is unclear. Methods used to address potential confounds associated with psychiatric comorbidities vary dramatically from study to study. Means of addressing comorbidities can range from excluding potential subjects with comorbidities, to including them and either adjusting results according to the presence of comorbidities (e.g. covarying out the effects of comorbidities), or simply reporting that the sample includes subjects with comorbidities without adjusting the results in any way. Furthermore, not all comorbid conditions are always addressed; one study may address comorbid depression and substance abuse, while another study may only address comorbid conduct or oppositional defiant disorder. This could potentially lead to neuropsychological heterogeneity driven by methodological variations in dealing with selective comorbidities rather than ADHD per se.

One comorbid disorder of ADHD that has a high likelihood of contributing to neuropsychological heterogeneity is the presence of a specific learning disorder (reading, spelling or arithmetic). The literature on ADHD has consistently documented that a substantial proportion of children with ADHD have learning disorders (Seidman et al., 2001). Rates of comorbid learning disorder vary depending on the definition and type of learning disorder, with estimates ranging from 10% to more than 90%, although a rate of approximately 30% using both reading and arithmetic as comorbid learning

disorders has been more realistically suggested (Willcutt et al., 2005). Establishing whether or not individuals within a sample have comorbid learning disorders is particularly important in ADHD because much of the available data (Seidman et al., 2006a; Willcutt et al., 2001) suggests that a substantial component of neuropsychological deficit in ADHD is explained by learning disorder comorbidity, and that having a learning disorder and ADHD may predispose children to significant executive dysfunctions. Therefore, factors such as no diagnostic assessment or learning disorder being misdiagnosed could contribute to the significant ADHD neuropsychological variability. Given these findings, it is critical that learning disorder is defined as consistently as possible across studies, and that learning disorder and other comorbidities are theoretically and statistically considered.

Interestingly, some studies have shown that ADHD children with a CD/ODD comorbidity actually out-perform individuals with ADHD only (see the conduct and oppositional defiant disorders section below for more details and discussion). It therefore cannot be assumed that the presence of any comorbidity will lead to poorer neuropsychological performance on tests. More research in this particular area is needed to disentangle the effects of each disorder (Schachar et al., 2000).

Whether levels of intelligence differ between ADHD children and comparative controls is another potentially confounding contributor to neuropsychological heterogeneity. On average, overall IQ scores tend to be lower in ADHD individuals across all ages (Frazier et al., 2004). Despite evidence that level of intelligence can affect research findings, there is inconsistency in whether investigations control for IQ in their analyses. The fact that many studies show that ADHD children have deficits in specific cognitive functions, even after controlling for IQ (Willcutt et al., 2005), suggests that at least some deficits are not a direct result of overall lower cognitive functioning. Nonetheless, to what degree it contributes to results in the literature is still unclear.

Finally, motor abnormalities are another potential source of neuropsychological heterogeneity. A substantial percentage of ADHD individuals demonstrate a range of both fine and gross motor abnormalities (see below). The extent to which subtle motor difficulties may contribute to impaired performance on timed tasks requiring motor control is unclear.

One could hypothesize that motor abnormalities, rather than more pure "cognitive" abnormalities, may contribute to poor or slowed performance on such neuropsychological tasks. Alternatively, it could also be proposed that these motor abnormalities are actually *driven* by deficits in cognitive functioning and are therefore part of the neuropsychology of ADHD rather than a confounding factor for neuropsychological testing. Although limited, some data suggest that at least some of these motor abnormalities are mediated by cognitive dysfunction. For example, in one ADHD sample, Klimkeit *et al.* (2005) showed impairments in motor *preparation* rather than *execution* suggesting that the motor impairments may be related to attentional/motivational problems rather than deficits in motor skills themselves. This is consistent with work by Pitcher *et al.* (2003), which showed that although inattentive and combined ADHD subtypes demonstrated motor abnormalities, the hyperactive/impulsive-only group did not. On the other hand, the substantial data on structural cerebellar abnormalities in ADHD children could provide an anatomical substrate for these to be more purely motor in nature.[2] More studies in this area are required in order to fully understand the interplay between cognitive and motor functioning in ADHD individuals and how this interplay may ultimately influence neuropsychological heterogeneity in ADHD.

Clinical neuropsychological assessment of ADHD

The research findings discussed above provide valuable information to assist the clinical neuropsychologist. The neuropsychological examination typically has three general aims (Seidman & Toomey, 1999): (1) the identification of neuropsychological deficits that assist in developing hypotheses regarding the presence, type and etiology of brain dysfunction; (2) the identification of strengths and weaknesses in various domains as a guide for treatment; and (3) the documentation and measurement of changes in cognition or level of functioning over time (if any). The first aim, comprising the identification of deficits, is most limited by the moderate levels of sensitivity and specificity of neuropsychological measurements commonly used.

In ADHD a diagnosis is made by taking a history and evaluating whether DSM-defined symptom criteria are met. In addition, the clinician may want to address the degree of formal attention or executive dysfunction that is present. This typically leads the examiner to evaluate vigilance (often using an attentional, Continuous Performance Test), response inhibition or interference (Stroop or Stop-Signal test) and organizational skills (the Rey–Osterrieth Complex Figure (ROCF); Seidman *et al.*, 1995; Teknos *et al.*, 2003). Because learning disabilities may co-exist with ADHD (Seidman *et al.*, 2001) and also influence long-term school outcome (Faraone *et al.*, 2001), it is often important to add a number of tests to aid their identification. Measures of phonological processing for assessment of dyslexia (Willcutt *et al.*, 2001), and/or measures of mathematical and spatial ability should be included to assess non-verbal learning disability (Seidman & Toomey, 1999).

More recently the importance of assessing within-subject or intra-subject variability has been acknowledged (Castellanos *et al.*, 2005), and therefore the examiner may also want to look at the trial-to-trial variability for children suspected of having ADHD. The individual case assessment requires a flexible, hypothesis-testing approach in which different assessment tools are used with different patients. Currently, no single test or battery can be recommended for a comprehensive evaluation of ADHD and its related neuropsychological dysfunctions. Because neuropsychological functioning is predictive of real-world functioning in ADHD and other disorders (Biederman *et al.*, 2004), its utility is widely appreciated as an addition to the assessment battery beyond simple diagnosis.

Neuropsychological assessment in preschoolers

Although a diagnosis of ADHD can be made in children even before the age of 3, there are relatively few studies examining neuropsychological functioning in preschoolers 3–5 years of age. Nonetheless, the available data provide a picture relatively consistent with observations and reports in later childhood and adolescence. Compared with healthy preschoolers, preschoolers with ADHD display more inhibitory control deficits and are more delay aversive (Sonuga-Barke *et al.*, 2002). They also perform more poorly on tasks of visual search cancellation, visual and/or auditory vigilance, motor control, working memory, goal-directed persistence and pre-academic skills including tests of memory, reasoning and conceptual development (see review by Valera & Seidman, 2006). Furthermore, there is some evidence that medication can be beneficial even in these early years. In a follow-up study, Byrne *et al.* (1998) demonstrated improved performance in 4–5-year-old ADHD preschoolers on a visual and auditory preschool vigilance test, as well as on a visual-search preschool cancellation test after treatment with stimulant medication.

There are also a number of neuropsychological studies of ADHD in "older preschoolers" aged 5–6 years (Berlin & Bohlin, 2002) and 5–7 years (Hanisch *et al.*, 2004). The results of these studies suggest the presence of executive function and inhibitory deficits in ADHD. As a group, the older ADHD preschool children perform significantly worse than controls on tasks of visuomotor ability, working memory and attention (Hanisch *et al.*, 2004).

Neuropsychological studies in children aged 6–12 years with ADHD

The neuropsychological functioning of elementary school-age ADHD children has been studied extensively since the early 1970s, beginning with the pioneering work by Douglas on vigilance deficits (Douglas, 1972). Numerous clinical studies (at least 100) have compared groups of ADHD children, typically aged 6–12 years, with normal controls and have generally shown group differences (Frazier *et al.*, 2004). Yet, while the hypothesis of executive function impairment has received substantial support, several studies have reported inconsistent deficits across different executive domains, whilst other studies have reported no executive dysfunctions (reviews in Barkley *et al.*, 1992; Sergeant *et al.*, 2002). Moreover, effect sizes are modest (Frazier *et al.*, 2004), usually ranging from 0.4–0.7 using Cohen's *d* (Willcutt *et al.*, 2005). As suggested earlier, this heterogeneity could reflect a true underlying neuropsychological heterogeneity of ADHD or methodological confounds across studies.

In general, investigations examining children with ADHD report below-average performance on various tasks of vigilance, verbal learning (particularly encoding), working memory and executive functions such as set-shifting, planning and organization, complex problem-solving and response inhibition (Barkley *et al.*, 1992; Fischer *et al.*, 1990; Pennington & Ozonoff, 1996; Seidman *et al.*, 1997). Deficits in response inhibition appear to be among the most

significant neuropsychological impairments (see meta-analysis by Willcutt *et al.*, 2005). These skills, requiring suppression of interference arising from conflicting information have been shown to be abnormal in large samples of ADHD boys and girls (Seidman *et al.*, 2005a). Notably, although the majority of neuropsychological studies of ADHD has been conducted with boys, it is now clear that girls with ADHD have neuropsychological deficits (Nigg *et al.*, 1998; Seidman *et al.*, 2006a) and that the severity and pattern of deficits is largely the same across genders (Seidman *et al.*, 2005a).

Timing and motor abnormalities in ADHD

Although not typically assessed in clinical neuropsychological assessments, there is now considerable evidence that ADHD children show abnormalities on tasks requiring precise timing (e.g. more difficulty maintaining an even rate of tapping or having difficulty identifying which time duration is longer). Studies on ADHD examining motor timing (paced finger tapping: Rubia *et al.*, 2003), duration discrimination (Toplak *et al.*, 2003), duration reproduction (Barkley *et al.*, 2001), verbal time estimation (Smith *et al.*, 2002) and anticipation tasks (Rubia *et al.*, 2003) tend to show that performance of ADHD children is either less accurate or more variable in their reaction time (RT) than that of control children, with an association between this increased variability in RT and attentional ratings (Rubia *et al.*, 1999). Furthermore, medication can significantly reduce these abnormalities (Rubia *et al.*, 2003).

As discussed above, up to 50% of ADHD children have been found to have motor difficulties (Pitcher *et al.*, 2002). Relative to control children, ADHD children have been found to perform more poorly on both fine and gross motor tasks including: goal-directed arm movements (Eliasson *et al.*, 2004), handwriting (Barkley, 1990), motor timing and force output (Pitcher *et al.*, 2002), "motor leg movement" (Nigg *et al.*, 1998), performance on the Purdue Pegboard Task (Pitcher *et al.*, 2003), dynamic balance and diadochokinesis[3] (Kroes *et al.*, 2002), manual dexterity skills (Piek *et al.*, 1999) and motor overflow (Denckla & Rudel, 1978). There is some evidence that ADHD subtype matters, as individuals in the inattentive or combined DSM-IV subgroup are more likely to have motor problems than are individuals in the hyperactive/impulsive subgroup (Piek *et al.*, 1999; Pitcher *et al.*, 2003).

The cause of these motor abnormalities and whether they are truly motor or affected by cognitive control is still under investigation. Whereas much of the data above may suggest that these motor disturbances are driven by pure motor deficits, other data suggest that some abnormalities are driven by attentional problems (Klimkeit *et al.*, 2005). Incorporating tests of timing or subtle motor abnormalities in testing sessions using common clinical neuropsychological tasks may help elucidate their selective contribution to neuropsychological impairment in ADHD.

Relating brain structure, function and neuropsychological dysfunctions

Lesion and neuropsychological findings have been the foundation for choosing brain regions of interest in both structural and functional neuroimaging studies in ADHD. To this end, the prefrontal cortex (PFC) and regions projecting to the PFC have been studied extensively. As the number of neuroimaging studies has grown, the regions of interest have expanded to include other areas, such as parietal regions for their association with attention, the nucleus accumbens for its known association with reward (e.g. some investigators, such as Sonuga-Barke and colleagues, have emphasized disturbances in processes such as reward anticipation in ADHD) and the cerebellum for its involvement in both motor and cognitive functioning.

Structural and functional neuroimaging data in ADHD have begun to provide a reasonably consistent picture about the brain regions involved with this disorder. Structural imaging data have commonly shown volumetric reductions in total cerebral volume, the cerebellum, the PFC, striatal regions (caudate and pallidum) and the splenium of the corpus callosum (for review see Seidman *et al.*, 2005a). Meta-analytic results of these structural imaging data indicate that frontal and cerebellar regions show the largest standardized mean difference scores, indicating that these regions show the greatest volumetric reductions relative to control individuals who do not have ADHD (Valera *et al.*, 2006). Functional imaging studies have demonstrated abnormalities in similar regions including prefrontal regions, the striatum, the dorsal anterior cingulate and cerebellum (for review see Bush *et al.*, 2005). Thus, the abnormalities identified by structural and functional imaging studies are consistent with what one might predict based on the neuropsychological deficits found in this population, namely, deficits in attention, working memory, response inhibition, planning and other executive functions, motor control and reward/motivation (Castellanos *et al.*, 2006).

The analysis of attention and executive functions into subcomponents, and the correlation of attentional functions with brain structure and function, supports the proposition that response inhibition and other executive deficits in ADHD are associated with specific components of neural networks underlying attention and executive functions. For example, abnormalities in a network of regions including the orbital frontal cortex, dorsal anterior cingulate, nucleus accumbens and cerebellar vermis may be specifically related to impulsivity problems in ADHD. However, there is currently limited research in this area in samples with ADHD. Casey *et al.* (1997) found that performance on three response inhibition tasks by children with ADHD only correlated with neuroanatomical regions previously associated with a fronto-striatal network; the structure of these regions was notably abnormal in this ADHD group (i.e. the PFC, caudate and globus pallidus, but not the putamen). The significant correlations between task performance and anatomical measures of the PFC and caudate nuclei were predominantly in the right hemisphere, supporting the role of right fronto-striatal circuitry in response inhibition and ADHD. Semrud-Clikeman *et al.* (2000) found a significant relationship between reversed caudate asymmetry and measures of inhibition (as measured by the Stroop) and externalizing behavior. Also, poorer performance on sustained attention tasks has been found to be related to smaller volume of right hemispheric white matter (Semrud-Clikeman *et al.*, 2000). Furthermore, there are now a growing number of functional imaging studies comparing ADHD youth and controls, which demonstrate abnormal activation patterns in relevant brain regions while performing executive function tasks (for review see Bush *et al.*, 2005). As neuroimaging findings are replicated across tasks and samples we will come closer to understanding the brain structure–function relationship in this disorder.

There is also some limited evidence that IQ and ADHD symptomatology are correlated with brain volume abnormalities. Castellanos *et al.* (1996) found that full-scale IQ score correlated significantly with total brain volume and with left and right prefrontal regions of boys with ADHD. Using the same sample, Berquin et al. (1998) found that full-scale IQ correlated with cerebellar volumes in ADHD. In another study of boys with ADHD, the area of the rostral body of the corpus callosum was significantly correlated with scores on the impulsivity/hyperactivity scale of the Conners parent and teacher questionnaires (Giedd et al., 1994). The only study of brain structure and cognition using only girls demonstrated that the pallidum, caudate and prefrontal brain volumes correlated significantly with ratings of ADHD severity and cognitive performance (Castellanos et al., 2001). The largest structural imaging study including both boys and girls by Castellanos et al. (2002) showed that volumes of frontal and temporal gray matter, caudate and cerebellum were significantly negatively correlated with global clinician ratings and ratings of attentional problems. The extant data, while limited, suggest IQ and ratings of ADHD symptomatology are associated with abnormal brain volumes in ADHD.

These data provide evidence for relatively widespread abnormalities throughout the brains of ADHD children. In order to move forward, we will need to move from the examination of individual brain regions to the examination of neural networks of cognitive functioning. This can be done with newer imaging techniques as well as more sophisticated means of analyzing data. For example, diffusion tensor imaging (DTI) can be used to assess the integrity of white matter fibers connecting functionally specialized areas of the brain. In the first DTI study in children, Ashtari et al. (2005) found abnormalities in a measure of white matter integrity in a cerebellar-prefrontal-striatal network.

Conduct and oppositional defiant disorders

Conduct disorder (CD) and oppositional defiant disorder (ODD) are disruptive behavior disorders diagnosed in childhood and adolescence. Most cases remit by adulthood, but adults showing these symptoms generally meet criteria for antisocial personality disorder. According to DSM–IV, the diagnosis of CD should be made when an individual under the age of 18 exhibits three of 15 behaviors from the following categories: (1) aggressive conduct that causes or threatens physical harm to other people or animals,

(2) non-aggressive conduct that causes property loss or damage, (3) deceitfulness or theft and (4) serious violations of rules. Oppositional defiant disorder is diagnosed when four of eight behaviors of defiance, disobedience or hostility are exhibited. For both disorders, such behaviors must be present in the past 12 months, with at least one behavior present in the past 6 months.

Oppositional defiant disorder is often thought of as a precursor to and a milder form of CD and the distinction between the two disorders is limited. This is reflected in the contrasting nosology between ICD-10's classification of an "ODD-subtype" of CD (World Health Organization, 1993), and DSM–IV's classification of two separate disorders. Also, DSM–IV specifies that ODD should not be diagnosed if criteria for CD are met, implying that the latter is a more severe case of the former. Because of the lack of distinction between the two disorders, most clinical research studies treat subjects with CD and ODD as one experimental group (Rowe et al., 2005).

The handful of behavioral studies addressing the neuropsychology of CD/ODD have concentrated on executive functions because of the similarities and high comorbidity of CD/ODD with ADHD, and because the defining impulsive, aggressive and socially inappropriate symptoms of CD/ODD can appear similar to deficits seen in patients with frontal lobe lesions. The research to date has yielded inconsistent results suggesting mild or no executive-function deficits in CD/ODD. As Pennington & Ozonoff (1996) have noted, the executive deficits found in some research may in fact be due to comorbid ADHD, or even subthreshold ADHD, and not to the CD/ODD diagnosis itself.

Most of the studies that include groups of children and adolescents with DSM diagnoses of CD/ODD, and that properly control for ADHD have found no significant executive function deficits. For example, in several studies of response inhibition, no evidence was found for a deficit in either the CD-only and/or CD+ADHD groups relative to controls (Dery et al., 1999; Schachar et al., 2000). This same pattern was true for a range of executive-function tasks including WCST, ROCF, Porteus mazes, or Trail Making A and B (see Clark et al., 2000; Dery et al., 1999; Kalff et al., 2002).

There have only been a few studies that provide support for executive-function deficits in CD/ODD (Giancola et al., 1998; Toupin et al., 2000).

A meta-analysis of response inhibition studies (Oosterlaan et al., 1998) found deficits in the CD/ODD group comparable with those found in ADHD children. The results, however, were more robust for the children with ADHD, and there was significant heterogeneity of results in the studies examining CD/ODD. The authors note that the findings for the CD/ODD groups should be taken with caution as there were "sharply conflicting findings obtained in each of the four studies" (p. 419).

Notably, the choice of sampling and diagnostic grouping seem to have an important impact on study results; particularly whether the analysis was conducted with a dimensional or categorical approach.[4] In support of the assertion of Pennington & Ozonoff (1996), it appears that the results indicating executive deficits in CD/ODD may have been driven, at least in part, by comorbidity of ADHD in the samples. Thus, most of the studies noted above that found executive-function deficits in CD/ODD, did not use a "pure" CD/ODD group, but using a dimensional approach, covaried for ADHD symptoms in their CD/ODD children (Giancola et al., 1998; Klorman et al., 1999; and methods were mixed in Oosterlaan et al., 1998 meta-analysis). In contrast, the studies that did compare children with CD/ODD-only with controls, a categorical approach, generally found no executive-function deficits (Clark et al., 2000; Dery et al., 1999; Kalff et al., 2002; Oosterlaan et al. 2005; Schachar et al., 2000). The only exception we found was Toupin et al. (2000), who reported executive deficits in CD/ODD when conducting both types of analyses on their sample.

It is interesting to note that several studies found that subjects with comorbid CD/ODD+ADHD performed better than ADHD-only subjects on several neurocognitive tests (Clark et al., 2000 on Six Elements Test and Haylings Sentence Completion Test; Klorman et al., 1999 on Tower of Hanoi; Oosterlaan et al., 2005 on Self-Ordered Pointing Test and Tower of London; Schachar et al., 2000 on estimated FSIQ and Stop-Signal task). This is an interesting and potentially counterintuitive finding as it seems to make more sense that one diagnosis on top of another one would result in more impairment than one diagnosis alone. These results imply that a better neuropsychological profile might be found in children and adolescents with both disorders. This led Schachar et al. (2000) to propose that the ADHD+CD diagnosis might be a phenocopy[5] of CD/ODD rather than a variant of ADHD. This finding is not consistent across our review, however, and should therefore be considered with caution. Additional research is needed to resolve this issue.

Neuropsychological studies assessing children and adolescents with CD/ODD on tasks outside of the executive domain are limited and, with the exception of one of three that we reviewed (Dery et al., 1999), tend to show small or no differences between CD/ODD groups and controls. Also, in contrast to what is found in ADHD, of four studies examining estimated full-scale IQ, only one (Oosterlaan et al., 2005) found significantly lower IQ scores for their CD sample compared to controls.

In summary, the evidence for neuropsychological impairments in CD/ODD is scarce in contrast to ADHD where robust impairments have been found in several domains of executive functioning. On classical executive-function assessment tests, a clinician would be more likely to see deficits in a child with pure ADHD than a child with pure CD/ODD. Importantly, however, neuropsychological testing alone is not currently a powerful enough tool to be able to diagnose either of these disorders, or to necessarily differentiate them from each other in any particular individual. More research is needed to delineate the dysfunctions that are specific to each disorder and determine if there are any dysfunctions that are impaired in all children with these diagnoses.

Autism-spectrum disorders

Autistic disorder is characterized by severe impairment in social interaction, communication and stereotyped behaviors. It is categorized in the DSM–IV as one of the pervasive developmental disorders, but many prefer to use "autistic spectrum disorders" (Tanguay, 2004). A large literature exists on core deficits (i.e. in social communication, language, face processing and Theory of Mind),[6] a review of which is beyond the scope of this chapter. Studies of the "classic" domains of neuropsychology in autism (autistic spectrum referred to herein as autism) are limited however, likely because the "islets" of abilities and disabilities can vary greatly between individuals and throughout development, making it difficult to produce an average "neuropsychological profile" of autism (Tager-Flusberg & Joseph, 2003). Also, the defining communication deficits in autism make for very difficult testing sessions, with testing being nearly impossible in the more severe cases who can be mentally retarded or have a complete lack of verbal skills. This has resulted in a selective literature based on "high functioning" autistics and individuals with Asperger's disorder.

In the domains of executive functions, children with autism show deficits in spatial working memory (Williams *et al.*, 2006), planning and mental flexibility, and inconsistent deficits on measures of inhibition (see Hill & Bird, 2006 for review). Abnormal patterns of shifting and allocating attention have also been reported (Liss *et al.*, 2006). The profile of attentional functioning in autism is complex, however, because highly focused hyper-attentive states are present for a restricted range of interests (see Murray *et al.*, 2005). Joint attention, the use of nonverbal communication with another person about a third entity, is often grossly deficient in autism (see Bruinsma *et al.*, 2004 for review). In the visuospatial domain, children with autism show a relative strength in block design and related tasks where attention to detail is an important skill. Attention to larger global aspects of stimuli when inhibition of the details is necessary is deficient. For example, there is a lack of "global precedence" when responding to a larger "global" number composed of smaller "local" numbers (Rinehart *et al.*, 2003). Memory recall has been found to be impaired in autism, but the level of complexity of the stimuli seems to be important, with autistics having relatively intact memory for single digits, but impairments in memory for complex visual and verbal information (Williams *et al.*, 2006). The literature seems to consistently point to a deficit in manipulation and integration of complex information across social, attentional and memory domains. There is currently debate in the literature as to whether or not this is due to a core deficit in executive function (Hill & Bird, 2006).

It has been suggested that the overlap in clinical symptoms between children with ADHD and those with autism is significant enough that there is an unclear boundary between the two disorders (Hattori *et al.*, 2006). Both populations show executive deficits, ADHD symptoms are found in a significant subset of the autistic population (Ogino *et al.*, 2005), and social and emotional processing has been found to be deficient in ADHD samples (Buitelaar *et al.*, 1999). It should be emphasized, however, that studies comparing ADHD with autistic-spectrum disorders generally include those on the less severe end of the autistic spectrum (i.e. high-functioning autistics and those with Asperger's disorder). Attention-deficit hyperactivity disorder has not been associated with such debilitating language and social interaction deficits as those seen in some of the more severe cases of autism.

In individuals with autism, the factors underlying poor performance on neuropsychological tests are unclear. This is probably because assessment tools often require skills that may be more fundamentally deficient in autism such as attentional distribution, sensory modulation and social interaction/communication with the tester (Kleinhans *et al.*, 2005). While children with autism can show deficits in many domains, it is difficult to know what core feature(s) underlie these deficits. Researchers will need to develop tests and testing situations that are amenable to children with severe impairments in social communication and that can parse out which deficits are due to which core features of the disorder.

Summary

This chapter provides the reader with a review of the neuropsychological deficits associated with ADHD, as well as a model commonly used to describe the cognitive deficits of the disorder. We also discuss the apparent neuropsychological heterogeneity of ADHD, and issues that may contribute to such heterogeneity. It is recommended that an integration of current cognitive models of ADHD is necessary in order to more accurately and fully characterize the neuropsychological deficits of this disorder. For more direct clinical application, suggestions are offered regarding the clinical evaluation of neurocognitive functioning in ADHD. Additionally, an overview of the structural and functional neuroimaging findings are presented to assist the reader in gaining an understanding of the neurobiological underpinnings of ADHD. We conclude the chapter with a brief review of the neuropsychological deficits associated with CD/ODD and autism-spectrum disorders as they relate to ADHD. Because ADHD is known to be a heterogeneous disorder with substantial psychiatric and cognitive comorbidity, this article will aid clinicians in developing a better framework for understanding their patients. It is in gaining this greater understanding that ADHD will be better understood and diagnosed, which will ultimately lead to the most efficient and efficacious treatment of this disorder.

Acknowledgments

This work was supported in part by grants from the National Institutes of Health (K23 MH071535–01A1, Dr. Valera), NIMH (R01-MH62152; Dr. Seidman) and the March of Dimes Foundation (Dr. Seidman). Thanks to Joseph Biederman, Alysa Doyle, Stephen Faraone, Ronna Fried and Michael Monuteaux for their contributions to this work.

Endnotes

1. Attention-deficit hyperactivity disorder also extends into adolescence and adulthood, but those data are beyond the scope of this chapter. However, we note that the neuropsychological deficits found in ADHD youth are largely the same as those found in adolescence and adulthood (Seidman, 2006).

2. Although it has long been known that the cerebellum is involved in motor processes, it is now also well established that the cerebellum is involved in cognitive processes. Therefore, it will be important to be more precise in our assessment of which specific cerebellar regions are abnormal and then begin to search for associations between cerebellar and both motor and cognitive abnormalities in ADHD individuals.

3. Diadochokinesis: The normal power of alternately bringing a limb into opposite positions, as flexion and extension or pronation and supination (The American Heritage Stedman's Medical Dictionary, 2002).

4. The categorical approach treats diagnoses as qualitatively different from each other with discrete boundaries, while the dimensional approach treats psychiatric disorders on a continuum, assuming they differ from each other only in degree of severity of the symptoms (see Sonuga-Barke, 1998 for a critical review of these approaches in child psychiatry).

5. Phenocopy: an environmentally induced, non-hereditary variation in an organism, closely resembling a genetically determined trait (The American Heritage Stedman's Medical Dictionary, 2002).

6. Theory of Mind is defined by Simon Baron-Cohen as "being able to infer the full range of mental states (beliefs, desires, intentions, imagination, emotions, etc.) that cause action. In brief, to be able to reflect on the contents of one's own and other's minds." (Baron-Cohen, 2000).

References

American Psychiatric Association (1994). *Diagnostic and Statistical Manual of Mental Disorders: DSM–IV* (4th edn.). Washington, DC: American Psychiatric Association.

Ashtari, M., Kumra, S., Bhaskar, S. L. *et al.* (2005). Attention-deficit/hyperactivity disorder: a preliminary diffusion tensor imaging study. *Biological Psychiatry*, **57**, 448–455.

Barkley, R. A. (1990). *Attention Deficit Hyperactivity Disorder: A Handbook for Diagnosis and Treatment.* New York, NY: Guilford Press.

Barkley, R. A. (1997). Behavioral inhibition, sustained attention, and executive functions: constructing a unifying theory of ADHD. *Psychological Bulletin*, **121**, 65–94.

Barkley, R. A., Grodzinsky, G. & DuPaul, G. J. (1992). Frontal lobe functions in attention deficit disorder with and without hyperactivity: a review and research report. *Journal of Abnormal Child Psychology*, **20**, 163–188.

Barkley, R. A., Murphy, K. & Bush, T. (2001). Time perception and reproduction in young adults with attention deficit hyperactivity disorder. *Neuropsychology*, **15**, 351–360.

Barnett, R., Maruff, P., Vance, A. *et al.* (2001). Abnormal executive function in attention deficit hyperactivity disorder: the effect of stimulant medication and age on spatial working memory. *Psychological Medicine*, **31**, 1107–1115.

Baron-Cohen, S. (2000). Theory of mind and autism: a fifteen year review. In S. Baron-Cohen, H. Tager-Flusberg & D. J. Cohen (Eds.), *Understanding Other Minds: Perspectives from Developmental Cognitive Neuroscience* (pp. 3–20). Oxford: Oxford University Press.

Berlin, L. & Bohlin, G. (2002). Response inhibition, hyperactivity, and conduct problems among preschool children. *Journal of Clinical Child and Adolescent Psychology*, **31**, 242–251.

Berquin, P. C., Giedd, J. N., Jacobsen, L. K. *et al.* (1998). Cerebellum in attention-deficit hyperactivity disorder: a morphometric MRI study. *Neurology*, **50**, 1087–1093.

Biederman, J., Monuteaux, M. C., Doyle, A. E. *et al.* (2004). Impact of executive function deficits and attention-deficit/hyperactivity disorder (ADHD) on academic outcomes in children. *Journal of Consulting and Clinical Psychology*, **72**(5), 757–766.

Bruinsma, Y., Koegel, R. L. & Koegel, L. K. (2004). Joint attention and children with autism: a review of the literature. *Mental Retardation and Developmental Disability Research and Reviews*, **10**, 169–175.

Buitelaar, J. K., van der Wees, M., Swaab-Barneveld, H. & van der Gaag, R. J. (1999). Theory of mind and emotion-recognition functioning in autistic spectrum disorders and in psychiatric control and normal children. *Developmental Psychopathology*, **11**, 39–58.

Bush, G., Valera, E. M. & Seidman, L. J. (2005). Functional neuroimaging of attention-deficit/hyperactivity disorder: a review and suggested future directions. *Biological Psychiatry*, **57**, 1273–1284.

295

Byrne, J. M., Bawden, H. N., DeWolfe, N. A. & Beattie, T. L. (1998). Clinical assessment of psychopharmacological treatment of preschoolers with ADHD. *Journal of Clinical and Experimental Neuropsychology*, **20**, 613–627.

Casey, B. J., Castellanos, F. X., Giedd, J. N. *et al.* (1997). Implication of right frontostriatal circuitry in response inhibition and attention-deficit/hyperactivity disorder. *Journal of the American Academy of Child and Adolescent Psychiatry*, **36**, 374–383.

Castellanos, F. X., Giedd, J. N., Berquin, P. C. *et al.* (2001). Quantitative brain magnetic resonance imaging in girls with attention-deficit/hyperactivity disorder. *Archives of General Psychiatry*, **58**, 289–295.

Castellanos, F. X., Giedd, J. N., Marsh, W. L. *et al.* (1996). Quantitative brain magnetic resonance imaging in attention-deficit hyperactivity disorder. *Archives of General Psychiatry*, **53**, 607–616.

Castellanos, F. X., Lee, P. P., Sharp, W. *et al.* (2002). Developmental trajectories of brain volume abnormalities in children and adolescents with attention-deficit/hyperactivity disorder. *Journal of the American Medical Association*, **288**, 1740–1748.

Castellanos, F. X., Sonuga-Barke, E. J., Milham, M. P. & Tannock, R. (2006). Characterizing cognition in ADHD: beyond executive dysfunction. *Trends in Cognitive Science*, **10**, 117–123.

Castellanos, F. X., Sonuga-Barke, E. J., Scheres, A. *et al.* (2005). Varieties of attention-deficit/hyperactivity disorder-related intra-individual variability. *Biological Psychiatry*, **57**, 1416–1423.

Clark, C., Prior, M. & Kinsella, G. J. (2000). Do executive function deficits differentiate between adolescents with ADHD and oppositional defiant/conduct disorder? A neuropsychological study using the Six Elements Test and Hayling Sentence Completion Test. *Journal of Abnormal Child Psychology*, **28**, 403–414.

Dalen, L., Sonuga-Barke, E. J., Hall, M. & Remington, B. (2004). Inhibitory deficits, delay aversion and preschool AD/HD: implications for the dual pathway model. *Neural Plasticity*, **11**, 1–11.

Denckla, M. B. & Rudel, R. G. (1978). Anomalies of motor development in hyperactive boys. *Annals of Neurology*, **3**, 231–233.

Dery, M., Toupin, J., Pauze, R., Mercier, H. & Fortin, L. (1999). Neuropsychological characteristics of adolescents with conduct disorder: association with attention-deficit-hyperactivity and aggression. *Journal of Abnormal Child Psychology*, **27**, 225–236.

Douglas, V. I. (1972). Stop, look and listen: the problem of sustained attention and impulse control in hyperactive and normal children. *Canadian Journal of Behavioral Science*, **4**, 259–282.

Doyle, A. E., Biederman, J., Seidman, L. J., Weber, W. & Faraone, S. V. (2000). Diagnostic efficiency of neuropsychological test scores for discriminating boys with and without attention deficit-hyperactivity disorder. *Journal of Consulting Clinical Psychology*, **68**, 477–488.

Eliasson, A. C., Rosblad, B. & Forssberg, H. (2004). Disturbances in programming goal-directed arm movements in children with ADHD. *Developmental Medicine and Child Neurology*, **46**, 19–27.

Faraone, S. V., Biederman, J., Monuteaux, M. C., Doyle, A. & Seidman, L. J. (2001). A psychometric measure of learning disability predicts educational failure four years later in boys with attention deficit hyperactivity disorder. *Journal of Attention Disorders*, **4**, 220–230.

Fischer, M., Barkley, R. A., Edelbrock, C. S. & Smallish, L. (1990). The adolescent outcome of hyperactive children diagnosed by research criteria: II. Academic, attentional, and neuropsychological status. *Journal of Consulting and Clinical Psychology*, **58**, 580–588.

Frazier, T. W., Demaree, H. A. & Youngstrom, E. A. (2004). Meta-analysis of intellectual and neuropsychological test performance in attention-deficit/hyperactivity disorder. *Neuropsychology*, **18**, 543–555.

Fuster, J. (1989). *The Prefrontal Cortex* (2nd edn.). New York, NY: Raven Press.

Giancola, P. R., Mezzich, A. C. & Tarter, R. E. (1998). Executive cognitive functioning, temperament, and antisocial behavior in conduct-disordered adolescent females. *Journal of Abnormal Psychology*, **107**, 629–641.

Giedd, J. N., Castellanos, F. X., Casey, B. J. *et al.* (1994). Quantitative morphology of the corpus callosum in attention deficit hyperactivity disorder. *American Journal of Psychiatry*, **151**, 665–669.

Grodzinsky, G. & Barkley, R. A. (1999). The predictive power of frontal lobe tests in the diagnosis of attention deficit hyperactivity disorder. *Clinical Neuropsychology*, **13**, 12–21.

Hanisch, C., Konrad, K., Gunther, T. & Herpertz-Dahlmann, B. (2004). Age-dependent neuropsychological deficits and effects of methylphenidate in children with attention-deficit/hyperactivity disorder: a comparison of pre- and grade-school children. *Journal of Neural Transmission*, **111**, 865–881.

Hattori, J., Ogino, T., Abiru, K. *et al.* (2006). Are pervasive developmental disorders and attention-deficit/hyperactivity disorder distinct disorders? *Brain Development*, **28**, 371–374.

Hill, E. L. & Bird, C. M. (2006). Executive processes in Asperger syndrome: patterns of performance in a multiple case series. *Neuropsychologia*.

Kalff, A. C., Hendriksen, J. G., Kroes, M. *et al.* (2002). Neurocognitive performance of 5- and 6-year-old children who met criteria for attention deficit/ hyperactivity disorder at 18 months follow-up: results from a prospective population study. *Journal of Abnormal Child Psychology*, 30, 589–598.

Kleinhans, N. Akshoomoff, N., & Delis, D. C. (2005). Executive functions in autism and Asperger's disorder: flexibility, fluency, and inhibition. *Developmental Neuropsychology*, 27, 379–401.

Klimkeit, E. I., Mattingley, J. B., Sheppard, D. M., Lee, P. & Bradshaw, J. L. (2005). Motor preparation, motor execution, attention, and executive functions in attention deficit/hyperactivity disorder (ADHD). *Child Neuropsychology*, 11, 153–173.

Klorman, R., Hazel-Fernandez, L. A., Shaywitz, S. E. *et al.* (1999). Executive functioning deficits in attention-deficit/hyperactivity disorder are independent of oppositional defiant or reading disorder. *Journal of the American Academy of Child and Adolescent Psychiatry*, 38, 1148–1155.

Kroes, M., Kalff, A. C., Steyaert, J. *et al.* (2002). A longitudinal community study: do psychosocial risk factors and child behavior checklist scores at 5 years of age predict psychiatric diagnoses at a later age? *Journal of the American Academy of Child and Adolescent Psychiatry*, 41, 955–963.

Liss, M., Saulnier, C., Fein, D. & Kinsbourne, M. (2006). Sensory and attention abnormalities in autistic spectrum disorders. *Autism*, 10, 155–172.

Logan, G. D., Schachar, R. J. & Tannock, R. (1997). Impulsivity and inhibitory control. *Psychological Science*, 8, 60–64.

Makris, N., Biederman, J., Valera, E. M. *et al.* (2007). Cortical thinning of the attention and executive function networks in adults with attention-deficit/hyperactivity disorder. *Cereb Cortex*, 17, 1364–1375.

Mattes, J. A. (1980). The role of frontal lobe dysfunction in childhood hyperkinesis. *Comprehensive Psychiatry*, 21, 358–369.

Murray, D., Lesser, M. & Lawson, W. (2005). Attention, monotropism and the diagnostic criteria for autism. *Autism*, 9, 139–156.

Nigg, J. T. (1999). The ADHD response-inhibition deficit as measured by the stop task: replication with DSM-IV combined type, extension, and qualification. *Journal of Abnormal Child Psychology*, 27, 393–402.

Nigg, J. T., Hinshaw, S. P., Carte, E. T. & Treuting, J. J. (1998). Neuropsychological correlates of childhood attention-deficit/hyperactivity disorder: explainable by comorbid disruptive behavior or reading problems? *Journal of Abnormal Psychology*, 107, 468–480.

Nigg, J. T., Willcutt, E. G., Doyle, A. E. & Sonuga-Barke, E. J. (2005). Causal heterogeneity in attention-deficit/ hyperactivity disorder: do we need neuropsychologically impaired subtypes? *Biological Psychiatry*, 57, 1224–1230.

Ogino, T., Hattori, J., Abiru, K. *et al.* (2005). Symptoms related to ADHD observed in patients with pervasive developmental disorder. *Brain Development*, 27, 345–348.

Oosterlaan, J., Logan, G. D. & Sergeant, J. A. (1998). Response inhibition in AD/HD, CD, comorbid AD/HD + CD, anxious, and control children: a meta-analysis of studies with the stop task. *Journal of Child Psychology and Psychiatry*, 39, 411–425.

Oosterlaan, J., Scheres, A. & Sergeant, J. A. (2005). Which executive functioning deficits are associated with AD/ HD, ODD/CD and comorbid AD/HD + ODD/CD. *Journal of Abnormal Child Psychology*, 33(1), 69–85.

Pennington, B. F. (2005). Toward a new neuropsychological model of attention-deficit/hyperactivity disorder: subtypes and multiple deficits. *Biological Psychiatry*, 57, 1221–1223.

Pennington, B. F. & Ozonoff, S. (1996). Executive functions and developmental psychopathology. *Journal of Child Psychology and Psychiatry*, 37, 51–87.

Piek, J. P., Pitcher, T. M. & Hay, D. A. (1999). Motor coordination and kinaesthesis in boys with attention deficit-hyperactivity disorder. *Developmental Medicine and Child Neurology*, 41, 159–165.

Pitcher, T. M., Piek, J. P. & Barrett, N. C. (2002). Timing and force control in boys with attention deficit hyperactivity disorder: subtype differences and the effect of comorbid developmental coordination disorder. *Human Movement Science*, 21, 919–945.

Pitcher, T. M., Piek, J. P. & Hay, D. A. (2003). Fine and gross motor ability in males with ADHD. *Developmental Medicine and Child Neurology*, 45, 525–535.

Pliszka, S. R. (2005). The neuropsychopharmacology of attention-deficit/hyperactivity disorder. *Biological Psychiatry*, 57, 1385–1390.

Rinehart, N. J., Bradshaw, J. L., Brereton, A. V. & Tonge, B. J. (2003). A clinical and neurobehavioural review of high-functioning autism and Asperger's disorder. *Australia and New Zealand Journal of Psychiatry*, 36, 762–770.

Rowe, R., Maughan, B., Costello, E. J. & Angold, A. (2005). Defining oppositional defiant disorder. *Journal of Child Psychology and Psychiatry*, 46, 1309–1316.

Rubia, K., Noorloos, J., Smith, A., Gunning, B. & Sergeant, J. (2003). Motor timing deficits in community and clinical boys with hyperactive behavior: the effect of methylphenidate on motor timing. *Journal of Abnormal Child Psychology*, **31**, 301–313.

Rubia, K., Overmeyer, S., Taylor, E. *et al.* (1999). Hypofrontality in attention deficit hyperactivity disorder during higher-order motor control: a study with functional MRI. *American Journal of Psychiatry*, **156**, 891–896.

Schachar, R., Mota, V. L., Logan, G. D., Tannock, R. & Klim, P. (2000). Confirmation of an inhibitory control deficit in attention-deficit/hyperactivity disorder. *Journal of Abnormal Child Psychology*, **28**, 227–235.

Seidman, L. J. (2006). Neuropsychological functioning in people with ADHD across the lifespan. *Clinical Psychology Review*, **26**, 466–485.

Seidman, L. J. & Toomey, R. (1999). The clinical use of psychological and neuropsychological tests. In A. Nicholi (Ed.), *Harvard Guide to Psychiatry* (3rd edn.), (pp. 40–64). Cambridge, MA: Harvard University Press.

Seidman, L. J., Benedict, K. B., Biederman, J. *et al.* (1995). Performance of children with ADHD on the Rey-Osterrieth complex figure: a pilot neuropsychological study. *Journal of Child Psychology and Psychiatry*, **36**, 1459–1473.

Seidman, L. J., Biederman, J., Faraone, S. V., Weber, W. & Ouellette, C. (1997). Toward defining a neuropsychology of attention deficit-hyperactivity disorder: performance of children and adolescents from a large clinically referred sample. *Journal of Consulting and Clinical Psychology*, **65**, 150–160.

Seidman, L. J., Biederman, J., Monuteaux, M. C., Doyle, A. E. & Faraone, S. V. (2001). Learning disabilities and executive dysfunction in boys with attention-deficit/hyperactivity disorder. *Neuropsychology*, **15**, 544–556.

Seidman, L. J., Biederman, J., Monuteaux, M. C. *et al.* (2005a). Impact of gender and age on executive functioning: do girls and boys with and without attention deficit hyperactivity disorder differ neuropsychologically in preteen and teenage years? *Developmental Neuropsychology*, **27**, 79–105.

Seidman, L. J., Biederman, J., Monuteaux, M. C., Weber, W. & Faraone, S. V. (2000). Neuropsychological functioning in nonreferred siblings of children with attention deficit/hyperactivity disorder. *Journal of Abnormal Psychology*, **109**, 252–265.

Seidman, L. J., Biederman, J., Valera, E. M. *et al.* (2006a). Neuropsychological functioning in girls with attention-deficit/hyperactivity disorder with and without learning disabilities. *Neuropsychology*, **20**, 166–177.

Seidman, L. J., Valera, E. M. & Makris, N. (2005b). Structural brain imaging of attention-deficit/hyperactivity disorder. *Biological Psychiatry*, **57**, 1263–1272.

Seidman, L. J., Valera, E. M., Makris, N. *et al.* (2006b). Dorsolateral prefrontal and anterior cingulate cortex volumetric abnormalities in adults with attention-deficit/hyperactivity disorder identified by magnetic resonance imaging. *Biological Psychiatry*.

Semrud-Clikeman, M. S., Steingard, R. J., Filipek, P. *et al.* (2000). Using MRI to examine brain-behavior relationships in males with attention deficit disorder with hyperactivity. *Journal of the American Academy of Child and Adolescent Psychiatry*, **39**, 477–484.

Sergeant, J. A., Geurts, H., Huijbregts, S., Scheres, A. & Oosterlaan, J. (2003). The top and bottom of ADHD: a neuropsychological perspective. *Neuroscience and Biobehavior Review*, **27**, 583–592.

Sergeant, J. A., Geurts, H. & Oosterlaan, J. (2002). How specific is a deficit of executive functioning for attention-deficit/hyperactivity disorder? *Behavioural Brain Research*, **130**, 3–28.

Smith, A., Taylor, E., Rogers, J. W., Newman, S. & Rubia, K. (2002). Evidence for a pure time perception deficit in children with ADHD. *Journal of Child Psychology and Psychiatry*, **43**, 529–542.

Sonuga-Barke, E. J. (1998). Categorical models of childhood disorder: a conceptual and empirical analysis. *Journal of Child Psychology and Psychiatry*, **39**, 115–133.

Sonuga-Barke, E. J. (2005). Causal models of attention-deficit/hyperactivity disorder: from common simple deficits to multiple developmental pathways. *Biological Psychiatry*, **57**, 1231–1238.

Sonuga-Barke, E. J., Dalen, L., Daley, D. & Remington, B. (2002). Are planning, working memory, and inhibition associated with individual differences in preschool ADHD symptoms? *Developmental Neuropsychology*, **21**, 255–272.

Still, G. (1902). The Goulstonian lectures on some abnormal psychical conditions in children. Lecture 1. *Lancet*, **1**, 1008–1012.

Tager-Flusberg, H. & Joseph, R. M. (2003). Identifying neurocognitive phenotypes in autism. *Philosophical Transactions of the Royal Society of London, Series B, Biological Sciences*, **358**(1430), 303–314.

Tanguay, P. E. (2004). Commentary: categorical versus spectrum approaches to classification in pervasive developmental disorders. *Journal of the American Academy of Child and Adolescent Psychiatry*, **43**, 181–182.

Teknos, K. S., Bernstein, J. H. & Seidman, L. J. (2003). Performance of attention-deficit/hyperactivity disordered children on the Rey–Osterrieth complex figure. In J. Knight & E. F. Kaplan (Eds.), *The Rey-Osterrieth Handbook*. Odessa, FL: Psychological Assessment Resources.

The American Heritage Stedman's Medical Dictionary (2002). New York, NY: Houghton Mifflin.

Toplak, M. E., Jain, U. & Tannock, R. (2005). Executive and motivational processes in adolescents with attention-deficit-hyperactivity disorder (ADHD). *Behavior and Brain Function*, **1**, 8.

Toplak, M. E., Rucklidge, J. J., Hetherington, R., John, S. C. & Tannock, R. (2003). Time perception deficits in attention-deficit/hyperactivity disorder and comorbid reading difficulties in child and adolescent samples. *Journal of Child Psychology and Psychiatry*, **44**, 888–903.

Toupin, J., Dery, M., Pauze, R., Mercier, H. & Fortin, L. (2000). Cognitive and familial contributions to conduct disorder in children. *Journal of Child Psychology and Psychiatry*, **41**, 333–344.

Valera, E. M., Faraone, S. V., Murray, K. E. & Seidman, L. J. (2006). Meta-analysis of structural imaging findings in attention-deficit/hyperactivity disorder. *Biol Psychiatry*.

Valera, E. M. & Seidman, L. J. (2006). Neurobiology of ADHD in preschoolers. *Infants and Young Children*, **19**, 94–108.

Willcutt, E. G., Doyle, A. E., Nigg, J. T., Faraone, S. V. & Pennington, B. F. (2005). Validity of the executive function theory of attention-deficit/hyperactivity disorder: a meta-analytic review. *Biological Psychiatry*, **57**, 1336–1346.

Willcutt, E. G., Pennington, B. F., Boada, R. *et al.* (2001). A comparison of the cognitive deficits in reading disability and attention-deficit/hyperactivity disorder. *Journal of Abnormal Psychology*, **110**, 157–172.

Williams, D. L., Goldstein, G. & Minshew, N. J. (2006). The profile of memory function in children with autism. *Neuropsychology*, **20**, 21–29.

World Health Organization (1993). *The International Classification of Mental and Behavioural Disorders: Diagnostic criteria for research* (ICD-10). Geneva: World Health Organization.

Zelazo, P. D. & Muller, U. (2004). Executive function in typical and atypical development. In U. Gaswami (Ed.), *Blackwell Handbook of Childhood Cognitive Development* (pp. 445–469). Malden, MA: Blackwell Publishing.

Chapter 20

A multidimensional neurobehavioral model of personality disorders

Richard A. Depue

From a scientific perspective, it is really no longer possible to accept the notion that personality disorders (PDs) represent distinct, categorical diagnostic entities. The behavioral features of PDs are not organized into discrete diagnostic entities, and multivariate studies of behavioral criteria fail to identify factors that resemble existing diagnostic constructs (Block, 2001; Ekselius *et al.*, 1994; Livesley, 2001; Livesley *et al.*, 1994). Indeed, just the opposite is observed: the behavioral features of PDs merge imperceptibly in a continous fashion across diagnostic categories, resulting in (1) significant overlap of behavioral features across categories and hence diagnostic comorbidity within individuals and (2) symptom heterogeneity within categories and hence frequent (and most common in some studies) application of the ambiguous diagnosis of "Personality disorders not otherwise specified" or PD NOS (Livesley, 2001; Saulsman & Page, 2004). Moreover, aside from schizotypy/schizotypic disorders (Korfine & Lenzenweger, 1995; Lenzenweger & Korfine, 1992), the existing latent class and taxometric analysis literature on PDs generally does *not* provide support for distinct entities for the majority of conditions in the PD realm in any compelling fashion (Haslam, 2003) and our reading of that literature suggests that even some provisional taxonic findings for borderline and antisocial PDs are open to doubt. It is, accordingly, not surprising that diagnostic membership is not significantly associated with predictive validity as to prognosis nor psychological or pharmacological treatments (Livesley, 2001). Such a state of affairs recently led Livesley (2001) to declare that "evidence on these points has accumulated to the point that it can no longer be ignored" (p. 278).

Such a state of affairs supports proponents of a dimensional approach to PDs, who note that (1) the behavioral features of PDs not only overlap diagnostic categories, but also merge imperceptibly with normality (Livesley, 2001; Saulsman & Page, 2004); and (2) the factorial structure of behavioral traits associated with PDs is similar in clinical and non-clinical samples (Livesley *et al.*, 1992; Reynolds & Clark, 2001). Furthermore, the higher-order structure of PD traits resembles four of the five major traits identified in the higher-order structure of normal personality (Clark & Livesley, 1994; Clark *et al.*, 1996; Reynolds & Clark, 2001). These findings suggest that PDs may be better understood as emerging at the extremes of personality dimensions that define the structure of behavior in the normal population (for reviews of this position see Costa & Widiger, 1994; Depue & Lenzenweger, 2005; Livesley, 2001; Reynolds & Clark, 2001; Saulsman & Page, 2004).

This realization has led to innumerable attempts to illustrate the association of personality traits with PD diagnostic categores. Most of these studies have relied on the so-called five-factor model of personality, which defines a structure characterized by the five higher-order traits of extraversion, neuroticism, agreeableness, conscientiousness and openness to experience. Although Reynolds & Clark (2001) demonstrated that four of these traits (openness shows no consistent relation to PDs; Saulsman & Page, 2004) account for a substantial proportion of the variance in interview-based ratings of DSM–IV PD diagnoses, a recent meta-analysis of similar studies demonstrated the limitation of the approach of correlating four traits with PDs (Saulsman & Page, 2004). The meta-analysis showed what most such studies illustrate: (1) the correlation of these four traits with PD categories is moderate to weak, (2) the complex "entity" of a PD category is defined by as little as one trait but never by

The Neuropsychology of Mental Illness, ed. Stephen J. Wood, Nicholas B. Allen and Christos Pantelis. Published by Cambridge University Press. © Cambridge University Press 2009.

four traits in a significant way and (3) single traits (e.g. neuroticism) characterize more than one, sometimes several, putatively distinct PDs. For example, how helpful is it to know that histrionic PD is characterized by moderately high extraversion but by no other trait; or, similarly, that dependent PD is associated with moderately high neuroticism but by no other trait. To what line of research or clinical intervention does that knowledge lead? Moreover, the traits relate more highly to PD categories that are studied in non-clinical samples, indicating that the traits may be less valuable in defining clinical entities. What the meta-analysis did reveal is that most PDs manifest, in common, higher trait levels of neuroticism and lower trait levels of agreeableness, meaning that most individuals with PDs are subject to negative emotionality and impaired affiliative or interpersonal behavior. Thus, again, when PD categories serve as the outcome variable, personality traits provide little in the way of power to discriminate between such categories. Overall, then, it is probably not unfair to conclude that such correlational studies have done little to inform the issue of continuity from personality systems to states of disorder, most of them having merely specified correlates of PDs and nothing more, and most of these studies lacked an underlying framework for understanding both personality and PDs.

The paradox in all of this is that, despite knowing that the PD diagnostic categories are unreliable and lack compelling construct and predictive validity, researchers cling to the approach of relating major personality traits, typically considered at the conceptual level of analysis one trait at a time, to *non-entities* of PDs. How can one learn something substantive by relating four higher-order traits to heterogeneous behavioral phenomena that are clustered conceptually (not statistically or theoretically) into diagnostic entities? As Livesley (2001) aptly notes, since PD diagnoses are so fundamentally flawed, it is not important to know whether each PD diagnosis can be accommodated by a dimensional model. Furthermore, the problem in this approach does not appear to be explained simply by use of a small number of broad traits. When the 30 facet scales of the NEO-PI were correlated with PD categories, only modest gains were achieved relative to the use of the four major traits (mean difference in $R^2 \sim 0.04$) (Dyce & O'Connor, 1998; Millon, 1997).

Perhaps one of the most crucial issues associated with a dimensional personality approach to PDs is

that the substantive meaning of the four major traits is not clear and generally has been a neglected topic (Block, 2001). Put differently, there is not a clear understanding as to which underlying neurobehavioral systems these traits reflect, which the behavioral genetic literature implies they must (Tellegen *et al.*, 1988). Accordingly, in this chapter we attempt to promote an alternative empirical and theoretical approach to PDs. First, we embrace the fact that PDs do not exist as *distinct entities* and, therefore, we refer to the behavioral manifestations that emerge at the extremes of personality dimensions as *personality disturbance* rather than disorders. We exclude schizotypal and paranoid personality disorders from our model, because there is evidence that they may be genetically related to schizophrenia (Kendler *et al.*, 1993; Lenzenweger & Loranger, 1989), representing an alternative manifestation of schizophrenia liability (Lenzenweger, 1998), and studies of the latent class structure of schizotypy show evidence that its underlying nature is more likely of a taxonic or qualitative nature (Korfine & Lenzenweger, 1995; Lenzenweger & Korfine, 1992; see also Haslam, 2003). The term *disorder*, though less formal and regimented than the term *disease*, nevertheless connotes a relatively coherent symptomatic entity that, with only more empirical attention, will be characterized by distinct boundaries and underlying dysfunction. We do not believe that, as PDs are currently conceived, such a state of scientific credibility will be achieved and hence warrant the use of the terms syndrome, disorder or disease. Second, we attempt to delineate the nature of the neurobehavioral systems that we postulate underlie the four major traits of personality. In so doing, we hope to provide a substantive meaning to the four major personality traits that supersedes the extant variation in trait labels and psychological concepts.

The implications of defining personality traits in terms of neurobehavioral systems leads to a third aspect of the chapter, where we derive a model of personality disturbance based on the *interaction* of these neurobehavioral systems. Though genetically speaking it may be possible to conceive of the neurobiological variables associated with neurobehavioral systems as subject to independent influences, it is impossible to imagine that neurobehavioral systems are independent at a functional level. Similarly, it is impossible to imagine that personality traits can be associated in an independent manner to PDs. Neurobehavioral systems, and the personality traits that reflect their influence, interact to produce complex behavior patterns – personality as a whole – in a multivariate fashion. Therefore, our model of personality disturbance rests on a foundation of multivariate interaction of neurobehavioral systems. Such an interaction may yield a phenotypic clustering of behavioral signs or symptoms that could be taken to suggest a demarcation, perhaps indicative of latent threshold effects in the neurobehavioral systems, but the observed clustering represents the end product of underlying continuous dimensional neurobehavioral systems. Such clusterings may be resolved with appropriate statistical methods such as finite mixture modeling. Furthermore, while it is true that our model is dimensional in nature, where personality disturbance lies at the extreme of normal, interacting personality dimensions, it is worth noting that no assumption is made herein that phenotypic dimensions of personality are genetically continuous. The phenotypic continuity could well represent several underlying *distinct* genotypic distributions, as may be the case even within the normal range of variation of some personality traits (Benjamin *et al.*, 1996; Ebstein *et al.*, 1996).

Neurobehavioral systems underlying higher-order personality traits

The higher-order structure of personality is converging on three to seven factors that account for the phenotypic variation in behavior (Digman, 1997; Tellegen & Waller, in press). Our model focuses on four higher-order traits which are robustly identified in the psychometric literature, and which we define with reference to coherent neurobehavioral systems. Higher-order traits resembling *extraversion* and *neuroticism* (anxiety) are identified in virtually every taxonomy of personality. Affiliation, termed *agreeableness* (Costa & McCrae, 1992; Goldberg & Rosolack, 1994) or *social closeness* (Tellegen & Waller, in press), has emerged more recently as a robust trait, and is comprised of affiliative or social tendencies, cooperativeness, and feelings of warmth and affection (Depue & Morrone-Strupinksy, 2005). Finally, some form of impulsivity, more recently termed *constraint* (Tellegen & Waller, in press) or *conscientiousness* (due to an emphasis on the unreliability and disorganization accompanying an impulsive disposition; Costa & McCrae, 1992; Goldberg & Rosolack, 1994), frequently emerges in factor studies.

Agentic extraversion and affiliation

The distinct aspects of the traits of agentic extraversion and affiliation are most effectively described in reference to social behavior. Social behavior is not a unitary characteristic, but rather has two major components (Depue, 2006). One component, *affiliation* or *social closeness*, reflects enjoying and valuing close interpersonal bonds, and being warm and affectionate; the other component, *agency*, reflects social dominance, assertiveness, exhibitionism and a subjective sense of potency in accomplishing goals. Thus, trait psychologists have proposed that affiliation and agency represent distinct dispositions (Depue & Collins, 1999; Depue & Morrone-Strupinsky, 2005; Tellegen & Waller, in press): whereas affiliation is clearly interpersonal in nature, agency represents a more general disposition that is manifest in a range of achievement-related, as well as interpersonal, contexts (Costa & McCrae, 1992; Goldberg & Rosolack, 1994; Tellegen & Waller, in press; Watson & Clark, 1997; Wiggins, 1991).

We have suggested that agentic extraversion and affiliation reflect the activity of two neurobehavioral systems involved in guiding behavior to *rewarding* goals (Depue & Collins, 1999; Depue & Strupinsky, 2005). Reward involves several dynamically interacting neurobehavioral processes occurring across two phases of goal acquisition (see Figure 20.1): *appetitive/approach* (reflecting individual differences in the strength of the agentic extraversion trait) and *consummatory* (reflecting individual differences in the strength of the affiliation or social closeness trait). Although both phases of reward are elicited by unconditioned incentive (reward-connoting) stimuli, their temporal onset, behavioral manifestations and putative neural systems differ (Berridge, 1999; Depue & Collins, 1999; Di Chiara & North, 1992; Wyvell & Berridge, 2000), and are dissociated in factor-analytic studies based on behavioral characteristics of animals (Pfaus *et al.*, 1999), just as agentic extraversion and affiliation are also dissociated in factor-analytic studies.

An appetitive/approach phase of goal acquisition represents the first step toward attaining biologically important goals (Hilliard *et al.*, 1998). It is based on a mammalian behavioral system that is activated by, and serves to bring an animal in contact with, unconditioned and conditioned rewarding incentive stimuli (Depue & Collins, 1999; Gray, 1973; Schneirla, 1959). This system is consistently described in all animals across phylogeny (Schneirla, 1959), and we define this

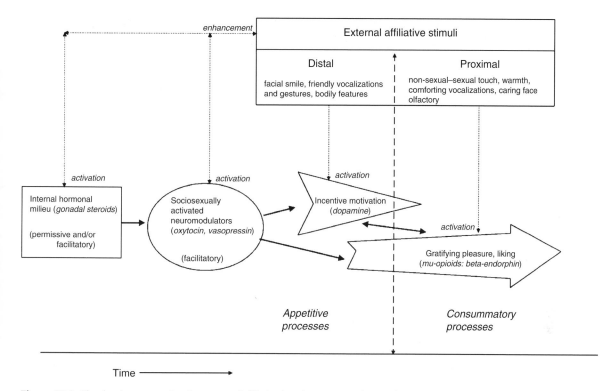

Figure 20.1. The development and maintenance of affiliative bonds across two phases of reward. Distal affiliative stimuli elicit an incentive-motivated approach to an affiliative goal, accompanied by strong emotional-motivational feelings of wanting, desire and positive activation. The approach phase not only ensures sociosexual interaction with an affiliative object, but also acquisition of a memory ensemble or network of the context in which approach, reward and goal acquisition occur. Next, proximal affiliative stimuli emanating from interaction with the affiliative object elicit strong feelings of consummatory reward, liking and physiological quiescence, all of which become associated with these stimuli as well as the context predictive of reward. As discussed below, dopamine encodes the incentive salience of contextual stimuli predictive of reward during the approach phase and, in collaboration with μ-opiate mediated consummatory reward, encodes the incentive salience of proximal stimuli directly linked to the affiliative object. The end result of this sequence of processes is an incentive-encoded affiliative memory network that continues to motivate approach toward and interaction with the affiliative object. Specialized processes ensure that affiliative stimuli are weighted as significant elements in the contextual ensembles representing affiliative memory networks. These specialized processes include the construction of a contextual ensemble via affiliative stimulus-induced opiate potentiation of dopamine processes, and the influence of permissive and/or facilitatory factors such as gonadal steroids, oxytocin and vasopressin on (1) sensory, perceptual and attentional processing of affiliative stimuli and (2) formation of social memories. See Depue & Morrone-Strupinsky (2005) for details.

system as *behavioral approach based on positive incentive motivation* (Depue & Collins, 1999).

The contrasting nature of the incentive motivational reward system and the consummatory reward system can be most efficiently described by using an affiliative object (e.g. a potential mate) as the rewarding goal object. In the appetitive/approach phase of securing a mate (see Figure 20.1), specific, *distal* affiliative stimuli of potential bonding partners – e.g. facial features and smiles, friendly vocalizations and gestures, and bodily features (Porges, 1998) – serve as unconditioned incentive stimuli based on their distinct patterns of sensory properties, such as smell, color, shape and temperature (Di Chiara & North,

1992; Hilliard *et al.*, 1998). These incentives are inherently evaluated as positive in valence, and activate incentive motivation, increased energy through sympathetic nervous system activity, and forward locomotion as a means of bringing individuals into close proximity (Di Chiara & North, 1992). Moreover, the incentive state is inherently rewarding, but in a highly activated manner, and animals will work intensively to obtain that reward without evidence of satiety (Depue & Collins, 1999).

In humans, activation of this incentive motivational system is associated with subjective feelings of desire, wanting, excitement, elation, enthusiasm, energy, potency and self-efficacy (Berridge, 1999;

Watson & Tellegen, 1985). This subjective experience of incentive motivation is concordant with the nature of the lower-order traits comprising the higher-order trait of agentic extraversion, including social dominance, achievement, endurance, persistence, efficacy, activity and energy. Therefore, we have proposed that agentic extraversion reflects the activity of a behavioral approach system based on *positive incentive motivation* (Depue, 2006; Depue & Collins, 1999; Depue & Morrone-Strupinsky, 2005).

When close proximity to a rewarding goal is achieved, the incentive-motivational approach system gives way to a consummatory phase of goal acquisition. In this phase, specific *interoceptive* and *proximal exteroceptive* stimuli related to critical primary biological aims elicit behavioral patterns that are relatively specific to those conditions (e.g. sexual, social or food-related; Hilliard *et al.*, 1998; Timberlake & Silva, 1995). Performance of these behavioral patterns is inherently rewarding (Berridge, 1999). In the case of potential mate acquisition, examples of affiliative behavioral patterns are courtship, gentle stroking and grooming, mating, and certain maternal patterns such as breast feeding, all of which may include facial, caressive tactile, gestural and certain vocal behaviors (Polan & Hofer, 1998). Tactile stimulation may be particularly effective in activating affiliative consummatory reward processes in animals and humans (Fleming *et al.*, 1994).

In contrast to the subjective state in an incentive motivational state of activation, desire and wanting, the expression of *consummatory* behavioral patterns is associated with intense feelings of pleasure, gratification, affection, and liking, plus physiological quiescence characterized by rest, sedation, anabolism and parasympathetic nervous system activity, thereby reinforcing the production and repetition of those behaviors (Berridge, 1999; Di Chiara & North 1992; Porges, 1998, 2001). Thus, whereas appetitive approach processes bring an individual into contact with incentive stimuli (a rewarding goal), consummatory processes bring behavior to a gratifying conclusion (Hilliard *et al.*, 1998).

The core content of affiliation or social closeness scales on personality inventories appears to reflect the operation of consummatory neurobehavioral processes in that the adjectives most closely associated with an affiliation trait are warm, affectionate and gratifying. Our hypothesis is two-fold: (1) that an affiliative/social closeness personality trait reflects individual differences

in the subjective experience of warmth and affection during interactions with other rewarding persons; and (2) that this experience of warmth and affection reflects an underlying *capacity to experience consummatory reward that is elicited by a broad array of proximal affiliative stimuli, such as gentle touch* (Depue, 2006; Depue & Morrone-Strupinsky, 2005). This capacity to experience consummatory reward is viewed as providing the key element utilized in additional psychobiological processes (such as associative learning) that permit the development and maintenance of longer-term social bonds that are characteristic of social organization in human and other primate societies (Gingrich *et al.*, 2000; Wang *et al.*, 1999). It is important to emphasize that a core capacity for affiliative consummatory reward is not viewed as a sufficient determinant of close social relationships, only as a necessary one, a *sine qua non* (see Depue, 2006; Depue & Morrone-Strupinsky, 2005 for full discussion).

Through Pavlovian associative learning, the experience of reward generated throughout both the appetitive/approach and consummatory phases is associated with previously affectively neutral stimulus contexts (objects, acts, events, places) in which pleasure occurred. Hence, across both phases of reward, conditioned incentive stimuli are formed that are subsequently predictive of reward (Berridge, 1999; Ostrowski, 1998; Timberlake & Silva, 1995). Thus, the acquisition and maintenance of a mate relationship, for example, depends closely on Pavlovian associative learning that links the subjective experience of reward generated in both approach (an activating reward) and consummatory (a calming sense of reward) phases of goal acquisition with (1) the salient contextual cues (including distal affiliative cues) that predict reward during the appetitive phase (e.g. features of a laboratory cage) and (2) a mate's individualistic cues associated directly with consummatory reward (e.g. individual characteristics of a sexually receptive female rat) (Domjan *et al.*, 2000). Taken together, the above processes support acquisition of affiliative or social memories, where contextual ensembles are formed and weighted in association with the reward provided by interaction with the potential mate.

Neurobiology of incentive motivation and affiliative reward

By drawing an association between traits and behavioral systems, i.e. agentic extraversion and incentive motivation, affiliation and consummatory reward, we are able to utilize the behavioral neurobiology animal literature to discern the neurobiology associated with these behavioral systems and, by analogy, with the personality traits of agentic extraversion and affiliation. As reviewed previously (Depue & Collins, 1999), animal research demonstrates that the positive incentive motivation and experience of reward that underlies a behavioral system of approach is dependent on the functional properties of the midbrain ventral tegmental area (VTA) dopamine (DA) projection system. Dopamine agonists or antagonists in the VTA or nucleus accumbens (NAS), which is a major terminal area of VTA DA projections, in rats and monkeys facilitate or markedly impair, respectively, a broad array of incentive motivated behaviors. Dopamine receptor cells, most numerously in the VTA, respond vigorously to and in proportion to the magnitude of both conditioned and unconditioned incentive stimuli and in anticipation of reward (Schultz et al., 1997).

In humans, incentive motivation is associated with both positive *emotional* feelings such as elation and euphoria, and *motivational* feelings of desire, wanting, craving, potency and self-efficacy. Neuroimaging studies of cocaine addicts found that during acute administration the intensity of a participant's subjective euphoria increased in a dose-dependent manner in proportion to cocaine binding to the DA uptake transporter (and hence to DA levels) in the striatum (Volkow et al., 1997). Moreover, cocaine-induced activity in the NAS was linked equally strongly (if not more strongly) to motivational feelings of desire, wanting and craving, as to the emotional experience of euphoric rush (Breiter et al., 1997). And the degree of amphetamine-induced DA release in healthy human ventral striatum assessed by PET was correlated strongly with feelings of euphoria (Drevets et al., 2001). Hence, taken together, the animal and human evidence demonstrates that the VTA DA–NAS pathway is a primary neural circuit for incentive motivation and its accompanying subjective state of reward.

With respect to consummatory reward and affiliative behavior, a broad range of evidence suggests a role for endogenous opiates. Endogenous opiate release or receptor binding is increased in rats, monkeys and humans by lactation and nursing, sexual activity, vaginocervical stimulation, maternal social interaction, brief social isolation, and grooming and other non-sexual tactile stimulation (see review

by Depue & Morrone-Strupinsky, 2005). Particularly important is the relation between opiates and grooming, because the primary function of primate grooming may well be to establish and maintain social bonds (Matheson & Bernstein, 2000). Perhaps most relevant to affiliative reward is the mu (μ)opioid receptor (OR) family, which is the main site of exogenously administered opiate drugs (e.g. morphine) and of endogenous endorphins (particularly, β-endorphin) (La Buda et al., 2000; Schlaepfer et al., 1998; Shippenberg & Elmer, 1998; Stefano et al., 2000; Wiedenmayer & Barr, 2000). Mu-opioid receptors also appear to be the main site for the effects of endogenous β-endorphins and endogenous morphine on the subjective feelings in humans of *increased* interpersonal warmth, euphoria, well-being and peaceful calmness, as well as of *decreased* elation, energy and incentive motivation (Schlaepfer et al., 1998; Shippenberg & Elmer, 1998; Stefano et al., 2000; Uhl et al., 1999). Importantly, μORs facilitate the rewarding effects associated with many motivated behaviors (Nelson & Panksepp, 1998; Niesink et al., 1996; Olive et al., 2001; Olson et al., 1997; Stefano et al., 2000; Strand, 1999). The rewarding effect of opiates may be especially mediated by μORs located in the NAS and VTA, both of which support self-administration of μOR agonists (Herz, 1998; Schlaepfer et al., 1998; Shippenberg & Elmer, 1998), and serve as unconditioned rewarding stimuli in producing a conditioned place preference, a behavioral measure of reward (Narita et al., 2000; Nelson & Panksepp, 1998; Shippenberg & Elmer, 1998). *Thus, DA and opiates appear to functionally interact in the NAS, but they apparently provide independent contributions to rewarding effects.* Indeed, transgenic mice lacking the μOR gene show no morphine-induced place preferences nor physical dependence from morphine consumption (Matthes et al., 1996; Simonin et al., 1998).

In sum, as illustrated in Figure 20.1, distal affiliative cues (e.g. friendly smiles and gestures, sexual features) serve as incentive stimuli that activate DA-facilitated incentive-reward motivation, desire, wanting and approach to affiliative objects. As these objects are reached, more proximal affiliative stimuli (e.g. pleasant touch) strongly activate μ-opiate release which promotes an intense state of pleasant reward, warmth, affection and physiological quiescence, and brings approach behavior to a gratifying conclusion. Throughout this entire sequence of goal acquisition, the contextual cues associated with approach to the goal, and the cues specifically related to the goal, are all associated with the experience of reward. It is beyond the scope of this chapter, but it is worth noting that DA and μ-opiates play a critical role in strengthening the association between these contextual cues and reward (Depue & Morrone-Strupinsky, 2005). Thus, these two neuromodulators are critical to establishing our preferences and memories for particular contexts and affiliative cues predictive of reward.

Finally, individual differences in agentic extraversion and affiliation are subject to strong genetic influence (Tellegen et al., 1988). If personality disturbance occurs in the region located at the extreme tails of individual difference distributions in the traits of agentic extraversion and affiliation, it is important to show that the neuromodulators associated with incentive motivation and affiliative reward are sources of individual differences in these behavioral systems. As reviewed elsewhere (Depue & Collins, 1999; Depue & Morrone-Strupinsky, 2005), studies show that genetic variation in DA and μOR properties in humans and rodents is (1) substantial, (2) an essential element in the variation in the rewarding value of DA and opiate agonists, and (3) critical in accounting for variation in the Pavlovian learning that underlies the association between contextual cues and reward, as occurs in partner and place preferences.

Anxiety or neuroticism

Anxiety and fear as two distinct behavioral systems

Fear is elicited by specific, discrete, explicit stimuli that threaten an organism's survival. These stimuli may be unconditioned or conditioned, and both types of stimuli elicit a rapid, high-amplitude escape response, if the context allows it, or a freezing response if escape is not possible. Thus, fear is a neurobehavioral system that provides for rapid action in order to escape or avoid threatening stimuli. However, there are many aversive circumstances that do not involve specific, discrete, explicit stimuli that evolutionarily have been neurobiologically linked to subjective fear and escape. That is, there are many situations in which specific aversive cues do not exist, but rather the stimulus conditions are associated with an elevated *potential* risk of danger or aversive consequences. In such cases, no explicit aversive stimuli are present to inherently activate escape circuitries. Nevertheless, the stimuli can be unconditioned in nature, as in darkness, open spaces, unfamiliarity and predator odors, or they can be

conditioned contextual cues (general textures, colors, relative spatial locations, sounds) that have been associated with previous exposure to specific aversive stimuli (Davis et al., 1997; Davis & Shi, 1999; Fendt et al., 2003). Conceptually, these stimuli are characterized in common by unpredictability and uncontrollability – or, more simply, uncertainty. In order to reduce the risk of danger in such circumstances, a behavioral system evolved that is *anxiety*. Anxiety is characterized by negative emotion or affect (anxiety, depression, hostility, suspiciousness, distress) that serves the purpose of informing the individual that, though no explicit, specific aversive stimuli are present, conditions are potentially threatening (White & Depue, 1999). This affective state, and the physiological arousal that accompanies it, continues or reverberates until the uncertainty is resolved. The trait literature supports the *independence* of anxiety and fear, which as personality traits are subject to distinct sources of genetic variation (Tellegen et al., 1988). As the averaged correlations derived from numerous studies show, the relation between the traits of neuroticism (anxiety) and of harm avoidance (fear) is essentially zero (Depue & Lenzenweger, 2005; White & Depue, 1999).

Neurobiology of anxiety

As reviewed elsewhere (Depue & Lenzenweger, 2005), anxiety is associated with prolonged activity of corticotrophin-releasing hormone (CRH) in the bed nucleus of the stria terminalis (BNST), which is a critical region within the extended amygdala. The significance of the prolonged effects of CRH in the BNST is that CRH and the BNST appear to be integrators of behavioral, neuroendocrine and autonomic responses to stressful circumstances (Leri et al., 2002; Pacak et al., 1995; Shaham et al., 2000).

The central CRH system is composed of CRH neurons located in many different subcortical brain regions (Strand, 1999). Whereas the majority of CRH neurons in the CNS do not mediate the effects of stress, some of the CRH-containing regions that are important in mediating stress effects are illustrated in Figure 20.2. As illustrated in Figure 20.2, the basolateral amygdala detects discrete aversive stimuli associated with the stressful circumstances and activates the extensive array of CRH neurons located in the central amygdala. These CRH neurons project to many brain regions that modulate emotion, memory and arousal, including the peripheral CRH neurons in

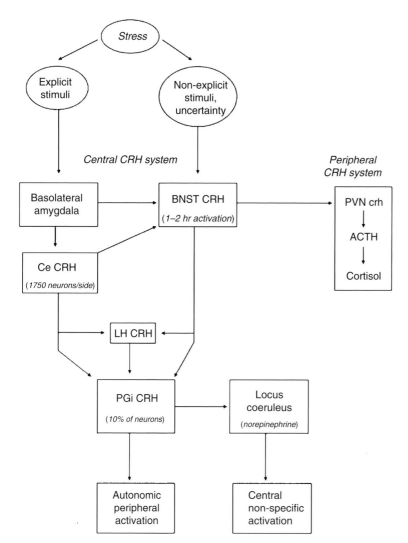

Figure 20.2. Components of the central and peripheral corticotrophin releasing-hormone (CRH) systems. Abbreviations: Ce = central amygdala nucleus, BNST = bed nucleus of the stria terminalis, LH = lateral hypothalamus, PGi = paragiganticocellularis, PVN = paraventricular nucleus of the hypothalamus, ACTH = corticotropic hormone from the anterior pituitary.

the paraventricular nucleus in the hypothalamus that facilitate cortisol release (Strand, 1999). Stress variables associated with context and uncertainty activate CRH neurons in the BNST, which have similar projection targets as the central amygdala (Erb et al., 2001; Macey et al., 2003; Shaham et al., 2000). Both the central amygdala and the BNST can activate CRH neurons in the lateral hypothalamus, a region that integrates central nervous system arousal. In turn, the lateral hypothalamic CRH projections modulate autonomic nervous system activity. Importantly, all three sources of CRH projections – the central amygdala, BNST and lateral hypothalamus – innervate CRH neurons in the paragiganticocellularis (PGi)

(Aston-Jones et al., 1996), which is located in the rostral ventrolateral area of the medulla. The PGi is a massive nucleus that provides major integration of central and autonomic arousal and, in turn, coordinates and triggers arousal responses to urgent stimuli via two main pathways eminating from its own population of CRH neurons, which make up 10% of PGi neurons (Aston-Jones et al., 1996). One CRH pathway modulates the autonomic nervous system and hence peripheral arousal effects via projections to the intermediolateral cell column of the spinal cord, activating sympathetic preganglionic autonomic neurons.

The other CRH pathway modulates central arousal effects via activation of the locus coeruleus

(LC), where PGi CRH innervation of the LC in humans and monkeys is dense (Aston-Jones et al., 1996). The LC is the major source of norepinephrine in the brain, and produces a non-specific emotional activation via broadly collateralizing axons to the central nervous system (Aston-Jones et al., 1996). This non-specific emotional activation pattern comprises a global urgent response system to unpredicted events and hence facilitates behavioral readiness, alerting (enhanced sensory processing) and attention (enhanced selection of stimuli) (Aston-Jones et al., 1996), which are characteristic of states of anxiety in highly stress-reactive rodents and monkeys (Blizard 1988; Redmond 1987). This central arousal can be enduring: PGi CRH activation of LC neurons endures and peaks 40 minutes after stimulation of the PGi (Aston-Jones et al., 1996). Not surprisingly, CRH administration in rodents, as well as in transgenic mice that have an overproduction of CRH centrally (but not peripherally), generates anxiogenic effects specifically via CRH2 receptors (Nie et al., 2004).

These findings taken together suggest that anxiety is essentially a stress response system that relies on a network of CRH neuron populations to modulate behaviorally relevant responses to the stressor. The most potent factors in determining the magnitude of a stressor are the very psychological factors that are eliciting stimuli of the anxiety system: uncontrollability, unpredictability, unfamiliarity, unavoidability and uncertainty. From the standpoint of trait anxiety or neuroticism, the strongest primary or facet scale in the higher-order factor of anxiety in Tellegen's personality questionnaire is termed *Stress reactivity* due to the stress-related content of items loading on the scale (Tellegen & Waller, in press).

In contrast to anxiety, the expression of fear involves activation of specific neural circuitries in longitudinal cell columns located in the periaqueductal gray area (PAG) of the midbrain. In the case of conditioned fear, activation of this PAG circuitry arises from afferents whose cell bodies are localized to the central nucleus of the amygdala. These central nucleus projections are activated themselves by neural groups in the basolateral amygdala that encode the association between neutral and aversive stimuli (i.e. conditioned fear). While there is no doubt that there are individual differences in the perception and expression of fear, the exact neurobiological influences that create these individual differences are not known, although

White & Depue (1999; White et al., 2006a, 2006b) have shown that variation in central noradrenergic functioning may be a strong contributor.

Non-affective constraint or impulsivity

Elicitation of behavior can be modeled neurobiologically by use of a minimum threshold construct, which represents a central nervous system weighting of the external and internal factors that contribute to the probability of response expression (Depue & Collins, 1999; Depue & Morrone-Strupinsky, 2005). External factors are characteristics of environmental stimulation, including magnitude, duration and psychological salience. Internal factors consist of both state (e.g. stress-induced endocrine levels) and trait biological variation. A response threshold is weighted most strongly by the joint function of two main variables: (1) magnitude of eliciting stimulation and (2) level of post-synaptic receptor activation of the neurobiological variable thought to contribute most variance to the behavioral process in question, such as DA to incentive motivation, μ-opiates to affiliative reward, and CRH to anxiety. The relation between these two variables is represented in Figure 20.3 as a trade-off function (White, 1986), where pairs of values (of stimulus magnitude and receptor activation) specify a diagonal representing the minimum threshold value for elicitation of a behavioral process.

As illustrated in Figure 20.3, we propose that non-affective constraint is the personality trait that reflects the greatest CNS weight on the construct of a minimum response threshold. As such, constraint exerts a general influence over the elicitation of any emotional behavior. In this model, other higher-order personality traits would thus reflect the influence of neurobiological variables that strongly contribute to the threshold for responding, such as DA in the facilitation of incentive motivated behavior, μ-opiates in the experience of affiliative reward, and CRH in the potentiation of anxiety.

The important question is what type of CNS variables could provide a major weighting of behavioral elicitation thresholds. Functional levels of neurotransmitters that provide a strong, relatively generalized *tonic inhibitory* influence on behavioral responding would be good candidates as significant modulators of a response elicitation threshold, and hence would likely account for a large proportion of the variance in the trait of non-affective constraint. We and others

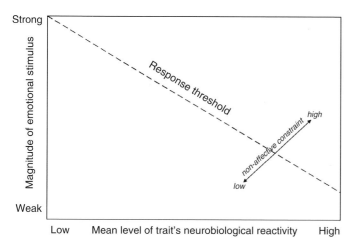

Figure 20.3. A minimum threshold for elicitation of a behavioral process (e.g. incentive motivation-positive affect, affiliative reward-affection, anxiety-negative affect) is illustrated as a trade-off function between eliciting stimulus magnitude (left vertical axis) and the mean level of a personality trait's neurobiological reactivity in a biological variable that strongly influences the expression of the trait (e.g. dopamine, µ-opiate, corticotropin-releasing hormone) (horizontal axis). Threshold effects due to modulation by non-affective constraint are also illustrated.

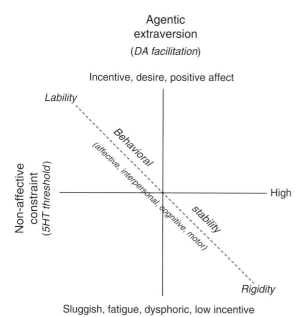

Figure 20.4. Combination of the higher-order personality traits of agentic extraversion and non-affective constraint. See text for details. DA = dopamine.

previously (Coccaro & Siever, 1991; Depue, 1995, 1996; Depue & Spoont, 1986; Nelson & Panksepp, 1998; Spoont, 1992; Zald & Depue, 2001; Zuckerman, 1994) and Lesch most recently (1998, 2006) suggested that serotonin (5HT), acting at multiple receptor sites in most brain regions, is such a modulator (Azmitia & Whitaker-Azmitia 1997; Tork 1990). As reviewed many times in animal and human literatures (Coccaro & Siever, 1991; Coccaro *et al.*, 1989; Depue,

1995, 1996; Depue & Spoont, 1986; Lesch, 1998, 2006; Spoont, 1992; Zald & Depue, 2001; Zuckerman, 1994), 5HT modulates a diverse set of functions – including emotion, motivation, motor, affiliation, cognition, food intake, sleep, sexual activity and sensory reactivity. Thus, 5HT plays a substantial modulatory role in general neurobiological functioning that affects many forms of motivated behavior. In this sense, non-affective constraint might be viewed as reflecting the influence of the CNS variable of 5HT, which we refer to later as *neural constraint*.

A vast body of animal and human evidence consistently associates *reduced* functioning of 5HT neurotransmission with *behavioral instability* or lability (Spoont, 1992). The *qualitative content* of unstable behavior will depend on which neurobehavioral–motivational system, or *affective* personality trait, is being elicited at any point in time (Depue & Collins, 1999; Zald & Depue, 2001), although differential strength of various personality traits will obviously produce relative predominance of particular affective behaviors *within individuals*. For instance, as illustrated in Figure 20.4, the interaction of agentic extraversion (DA facilitation) with non-affective constraint (5HT inhibition) creates a diagonal dimension of *behavioral stability* that applies equally to affective, cognitive, interpersonal, motor and incentive processes (Depue & Spoont, 1986; Luciana *et al.*, 1998; Spoont, 1992; Zald & Depue, 2001). The diagonal represents the line of greatest variance in stability, ranging from lability in the upper left quadrant of the two-space (low 5HT, high DA) to rigidity in the lower right (high 5HT, low DA).

309

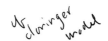

A model of personality disturbance

Illustration of the interactions of two traits taken at a time, as above, is informative, but of course underestimates the complexity of reality. The neurobehavioral systems underlying all of the higher-order traits interact. Therefore, we conceive of personality disturbance as *emergent* phenotypes arising from the interaction of the above neurobehavioral systems underlying major personality traits.

Our multidimensional model is illustrated in Figure 20.5. In the model, the axes are defined by neurobehavioral systems rather than by traits, because traits are only approximate, fallible estimates of these systems, and trait measures vary in content and underlying constructs. In Figure 20.5, positive *incentive motivation* (underlying agentic extraversion) and anxiety (underlying neuroticism or trait anxiety) are modeled as a ratio of their relative strength, because the opposing nature of their eliciting stimuli affects behavior in a reciprocal manner, such that the *elicitation* or *expression* of one system is influenced by the strength of the other (Gray, 1973). As discussed above, the interaction of these two systems strongly influences the style of an individual's emotional behavior. The affiliative reward dimension (underlying trait affiliation) in the model largely influences the interpersonal domain, whereas the neural constraint (underlying the trait of non-affective constraint) dimension modulates the expressive features of the other systems. Due to the limitation of graphing more than three dimensions, it should be noted that the model includes two other systems/traits that we

suggest influence the manifestation of personality disturbance. We believe a dimension of affective aggression: fear is necessary to account for the full range of antisocial (high aggression: low fear) behavior, and that a dimension of separation anxiety/rejection sensitivity strongly contributes to dependent-, avoidant- and borderline-like disturbance (all high on this dimension). Taken together, then, the model proposes that the interaction of at least six neurobehavioral systems underlying dimensional personality traits are necessary to account for the emergent phenotypes observed in personality disturbance.

Three significant features of the model that are illustrated in Figure 20.5 are worth emphasizing. First, the phenotypic expression of personality disturbance, represented by the gray-shaded *reaction surface* in the figure (accounting for ~10% of the population; Lenzenweger *et al.*, 1997; Livesley, 2001; Torgersen *et al.*, 2001), is continuous in nature, changing in character gradually but seamlessly across the surface in a manner that reflects the changing product of the mulitdimensional interactions. It may be that certain areas of the surface are associated with increased probability (risk) of certain features of personality disturbance, and this is represented in the right-back area of the figure as an elevation in the surface that is continous rather than distinct in contour. Thus, this representation is not meant to imply that a distinct disorder or category exists in that particular area of the surface. Second, the extent and positioning of the reaction surface is weighted most heavily by increasing anxiety, decreasing neural constraint and decreasing affiliative reward. This weighting is also reflected in the lines with directional arrows overlaying the gray surface in the figure, which illustrate increasing negative emotionality, lability, and interpersonal impairment. These three factors were found to be the most common characteristics of all personality disorders in the meta-analysis of Saulsman & Page (2004), thereby empirically supporting their emphasis in our model. Third, viewing personality disturbance as a *reaction* surface implies that the magnitude of disturbance at any point on the surface is variable, waxing and waning with fluctuations in environmental circumstances, stressors, and interpersonal disruptions, both within and across persons over time. Indeed, we recently demonstrated in a longitudinal assessment of the stability of formally defined personality disorders that phenotypic intensity varied markedly over time,

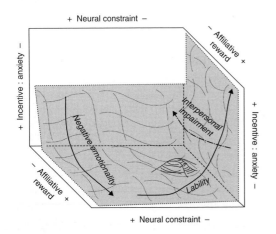

Figure 20.5. A multidimensional model of personality disturbance. See text for details.

thereby affecting the presence/absence of diagnostic status as well as level of symptomatology (Lenzenweger *et al.*, 2004).

Implications of the model

Several implications of the model can be outlined. First, the model may help to explain sex differences in some forms of personality disturbance. The increased prevalence of males with antisocial behavior may reflect the higher mean of males in the population on the trait of aggression : fear and a lower mean on non-affective constraint (including 5HT functioning; Spoont, 1992). Additionally, the increased prevalence of females in clinical populations with borderline- and dependent-like personality disturbance may reflect a combination of (1) their higher mean on both trait anxiety (borderline) and separation distress (dependent), (2) their higher mean on affiliation, thereby increasing the need for social relationships whose loss is feared, (3) their lower mean on agentic extraversion, particularly social dominance, hence enhancing the predominance of high levels of trait anxiety, and (4) their lower mean on aggression : fear, hence decreasing the prevalence of antisocial behavior (Depue & Collins, 1999; Kohnstamm, 1989; Tellegen & Waller, in press).

Second, the model suggests that research on the lines of causal neurobiological influence within the structure of *normal* personality will need to be a primary focus if the neurobiological nature of personality disturbance is to be fully understood. At present, there is a paucity of systematic research in this domain (Depue & Collins, 1999; Depue & Morrone-Strupinsky, 2005). Third, the multidimensional nature of the model indicates that univariate biological research in personality disturbance will inadequately discover the neurobiological nature of personality disturbance. Thus, not only is multivariate assessment suggested, but methods of *combinatorial* representation of those multiple variables – as in profile, finite mixture modeling, latent class, discriminant function and multivariate taxonomic analyses – will need to be more fully integrated in this area of research. Finally, the trend in development of neurotransmitter-specific drugs may not fully complement the pharmocotherapy requirements of personality disturbance. If personality disturbance represents emergent phenotypes of multiple, interacting neurobehavioral systems, then (1) basic research on the

pharmacological modulation of neurobehavioral systems and (2) clinical research on multi-regiment pharmacotherapy is greatly needed.

Acknowledgments
Supported by NIMH Research Grant MH55347 awarded to R. A. Depue.

References
Aston-Jones, G., Rajkowski, J., Kubiak, P, Valentino, R. & Shiptley, M. (1996). Role of the locus coeruleus in emotional activation. In G. Holstege, R. Bandler & C. Saper (Eds.), *The Emotional Motor System* (pp. 254–279). New York, NY: Elsevier.

Azmitia, E. & Whitaker-Azmitia, P. (1997). Development and adult plasticity of serotonergic neurons and their target cells. In H. Baumgarten & M. Gothert (Eds.), *Serotonergic Neurons and 5HT Receptors in the CNS* (Vol 129, pp. 1–39). New York, NY: Springer.

Benjamin, J., Li, L., Patterson, C. *et al.* (1996). Population and familial association between the D4 dopamine receptor gene and measures of novelty seeking. *Nature Genetics*, **12**, 81–84.

Berridge, K. C. (1999). Pleasure, pain, desire, and dread: hidden core processes of emotion. In D. Kahneman, E. Diener & N. Schwarz (Eds.), *Well-Being: The Foundations of Hedonic Psychology* (pp. 525–557). New York, NY: Russell Sage Foundation.

Blizard, D. A. (1988). The locus ceruleus: a possible neural focus for genetic differences in emotionality. *Experientia*, **44**, 491–495.

Block, J. (2001). Millennial contrarianism: the five-factor approach to personality description 5 years later. *Journal of Personality*, **69**, 98–107.

Breiter, H. C., Gollub, R. L., Weisskoff, R. M. *et al.* (1997). Acute effects of cocaine on human brain activity and emotion. *Neuron*, **19**, 591–611.

Clark, L. A. & Livesley, W. J. (1994). Two approaches to identifying the dimensions of personality disorder. In P. T. Costa, Jr., T. A. Widiger (Eds.), *Personaltiy Disorders and the Five Factor Model of Personality*. Washington, DC: American Psychological Association.

Clark, L. A., Livesley, W. J., Schroeder, M. L. & Irish, S. L. (1996). Convergence of two systems for assessing personality disorder. *Psychological Assessment*, **8**, 294–303.

Coccaro, E. & Siever, L. (1991). *Serotonin and Psychiatric Disorders*. Washington, DC: American Psychiatric Association Press.

Coccaro, E., Siever, L., Klar, H. *et al.* (1989). Serotonergic studies in patients with affective and personality disorders. *Archives of General Psychiatry*, **46**, 587–599.

Costa, P. & McCrae, R. (1992). *Revised NEO Personality Inventory (NEO-PI-R) and NEO Five-Factor Inventory (NEO-FFI) Professional Manual*. Odessa, FL: Psychological Assessment Resources.

Davis, M. & Shi, C. (1999). The extended amygdala: are the central nucleus of the amygdala and the bed nucleus of the stria terminalis differentially involved in fear versus anxiety. *Annals of the New York Academy of Sciences*, **877**, 281–291.

Davis, M., Walker, D. & Lee, Y. (1997). Roles of the amygdala and bed nucleus of the stria terminalis in fear and anxiety measured with the acoustic startle reflex. *Annals of the New York Academy of Sciences*, **821**, 305–331.

Depue, R. (1995). Neurobiological factors in personality and depression. *European Journal of Personality*, **9**, 413–439.

Depue, R. (1996). Neurobiology and the structure of personality: implications for the personality disorders. In J. Clarkin & M. Lenzenweger (Eds.), *Major Theories of Personality Disorders*. New York, NY: Guilford Press.

Depue, R. (2006). Interpersonal behavior and the structure of personality: neurobehavioral foundation of agentic extraversion and affiliation. In T. Canli (Ed.), *Biology of Personality and Individual Differences* (pp. 34–68). New York, NY: Guilford Press.

Depue, R. A. & Collins, P. F. (1999). Neurobiology of the structure of personality: dopamine, facilitation of incentive motivation, and extraversion. *Behavioral and Brain Sciences*, **22**, 491–569.

Depue, R. A. & Lenzenweger, M. F. (2005). Neurobiology and personality disorders. In M. F. Lenzenweger & J. Clarkin (Eds.), *Theories of Personality Disorders* (2nd edn), (pp. 93–145). New York, NY: Guilford Press.

Depue, R. A. & Morrone-Strupinsky (2005). A neurobehavioral model of affiliative bonding: implications for coneptualizing a human trait of affiliation. *Behavioral and Brain Sciences*, **28**, 313–395.

Depue, R. & Spoont, M. (1986). Conceptualizing a serotonin trait: a behavioral dimension of constraint. *Annals of the New York Academy of Sciences*, **487**, 47–62.

Di Chiara, G. & North, R. A. (1992). Neurobiology of opiate abuse. *Trends in the Physiological Sciences*, **13**, 185–193.

Digman, J. M. (1997). Higher-order factors of the big five. *Journal of Personality and Social Psychology*, **73**, 1246–1256.

Domjan, M., Cusato, B. & Villarreal, R. (2000). Pavlovian feed-forward mechanisms in the control of social behavior. *Behavioral and Brain Sciences*, **23**, 1–29.

Drevets, W. C., Gautier, C., Price, J. C. *et al.* (2001). Amphetamine-induced dopamine release in human ventral striatum correlates with euphoria. *Biological Psychiatry*, **49**, 81–96.

Dyce, J. A. & Connor, B. P. (1998). Personality disorders and the five-factor model: a test of facet-level predictions. *Journal of Personality Disorders*, **12**, 31–45.

Ebstein, R., Novick, O., Umansky, R. *et al.* (1996). Dopamine D4 receptor (DRD4) exon III polymorphism associated with the human personality trait of novelty seeking. *Nature Genetics*, **12**, 78–80.

Ekselius, L., Lindstrom, E., von Knorring, L., Bodlund, O., & Kullgren, G. (1994). A principal component analysis of the DSM-III R axis II personality disorders. *Journal of Personality Disorders*, **8**, 140–148.

Erb, S., Salmaso, N., Rodaros, D. & Stewart, J. (2001). A role for the CF-containing pathway from central nucleus of the amygdala to the bed nucleus of the stria terminalis in the stress-induced reinstatement of cocaine seeking in rats. *Psychopharmacology*, **158**, 360–365.

Fendt, M., Endres, T. & Apfelbach, R. (2003). Temporary inactivation of the bed nucleus of the stria terminalis but not of the amygdala blocks freezing induced by trimethylthiazoline, a component of fox feces. *Journal of Neuroscience*, **23**, 23–28.

Fleming, A. S., Korsmit, M. & Deller, M. (1994). Rat pups are potent reinforcers to the maternal animal: effects of experience, parity, hormones, and dopamine function. *Psychobiology*, **22**, 44–53.

Gingrich, B., Liu, Y., Cascio, C., Wang, Z. & Insel., T. R. (2000). Dopamine D2 receptors in the nucleus accumbens are important for social attachment in female prairie voles (*Microtus ochrogaster*). *Behavioral Neuroscience*, **114**, 173–183.

Goldberg, L. & Rosolack, T. (1994). The big five factor structure as an integrative framework. In C. Halverson, G. Kohnstamm & R. Marten (Eds.), *The Developing Structure of Temperament and Personality from Infancy to Adulthood*. Hillsdale, NJ: Lawrence Erlbaum Associates.

Gray, J. A. (1973). Causal theories of personality and how to test them. In J. R. Royce (Ed.), *Multivariate Analysis and Psychological Theory*. Academic Press.

Haslam, N. (2003). The dimensional view of personality disorders: a review of the taxometric evidence. *Clinical Psychology Review*, **23**, 75–93.

Herz, A. (1998). Opioid reward mechanisms: a key role in drug abuse? *Canadian Journal of Physiology and Pharmacology*, **76**, 252–258.

Hilliard, S., Domjan, M., Nguyen, M. & Cusato, B. (1998). Dissociation of conditioned appetitive and consummatory sexual behavior: satiation and extinction tests. *Animal Learning and Behavior*, **26**, 20–33.

Kendler, K. S., McGuire, M., Gruenberg, A. M. *et al.* (1993). The Roscommon Family Study: III. Schizophrenia-related personality disorders in relatives. *Archives of General Psychiatry*, **50**, 781–788.

Kohnstamm, G. (1989). Temperament in childhood: cross-cultural and sex differences. In G. Kohnstamm, J. Bates & M. Rothbart (Eds.), *Temperament in Childhood*. New York, NY: Wiley.

Korfine, L. & Lenzenweger, M. F. (1995). The taxonicity of schizotypy: a replication. *Journal of Abnormal Psychology*, **104**, 26–31.

Kranzler, H. R. (2000). Pharmacotherapy of alcoholism: gaps in knowledge and opportunities for research. *Acohol and Alcoholism*, **35**, 537–547.

La Buda, C., Sora, I., Uhl, G. & Fuchs (2000). Stress-induced analgesia in mu-opioid receptor knockout mice reveals normal function of the delta-opioid receptor system. *Brain Research*, **869**, 1–10.

Lenzenweger, M. F. (1998). Schizotypy and schizotypic psychopathology: mapping an alternative expression of schizophrenia liability. In M. F. Lenzenweger & R. H. Dworkin (Eds.), *Origins and Development of Schizophrenia: Advances in Experimental Psychopathology* (pp. 93–121). Washington, DC: American Psychological Association.

Lenzenweger, M. F. & Korfine, L. (1992). Confirming the latent structure and base rate of schizotypy: a taxometric analysis. *Journal of Abnormal Psychology*, **101**, 567–571.

Lenzenweger, M. F. & Loranger, A. W. (1989). Detection of familial schizophrenia using a psychometric measure of schizotypy. *Archives of General Psychiatry*, **46**, 902–907.

Lenzenweger, M. F., Johnson, M. D. & Willett, J. B. (2004). Individual growth curve analysis illuminates stability and change in personality disorder features: the longitudinal study of personality disorders. *Archives of General Psychiatry*, **61**, 1015–1024.

Lenzenweger, M. F., Loranger, A. W., Korfine, L. & Neff, C. (1997). Detecting personality disorders in a nonclinical population: application of a two-stage procedure for case identification. *Archives of General Psychiatry*, **54**, 345–351.

Leri, F., Flores, J., Rodaros, D. & Stewart, J. (2002). Blockade of stress-induced but not cocaine-induced reinstatement by infusion of noradrenergic antagonists into the bed nucleus of the stria terminalis or the central nucleus of the amygdala. *Journal of Neuroscience*, **22**, 5713–5718.

Lesch, K.-P. (1998). Serotonin transporter and psychiatric disorders. *The Neuroscientist*, **4**, 25–34.

Lesch, K.-P. (2006). Serotonin transporter and behavior. In T. Canli (Ed.), *Biology of Personality and Individual Differences* (pp. 92–117). New York: NY: Guilford Press.

Livesley, W. J. (2001). Commentary on reconceptualizing personality disorder categories using trait dimensions. *Journal of Personality*, **69**, 277–286.

Livesley, W. J., Jackson, D. N. & Schroeder, M. L. (1992). Factorial structure of traits delineating personality disorders in clinical and general population samples. *Journal of Abnormal Psychology*, **101**, 432–440.

Livesley, W. J., Schroeder, M. L., Jackson, D. N. & Jang, K. L. (1994). Categorical distinctions in the study of personality disorder: implication for classification. *Journal of Abnormal Psychology*, **103**, 6–17.

Luciana, M., Collins, P. & Depue, R. (1998). Opposing roles for dopamine and serotonin in the modulation of human spatial working memory functions. *Cerebral Cortex*, **8**, 218–226.

Macey, D., Smith, H., Nader, M. & Porrino, L. (2003). Chronic cocaine self-administration upregulates the norepinephrine transporter and alters functional activity in the bed nucleus of the stria terminalis of the Rhesus monkey. *Journal of Neuroscience*, **23**, 12–16.

Matheson, M. D. & Bernstein, I. S. (2000). Grooming, social bonding, and agonistic aiding in rhesus monkeys. *American Journal of Primatology*, **51**, 177–186.

Matthes, H. W., Maldonado, R., Simonin, F. *et al.* (1996). Loss of morphine-induced analgesia, reward effect and withdrawal symptoms in mice lacking the μ-opioid-receptor gene. *Nature*, **383**, 819–823.

Millon, T. (1997). *The Millon Inventories: Clinical and Personality Assessment*. New York, NY: Guilford Press.

Narita, M., Aoki, T. & Suzuki, T. (2000). Molecular evidence for the involvement of NR2B subunit containing N-methyl-D-aspartate receptors in the development of morphine-induced place preference. *Neuroscience*, **101**, 601–606.

Nelson, E. E. & Panksepp, J. (1998). Brain substrates of infant-mother attachment: contributions of opioids, oxytocin, and norepinephrine. *Neuroscience and Biobehavioral Reviews*, **22**, 437–452.

Nie, Z., Schweitzer, P., Roberts, A. *et al.* (2004). Ethanol augments GABAergic transmission in the central amygdala via CRF1 receptors. *Science*, **303**, 1512–1514.

Niesink, R. J. M., Vanderschuen, L. J. M. J. & van Ree, J. M. (1996). Social play in juvenile rats in utero exposure to morphine. *Neurotoxicology*, **17**, 905–912.

Olive, M., Koenig, H., Nannini, M. & Hodge, C. (2001). Stimulation of endorphin neurotransmission in the nucleus accumbens by ethanol, cocaine, and amphetamine. *Journal of Neuroscience*, **21**, 1–5.

Olson, G., Olson, R. & Kastin, A. (1997). Endogenous opiates: 1996. *Peptides*, **18**, 1651–1688.

Ostrowski, N. L. (1998). Oxytocin receptor mRNA expression in rat brain: implications for behavioral

313

integration and reproductive success. *Psychoneuroendocrinology*, 23, 989–1004.

Pacak, K., McCarty, R., Palkovits, M., Kopin, I. & Goldstein, D. (1995). Effects of immobilization on in vivo release of norepinephrine in the bed nucleus of the stria terminalis in conscious rats. *Brain Research*, **688**, 242–246.

Pfaus, J. G., Smith, W. J. & Coopersmith, C. B. (1999). Appetitive and consummatory sexual behaviors of female rats in bilevel chambers: I. A correlational and factor analysis and the effects of ovarian hormones. *Hormones and Behavior*, **35**, 224–240.

Polan, H. J. & Hofer, M. A. (1998). Olfactory preference for mother over home nest shavings by newborn rats. *Developmental Psychobiology*, **33**, 5–20.

Porges, S. (1998). Love: an emergent property of the mamalian autonomic nervous system. *Psychoneuroendocrinology*, **23**, 837–861.

Porges, S. (2001). The polyvagal theory: phylogenetic substrates of a social nervous system. *International Journal of Psychophysiology*, **42**, 123–146.

Redmond, D. E. (1987). Studies of the nucleus locus coeruleus in monkeys and hypotheses for neuropsychopharmacology. In J. Y. Meltzer (Ed.), *Psychopharmacology: The Third Generation of Progress* (pp. 967–975). New York, NY: Raven Press.

Reynolds, S. K. & Clark, L. A. (2001). Predicting dimensions of personality disorder from domains and facets of the five-factor model. *Journal of Personality*, **69**, 199–222.

Saulsman, L. M. & Page, A. C. (2004). The five-factor model and personality disorder empirical literature: a meta-analytic review. *Clinical Psychology Review*, **23**, 1055–1085.

Schlaepfer, T. E., Strain, E. C., Greenberg, B. D. *et al.* (1998). Site of opioid action in the human brain: mu and kappa agonists' subjective and cerebral blood flow effects. *American Journal of Psychiatry*, **155**, 470–473.

Schneirla, T. (1959). An evolutionary and developmental theory of biphasic processes underlying approach and withdrawal. In M. Jones (Ed.), *Nebraska Symposium on Motivation*. University of Nebraska Press.

Schultz, W., Dayan, P. & Montague, P. (1997). A neural substrate of prediction and reward. *Science*, **275**, 1593–1595.

Shaham, Y., Erb, S. & Stewart, J. (2000). Stress-induced relapse to heroin and cocaine seeking in rats: a review. *Brain Research Reviews*, **33**, 13–33.

Shippenberg, T. S. & Elmer, G. I. (1998). The neurobiology of opiate reinforcement. *Critical Reviews in Neurobiology*, **12**, 267–303.

Simonin, F., Valverde, O., Smadja, C. *et al.* (1998). Disruption of the kappa-opioid receptor gene in mice enhances sensitivity to chemical visceral pain, impairs

pharmacological actions of the selective kappa-agonist U-50,488H and attenuates morphine withdrawal. *EMBO Journal* 17, 886–897.

Spoont, M. (1992). Modulatory role of serotonin in neural information processing: implications for human psychopathology. *Psychological Bulletin*, 112, 330–350.

Stefano, G., Goumon, Y., Casares, F. *et al.* (2000). Endogenous morphine. *Trends in Neuroscience*, 23, 436–442.

Strand, F. L. (1999). *Neuropeptides: Regulators of Physiological Processes*. Cambridge, MA: MIT Press.

Tellegen, A., Lykken, D. T., Bouchard, T. J. *et al.* (1988). Personality similarity in twins reared apart and together. *Journal of Personality and Social Psychology*, 54, 1031–1039.

Tellegen, A. & Waller, N. G. (in press). Exploring personality through test construction: development of the multidimensional personality questionnaire. In S. Briggs & J. Cheek (Eds.), *Personality Measures: Development and Evaluation* (Vol. 1). New York, NY: JAI Press.

Timberlake, W. & Silva, K. (1995). Appetitive behavior in ethology, psychology, and behavior systems. In N. Thompson (Ed.), *Perspectives in Ethology*, (Vol. 11 *Behavioral Design*, pp. 211–253). New York, NY: Plenum.

Torgersen, S., Kringlen, E. & Cramer, V. (2001). The prevalence of personality disorders in a community sample. *Archives of General Psychiatry*, 58, 590–596.

Tork, I. (1990). Anatomy of the serotonergic system. *Annals of the New York Academy of Sciences*, **600**, 9–32.

Uhl, G. R., Sora, I. & Wang, Z. (1999). The μ opiate receptor as a candidate gene for pain: polymorphisms, variations in expression, nociception, and opiate responses. *Proceedings of the National Academy of Sciences*, **96**, 7752–7755.

Volkow, N., Wang, G., Fischman, M. *et al.* (1997). Relationship between subjective effects of cocaine and dopamine transporter occupancy. *Nature*, **386**, 827–829.

Wang, Z., Yu, G., Cascio, C. *et al.* (1999). Dopamine D2 receptor-mediated regulation of partner preferences in female prairie voles (*Microtus ochrogaster*): a mechanism for pair bonding? *Behavioral Neuroscience*, **113**, 602–611.

Watson, C. & Clark, L. (1997). Extraversion and its positive emotional core. In S. Briggs, W. Jones & R. Hogan (Eds.), *Handbook of Personality Psychology*. New York, NY: Academic Press.

Watson, D. & Tellegen, A. (1985). Towards a consensual structure of mood. *Psychological Bulletin*, **98**, 219–235.

White, N. (1986). Control of sensorimotor function by dopaminergic nigrostriatal neurons: influence on eating and drinking. *Neuroscience and Biobehavioral Reviews*, **10**, 15–36.

White, T. L. & Depue, R. A. (1999). Differential association of traits of fear and anxiety with norepinephrine- and dark-induced pupil reactivity. *Journal of Personality and Social Psychology*, **77**, 863–877.

White, T. L., Lott, D. & de Wit, H. (2006a). Personality and the subjective effects of acute amphetamine in healthy volunteers. *Neuropsychopharmacology*, **31**, 1064–1074.

White, T. L., Grover, V. K. & de Wit, H. (2006b). Cortisol effects of D-amphetamine relate to traits of fearlessness and aggression but not anxiety in healthy humans. *Pharmacology, Biochemistry and Behavior*, **82**, 523–543.

Wiedenmayer, C. & Barr, G. (2000). Mu opioid receptors in the ventrolateral periaqueductal gray mediate stress-induced analgesia but not immobility in rat pups. *Behavioral Neuroscience*, **114**, 125–138.

Wiggins, J. (1991). Agency and communion as conceptual coordinates for the understanding and measurement of interpersonal behavior. In D. Cicchetti & W. Grove (Eds.), *Thinking Clearly about Psychology: Essays in Honor of Paul Everett Meehl* (pp. 89–113). Minneapolis, MN: University of Minnesota Press.

Wyvell, C. L. & Berridge, K. C. (2000). Intra-accumbens amphetamine increases the conditioned incentive salience of sucrose reward: Enhancement of reward "wanting" without enhanced "liking" or response reinforcement. *Journal of Neuroscience*, **20**, 8122–8130.

Zald, D. & Depue, R. (2001). Serotonergic modulation of positive and negative affect in psychiatrically healthy males. *Personality and Individual Differences*, **30**, 71–86.

Zuckerman, M. (1994). An alternative five-factor model for personality. In C. Halverson, G. Kohnstamm & R. Marten (Eds.), *The Developing Structure of Temperament and Personality from Infancy to Adulthood*. Hillsdale, NJ: Lawrence Erlbaum Associates.

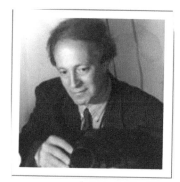

Richard A Depue

Neuropsychology in eating disorders

Laura Southgate, Kate Tchanturia and Janet Treasure

Overview of the literature

In our recent systematic review of neuropsychological function in anorexia nervosa (AN) and bulimia nervosa (BN) (Southgate *et al.*, 2006), we highlighted the limitations associated with the literature, including the inadequacies of existing theories or models (Southgate *et al.*, 2006; Tchanturia *et al.*, 2005a), as well as the paucity of research replicating previous findings. This latter issue may be due to methodological limitations inherent in this literature, ranging from poor reporting of sample characteristics, to issues associated with study design and the variety of tests employed. As a result of these factors, the conclusions that can be drawn from existing literature are greatly limited and unclear.

In current literature, eating disorders (EDs) have been associated with anomalous cognitive functioning that extends across many domains, including attention, memory, executive functions, motor control and visuospatial processing. However, general intellectual ability in this clinical group has consistently been found to be in the average to high average range. Selective deficits have therefore been reported in the presence of preserved, and in some cases superior, functioning in other cognitive domains.

Diagnostic issues may contribute towards this confusing and sometimes contradictory literature. DSM–IV recognizes two subtypes of AN based on eating pathology (American Psychiatric Association, 1994). Patients with "restricting type" (RAN) control their weight through food restriction alone, whereas those with "binge-eating/purging type" (BPAN) also engage in binge-eating with compensatory purging behaviors to reduce weight gain. The validity of these subtypes has been endorsed in the vast personality literature, with heightened impulsivity reported in participants with BPAN compared with those with pure RAN (Claes *et al.*, 2002). Neurophysiological differences have also been suggested, with different patterns of regional cerebral blood flow reported across the different subgroups of AN when participants are asked to imagine food (Naruo *et al.*, 2000). However, the data appear inconsistent with regards to neuropsychological function across the current diagnostic subtypes of AN. Both similarities (Strupp *et al.*, 1986; in set shifting, Tchanturia *et al.*, 2004a) and differences (in impulsive vs reflective cognitive styles, Toner *et al.*, 1987; in decision-making, Cavedini *et al.*, 2004) in neuropsychological performance have been reported across individuals with RAN and BPAN.

Of greatest concern with regards to the validity of the current diagnostic system is the evidence that ED diagnoses are not temporally stable. Migration across the subtypes of AN (Eddy *et al.*, 2002) and diagnostic categories of AN, BN and eating disorder not otherwise specified (EDNOS) is often found (Fairburn & Harrison, 2003). Traits are thought to characterize variation in developmental and biological indices more accurately than diagnostic distinctions (Collier & Treasure, 2004; Steiger, 2004). The more recent use of mathematical modeling with dimensional personality data is proving to have utility in the determination of homogeneous clinical ED phenotypes. Remarkable similarity has been uncovered in the grouping of participants based upon personality in both control and ED groups using cluster and latent profile analysis. Three to four clusters of personality typology are consistently revealed, with considerable overlap in their content across studies employing diverse methodologies and materials (Espelage *et al.*, 2002; Goldner *et al.*, 1999; Livesley *et al.*, 1998; Westen & Harnden-Fischer, 2001; Wonderlich *et al.*,

The Neuropsychology of Mental Illness, ed. Stephen J. Wood, Nicholas B. Allen and Christos Pantelis. Published by Cambridge University Press. © Cambridge University Press 2009.

2005). The clusters distinguish perfectionistic, inhibited groups from more impulsive, disinhibited participants. Thus the methodology of solely grouping participants based upon the clinical diagnosis of "AN," as found in the majority of the neuropsychological studies published to date, may be unsatisfactory.

Another major problem in the interpretation of ED research is the delineation of state and trait features; this is particularly relevant in these disorders, as there are acute changes in patients' physical state. A common methodological technique used to examine illness state and trait features is to investigate the behavior of interest in recovered participants. This occurs with the assumption that the presence of specific state features, independent of the presence of acute illness, may be representative of an illness trait. The identification of enduring traits (thus assumed to be present premorbidly) is important, as they may be involved in vulnerability to the disorder. However, there are methodological limitations regarding the definition of "recovery," as there is still uncertainty as to whether those who achieve "recovery" can be regarded as representative of the ED population as a whole. If not, then findings will be limited to a subgroup of the ED population.

With regards to cross-sectional neuropsychological data in eating disorders, Jones et al. (1991) reported that individuals in an acute illness state exhibited mild cognitive impairment in the domains of focusing/execution, memory, verbal and visuospatial processing; these deficits were not identified in recovered AN participants (who had maintained a "weight-restored status" for at least 6 months prior to participation). In contrast, there are reports that set-shifting deficits in AN are not limited to acute illness states (Holliday et al., 2005; Steinglass et al., 2006; Tchanturia et al., 2002, 2004b). The persistence of problems in cognitive and perceptual set shifting in recovered individuals suggests that these features could represent stable traits of disorder. The criteria for recovered status in our three studies were more stringent, requiring participants to have fulfilled the criteria for AN in the past but having maintained a normal body mass index (BMI 19–25; weight in kilos divided by height in meters squared) with regular menstruation for at least a year and to have maintained normal eating patterns (Holliday et al., 2005; Tchanturia et al., 2002, 2004b). Including a group of former patients with "long-term recovery" enhances the likelihood that these participants had achieved a healthy nutritional status, thus removing the confounding influence of severe metabolic imbalance.

Longitudinal studies to investigate the effect of weight gain on cognitive functions in AN have again produced conflicting reports. The most consistent improvements in cognition reported across studies concern attention, speed of information processing and problem-solving (Kingston et al., 1996; Kohlmeyer et al., 1983; Lauer et al., 1999; Moser et al., 2003; Szmukler et al., 1992). However these significant gains may not be global; for example, Kingston et al. (1996) highlight persistent impairment in memory and visuospatial processing domains amongst individuals who show improvement in attentional capacity. Deficits in recall, reaction time and motor speed (Green et al., 1996), somatosensory processing (Grunwald et al., 2002) and set shifting (Tchanturia et al., 2004b) are not affected by weight gain. Whilst it may be tempting to suggest that these deficits represent enduring features of disorder, it is important to note that the mean participant BMIs are still below what may be considered a "normal healthy range" (BMI 19–25) in the latter three studies. Thus it remains to be seen whether performance in such cognitive domains would improve with further weight restoration. Gillberg et al. (1994, 1996) found the persistence of dysdiadochokinesis alongside poor performance on the object assembly task (visuospatial processing) following weight recovery well into the healthy range, indicative of a neurological impairment in AN independent of nutritional status.

As discussed in the following section, despite the research limitations some recurrent themes in the AN literature have been identified. These have provided insight into potential areas of anomalous cognitive functioning in eating disorders, which involve trait-related strengths and weaknesses in information processing, specifically reduced cognitive flexibility and a preferential bias towards local/detail level processing. These vulnerabilities occur in the key domains of the "social information processing network," a model developed to explain the elevated incidence of affective and anxiety disorders during adolescence (Nelson et al., 2005).

Specificity of neuropsychological functioning

A careful description of the developmental phenotype with an emphasis on those factors that represent trait rather than a state vulnerability is critical in order to make further progress in our understanding of the underlying neurobiology and etiology of eating disorders. Following a focused, hypothesis-driven approach, the pattern of information processing anomalies that we have found in people with AN are consistent with potential endophenotypes of disorder.

There is considerable evidence that argues that AN is part of the obsessive-compulsive spectrum of disorders (Hollander & Wong, 1995). Disorders identified as belonging to this spectrum are proposed to lie along a continuum of compulsivity and impulsivity and are characterized by the presence of intrusive thoughts, impulses and compulsive behaviors (Hollander & Benzaquen, 1997).

In addition to similarities in symptomatology, Murphy et al. (2004) reported similar neuropsychological deficits between AN and OCD participants in a conditional associative learning task. Both groups showed selective impairment in learning conditional associations with emotionally neutral stimuli, with normal performance when presented with individually threatening stimuli (i.e. illness-related words). It was proposed that the preserved learning ability seen when the tasks involved threatening stimuli could be attributed to hyperactivity of the "Behavioral Inhibition System" (Gray & McNaughton, 2000), resulting in superior task performance due to increased arousal and attention to such stimuli (Murphy et al., 2002). Comparable deficits in organizational strategies have also been highlighted across AN and OCD participants (Sherman et al., 2006). Such findings support the hypothesis of a common neurobiological dysfunction in these two disorders (Hollander, 1993).

People with AN and BN display characteristics that are in line with features of obsessive-compulsive personality disorder (OCPD), defined as "a pervasive pattern of preoccupation with orderliness, perfectionism, mental and interpersonal control" (DSM–IV) which may be demonstrated by (1) a preoccupation with details, lists, order, (2) perfectionism that interferes with task completion, (3) excessive devotion to a task, exclusive of leisure and friends and (4) inflexible, rigid and stubborn mental set (Halmi, 1999). Empirical evidence suggests that obsessive-compulsive personality traits are significant vulnerability factors in the complex etiology of eating disorders. First, they have been found to be precursors to illness (Anderluh et al., 2003; Fairburn et al., 1999; Rastam, 1992). Second, they remain after recovery (Kaye et al.,

1998). Third, they are present in relatives of ED probands (Lilenfeld et al., 1998). Finally they are associated with illness outcome (Rastam et al., 2003; Steinhausen, 2002; Sutandar-Pinnock et al., 2003). There is a paucity of research examining whether the characteristic traits highlighted above have information-processing parallels; that is, whether biological traits analogous to those relating to personality and behavior exist. In recent years, the work of our department has followed a hypothesis-driven approach, focusing upon this potential link (Tchanturia et al., 2005a).

Cognitive flexibility

Set shifting is an essential component of cognitive and behavioral flexibility. It involves the ability to direct attention away from a previously relevant stimulus dimension towards one that was previously irrelevant, thus allowing the adaptation of behavior in line with changing demands of the environment (Miyake et al., 2000). Problems in set shifting may underlie several different cognitive deficits including cognitive inflexibility (e.g. concrete and rigid approaches to problem-solving and stimulus bound behavior) and response inflexibility (e.g. perseverative or stereotyped behaviors). Using a broad battery of tasks, we have repeatedly demonstrated deficits in set shifting amongst participants in the acute and recovered stage of illness (Holliday et al., 2005; Tchanturia et al., 2001, 2002, 2004a, 2004b) and in healthy sisters, introducing the possibility that this feature may be an endophenotype of disorder (Holliday et al., 2005). Set-shifting deficits have been repeatedly identified in the ED literature. In a systematic review and meta-analysis of the 15 published studies comparing the performance of current AN samples with that of healthy controls in tests of cognitive flexibility (e.g. Brixton Task, Cambridge Automated Neuropsychological Test Battery (CANTAB) set shift, Trail Making Test, Wisconsin Card Sorting Test), the magnitude of difference in performance between groups (effect size) is most frequently in the ranges of "medium" (0.40–0.75) to "large" (0.75–1.10) (Roberts et al., 2007).

The parallel between reduced cognitive flexibility seen amongst individuals with eating disorders in laboratory measures and the personality and symptom profiles seen clinically are clear. This cognitive profile may play a role in the maintenance of disorder and thus the limited efficacy current intervention strategies have in the treatment of AN in particular (Wilson *et al.*, 2007; National Institute for Clinical Excellence – NICE, 2004).

Central coherence

The term "central coherence" was introduced by Frith (1989) to refer to the natural tendency to process incoming information in context, which includes integrating features to derive an overall gestalt. "Weak central coherence," therefore, refers to a cognitive style in which information remains fragmented as opposed to integrated, with processing occurring at the level of "detail" as opposed to "whole." Weak central coherence theory has been successful in explaining the cognitive processing style associated with autism, accounting for both the strengths and weaknesses observed (Happe, 1999). It may therefore be part of a "broader autism phenotype," being found subclinically in fathers of autistic probands (Happe *et al.*, 2001).

Gillberg *et al.* (1996) have proposed that some people with AN lie within the autistic spectrum of disorders. Within a community sample of teenage-onset AN, 30% displayed an "empathy disorder" (including Asperger's syndrome and other autistic-like conditions), that were still present in some individuals 10 years after ED onset (Rastam *et al.*, 2003). Traits relating to problems in social interaction were found to predict poor psychosocial outcome better than the ED or other comorbid diagnoses (Rastam *et al.*, 2003).

Autistic-spectrum traits have also been identified in the neuropsychological domain. Performance across visuospatial tasks suggest that participants with AN display weak central coherence (Gillberg *et al.*, 1996). Whilst deficits have been observed in tasks requiring global information processing (Object Assembly; Wechsler Adult Intelligence Scale-III), AN participants performed as well as controls in Block Design. This is thought to be attributed to a piecemeal processing style, as seen in individuals with autism, which would improve their performance (Happe, 1999). A preference for piecemeal rather than global information processing in AN may explain performance deficits in tasks that require the processing of a global design rather than local aspects of stimuli such as the Rey Complex Figure (Jones *et al.*, 1991; Kingston *et al.*, 1996; Lopez *et al.*, 2008a; Sherman *et al.*, 2006) and a version of the Bender Gestalt Test (Bowers, 1994), and also the superior performance seen in the Matching Familiar Figures

Test (Southgate *et al.*, 2008). Sherman *et al.* (2006) highlight that, as in OCD, AN participants are impaired in the organizational strategy used to copy the Rey figure, and that this is directly linked with the subsequent deficits in immediate and delayed figure recall. Thus it appears that cognitive style may account for both optimal and impaired performance across different visuospatial tasks, depending on their processing requirements. Further work is underway in our department to explore this intriguing hypothesis in more detail (Lopez *et al.*, 2008b, 2009).

Parallels can be seen between the concept of central coherence and the suggestion that AN is associated with "hyperarousal," (Galderisi *et al.*, 2003). This phenomenon has been described as the narrowing of the focus of attention onto the detail of the task to such a degree that it is performed with little awareness, processing or integration of extraneous variables. This results in enhanced performance in effortful tasks to the detriment of incidental learning (Galderisi *et al.*, 2003; Strupp *et al.*, 1986).

The concept of weak central coherence as the preferential cognitive style in eating disorders may be reflected in the psychopathology. Those who suffer with eating disorders are so focused on maintaining their maladaptive behaviors that they are unable to see the "bigger picture" and the severe consequences of them. Extreme perfectionism and "attention to detail" is manifest in their eating behavior, as well as other facets of their life including academic, work and home life. Furthermore, this cognitive style may account for the disturbance of body image in the absence of an apparent visuospatial disorder (Gillberg *et al.*, 1996). The bias toward local over global information processing may be relevant in the perceptual domain, focusing on individual features of the body as opposed to integrating them into a "whole." The preferential, continual focus on the individual parts of the body (e.g. stomach, thighs) as opposed to the gestalt, could lead to a distortion of perception, resulting in claims of "fat" or "disproportionate" body features even in individuals who are emaciated.

A neurodevelopmental model

Gillberg *et al.* (1994) argued that the eating disorders, in particular AN, should be considered to be neurodevelopmental disorders. They note the presence of neurological soft signs like dysdiadochokinesis, suggesting that this characteristic might mirror some inherent underlying immaturity or other abnormality of the central nervous system. We have recently updated our neurodevelopmental model of eating disorders, incorporating evidence from the neuropsychological and neuroimaging literature (Connan et al., 2003; Southgate et al., 2005). In the latter model we consider two components of adolescent brain development: (1) collaborative brain function (Luna & Sweeney, 2004) and (2) the "social information processing network" (Nelson et al., 2005), which are marked by the development of sustained inhibitory control and enhanced reflective capabilities, and may be of relevance to AN.

Collaborative brain function

Adolescence marks a critical period in brain development, with changes in the organizational processes of brain function. Myelination and synaptic pruning are two developmental processes considered to ' "support the collaboration of a widely distributed circuitry, integrating regions that support top-down cognitive control of behavior" ' (Luna & Sweeney, 2004, p. 296). The improvement of connections between the prefrontal cortex and important subcortical structures, such as the basal ganglia and thalamus, allows the modulation of subcortical regions by the executive area of the brain. This, therefore, represents the emergence of "collaborative brain function." Functionally, this maturation serves to make inhibitory and reflective processes more efficient and consistent.

We propose that, in eating disorders, the persistence of a state of highly demanding emotional distress, which is brought about by the poor regulation of the stress response and the modification of the hypothalamic–pituitary–adrenal axis (Connan et al., 2003), interrupts the developmental transition from localized to distributed brain function. Therefore, the preferential cognitive style relating to weak central coherence may be associated with reduced connectivity throughout the brain (Happe & Frith, 2006). Furthermore, secondary effects of eating disorders such as poor nutritional status can also interrupt normal maturational processes in the brain and disrupt the progression of hormonal changes. In the absence of efficient brain integration, behavior may be captured by internal or external stimuli endorsing immediately rewarding tendencies, despite these being less adaptive in the long term. This can lead to the maintenance of maladaptive behaviors.

Empirical support for the disruption of the development of collaborative brain function has been found in the neuroimaging literature, with reports of hypoperfusion (Chowdhury et al., 2003) and functional anomalies in response to illness-related cues (Ellison et al., 1998; Uher et al., 2003; Uher et al., 2004; Uher et al., 2005). These studies have illustrated abnormal activation in those areas of the brain relating to affective processing and the control and planning of behavior (for review, see Treasure & Uher, 2004).

The "social information processing network"

Adolescence is a critical phase in the development of the "social information processing network" (SIPN; Nelson et al., 2005). This model suggests that changes in the neurohumoral milieu impact on the "affective node" and subsequently the assignment of emotional significance; changes in connectivity as a result of neurodevelopmental maturation impact on the "cognitive regulatory node" and subsequently its higher-order processes (Nelson et al., 2005). "Mismatch" between the development of the cognitive and affective node is thought to result in the onset of behavioral difficulties in some individuals. Thus social hassles and trauma during adolescence can have a profound effect because the ability to regulate, contextualize and plan an effective coping response is immature.

Eating disorders are often triggered by interpersonal problems (Schmidt et al., 1997, 1999) and it is possible that immaturity and transitions in the SIPN form the neural context in which eating disorders develop. Hypersensitivity of the affective node can lead to heightened emotional responsiveness in situations concerning motivation, self-esteem, acceptance and rejection. The literature pertaining to neurodevelopmental anomalies in eating disorders highlights the potential for a mismatch in the SIPN to occur, thus being implicated in either the development or maintenance of eating disorders. The interaction between the affective and cognitive regulatory nodes of the SIPN is of central importance to this model, and empirical evidence appears in line with a disturbance in emotion processing and cognitive control in eating disorders.

Examination of affective processing in eating disorders suggests the presence of poor emotional intelligence, with "alexithymia" (an inability to experience and express emotions and to discriminate between emotional states and bodily sensations) and weak performance in laboratory tests of emotion recognition (Kucharska-Pietura *et al.*, 2004; Schmidt *et al.*, 1993; Zonnevylle-Bendek *et al.*, 2004). Preliminary studies from our group using the startle eye blink modulation to investigate reflexive motivational responding to general and disorder-specific cues also suggest that there is a disturbance in affective processing (Friederich *et al.*, 2006). Interestingly, in people with AN, none of the cues used (pleasant [excluding erotic images], food, thin bodies and body checking) attenuated the startle response. This suggests pervasive anhedonia and a failure of the reward system and the experience of pleasure.

The ability to make effective judgments between short- and long-term rewards as exemplified by the Iowa Gambling Task is also considered to be a marker of functional emotional processing (Bechara *et al.*, 1994). The aim of this task is to anticipate risk, which is an important cognitive and emotional component of decision-making. Damasio's somatic marker hypothesis states that emotional feedback facilitates judgments about risk (Damasio, 1996). Impairments in this task reflect an inability to advantageously assess future consequences. People with acute AN perform poorly on this task (Cavedini *et al.*, 2004; Tchanturia *et al.*, 2007). In a study by Tchanturia *et al.* (2007), poor performance and a blunted anticipatory skin conductance response before making high-risk (disadvantageous) choices was identified. These data appear in line with the somatic marker hypothesis (Damasio, 1996), supporting the significance of the interaction between the affective and cognitive regulatory nodes of the SIPN in AN.

Collectively, this preliminary evidence suggests that people with eating disorders have abnormalities in emotional processing and in the appetitive responses that result from reward pathways, implicating dopaminergic mechanisms. Earlier in the chapter, we reviewed the anomalies in the proposed central functions of the cognitive regulation node, with markers of poor cognitive inhibition in the flexibility/set-shifting domain, and "weak central coherence." These performance patterns suggest that behavior is not adapted according to the overall goal of the tasks. Thus recent findings suggest that abnormalities in the development of the emotional and cognitive nodes of the social brain may underpin AN, possibly contributing to both causal and perpetuating factors. This model has implications for the development of novel approaches to the treatment.

Application of knowledge

Our group has argued that these anomalies in emotional and information processing are key maintaining factors in anorexia nervosa (Schmidt & Treasure, 2006) and we have developed a model of treatment which specifically addresses these (Treasure *et al.*, 2005). We are currently investigating whether some of the core vulnerabilities in information processing may respond to cognitive remediation (Tchanturia *et al.*, 2005b).

Cognitive remediation therapy (CRT) is an approach that helps the patient to engage in stimulating and positive mental activities without the burden or complexity of confronting issues or emotions that relate to their eating disorder (Davies & Tchanturia, 2005). The key tenets of CRT are that (1) practice in a cognitive skill will improve the performance of and confidence in using that skill and (2) by practicing a cognitive process, networks in the brain will be activated and lesser-used areas will be increasingly involved. Cognitive remediation therapy has proven therapeutic value when used with patients with schizophrenia, improving executive functioning and engagement in therapy (Wykes & Reeder, 2005).

Our work in progress focuses on increasing cognitive flexibility and looking at the wider picture ("seeing the wood from the trees"), reducing the natural tendency for extreme attention to detail. It is hypothesized that the cognitive skills practiced within CRT will help people with eating disorders learn to have an approach to life which uses strengths rather than a skewed approach in which they can only play their dominant hand. This approach may prepare an individual for more general psychotherapy. Single case studies using this therapeutic approach in AN report favorable outcomes (Davies & Tchanturia, 2005; Tchanturia *et al.*, 2006).

Concluding comment

The literature suggests that cognitive anomalies in eating disorders are not simply a consequence of illness state, but are probably of etiological significance. Future research is needed to validate our model of eating disorders, with careful methodological design to address the many complex issues highlighted earlier. The varied populations, different illness stages and experimental procedures used need to be clearly defined. In-depth exploration into the neuropsychological profile of eating disorders will allow clinical interventions to be tailored according to the specific processing style. We have described how neuroscience can be integrated into treatment models (Baldock & Tchanturia 2007; Southgate *et al.*, 2005; Treasure *et al.*, 2005) and it will be seen whether this experimentally informed approach improves outcome for these conditions.

Acknowledgments

Laura Southgate was supported by the Nina Jackson Eating Disorders Research PhD fellowship, in conjunction with the Psychiatry Research Trust (registered charity no. 284286). The Wellcome Trust, Psychiatry Research Trust, BIAL Foundation (grant nos. 88/02: 61/04) and the European Commission Framework 5 Project "Factors in Healthy Eating" QLK1-1999-916 have supported Kate Tchanturia and different neuroscience projects within our research group.

References

American Psychiatric Association (1994). *Diagnostic and Statistical Manual of Mental Disorders* (4th edn.) (*DSM–IV*). Washington.

Anderluh, M. B., Tchanturia, K., Rabe-Hesketh, S. & Treasure, J. (2003). Childhood obsessive-compulsive personality traits in adult women with eating disorders: defining a broader eating disorder phenotype. *American Journal of Psychiatry*, **160**, 242–247.

Baldock, E. & Tchanturia, K. (2007). Translating laboratory research into clinical practice: foundations, functions and future of cognitive remediation therapy for anorexia nervosa. *Therapy*, **4**, 285–293.

Bechara, A., Damasio, A. R., Damasio, H. & Anderson, S. W. (1994). Insensitivity to future consequences following damage to human prefrontal cortex. *Cognition*, **50**, 7–15.

Bowers, W. A. (1994). Neuropsychological impairment among anorexia nervosa and bulimia patients. *Eating Disorders: The Journal of Treatment and Prevention*, **2**, 42–46.

Cavedini, P., Bassi, T., Ubbiali, A. *et al.* (2004). Neuropsychological investigation of decision-making in anorexia nervosa. *Psychiatry Research*, **127**, 259–266.

Chowdhury, U., Gordon, I., Lask, B. *et al.* (2003). Early-onset anorexia nervosa: is there evidence limbic system imbalance? *International Journal of Eating Disorders*, **33**, 388–396.

Claes, L., Vandereycken, W. & Vertommen, H. (2002). Impulsive and compulsive traits in eating disordered patients compared with controls. *Personality and Individual Differences*, **32**, 707–714.

Collier, D. A. & Treasure, J. L. (2004). The aetiology of eating disorders. *British Journal of Psychiatry*, **185**, 363–365.

Connan, F., Campbell, I. C., Katzman, M., Lightman, S. L. & Treasure, J. (2003). A neurodevelopmental model for anorexia nervosa. *Physiology and Behavior*, **79**, 13–24.

Damasio, A. R. (1996). The somatic marker hypothesis and the possible functions of the prefrontal cortex. *Philosophical Transactions of the Royal Society of London Series B Biological Sciences*, **351**, 1413–1420.

Davies, H. & Tchanturia, K. (2005). Cognitive remediation therapy as an intervention for acute anorexia nervosa: a case report. *European Eating Disorders Review*, **13**, 311–316.

Eddy, K. T., Keel, P. K., Dorer, D. J. *et al.* (2002). Longitudinal comparison of anorexia nervosa subtypes. *International Journal of Eating Disorders*, **31**, 191–201.

Ellison, Z., Foong, J., Howard, R. *et al.* (1998). Functional anatomy of calorie fear in anorexia nervosa. *Lancet*, **352**, 1192.

Espelage, D. L., Mazzeo, S. E., Sherman, R. & Thompson, R. (2002). MCMI-II profiles of women with eating disorders: a cluster analytic investigation. *Journal of Personality Disorders*, **16**, 453–463.

Fairburn, C. G., Cooper, Z., Doll, H. A. & Welch, S. L. (1999). Risk factors for anorexia nervosa: three integrated case-control comparisons. *Archives of General Psychiatry*, **56**, 468–476.

Fairburn, C. G. & Harrison, P. J. (2003). Eating disorders. *Lancet*, **361**, 407–416.

Friederich, H. C., Kumari, V., Uher, R. *et al.* (2006). Differential motivational responses to food and pleasurable cues in anorexia and bulimia nervosa: a startle reflex paradigm. *Psychological Medicine*, **36**, 1327–1335.

Frith, U. (1989). *Autism: Explaining the Enigma*. Oxford: Blackwell Science.

Galderisi, S., Mucci, A., Monteleone, P. *et al.* (2003). Neurocognitive functioning in subjects with eating disorders: the influence of neuroactive steroids. *Biological Psychiatry*, **53**, 921–927.

Gillberg, C., Rastam, M. & Gillberg, I. C. (1994). Anorexia nervosa: physical health and neurodevelopment at 16 and 21 years. *Developmental Medicine and Child Neurology*, **36**, 567–575.

Gillberg, I. C., Gillberg, C., Rastam, M. & Johansson, M. (1996). The cognitive profile of anorexia nervosa: a comparative study including a community-based sample. *Comprehensive Psychiatry*, **37**, 23–30.

Goldner, E. M., Srikameswaran, S., Schroeder, M. L., Livesley, W. J. & Birmingham, C. L. (1999). Dimensional assessment of personality pathology in patients with eating disorders. *Psychiatry Research*, **85**, 151–159.

Gray, J. A. & McNaughton, N. (2000). *The Neuropsychiatry of Anxiety: An Enquiry into the Functions of the Septo-hippocampal System* (2nd edn.). New York, NY: Oxford University Press.

Green, M. W., Elliman, N. A., Wakeling, A. & Rogers, P. J. (1996). Cognitive functioning, weight change and therapy in anorexia nervosa. *Journal of Psychiatric Research*, **30**, 401–410.

Grunwald, M., Ettrich, C., Busse, F. *et al.* (2002). Angle paradigm – a new method to measure right parietal dysfunctions in anorexia nervosa. *Archives of Clinical Neuropsychology*, **17**, 485–496.

Halmi, K. (1999). Obsessive compulsive traits and behaviours in anorexia nervosa. In L. Bellodi & F. Brambilla (Eds.), *Eating Disorders and Obsessive Compulsive Disorder: An Etiopathogenetic Link* (pp. 4–13). Turin, Italy: Centro Scientifico Editore.

Happe, F. (1999). Autism: cognitive deficit or cognitive style? *Trends in Cognitive Sciences*, **3**, 216–222.

Happe, F. & Frith, U. (2006). The weak coherence account: detail focused cognitive style in autism spectrum disorders. *Journal of Autism and Developmental Disorders*, **36**, 5–25.

Happe, F., Briskman, J. & Frith, U. (2001). Exploring the cognitive phenotype of autism: Weak 'central coherence' in parents and siblings of children with autism: 1. Experimental tests. *Journal of Child Psychology, Psychiatry and Allied Disciplines*, **42**, 299–307.

Hollander, E. (1993). Obsessive-compulsive spectrum disorders: an overview. *Psychiatric Annals*, **23**, 355–358.

Hollander, E. & Benzaquen, S. D. (1997). The obsessive-compulsive spectrum disorders. *International Review of Psychiatry*, **9**, 99–109.

Hollander, E. & Wong, C. M. (1995). Obsessive-compulsive spectrum disorders. *Journal of Clinical Psychiatry*, **56** (suppl. 4), 3–6.

Holliday, J., Tchanturia, K., Landau, S., Collier, D. A. & Treasure, J. (2005). Is impaired set shifting an endophenotype of anorexia nervosa. *American Journal of Psychiatry*, **162**, 2269–2275.

Jones, B. P., Duncan, C. C., Brouwers, P. & Mirsky, A. F. (1991). Cognition in eating disorders. *Journal of Clinical and Experimental Neuropsychology*, **13**, 711–728.

Kaye, W. H., Greeno, C. G., Moss, H. *et al.* (1998). Alterations in serotonin activity and psychiatric symptoms after recovery from bulimia nervosa. *Archives of General Psychiatry*, **55**, 927–935.

Kingston, K., Szmuckler, G., Andrews, D., Tress, B. & Desmond, P. (1996). Neuropsychological and structural brain changes in anorexia nervosa before and after refeeding. *Psychological Medicine*, **26**, 15–28.

Kohlmeyer, K., Lehmkuhl, G. & Poutska, F. (1983). Computed tomography of anorexia nervosa. *AJNR*, **4**, 437–438.

Kucharska-Pietura, K., Nickolaou, V., Marsiak, M. & Treasure, J. (2004). The recognition of emotion in the faces and voice of anorexia nervosa. *International Journal of Eating Disorders*, **35**, 42–47.

Lauer, C. J., Gorzewski, B., Gerlingloff, M., Backmund, H. & Zihl, J. (1999). Neuropsychological assessments before and after treatment in patients with anorexia nervosa and bulimia nervosa. *Journal of Psychiatric Research*, **33**, 129–138.

Lilenfeld, L. R., Kaye, W. H., Greeno, C. G. *et al.* (1998). A controlled family study of anorexia nervosa and bulimia nervosa: psychiatric disorders in first-degree relatives and effects of proband comorbidity. *Archives of General Psychiatry*, **55**, 603–610.

Livesley, W. J., Jang, K. L. & Vernon, P. A. (1998). Phenotypic and genetic structure of traits delineating personality disorder. *Archives of General Psychiatry*, **55**, 941–948.

Lopez, C., Tchanturia, K., Stahl, D. *et al.* (2008a). An examination of the concept of central coherence in women with anorexia nervosa. *International Journal of Eating Disorders*, **41**, 143–152.

Lopez, C., Tchanturia, K., Stahl, D. & Treasure, J. (2008b). Central coherence in eating disorders: a systematic review. *Psychological Medicine*, **38**, 1393–1404.

Lopez, C., Tchanturia, K., Stahl, D. & Treasure, J. (2009). Weak central coherence in eating disorders: a step towards looking for an endophenotype of eating disorders. *Journal of Clinical and Experimental Neuropsychology*, **31**, 117–125.

Luna, B. & Sweeney, J. A. (2004). The emergence of collaborative brain function. *Annals of the New York Academy of Sciences*, **1021**, 296–309.

Miyake, A., Friedman, N. P., Emerson, M. J., Witzki, A. H. & Howerter, A. (2000). The unity and diversity of executive functions and their contributions to complex "frontal lobe" tasks: a latent variable analysis. *Cognitive Psychology*, **41**, 49–100.

Moser, D. J., Benjamin, M. L., Bayless, J. D. *et al.* (2003). Neuropsychological functioning pretreatment and posttreatment in an inpatient eating disorders program. *International Journal of Eating Disorders*, **33**, 64–70.

Murphy, R., Nutzinger, D. O., Paul, T. & Leplow, B. (2002). Dissociated conditional-associative learning in anorexia nervosa. *Journal of Clinical and Experimental Neuropsychology*, **24**, 176–186.

Murphy, R., Nutzinger, D. O., Paul, T. & Leplow, B. (2004). Conditional-associative learning in eating disorders: a comparison with OCD. *Journal of Clinical and Experimental Neuropsychology*, **26**, 190–199.

Naruo, T., Nakabeppu, Y., Sagiyama, K. I. *et al.* (2000). Characteristic regional cerebral blood flow patterns in anorexia nervosa patients with binge/purge behavior. *American Journal of Psychiatry*, **157**, 1520–1522.

National Institute for Clinical Excellence – NICE (2004). Core Interventions for the treatment and management of anorexia nervosa, bulimia nervosa and related eating disorders. http://www.nice.org.uk/nicemediapdf/CG9FullGuideline.pdf [On-line].

Nelson, E. E., Liebenluft, E., McClure, E. B. & Pine, D. S. (2005). The social re-orientation of adolescence: a neuroscience perspective on the process and its relation to psychopathology. *Psychological Medicine*, **35**, 163–174.

Rastam, M. (1992). Anorexia nervosa in 51 Swedish adolescents: premorbid problems and comorbidity. *Academy of Child and Adolescent Psychiatry*, **31**, 819–829.

Rastam, M., Gillberg, C. & Wentz, E. (2003). Outcome of teenage-onset anorexia nervosa in a Swedish community-based sample. *European Child and Adolescent Psychiatry*, **12** (suppl. 1), i78–i90.

Roberts, M., Tchanturia, K., Stahl, D., Southgate, L. & Treasure, J. (2007). A systematic review and meta-analysis of set-shifting ability in eating disorders. *Psychological Medicine*, **37**, 1075–1084.

Schmidt, U., Jiwany, A. & Treasure, J. (1993). A controlled study of alexithymia in eating disorders. *Comprehensive Psychiatry*, **34**, 54–58.

Schmidt, U., Tiller, J., Blanchard, M., Andrews, B. & Treasure, J. (1997). Is there specific trauma precipitating anorexia nervosa? *Psychological Medicine*, **27**, 523–530.

Schmidt, U. & Treasure, J. (2006). Anorexia nervosa valued and visible: a cognitive-interpersonal maintenence model and its implications for research and practice. *British Journal of Clinical Psychology*, **45**, 343–366.

Schmidt, U., Troop, N. A. & Treasure, J. L. (1999). Events and the onset of eating disorders: correcting an "age-old" myth. *International Journal of Eating Disorders*, **25**, 83–88.

Sherman, B. J., Savage, C. R., Eddy, K. T. *et al.* (2006). Strategic memory in adults with anorexia nervosa: are there similarities to obsessive compulsive spectrum disorders? *International Journal of Eating Disorders*, **39**, 468–476.

Southgate, L. (2005). *Response inhibition in anorexia nervosa and bulimia nervosa: An exploration of neuropsychological functions and their association with personality traits and behaviours.* PhD dissertation. Kings College London, Institute of Psychiatry.

Southgate, L., Tchanturia, K. & Treasure, J. (2005). Building a model of the aetiology of eating disorders by translating experimental neuroscience into clinical practice. *Journal of Mental Health*, **14**, 553–566.

Southgate, L., Tchanturia, K. & Treasure, J. (2006). Neuropsychological studies in eating disorders: a review. In P. Swain (Ed.), *Eating Disorders: New Research* (pp. 1–69) New York, NY: Nova Publishers.

Southgate, L., Tchanturia, K. & Treasure, J. (2008). Information processing bias in anorexia nervosa. *Psychiatry Research*, **160**, 221–227.

Steiger, H. (2004). Eating disorders and the serotonin connection: state, trait and developmental effects. *Journal of Psychiatry and Neuroscience*, **29**, 20–29.

Steinglass, J., Walsh, B. T. & Stern, Y. (2006). Set shifting deficit in anorexia nervosa. *Journal of the International Neuropsychological Society*, **12**, 431–435.

Steinhausen, H. C. (2002). The outcome of anorexia nervosa in the 20th century. *American Journal of Psychiatry*, **159**, 1284–1293.

Strupp, B. J., Weingartner, H., Kaye, W. & Gwirtsman, H. (1986). Cognitive processing in anorexia nervosa: a disturbance in automatic information processing. *Neuropsychobiology*, **15**, 89–94.

Sutandar-Pinnock, K., Woodside, D. B., Carter, J. C., Olmsted, M. P. & Kaplan, A. S. (2003). Perfectionism in anorexia nervosa: a 6–24-month follow-up study. *International Journal of Eating Disorders*, **33**, 225–229.

Szmukler, G. I., Andrewes, D., Kingston, K. & Chen, L. (1992). Neuropsychological impairment in anorexia nervosa: before and after refeeding. *Journal of Clinical and Experimental Neuropsychology*, **14**, 347–352.

Tchanturia, K., Anderluh, M. B., Morris, R. G. *et al.* (2004a). Cognitive flexibility in anorexia nervosa and bulimia nervosa. *Journal of the International Neuropsychological Society*, **10**, 513–520.

Tchanturia, K., Campbell, I., Morris, R. G. & Treasure, J. (2005). Neuropsychological studies in anorexia nervosa. *International Journal of Eating Disorders*, **37** (Suppl.), S72–S76.

Tchanturia, K., Davies, H., Schmidt, U. & Treasure, J. (2005). *Cognitive Remediation Flexibility Module for Anorexia Nervosa.* London: Kings College London, Institute of Psychiatry.

Tchanturia, K., Liao, T., Uher, R. *et al.* (2007). An investigation of decision making in people with anorexia nervosa using Iowa Gambling task and skin conductance measurements. *Journal of the International Neuropsychological Society*, **13**, 635–641.

Tchanturia, K., Morris, R. G., Brecelj Anderluh, M. *et al.* (2004b). Set shifting in anorexia nervosa: an examination before and after weight gain, in full recovery and relationship to childhood and adult OCPD traits. *Journal of Psychiatric Research*, **38**, 545–552.

Tchanturia, K., Morris, R. G., Surguladze, S. & Treasure, J. (2002). An examination of perceptual and cognitive set shifting tasks in acute anorexic nervosa and following recovery. *Eating and Weight Disorders*, **7**, 312–315.

Tchanturia, K., Serpell, L., Troop, N. & Treasure, J. (2001). Perceptual illusions in eating disorders: rigid and fluctuating styles. *Journal of Behavior Therapy and Experimental Psychiatry*, **32**, 107–115.

Tchanturia, K., Whitney, J. & Treasure, J. (2006). Can cognitive exercises help treat anorexia nervosa? A case report. *Eating and Weight Disorders*, **11**, 112–117.

Toner, B. B., Garfinkel, P. E. & Garner, D. M. (1987). Cognitive style of patients with bulimic and diet-restricting anorexia nervosa. *American Journal of Psychiatry*, **144**, 510–512.

Treasure, J., Tchanturia, K. & Schmidt, U. (2005). Developing a model of the treatment for eating disorder: using neuroscience research to examine the how rather than the what of change. *Counselling and Psychotherapy Research*, **5**, 187–190.

Treasure, J. & Uher, R. (2004). Neuroimaging of the eating disorders. In *Clinical Handbook of Eating Disorders: An Integrated Approach* (pp. 297–322). New York: Marcel Dekker.

Uher, R., Brammer, M. J., Murphy, T. *et al.* (2003). Recovery and chronicity in anorexia nervosa: brain activity associated with differential outcomes. *Biological Psychiatry*, **54**, 934–942.

Uher, R., Murphy, T., Brammer, M. J. *et al.* (2004). Medial prefrontal cortex activity associated with symptom provocation in eating disorders. *American Journal of Psychiatry*, **161**, 1238–1246.

Uher, R., Murphy, T., Friederich, H.-C. *et al.* (2005). Functional neuroanatomy of body shape perception in healthy and eating disordered women. *Biological Psychiatry*, **58**, 990–997.

Westen, D. & Harnden-Fischer, J. (2001). Personality profiles in eating disorders: rethinking the distinction between axis I and axis II. *American Journal of Psychiatry*, **158**, 547–562.

Wilson, G. T., Grilo, C. M. & Vitousek, K. M. (2007). Psychological treatment of eating disorders. *American Psychologist*, **62**, 216.

Wonderlich, S., Crosby, R., Joiner, T. *et al.* (2005). Personality subtyping and bulimia nervosa: psychopathological and genetic correlates. *Psychological Medicine*, **35**, 1–9.

Wykes, T. & Reeder, C. (2005). *Cognitive Remediation Therapy for Schizophrenia. Theory and Practice.* London: Routledge Taylor & Francis Group.

Zonnevylle-Bendek, M. J. S., van Goozen, S. H. M., Cohen-Kettenis, P. T. *et al.* (2004). Emotional functioning in anorexia nervosa patients: adolescents compared to adults. *Depression and Anxiety*, **19**, 35–42.

Chapter 22

Neurobiological and neuropsychological pathways into substance abuse and addictive behavior

Murat Yücel, Dan I. Lubman, Nadia Solowij and Warrick J. Brewer

Introduction and overview

"Addiction," derived from the Latin verb *addicere* (meaning "to enslave"), is characterized by the apparent "loss of control" or autonomy over one's behavior. Indeed, the continued use of substances by addicted individuals, despite an apparent awareness of the adverse negative consequences, suggests that addictive behavior may involve deficits in inhibitory control, decision-making and the regulation of affect (Bechara *et al.*, 2001; Fillmore, 2003; Goldstein & Volkow, 2002; Grant *et al.*, 2000; Jentsch & Taylor, 1999; Lubman *et al.*, 2004; Yücel & Lubman, 2007). Recent neuropsychological and neuroimaging studies across a variety of substance-using populations support this notion, implicating impairments in frontal cortical systems critically involved in executive control (Everitt *et al.*, 2001; Rogers & Robbins, 2001). However, an important question that remains is why only a minority of individuals who experiment with addictive substances develop problematic substance-use patterns. This chapter explores this issue from a neuropsychological perspective, specifically focusing on the neuropsychological aspects of addictive behavior (including neuroimaging findings where relevant) under three main sections:

(1) *Neuropsychological sequelae of specific substances and their role in addictive behaviors.* This section will briefly discuss the evidence for specific neuropsychological and neurobiological effects of several major classes of substances including alcohol, cannabis, inhalants, stimulants, opiates and ecstasy. The section ends with a summary of the major findings across the various substances, highlighting consistent evidence for problems in prefrontally mediated functions (such as inhibitory control, decision-making and affect regulation).

(2) *Premorbid neuropsychological vulnerability to addictive behaviors.* Here we discuss how early difficulties in prefrontally mediated tasks of behavioral regulation can render the individual at risk for developing an addictive disorder. There is also a discussion of how problems in neurobehavioral disinhibition may manifest and be exacerbated by genetic polymorphisms, personality traits and comorbid disorders (medical, neurological or psychiatric), resulting in an increased vulnerability to addictive behavior.

(3) *Adolescence: a key neurodevelopmental period of vulnerability.* This section focuses on the changes that occur in the adolescent brain. We discuss how premorbid vulnerabilities may impact upon this critical period of development.

Finally, we summarize how substance-associated neuropsychological impairments may interact with premorbid neuropsychological vulnerabilities and the adolescent period to render an individual at increased risk for addictive disorders.

Neuropsychological sequelae of specific drugs and their role in addictive behavior

Alcohol

The most consistent findings of neuropsychological impairment in heavy and long-term drinkers of alcohol are in the domains of attention, short-term memory, visuospatial abilities, postural stability and executive functions (such as problem-solving, mental flexibility, judgment, working memory, response inhibition and decision-making), with a relative sparing of declarative memory, language skills and primary motor and perceptual abilities (Bowden-Jones et al., 2005; Corral-Varela & Cadaveira, 2002; Fishbein et al., 2006; Goudriaan et al., 2006; Scheurich, 2005). The link between lifetime exposure and the development of cognitive problems is unclear. While some research findings suggest that cognitive performance worsens in direct proportion to the frequency and duration of drinking (Beatty et al., 2000; Parsons, 1998), other findings suggest that cognitive deficits may be detectable only in those who have been drinking regularly for at least 10 years (Eckardt et al., 1998; Parsons & Nixon, 1998). These contrasting findings highlight the need for further research to determine how patterns of alcohol use are related to cognitive impairment, especially in light of some evidence to suggest that long-term, light-to-moderate social drinkers have also been found to have cognitive deficits (Parsons, 1998).

The nature of the neuropsychological deficits observed in long-term drinkers is consistent with disruption to the fronto-temporal, fronto-parietal and cerebellar brain systems. Indeed, structural MRI reveals a consistent association between heavy drinking and structural neuronal injury and volume loss that is more extensive in the frontal lobe, temporal lobe and cerebellum (Mann et al., 2001; Pfefferbaum et al., 1997). Results of autopsy studies show that individuals with a history of chronic alcohol consumption have smaller, lighter and more shrunken brains than non-alcoholic adults of the same age and gender (Hommer et al., 1996, 2001). However, the evidence for this is not always consistent (Hommer, 2003; Wang et al., 2003).

Some alcohol-related cognitive impairment and structural brain deficits can be reversed with abstinence over a period of several months to years (Corral-Varela & Cadaveira, 2002). Compared with treated alcoholics who subsequently relapsed to drinking, abstinence-associated improvements have been documented in neuropsychological functions such as working memory, visuospatial functioning and attention, and are accompanied by significant increases in brain volume (Sullivan et al., 2000a, 2000b; Volkow et al., 1994).

Cannabis

Neuropsychological studies of chronic cannabis users in the unintoxicated state have demonstrated impaired performance on a variety of attention, memory and executive function tasks (Bolla et al., 2002; Fletcher et al., 1996; Pope & Yurgelun-Todd, 1996; Pope et al., 2001, 2003; Solowij et al., 2002). Deficits have been attributed to duration of cannabis use (Solowij et al., 2002), frequency of cannabis use (Pope et al., 2001) or cumulative dosage effects (Bolla et al., 2002). For example, impaired verbal learning and memory performance was found in heavy cannabis users but not light users, regardless of duration of cannabis use (Pope & Yurgelun-Todd, 1996; Pope et al., 2001); comparable findings were also reported in long-term but not short-term cannabis users (e.g. 34 vs 8 years of use (Fletcher et al., 1996); 24 vs 10 years of use (Solowij et al., 2002)), even when both groups were using cannabis on a near daily basis (Solowij et al., 2002). Performance on executive tests, such as the Stroop task (Eldreth et al., 2004), is not consistently impaired in cannabis users, but performance decrements have nevertheless been shown to be related to duration of use (Solowij et al., 2002), or dose interacting with lower IQ (Bolla et al., 2002). Few studies have sought to specifically tease out differential impairments associated with varying patterns of cannabis use (e.g. heavy daily use for short periods vs light weekly use for long periods). Solowij et al. (1995) showed that the ability to focus attention and filter out irrelevant information was progressively impaired with increasing years of cannabis use, while speed of information processing was impaired with increasing frequency of use (days per month).

Recent neuroimaging studies of cannabis users demonstrate impaired performance in attention, verbal memory (Block et al., 2000; Solowij et al., 2004), working memory (Kanayama et al., 2004), response inhibition (Eldreth et al., 2004; Gruber & Yurgelun-Todd, 2005; Smith et al., 2004) and decision-making tasks (Bolla et al., 2005), with concomitant alterations in blood flow, activation or brain-tissue density primarily in prefrontal cortical, anterior cingulate, basal ganglia, cerebellar and hippocampal regions. For example, Matochik et al. (2005) found gray and white matter density changes in 28-day abstinent cannabis users in the medial temporal regions, and some of the density changes were associated with duration of cannabis use. Moreover, altered frontal cortical activation is apparent in cannabis users despite normal Stroop task performance (Eldreth et al., 2004; Gruber & Yurgelun-Todd, 2005), suggesting that there may be disturbances in brain physiology that are not as yet apparent behaviorally.

The extent of persistence of effects or recovery of function following abstinence is also uncertain, with some studies suggesting no recovery after 25–28 days abstinence (Bolla et al., 2002, 2005; Eldreth et al., 2004), whilst others report full recovery after 28 days abstinence (Pope et al., 2001) and partial early recovery after 2 years abstinence (Solowij et al., 1995).

Inhalants

While the toxic effects of chronic inhalant abuse are well described (Lubman et al., 2006; Rosenberg et al., 2002), there is only a small research literature examining the neurobiological and neuropsychological effects of voluntary exposure to this class of drugs (Brust, 1993; Fiedler et al., 2003; Lubman et al., 2006). One of the earliest neuropsychological investigations of inhalant abuse showed that inhalant abusers (mainly those abusing metallic paints) had deficits in motor coordination, learning, memory, executive functioning and overall verbal intelligence (Berry et al., 1977; Maruff et al., 1998). Cairney and colleagues have conducted a number of studies examining the effects of petrol sniffing on cognitive outcomes (Cairney et al., 2002, 2004b, 2004a). They report that petrol sniffers (mean age 30 years) who have recovered from lead encephalopathy continue to demonstrate considerable neurological and cognitive impairments, including impaired visual attention, visual recognition memory and visual paired associate learning. Petrol sniffers who had not suffered lead encephalopathy demonstrated only mild deficits. One of the largest investigations examining the effects of inhalant use on neuropsychological functioning in adolescents was conducted by Chadwick et al. (1989). Those who had used volatile substances performed significantly worse on tests of vocabulary and impulsivity, and had significantly lower verbal and full-scale IQ. However, these differences were no longer significant when background social disadvantage was taken into account, although it is important to note that the inhalant group consisted of primarily experimental or recreational users.

From a neurobiological perspective, there is more conclusive evidence that inhalant exposure is associated with adverse consequences. A recent study comparing 55 inhalant abusers (mean age 30 years) and 61 cocaine abusers (mean age 29 years) found substantial brain abnormalities (especially in subcortical and white matter regions) and cognitive impairment within both groups (Rosenberg et al., 2002). However, the structural brain abnormalities were more common (44% vs 25%) and more extensive in the inhalant-using group. In addition, this group performed significantly worse on tests of working memory and tests requiring focused attention, planning and problem-solving. Interestingly, even within the inhalant-using group, solvent abusers had more extensive and severe abnormalities in brain white matter than other inhalant users, and these abnormalities were associated with greater cognitive impairment. For example, the 12% of solvent abusers who had diffuse moderate to severe white matter abnormalities had a mean verbal IQ score that was nearly 20% lower than the already low average score registered by the rest of the inhalant group. Thus, it appears that the nature and extent of neurobiological and neuropsychological impairment is associated with the length and chronicity of the abuse, as well as the type/composition of the volatile substance. Similar findings have been observed in other neurobiological and neuroimaging studies of chronic solvent exposure in occupational settings (Yamanouchi et al., 1995, 1997).

Very few studies have specifically investigated recovery of function after prolonged exposure to inhalants. Cairney et al. (2004b, 2005) found significant improvements in previously identified neurobehavioral impairments following 2 years of abstinence. In fact, in many cases these deficits normalized completely. However, while those with the greatest levels of impairment showed the greatest degree of improvement with abstinence, they were less likely to recover completely.

Opiates

Research on the long-term neuropsychological effects of chronic opiate abuse has been relatively limited. Davis and colleagues reported that 60% of individuals currently abusing opiates had impairments of at least two standard deviations below published norms on two or more neuropsychological tests, a significantly higher incidence than found in matched controls with no history of drug abuse (Davis et al., 2002). In particular, deficits were identified in impulse control in those with a history of 5 or more years of heroin use. Similarly, Pau et al. (2002) examined the impact of heroin on frontal executive functioning in three cognitive domains, namely attention, impulse control and mental flexibility. They found that heroin abuse had adverse effects on impulse control but not attention or mental flexibility. Other studies have reported more diffuse deficits across the domains of attention, working memory, memory and executive function in chronic opiate abusers (Guerra *et al.*, 1987; Lee & Pau, 2002; Ornstein *et al.*, 2000; Pau *et al.*, 2002; Rogers *et al.*, 1999). Ornstein and colleagues found that heroin addicts were impaired on performance of cognitive tasks (e.g. learning, spatial working memory, strategic thinking) known to be sensitive to cortical damage (including selective lesions of the temporal and frontal lobes) (Ornstein *et al.*, 2000). Darke *et al.* (2000) reported that methadone-maintained heroin addicts performed more poorly on all neuropsychological domains tested, including attention (information processing speed, attentional capacity), memory (visual and verbal learning and memory) and executive functioning (problem-solving) compared with matched controls.

Chronic opiate- and amphetamine-using populations have been shown to have disturbances in prefrontal cortical activity, which was associated with performance on a task involving a decisional conflict between an unlikely high-reward option and a likely low-reward option (Ersche *et al.*, 2005). Moreover, this disturbance was observed in a group of drug users who had been abstinent for at least 1 year. Further support for prefrontal dysfunction comes from the large structural imaging study of Lyoo *et al.* (2006), which investigated gray matter density across the brain in 63 opiate-dependent subjects and 46 matched controls. These authors found that relative to controls, the opiate-dependent group exhibited significantly decreased gray-matter in the prefrontal, as well as superior temporal cortex, insula and fusiform gyrus. Another study by Kivisaari *et al.* (2004) in long-term opiate users found that the sylvian fissures and ventricles were wider in opiate-dependent subjects than in controls, which may be related to brain atrophy within frontal and temporal lobes.

Studies evaluating the persistence of cognitive deficits amongst abstinent opiate addicts remain mixed. A number of studies have found that abstinent groups of recovering addicts have no significant cognitive deficits (Davis *et al.*, 2002; Guerra *et al.*, 1987). Guerra *et al.* (1987) reported that individuals with current heroin abuse demonstrated deficits in attention, working memory, episodic memory and verbal fluency, which normalized 7–14 days following rapid detoxification. However, two other studies of abstinent heroin users (8 and 14 months, respectively)

reported ongoing deficits in executive function (Lee & Pau, 2002; Pau *et al.*, 2002). Using a more sophisticated battery of experimental neuropsychological tests, Ersche *et al.* (2006) reported that opiate-dependent individuals demonstrated marked impairments in spatial planning, paired associate learning and visual pattern recognition compared with matched controls. Performance of former opiate users (abstinent for 8 years on average) was not statistically different from current users on any measure, suggesting that the deficits observed did not simply reflect the current effects of drug use. These findings are in keeping with other studies describing prefrontal dysfunction in chronic drug users (Bechara *et al.*, 2001; Goldstein & Volkow, 2002; Jentsch & Taylor, 1999; Lubman *et al.*, 2004; Yücel & Lubman, 2007).

Psychostimulants (cocaine, amphetamine/methamphetamine)

Few studies have explicitly attempted to examine cognitive functioning amongst methamphetamine users. Some researchers point to studies that suggest memory and executive problems, whilst others maintain that no firm evidence for a link exists (Maxwell, 2005). Recent studies of chronic amphetamine/methamphetamine abusers have shown that they perform poorly on decision-making tasks that involve regions of the frontal cortex (specifically the ventromedial prefrontal cortex), such that they make disadvantageous decisions that reflect valuing short-term gain over longer-term losses (Nordahl *et al.*, 2003; Rogers *et al.*, 1999). Methamphetamine users also appear to be more distractible and are unable to suppress processing task-irrelevant information (Nordahl *et al.*, 2003), which is consistent with their clinical presentation. Other work has also shown cognitive deficits related to processing speed, learning, delayed recall and inhibitory control and working memory (Gonzalez *et al.*, 2004; Rippeth *et al.*, 2004; Salo *et al.*, 2002). Another recent study found methamphetamine abuse to be associated with deficient strategic (i.e. executive) control of verbal encoding and retrieval, which is consistent with the proposed sequelae of methamphetamine-related prefronto-striatal circuit neurotoxicity (Woods *et al.*, 2005). Interestingly, comorbid cannabis use does not appear to exacerbate methamphetamine neurotoxicity, but rather has been suggested to have neuroprotective actions (Gonzalez *et al.*, 2004).

Neuropsychological studies of chronic cocaine users, like chronic amphetamine users, also demonstrate higher-order cognitive impairments (e.g. inhibitory dysregulation) that is consistent with abnormal blood flow in frontal brain regions (Strickland et al., 1993). Several studies have reported that cocaine abuse is associated with decrements on neurobehavioral tests measuring executive control, visuoperception, psychomotor speed, manual dexterity, verbal learning and memory (Bolla et al., 1999; Rogers & Robbins, 2001). Ardila et al. (1991) found that neuropsychological test scores were correlated with lifetime amount of cocaine used, suggesting a direct relationship between cocaine abuse and cognitive impairment.

Neuroimaging studies of methamphetamine users have shown abnormalities of brain function relative to healthy controls including alterations of frontal, temporal and subcortical metabolism (Gouzoulis-Mayfrank et al., 1999; Iyo et al., 1997; Volkow et al., 2001a, 2001b, 2001c). Changes in neuronal biochemistry that are suggestive of neuronal injury have also been found in the frontal cortex and basal ganglia (Ernst et al., 2000). Using proton magnetic resonance spectroscopy (1H-MRS), Ernst et al. (2000) reported abnormally low levels of the neuronal marker N-acetylaspartate (NAA) in the basal ganglia of abstinent methamphetamine-dependent subjects. They also observed an inverse association between prefrontal white-matter NAA values and years of use, implying direct effects of this drug on neuronal integrity of the prefrontal tissue. Similar findings have been reported in the anterior cingulate cortex (Nordahl et al. 2002, 2005). Recent neuroimaging studies have shown that frontal and temporal lobe white matter continues to increase into the fifth decade of life (Bartzokis et al., 2000). However, Bartzokis and colleagues found that cocaine-dependent subjects (aged 19 to 47) do not demonstrate the normal pattern of age-related increases in white matter within these brain regions (Bartzokis et al., 2000), suggesting that continued cocaine use may arrest normal white matter maturation.

Examination of cognitive function in abstinent cocaine-dependent individuals after both 6 weeks and 6 months abstinence reveals persistent cognitive impairment across a wide range of functions compared with controls at both time points. Further, a close relationship between the degree of neuropsychological impairments and dosage (i.e. quantity and dosage of peak usage) has also been reported (Di Sclafani et al., 2002). Consistent with their neuropsychological findings, the authors also found that cocaine-induced brain volumetric reduction in the prefrontal cortex persists after 6 weeks of abstinence (Fein et al., 2002).

MDMA (N-methyl-3,4-methylenedioxy-amphetamine, ecstasy)

A number of persisting cognitive problems have been attributed to regular MDMA use and suggest underlying serotonergic dysfunction (Gouzoulis-Mayfrank & Daumann, 2006; McGuire, 2000; Montoya et al., 2002). For example, impairments in memory (both visual and verbal) have been shown to correlate with in vivo measurements of brain serotonin function and levels of 5-HIAA in cerebrospinal fluid (CSF), as well as relating to the level of previous MDMA use (i.e. are dose related) (Bolla et al., 1998). Other neuropsychological deficits that have been reported in regular ecstasy users include impairments of executive function and self-control (i.e. decreased inhibitory control and increased impulsivity) (McCardle et al., 2004; Morgan et al., 2005). McCardle et al. (2004) found that MDMA users exhibit difficulties in coding information into long-term memory, have impaired verbal learning, are more easily distracted and are less efficient at focusing attention on complex tasks. Interestingly, Spatt and colleagues have described a case of profound amnesia, associated with bilateral brain changes on MRI, following a single exposure to MDMA (Spatt et al., 1997).

Although cognitive deficits among MDMA users have been well documented, little is known of the neurobiological sequelae of MDMA use. In one study, MDMA use in adolescence was associated with difficulties in the ability to focus and divide attention, as well as abnormal hippocampal activity during performance of a working-memory task (Jacobsen et al., 2004). Other functional MRI studies have found abnormal fronto-temporal, parietal and subcortical activity during performance of working-memory tasks (Daumann et al., 2001, 2003, 2004, 2005). Additionally, Daumann et al. (2003) found that relative to a group of controls and currently abstinent but previously moderate users, currently abstinent but previously heavy users showed more prominent frontal and temporal lobe activation abnormalities during performance of a working-memory task.

Structural MRI findings amongst MDMA polydrug users include evidence of diffuse gray matter reductions across the cortex, cerebellum and brainstem (Cowan *et al.*, 2003).

Little is known about the possible persistent neuropsychological effects of extensive MDMA use. However, there is tentative evidence that these cognitive deficits persist for at least 6 months after abstinence, whereas anxiety and hostility remit after a year of abstinence (Gouzoulis-Mayfrank & Daumann, 2006; Morgan *et al.*, 2002). Morgan *et al.* (2002) compared four groups of participants: current regular recreational MDMA users, ex-regular MDMA users who had abstained from using the drug for an average of 2 years, polydrug users who had never taken MDMA, and drug-naïve controls. They found that both current and ex-MDMA users exhibited elevated psychopathology and behavioral impulsivity compared with polydrug users and drug-naïve controls, but current MDMA users exhibited a broader range of psychopathology than ex-users. Both groups of MDMA users also exhibited impaired working memory and verbal recall performance compared with drug-naïve controls. These findings suggest that selective impairments of neuropsychological performance associated with regular MDMA use are not reversed by prolonged abstinence. This is consistent with evidence that MDMA may affect brain serotonergic systems in human users. Other studies have also found altered neural activations suggestive of prefrontal neuronal injury in abstinent MDMA users during performance of working-memory tasks (Daumann *et al.*, 2004).

Summary of findings

In summary, the findings suggest that chronic substance abuse across a wide range of addictive substances can adversely affect neuropsychological functioning. While there is marked inter-individual variability in the patterns of substance use (e.g. duration, frequency, dosage), almost all substances have been found to affect the domains of attention, learning and memory, visuospatial abilities and executive functioning. Similarly, the neurobiological findings from structural, functional and spectroscopic MRI studies suggest dysfunction in neural systems that subserve these functions, particularly the fronto-temporal circuitry. The findings of impaired inhibitory control (variously referred to as response inhibition, inhibitory regulation, self-control or impulsivity), working memory and decision-making, together with prefrontal imaging abnormalities, appear to be the most consistent findings across studies and substances.

It is important to note, however, that pathways into addiction are invariably complex, which makes it hard to disentangle the neuropsychological effects of substance abuse from associated risk factors. For example, while the study by Chadwick *et al.* (1989) identified a number of neuropsychological deficits amongst inhalant-using teenagers, these were not significantly different from non-users when background social disadvantage was controlled. Similarly Darke *et al.* (2000), in their study of methadone-maintained opiate users, noted that the methadone group had high rates of poly-substance use, overdose, head injury and comorbid psychopathology. The authors found that the neuropsychological deficits identified were more characteristic of those with associated comorbidities, further raising issues regarding the specificity of findings reported. We still have only a limited understanding of the role of these associated factors in the nature and extent of neuropsychological deficits observed.

Another related issue in the field is our limited understanding of the degree to which the observed neuropsychological deficits are pre-existing (i.e. present prior to any substance abuse) and indeed predispose to addictive behavior. While in some instances, these deficits have been found to be dose-dependent, implying that they are a direct consequence of drug exposure, the fact that most studies are cross-sectional in nature means that it is not possible to categorically determine whether the identified deficits are a consequence of the drugs specifically, relate to pre-existing vulnerabilities, or are a combination of both. More recent research is attempting to tease these issues apart. The next section will focus on how early behavioral dysregulation, psychopathology and genetic polymorphisms may each be associated with disturbances to normal neuropsychological functioning, leaving the individual at risk of developing an addictive disorder.

Premorbid neuropsychological vulnerability to addictive behaviors
Risk-taking behavior

Initiation of substance use typically occurs during adolescence, a critical period of neural, cognitive (as reviewed below), emotional and social development.

Notably, adolescence is a period during which there is increased affective reactivity together with significant but more protracted neural maturation (Giedd et al., 1999; Gogtay et al., 2004; Paus, 2005; Paus et al., 1999; Steinberg, 2005). This occurs in areas associated with core executive and self-regulatory skills, including inhibitory control and affect-regulation (reviewed in more detail in the next section; see also chapter 8). The developmental delay between increases in emotional arousability during early adolescence, and the subsequent maturation of neurobiological systems subserving self-regulatory competence that continues into late adolescence or early adulthood, results in a developmentally normative "mismatch." Adolescents are therefore left with a limited capacity for regulating strong affective and behavioral impulses. This, in turn, increases the likelihood of adolescents engaging in more impulsive, emotive and risky decisions, which often involve experimentation and social use of drugs and alcohol, the incidence of which sharply increases during adolescence (Steinberg, 2004, 2005). However, some individuals appear to have a greater "mismatch" than others and this may provide important clues as to whether the individual is more vulnerable to behavioral dysregulation and addictive behaviors.

Behavioral dysregulation

While a certain degree of behavioral dysregulation can be considered a normal part of adolescence, current research shows that some young individuals are significantly more impaired in this regard. These individuals have been shown to not only be more vulnerable to experiment with and use substances socially, but also to develop addictive behaviors. For example, Tarter and colleagues (Kirisci et al., 2004; Tarter et al., 2003) recently conducted a cross-sectional and longitudinal analysis of children at low-risk and high-risk of substance use (on the basis of parental substance-use history) and found that deficits in behavioral regulation (referred to as "neurobehavioral inhibition") at age 16 in the high-risk children predicted a substance-use disorder (SUD) at age 19 with 85% accuracy. Their measure of behavioral regulation was derived using primarily prefrontal tests of cognition (e.g. Stroop interference task, Porteus mazes, motor restraint), affect (a temperament survey) and behavior (number of behavioral disorder symptoms). The indices derived from these

areas converge with other evidence to suggest that behavioral dysregulation is a key component of liability to addictive behavior.

Behavioral and mental health disorders

Childhood and adolescence is also a time during which the incidence of behavioral and mental health disorders rises sharply (Lewinsohn et al., 1993). Young people who have behavioral problems early (e.g. a difficult temperament in infancy, or childhood oppositional, aggressive or impulsive behaviors) are at increased risk of developing SUDs, especially males (Lewinsohn et al., 1993). Childhood diagnoses of oppositional defiant disorder, conduct disorder and attention-deficit hyperactivity disorder are also well-established risk factors for youth SUD (Button et al., 2006; Conway et al., 2006; Hasin et al., 2005; Kantojarvi et al., 2006). In addition, a number of mental health disorders are also associated with the development of problematic substance use. Disorders such as depression, anxiety, schizophrenia, bipolar disorder and obsessive-compulsive disorder have high rates of comorbid substance use (Bogenschutz & Nurnberg, 2000; Brady & Sinha, 2005; Hides et al., 2004; Swartz et al., 2006). Given that deficits in inhibitory control and affect regulation are often found across many of these disorders, together with disruption to brain regions subserving these functions (e.g. prefrontal and temporal areas), it is possible that they form a key component of liability to not only behavioral and mental health disorders, but also to addictive behavior.

Personality disorders

Certain personality characteristics may also influence an individual's decision to use drugs, as well as their liability to addictive behavior. Indeed, previously identified inhibitory-control and affect-regulation difficulties may be components of a premorbid personality style rather than the result of state-related cognitive-affective processes. To this end, there is a growing literature on temperament and personality as risk factors for SUDs and addiction. These studies highlight a relationship between measures of impulsivity and related constructs (such as risk-taking, sensation-seeking) in childhood and the development of later SUDs in adulthood (Tarter et al., 2003). In fact, studies of both adolescents and adults consistently report an association between impulsivity (e.g. acting in a sudden and unplanned manner, acting without having all the necessary information or failing to think through the pros and cons of a decision) and substance-related problems (Acton, 2003; Dawe et al., 2004; Stepp et al., 2005). More recently, researchers have suggested that it is a specific domain of impulsivity, termed "rash-spontaneous impulsivity" (the tendency to act rashly and without consideration of consequences; see Dawe et al., 2004) that is more directly associated with SUD.

Other personality traits such as negative affectivity/neuroticism have also been identified as risk factors for SUD. Negative affect/neuroticism is characterized by a general tendency to experience life as more negative, difficulty in controlling one's mood (i.e. difficulties with affect regulation), and/or being less tolerant to stressful life events. There is growing evidence to suggest that adolescent SUD may not only result in disinhibited behavior or impulsivity (reviewed above), but may in fact reflect an attempt to reduce negative affectivity (Chassin et al., 1993, 2004). From a neurobiological and neuropsychological perspective, this inability to internally regulate moods and the over-reliance upon external agents, such as psychoactive substances, suggests inappropriate neural (particularly prefrontal) and cognitive modulation of emotions (Whittle et al., 2006).

Genetic polymorphisms

Genetic factors appear to account for 30–60% of the overall variance in risk for developing a drug addiction (Kreek et al., 2005). While the precise mechanisms underlying this relationship remain unclear, recent work implicates the role of specific genetic polymorphisms. For example, studies investigating the catechol-O-methyltransferase (COMT) gene, which affects how long dopamine acts in the synapses of the prefrontal cortex, suggests that specific polymorphisms are less common in addicted populations. The methionine polymorphism, which results in a slower breakdown of prefrontal dopamine, is associated with better prefrontal cortical function (including working memory and inhibitory control) in both children (Diamond et al., 2004) and adults (Egan et al., 2001; Malhotra et al., 2002). Interestingly, the polymorphism is significantly less common in drug-addicted populations, suggesting that this particular genetic vulnerability may be mediated by its effects on prefrontally mediated cognitive functioning (Beuten et al., 2006; Li et al., 2004).

Summary of findings

Adolescence is a critical period of development, characterized by gradually maturing self-regulatory skills. The immaturity of these cognitive skills, compounded by increased emotional arousability at this time, may at least in part explain why adolescence represents such a period of vulnerability for risk-taking behavior, including experimentation and social use of drugs and alcohol. These developmental processes may be exaggerated in some individuals and partly underlie increased risk for behavioral and mental health disorders that also emerge during this period, together with associated neuropsychological impairments. In turn, behavioral and mental health problems, together with certain personality traits have been identified as major risk factors for SUDs. Given that deficits in inhibitory control and affect regulation are often found across many of these disorders, together with disruption to brain regions subserving such functions (e.g. prefrontal and temporal areas), it is possible that they represent a common component of a liability to SUDs and addictive behaviors more generally. Genetic factors that affect prefrontal cortical functioning may also further increase behavioral dysregulation and vulnerability to addiction.

Adolescence: a key neurodevelopmental period of vulnerability

Remodeling the prefrontal cortex and maturing executive abilities

As noted above, one critical characteristic of human brain development is an initial overproduction of gray matter, followed by a period of *pruning* during adolescence (Giedd et al., 1999; Gogtay et al., 2004; Paus, 2005; Paus et al., 1999). This latter process results in a marked decline in synaptic connections, such that only synapses integral for optimal functioning are retained. Pruning is accompanied by *myelination*, a process that also makes the brain's operations more efficient, sometimes by 100-fold. Myelination does not occur concurrently in all brain regions – there is a graded progression of maturation with posterior and deep brain structures (regions responsible for more primitive functions) maturing earlier, while the medial and lateral frontal areas (regions responsible for higher-cognitive functions) continue to develop well into adolescence and young adulthood. As such, while overall brain weight is not changing markedly as a result of the pruning of gray matter and the development of white matter, the composition of the brain is changing considerably during adolescence – often referred to as a 'remodeling' of the brain. Importantly, this remodeling associated with developmental maturation within frontal, temporal and parietal structures, mirrors the development of more complex cognitive (e.g. inhibitory/impulse control, working memory, decision-making and other cognitive processes that encompass the executive suite), as well as affective abilities (e.g. capacity to regulate motivational drive, affect and social cognition) (Giedd *et al.*, 1999; Gogtay *et al.*, 2004; Paus, 2005; Paus *et al.*, 1999). Given that the prefrontal cortex undergoes dramatic developmental changes from adolescence to adulthood, drug administration during adolescence may have greater impact on behaviors, which are mediated by this region. Indeed, there is limited but growing evidence that adolescents appear to be more vulnerable than adults to the adverse neuropsychological and neurobiological effects of substance use (Scheier & Botvin, 1995). Some evidence for this comes from studies of teenage alcohol and cannabis use.

Alcohol and its effects on adolescent brain development

Adolescents who misuse alcohol show greater neuropsychological deficits on learning, memory and executive brain function than adults who misuse alcohol, a finding that might stem from the adverse effects of alcohol on the development and maturation of brain regions such as the hippocampus and prefrontal cortices. For example, De Bellis and colleagues compared the hippocampal volumes of adolescents and young adults with alcohol-use disorders (aged 13–21 years) to those of healthy matched controls (De Bellis *et al.*, 2000). They found that the size of the hippocampus was significantly smaller in subjects with alcohol problems, and that its volume positively correlated with age of first use and negatively correlated with duration of use. More recently, they reported that adolescents with alcohol-use disorders had smaller prefrontal cortices and white matter volumes compared with matched controls (De Bellis *et al.*, 2005). Further, prefrontal cortical volumes significantly correlated with measures of alcohol consumption. While interpretation of these studies is limited by their cross-sectional nature and the high rates of other types of psychopathology among the participants with alcohol-use disorders, they suggest that adolescents may be particularly vulnerable to the effects of alcohol on learning, memory and executive brain function.

Cannabis and its effects on adolescent brain development

With respect to cannabis, early-onset cannabis users have also been found to have smaller whole brain volume, lower percent cortical gray matter, higher percent white matter, and increased resting cerebral blood flow compared with late-onset users (Wilson *et al.*, 2000). There is growing evidence that individuals who initiate cannabis use at an early age, when the brain is still developing, might be more vulnerable to lasting neuropsychological deficits than individuals who begin using later in life. Early-onset cannabis use (prior to age 16 or 17), but not late-onset cannabis use (after age 17), was shown to impair attentional processes measured by reaction time during visual scanning (Ehrenreich *et al.*, 1999), visual search and short-term memory (Huestegge *et al.*, 2002), and resulted in greater reduction of P300 amplitudes in an attention task (Kempel *et al.*, 2003). Cannabis users who had commenced use prior to age 17 were more impaired than late-onset cannabis users on measures of learning and executive functions (Pope *et al.*, 2003) and were the least likely to show recovery of cognitive functions after 28 days abstinence (Harrison *et al.*, 2002). Jacobsen *et al.* (2004) found that adolescent cannabis users showed impaired performance on executive tasks such as the Continuous Performance Task and in an n-back working-memory task, which was accompanied by failure to deactivate the right hippocampus (measured by fMRI).

Summary of findings

There is emerging evidence that early-onset alcohol and cannabis use is associated with a range of later negative outcomes. However, it is not clear whether those who initiated substance use early have pre-existing neuropsychological deficits or whether any reported deficits are a direct consequence of early-onset substance use. Recent animal work supports the latter notion, with studies finding that adolescence may be associated with an increased sensitivity to the neurotoxic properties of addictive drugs. However, it is likely that any additional pre-existing compromise to the behavioral-regulatory system (e.g. through associated psychopathology or genetic polymorphisms) may further widen the "mismatch" between developmental trajectories, leading to greater behavioral dysregulation and vulnerability to addictive behaviors.

Summary and conclusions

There is now a large body of evidence suggesting that addicted individuals have neuropsychological impairments in the domains of attention, learning/memory and executive functioning, as well as associated neurobiological abnormalities involving fronto-temporal and basal ganglia circuits. In some instances, these deficits have been found to be dose-dependent, implying that they are a direct consequence of prolonged drug exposure. However, the nature and extent of these deficits and the factors mediating them (e.g. patterns of drug use, polysubstance abuse, comorbidities) are still not fully clear. The fact that most studies are cross-sectional in nature means that it is not possible to categorically determine whether the identified deficits are a consequence of the drugs specifically, whether they relate to pre-existing vulnerabilities, or are a combination of both.

While more recent research is attempting to elucidate these issues of cause and effect, there is consistent evidence from research conducted in other disciplines to suggest that behavioral, personality and mental health problems often manifest prior to SUD onset, suggesting that they are either specific risk factors for the development of SUDs, or share common risk factors. Indeed, inhibitory-control deficits are not only central to drug dependence/addiction but also to many behavioral, personality and mental health problems. This notion is also consistent with epidemiological data demonstrating that many of these conditions frequently co-occur, as well as neurobiological data showing overlapping abnormalities of the prefrontal, anterior cingulate, orbitofrontal and hippocampal regions – regions critically involved in inhibitory-control of behavior. In addition, recent genetic studies suggest a link between genetic predisposition and impaired cognitive functioning, with the notion that certain polymorphisms are significantly more common in drug-addicted populations.

Finally, brain regions subserving inhibitory control of behavior do not fully mature until midway through the third decade of life. Emerging evidence from alcohol and cannabis using populations suggests that early-onset substance use is associated with increased risk for a range of adverse outcomes. While the mechanisms that underlie this relationship are not fully understood, recent advances in developmental neuroscience, together with emerging literature on early-onset substance use, suggest that the adolescent brain may be more vulnerable to the effects of psychoactive drugs because of the unique and critical neurodevelopmental processes that are occurring during this period (e.g. maturation of inhibitory control and associated brain regions/connections).

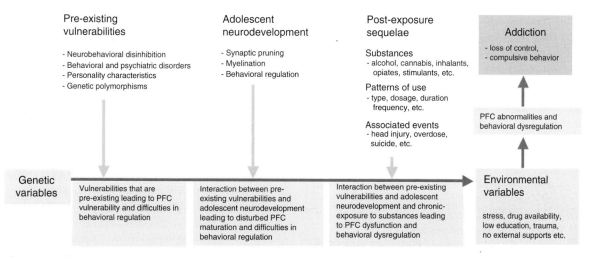

Figure 22.1. Illustrations of how substance-associated neuropsychological sequelae may interact with adolescent neurodevelopment and pre-existing vulnerabilities rendering the individual at increasing risk for addictive disorders. PFC = prefrontal cortex.

So why do only a minority of individuals who experiment with alcohol and drugs develop problematic substance-use patterns? As illustrated in Figure 22.1, the pathways leading to drug addiction are likely to be both multi-faceted and complex. It seems probable that there is an intricate relationship between pre-existing neuropsychological vulnerabilities (described above), the age of initiation of substance use (or neurodevelopmental maturity), patterns of substance use (type, dosage, duration, frequency) and associated events (head injury, overdose, suicide). Clearly, each of these areas can impact upon the development and functional integrity of the prefrontal cortex (PFC), which is postulated to play an important role in the initiation and maintenance of drug-use behavior. Such adverse effects are likely to render the individual at increased risk for making decisions that are impulsive, focused on short-term gains, and lack inhibitory control. It is therefore not surprising that affected individuals find it difficult to regulate their drug-seeking and drug-taking behavior and frequently relapse. However, the nature and extent of the impact on PFC integrity is likely to depend on a number of factors from genetic through to environmental variables. Such relationships need further investigation, especially as neuropsychological studies comprehensively exploring these notions in a prospective and longitudinal manner have been limited to date. Nevertheless, this is an exciting time in drug-addiction research. There are currently several prospective, multi-method, multi-modal studies being conducted internationally that capture the relevant variables identified to date. These studies will soon provide further insights into the neuropsychological and neurobiological pathways that increase risk for the development of addictive behavior.

References

Acton, G. S. (2003). Measurement of impulsivity in a hierarchical model of personality traits: implications for substance use. *Substance Use and Misuse*, **38**, 67–83.

Ardila, A., Rosselli, M. & Strumwasser, S. (1991). Neuropsychological deficits in chronic cocaine abusers. *International Journal of Neuroscience*, **57**, 73–79.

Bartzokis, G., Beckson, M., Lu, P. H. *et al.* (2000). Age-related brain volume reductions in amphetamine and cocaine addicts and normal controls: implications for addiction research. *Psychiatry Research*, **98**, 93–102.

Beatty, W. W., Tivis, R., Stott, H. D., Nixon, S. J. & Parsons, O. A. (2000). Neuropsychological deficits in sober alcoholics: influences of chronicity and recent alcohol consumption. *Alcoholism, Clinical and Experimental Research*, **24**, 149–54.

Bechara, A., Dolan, S., Denburg, N. *et al.* (2001). Decision-making deficits, linked to a dysfunctional ventromedial prefrontal cortex, revealed in alcohol and stimulant abusers. *Neuropsychologia*, **39**, 376–389.

Berry, G., Heaton, R. & Kirby, M. (1977). Neuropsychological deficits of chronic inhalant abusers. In B. Rumac. & A. Temple (Eds.), *Management of the Poisoned Patient* (pp. 9–31). Princeton, NJ: Science Press.

Beuten, J., Payne, T. J., Ma, J. Z. & Li, M. D. (2006). Significant association of catechol-O-methyltransferase (COMT) haplotypes with nicotine dependence in male and female smokers of two ethnic populations. *Neuropsychopharmacology*, **31**, 675–684.

Block, R. I., O'Leary, D. S., Ehrhardt, J. C. *et al.* (2000). Effects of frequent marijuana use on brain tissue volume and composition. *Neuroreport*, **11**, 491–496.

Bogenschutz, M. P. & Nurnberg, H. G. (2000). Theoretical and methodological issues in psychiatric comorbidity. *Harvard and Review of Psychiatry*, **8**, 18–24.

Bolla, K. I., Brown, K., Eldreth, D., Tate, K. & Cadet, J. L. (2002). Dose-related neurocognitive effects of marijuana use. *Neurology*, **59**, 1337–1343.

Bolla, K. I., Eldreth, D. A., Matochik, J. A. & Cadet, J. L. (2005). Neural substrates of faulty decision-making in abstinent marijuana users. *Neuroimage*, **26**, 480–492.

Bolla, K. I., Mccann, U. D. & Ricaurte, G. A. (1998). Memory impairment in abstinent MDMA ("Ecstasy") users. *Neurology*, **51**, 1532–1537.

Bolla, K. I., Rothman, R. & Cadet, J. L. (1999). Dose-related neurobehavioral effects of chronic cocaine use. *Journal of Neuropsychiatry and Clinical Neuroscience*, **11**, 361–369.

Bowden-Jones, H., McPhillips, M., Rogers, R., Hutton, S. & Joyce, E. (2005). Risk-taking on tests sensitive to ventromedial prefrontal cortex dysfunction predicts early relapse in alcohol dependency: a pilot study. *Journal of Neuropsychiatry and Clinical Neuroscience*, **17**, 417–420.

Brady, K. T. & Sinha, R. (2005). Co-occurring mental and substance use disorders: the neurobiological effects of chronic stress. *American Journal of Psychiatry*, **162**, 1483–1493.

Brust, J. (1993). *Neurological Aspects of Substance Abuse*. Boston, MA: Butterworth-Heinemann.

Button, T. M., Hewitt, J. K., Rhee, S. H. *et al.* (2006). Examination of the causes of covariation between conduct disorder symptoms and vulnerability to drug dependence. *Twin Research and Human Genetics*, **9**, 38–45.

Cairney, S., Maruff, P., Burns, C. & Currie, B. (2002). The neurobehavioural consequences of petrol (gasoline) sniffing. *Neuroscience and Biobehavior Review*, **26**, 81–89.

Cairney, S., Maruff, P., Burns, C. B., Currie, J. & Currie, B. J. (2004a). Neurological and cognitive impairment associated with leaded gasoline encephalopathy. *Drug and Alcohol Dependence*, **73**, 183–188.

Cairney, S., Maruff, P., Burns, C. B., Currie, J. & Currie, B. J. (2004b). Saccade dysfunction associated with chronic petrol sniffing and lead encephalopathy. *Journal of Neurologyery Neurosurgery and Psychiatry*, **75**, 472–476.

Cairney, S., Maruff, P., Burns, C. B., Currie, J. & Currie, B. J. (2005). Neurological and cognitive recovery following abstinence from petrol sniffing. *Neuropsychopharmacology*, **30**, 1019–1027.

Chadwick, O., Anderson, R., Bland, M. & Ramsey, J. (1989). Neuropsychological consequences of volatile substance abuse: a population based study of secondary school pupils. *British Medical Journal*, **298**, 1679–1683.

Chassin, L., Fora, D. B. & King, K. M. (2004). Trajectories of alcohol and drug use and dependence from adolescence to adulthood: the effects of familial alcoholism and personality. *Journal of Abnormal Psychology*, **113**, 483–498.

Chassin, L., Pillow, D. R., Curran, P. J., Molina, B. S. & Barrera, M., Jr. (1993). Relation of parental alcoholism to early adolescent substance use: a test of three mediating mechanisms. *Journal of Abnormal Psychology*, **102**, 3–19.

Conway, K. P., Compton, W., Stinson, F. S. & Grant, B. F. (2006). Lifetime comorbidity of DSM-IV mood and anxiety disorders and specific drug use disorders: results from the National Epidemiologic Survey on Alcohol and Related Conditions. *Journal of Clinical Psychiatry*, **67**, 247–257.

Corral-Varela, M. & Cadaveira, F. (2002). Neuropsychological aspects of alcohol dependence: the nature of brain damage and its reversibility. *Reviews in Neurology*, **35**, 682–687.

Cowan, R. L., Lyoo, I. K., Sung, S. M. *et al.* (2003). Reduced cortical gray matter density in human MDMA (Ecstasy) users: a voxel-based morphometry study. *Drug and Alcohol Dependence*, **72**, 225–235.

Darke, S., Sims, J., Mcdonald, S. & Wickes, W. (2000). Cognitive impairment among methadone maintenance patients. *Addiction*, **95**, 687–695.

Daumann, J., Fischermann, T., Heekeren, K. *et al.* (2005). Memory-related hippocampal dysfunction in poly-drug ecstasy (3,4-methylenedioxymethamphetamine) users. *Psychopharmacology (Berlin)*, **180**, 607–611.

Daumann, J., Jr., Fischermann, T., Heekeren, K., Thron, A. & Gouzoulis-Mayfrank, E. (2004). Neural mechanisms of working memory in ecstasy (MDMA) users who continue or discontinue ecstasy and amphetamine use: evidence from an 18-month longitudinal functional magnetic resonance imaging study. *Biological Psychiatry*, **56**, 349–355.

Daumann, J., Pelz, S., Becker, S., Tuchtenhagen, F. & Gouzoulis-Mayfrank, E. (2001). Psychological profile of abstinent recreational ecstasy (MDMA) users and significance of concomitant cannabis use. *Human Psychopharmacology*, **16**, 627–633.

Daumann, J., Schnitker, R., Weidemann, J. *et al.* (2003). Neural correlates of working memory in pure and polyvalent ecstasy (MDMA) users. *Neuroreport*, **14**, 1983–1987.

Davis, P. E., Liddiard, H. & Mcmillan, T. M. (2002). Neuropsychological deficits and opiate abuse. *Drug and Alcohol Dependence*, **67**, 105–108.

Dawe, S., Gullo, M. J. & Loxton, N. J. (2004). Reward drive and rash impulsiveness as dimensions of impulsivity: implications for substance misuse. *Addictive Behavior*, **29**, 1389–1405.

De Bellis, M. D., Clark, D. B., Beers, S. R. *et al.* (2000). Hippocampal volume in adolescent-onset alcohol use disorders. *American Journal of Psychiatry*, **157**, 737–744.

De Bellis, M. D., Narasimhan, A., Thatcher, D. L. *et al.* (2005). Prefrontal cortex, thalamus, and cerebellar volumes in adolescents and young adults with adolescent-onset alcohol use disorders and comorbid mental disorders. *Alcoholism, Clinical and Experimental Research*, **29**, 1590–1600.

Di Sclafani, V., Tolou-Shams, M., Price, L. J. & Fein, G. (2002). Neuropsychological performance of individuals dependent on crack-cocaine, or crack-cocaine and alcohol, at 6 weeks and 6 months of abstinence. *Drug and Alcohol Dependence*, **66**, 161–171.

Diamond, A., Briand, L., Fossella, J. & Gehlbach, L. (2004). Genetic and neurochemical modulation of prefrontal cognitive functions in children. *American Journal of Psychiatry*, **161**, 125–132.

Eckardt, M. J., File, S. E., Gessa, G. L. *et al.* (1998). Effects of moderate alcohol consumption on the central nervous system. *Alcoholism, Clinical and Experimental Research*, **22**, 998–1040.

Egan, M. F., Goldberg, T. E., Kolachana, B. S. *et al.* (2001). Effect of COMT Val108/158 Met genotype on frontal lobe function and risk for schizophrenia. *Proceedings of the National Academy of Sciences USA*, **98**, 6917–6922.

Ehrenreich, H., Rinn, T., Kunert, H. J. *et al.* (1999). Specific attentional dysfunction in adults following early start of cannabis use. *Psychopharmacology (Berlin)*, **142**, 295–301.

Eldreth, D. A., Matochik, J. A., Cadet, J. L. & Bolla, K. I. (2004). Abnormal brain activity in prefrontal brain regions in abstinent marijuana users. *Neuroimage*, **23**, 914–920.

Ernst, T., Chang, L., Leonido-Yee, M. & Speck, O. (2000). Evidence for long-term neurotoxicity associated with methamphetamine abuse: a 1H MRS study. *Neurology*, **54**, 1344–1349.

Ersche, K. D., Clark, L., London, M., Robbins, T. W. & Sahakian, B. J. (2006). Profile of executive and memory function associated with amphetamine and opiate dependence. *Neuropsychopharmacology*, **31**, 1036–1047.

Ersche, K. D., Fletcher, P. C., Lewis, S. J. *et al.* (2005). Abnormal frontal activations related to decision-making in current and former amphetamine and opiate dependent individuals. *Psychopharmacology (Berlin)*, **180**, 612–623.

Everitt, B. J., Dickinson, A. & Robbins, T. W. (2001). The neuropsychological basis of addictive behaviour. *Brain Research Brain Research Reviews*, **36**, 129–138.

Fein, G., Di Sclafani, V. & Meyerhoff, D. J. (2002). Prefrontal cortical volume reduction associated with frontal cortex function deficit in 6-week abstinent crack-cocaine dependent men. *Drug and Alcohol Dependence*, **68**, 87–93.

Fiedler, N., Weisel, C., Lynch, R. *et al.* (2003). Cognitive effects of chronic exposure to lead and solvents. *American Journal of Industrial Medicine*, **44**, 413–423.

Fillmore, M. T. (2003). Drug abuse as a problem of impaired control: current approaches and findings. *Behavioral and Cognitive Neuroscience Reviews*, **2**, 179–197.

Fishbein, D. H., Herman-Stahl, M., Eldreth, D. *et al.* (2006). Mediators of the stress-substance-use relationship in urban male adolescents. *Prevention Science*, **7**, 113–126.

Fletcher, J. M., Page, J. B., Francis, D. J. *et al.* (1996). Cognitive correlates of long-term cannabis use in Costa Rican men. *Archives of General Psychiatry*, **53**, 1051–1057.

Giedd, J. N., Blumenthal, J., Jeffries, N. O. *et al.* (1999). Brain development during childhood and adolescence: a longitudinal MRI study. *Nature Neuroscience*, **2**, 861–863.

Gogtay, N., Giedd, J. N., Lusk, L. *et al.* (2004). Dynamic mapping of human cortical development during childhood through early adulthood. *Proceedings of the National Academy of Sciences USA*, **101**, 8174–8179.

Goldstein, R. Z. & Volkow, N. D. (2002). Drug addiction and its underlying neurobiological basis: neuroimaging evidence for the involvement of the frontal cortex. *American Journal of Psychiatry*, **159**, 1642–1652.

Gonzalez, R., Rippeth, J. D., Carey, C. L. *et al.* (2004). Neurocognitive performance of methamphetamine users discordant for history of marijuana exposure. *Drug and Alcohol Dependence*, **76**, 181–190.

Goudriaan, A. E., Oosterlaan, J., De Beurs, E. & Van Den Brink, W. (2006). Neurocognitive functions in pathological gambling: a comparison with alcohol dependence, Tourette syndrome and normal controls. *Addiction*, **101**, 534–547.

Gouzoulis-Mayfrank, E. & Daumann, J. (2006). Neurotoxicity of methylenedioxyamphetamines (MDMA; ecstasy) in humans: how strong is the evidence for persistent brain damage? *Addiction*, **101**, 348–361.

Gouzoulis-Mayfrank, E., Schreckenberger, M., Sabri, O. *et al.* (1999). Neurometabolic effects of psilocybin, 3,4-methylenedioxyethylamphetamine (MDE) and d-methamphetamine in healthy volunteers. A double-blind, placebo-controlled PET study with [18F]FDG. *Neuropsychopharmacology*, **20**, 565–581.

Grant, S., Contoreggi, C. & London, E. D. (2000). Drug abusers show impaired performance in a laboratory test of decision making. *Neuropsychologia*, **38**, 1180–1187.

Gruber, S. A. & Yurgelun-Todd, D. A. (2005). Neuroimaging of marijuana smokers during inhibitory processing: a pilot investigation. *Brain Research Cognitive Brain Research*, **23**, 107–118.

Guerra, D., Sole, A., Cami, J. & Tobena, A. (1987). Neuropsychological performance in opiate addicts after rapid detoxification. *Drug and Alcohol Dependence*, **20**, 261–270.

Harrison, G. P., Jr., Gruber, A. J., Hudson, J. I., Huestis, M. A. & Yurgelun-Todd, D. (2002). Cognitive measures in long-term cannabis users. *Journal of Clinical Pharmacology*, **42**, 41S–47S.

Hasin, D. S., Goodwin, R. D., Stinson, F. S. & Grant, B. F. (2005). Epidemiology of major depressive disorder: results from the National Epidemiologic Survey on Alcoholism and Related Conditions. *Archives of General Psychiatry*, **62**, 1097–1106.

Hides, L., Lubman, D. I. & Dawe, S. (2004). Models of co-occurring substance misuse and psychosis: are personality traits the missing link? *Drug and Alcohol Review*, **23**, 425–432.

Hommer, D. W. (2003). Male and female sensitivity to alcohol-induced brain damage. *Alcohol Research and Health*, **27**, 181–185.

Hommer, D., Momenan, R., Kaiser, E. & Rawlings, R. (2001). Evidence for a gender-related effect of alcoholism on brain volumes. *American Journal of Psychiatry*, **158**, 198–204.

Hommer, D., Momenan, R., Rawlings, R. *et al.* (1996). Decreased corpus callosum size among alcoholic women. *Archives of Neurology*, **53**, 359–363.

Huestegge, L., Radach, R., Kunert, H. J. & Heller, D. (2002). Visual search in long-term cannabis users with early age of onset. *Progress in Brain Research*, **140**, 377–394.

Iyo, M., Namba, H., Yanagisawa, M. *et al.* (1997). Abnormal cerebral perfusion in chronic methamphetamine abusers: a study using 99MTc-HMPAO and SPECT. *Progress in Neuropsychopharmacology and Biological Psychiatry*, **21**, 789–796.

Jacobsen, L. K., Mencl, W. E., Pugh, K. R., Skudlarski, P. & Krystal, J. H. (2004). Preliminary evidence of hippocampal dysfunction in adolescent MDMA ("ecstasy") users: possible relationship to neurotoxic effects. *Psychopharmacology (Berlin)*, **173**, 383–390.

Jentsch, J. D. & Taylor, J. R. (1999). Impulsivity resulting from frontostriatal dysfunction in drug abuse: implications for the control of behavior by reward-related stimuli. *Psychopharmacology (Berlin)*, **146**, 373–390.

Kanayama, G., Rogowska, J., Pope, H. G., Gruber, S. A. & Yurgelun-Todd, D. A. (2004). Spatial working memory in heavy cannabis users: a functional magnetic resonance imaging study. *Psychopharmacology (Berlin)*, **176**, 239–247.

Kantojarvi, L., Veijola, J., Laksy, K. *et al.* (2006). Co-occurrence of personality disorders with mood, anxiety, and substance use disorders in a young adult population. *Journal of Personality Disorders*, **20**, 102–112.

Kempel, P., Lampe, K., Parnefjord, R., Hennig, J. & Kunert, H. J. (2003). Auditory-evoked potentials and selective attention: different ways of information processing in cannabis users and controls. *Neuropsychobiology*, **48**, 95–101.

Kirisci, L., Tarter, R. E., Vanyukov, M., Reynolds, M. & Habeych, M. (2004). Relation between cognitive distortions and neurobehavior disinhibition on the development of substance use during adolescence and substance use disorder by young adulthood: a prospective study. *Drug and Alcohol Dependence*, **76**, 125–133.

Kivisaari, R., Kahkonen, S., Puuskari, V. *et al.* (2004). Magnetic resonance imaging of severe, long-term, opiate-abuse patients without neurologic symptoms may show enlarged cerebrospinal spaces but no signs of brain pathology of vascular origin. *Archives of Medical Research*, **35**, 395–400.

Kreek, M. J., Nielsen, D. A., Butelman, E. R. & Laforge, K. S. (2005). Genetic influences on impulsivity, risk taking, stress responsivity and vulnerability to drug abuse and addiction. *Nature Neuroscience*, **8**, 1450–1457.

Lee, T. M. & Pau, C. W. (2002). Impulse control differences between abstinent heroin users and matched controls. *Brain Injury*, **16**, 885–889.

Lewinsohn, P. M., Hops, H., Roberts, R. E., Seeley, J. R. & Andrews, J. A. (1993). Adolescent psychopathology: I. Prevalence and incidence of depression and other DSM-III-R disorders in high school students. *Journal of Abnormal Psychology*, **102**, 133–144.

Li, T., Chen, C. K., Hu, X. *et al.* (2004). Association analysis of the DRD4 and COMT genes in methamphetamine abuse. *American Journal of Medical Genetics B Neuropsychiatry and Genetics*, **129**, 120–124.

Lubman, D. I., Hides, L. & Yucel, M. (2006). Inhalant abuse in youth: time for a coordinated response. *Medical Journal of Australia*, **185**(6), 327–330.

Lubman, D. I., Yucel, M. & Pantelis, C. (2004). Addiction, a condition of compulsive behaviour? Neuroimaging and neuropsychological evidence of inhibitory dysregulation. *Addiction*, **99**, 1491–1502.

Lyoo, I. K., Pollack, M. H., Silveri, M. M. *et al.* (2006). Prefrontal and temporal gray matter density decreases in opiate dependence. *Psychopharmacology (Berlin)*, **184**, 139–144.

Malhotra, A. K., Kestler, L. J., Mazzanti, C. *et al.* (2002). A functional polymorphism in the COMT gene and performance on a test of prefrontal cognition. *American Journal of Psychiatry*, **159**, 652–654.

Mann, K., Agartz, I., Harper, C. *et al.* (2001). Neuroimaging in alcoholism: ethanol and brain damage. *Alcoholism, Clinical and Experimental Research*, **25**, 104S–109S.

Maruff, P., Burns, C. B., Tyler, P., Currie, B. J. & Currie, J. (1998). Neurological and cognitive abnormalities associated with chronic petrol sniffing. *Brain*, **121** (Pt 10), 1903–1917.

Matochik, J. A., Eldreth, D. A., Cadet, J. L. & Bolla, K. I. (2005). Altered brain tissue composition in heavy marijuana users. *Drug and Alcohol Dependence*, **77**, 23–30.

Maxwell, J. A. (2005). Emerging research on methamphetamine. *Current Opinion in Psychiatry*, **18**, 235–242.

McCardle, K., Luebbers, S., Carter, J. D., Croft, R. J. & Stough, C. (2004). Chronic MDMA (ecstasy) use, cognition and mood. *Psychopharmacology (Berlin)*, **173**, 434–439.

McGuire, P. (2000). Long term psychiatric and cognitive effects of MDMA use. *Toxicology Letters*, **112–113**, 153–156.

Montoya, A. G., Sorrentino, R., Lukas, S. E. & Price, B. H. (2002). Long-term neuropsychiatric consequences of "ecstasy" (MDMA): a review. *Harvard Review of Psychiatry*, **10**, 212–220.

Morgan, M. J., Impallomeni, L. C., Pirona, A. & Rogers, R. D. (2005). Elevated impulsivity and impaired decision-making in abstinent ecstasy (MDMA) users compared to polydrug and drug-naive controls. *Neuropsychopharmacology*, **31**(7), 1562–1573.

Morgan, M. J., Mcfie, L., Fleetwood, H. & Robinson, J. A. (2002). Ecstasy (MDMA): are the psychological problems associated with its use reversed by prolonged abstinence? *Psychopharmacology (Berlin)*, **159**, 294–303.

Nordahl, T. E., Salo, R. & Leamon, M. (2003). Neuropsychological effects of chronic methamphetamine use on neurotransmitters and cognition: a review. *Journal of Neuropsychiatry and Clinical Neuroscience*, **15**, 317–325.

Nordahl, T. E., Salo, R., Natsuaki, Y. *et al.* (2005). Methamphetamine users in sustained abstinence: a proton magnetic resonance spectroscopy study. *Archives of General Psychiatry*, **62**, 444–452.

Nordahl, T. E., Salo, R., Possin, K. *et al.* (2002). Low N-acetyl-aspartate and high choline in the anterior cingulum of recently abstinent methamphetamine-dependent subjects: a preliminary proton MRS study. Magnetic resonance spectroscopy. *Psychiatry Research*, **116**, 43–52.

Ornstein, T. J., Iddon, J. L., Baldacchino, A. M. *et al.* (2000). Profiles of cognitive dysfunction in chronic amphetamine and heroin abusers. *Neuropsychopharmacology*, **23**, 113–126.

Parsons, O. A. (1998). Neurocognitive deficits in alcoholics and social drinkers: a continuum? *Alcoholism, Clinical and Experimental Research*, **22**, 954–961.

Parsons, O. A. & Nixon, S. J. (1998). Cognitive functioning in sober social drinkers: a review of the research since 1986. *Journal of Studies on Alcoholism*, **59**, 180–190.

Pau, C. W., Lee, T. M. & Chan, S. F. (2002). The impact of heroin on frontal executive functions. *Archives of Clinical Neuropsychology*, **17**, 663–670.

Paus, T. (2005). Mapping brain maturation and cognitive development during adolescence. *Trends in Cognitive Science*, **9**, 60–68.

Paus, T., Zijdenbos, A., Worsley, K. *et al.* (1999). Structural maturation of neural pathways in children and adolescents: in vivo study. *Science*, **283**, 1908–1911.

Pfefferbaum, A., Sullivan, E. V., Mathalon, D. H. & Lim, K. O. (1997). Frontal lobe volume loss observed with magnetic resonance imaging in older chronic alcoholics. *Alcoholism, Clinical and Experimental Research*, **21**, 521–529.

Pope, H. G., Jr. & Yurgelun-Todd, D. (1996). The residual cognitive effects of heavy marijuana use in college students. *Journal of the American Medical Association*, **275**, 521–527.

Pope, H. G., Jr., Gruber, A. J., Hudson, J. I. *et al.* (2003). Early-onset cannabis use and cognitive deficits: what is the nature of the association? *Drug and Alcohol Dependence*, **69**, 303–310.

Pope, H. G., Jr., Gruber, A. J., Hudson, J. I., Huestis, M. A. & Yurgelun-Todd, D. (2001). Neuropsychological performance in long-term cannabis users. *Archives of General Psychiatry*, **58**, 909–915.

Rippeth, J. D., Heaton, R. K., Carey, C. L. *et al.* (2004). Methamphetamine dependence increases risk of neuropsychological impairment in HIV infected persons. *Journal of the International Neuropsychology Society*, **10**, 1–14.

Rogers, R. D., Everitt, B. J., Baldacchino, A. *et al.* (1999). Dissociable deficits in the decision-making cognition of chronic amphetamine abusers, opiate abusers, patients with focal damage to prefrontal cortex, and tryptophan-depleted normal volunteers: evidence for monoaminergic mechanisms. *Neuropsychopharmacology*, **20**, 322–339.

Rogers, R. D. & Robbins, T. W. (2001). Investigating the neurocognitive deficits associated with chronic drug misuse. *Current Opinion in Neurobiology*, **11**, 250–257.

Rosenberg, N. L., Grigsby, J., Dreisbach, J., Busenbark, D. & Grigsby, P. (2002). Neuropsychologic impairment and MRI abnormalities associated with chronic solvent abuse. *Journal of Toxicology Clinical and Toxicology*, **40**, 21–34.

Salo, R., Nordahl, T. E., Possin, K. *et al.* (2002). Preliminary evidence of reduced cognitive inhibition in methamphetamine-dependent individuals. *Psychiatry Research*, **111**, 65–74.

Scheier, L. M. & Botvin, G. J. (1995). Effects of early adolescent drug use on cognitive efficacy in early-late adolescence: a developmental structural model. *Journal of Substance Abuse*, **7**, 379–404.

Scheurich, A. (2005). Neuropsychological functioning and alcohol dependence. *Current Opinion in Psychiatry*, **18**, 319–323.

Smith, A., Fried, P., Hogan, M. & Cameron, I. (2004). The effects of prenatal and current marijuana exposure on response inhibition: a functional magnetic resonance imaging study. *Brain and Cognition*, **54**, 147–149.

Solowij, N., Michie, P. T. & Fox, A. M. (1995). Differential impairments of selective attention due to frequency and duration of cannabis use. *Biological Psychiatry*, **37**(10), 731–739.

Solowij, N., Respondek, C. & Ward, P. (2004). Functional magnetic resonance imaging indices of memory function in long-term cannabis users. In *2004 Symposium on the Cannabinoids* (p. 89). Burlington, VT: International Cannabinoid Research Society.

Solowij, N., Stephens, R. S., Roffman, R. A. *et al.* (2002). Cognitive functioning of long-term heavy cannabis users seeking treatment. *Journal of the American Medical Association*, **287**, 1123–1131.

Spatt, J., Glawar, B. & Mamoli, B. (1997). A pure amnestic syndrome after MDMA ("ecstasy") ingestion. *Journal of Neurology, Neurosurgery and Psychiatry*, **62**, 418–419.

Steinberg, L. (2004). Risk taking in adolescence: what changes, and why? *Annals of the New York Academy of Sciences*, **1021**, 51–58.

Steinberg, L. (2005). Cognitive and affective development in adolescence. *Trends in Cognitive Science*, **9**, 69–74.

Stepp, S. D., Trull, T. J. & Sher, K. J. (2005). Borderline personality features predict alcohol use problems. *Journal of Personality Disorders*, **19**, 711–722.

Strickland, T. L., Mena, I., Villanueva-Meyer, J. et al. (1993). Cerebral perfusion and neuropsychological consequences of chronic cocaine use. *Journal of Neuropsychiatry and Clinical Neuroscience*, **5**, 419–427.

Sullivan, E. V., Rosenbloom, M. J., Lim, K. O. & Pfefferbaum, A. (2000a). Longitudinal changes in cognition, gait, and balance in abstinent and relapsed alcoholic men: relationships to changes in brain structure. *Neuropsychology*, **14**, 178–188.

Sullivan, E. V., Rosenbloom, M. J. & Pfefferbaum, A. (2000b). Pattern of motor and cognitive deficits in detoxified alcoholic men. *Alcoholism, Clinical and Experimental Research*, **24**, 611–621.

Swartz, M. S., Wagner, H. R., Swanson, J. W. et al. (2006). Substance use in persons with schizophrenia: baseline prevalence and correlates from the NIMH CATIE study. *Journal of Nervous and Mental Diseases*, **194**, 164–172.

Tarter, R. E., Kirisci, L., Mezzich, A. et al. (2003). Neurobehavioral disinhibition in childhood predicts early age at onset of substance use disorder. *American Journal of Psychiatry*, **160**, 1078–1085.

Volkow, N. D., Chang, L., Wang, G. J. et al. (2001a). Low level of brain dopamine D2 receptors in methamphetamine abusers: association with metabolism in the orbitofrontal cortex. *American Journal of Psychiatry*, **158**, 2015–2021.

Volkow, N. D., Chang, L., Wang, G. J. et al. (2001b). Loss of dopamine transporters in methamphetamine abusers recovers with protracted abstinence. *Journal of Neuroscience*, **21**, 9414–9418.

Volkow, N. D., Chang, L., Wang, G. J. et al. (2001c). Association of dopamine transporter reduction with psychomotor impairment in methamphetamine abusers. *American Journal of Psychiatry*, **158**, 377–382.

Volkow, N. D., Wang, G. J., Hitzemann, R. et al. (1994). Recovery of brain glucose metabolism in detoxified alcoholics. *American Journal of Psychiatry*, **151**, 178–183.

Wang, G. J., Volkow, N. D., Fowler, J. S. et al. (2003). Alcohol intoxication induces greater reductions in brain metabolism in male than in female subjects. *Alcoholism, Clinical and Experimental Research*, **27**, 909–917.

Whittle, S., Allen, N. B., Lubman, D. I. & Yucel, M. (2006). The neurobiological basis of temperament: towards a better understanding of psychopathology. *Neuroscience and Biobehavior Reviews*, **30**, 511–525.

Wilson, W., Mathew, R., Turkington, T. et al. (2000). Brain morphological changes and early marijuana use: a magnetic resonance and positron emission tomography study. *Journal of Addictive Diseases*, **19**, 1–22.

Woods, S. P., Rippeth, J. D., Conover, E. et al. (2005). Deficient strategic control of verbal encoding and retrieval in individuals with methamphetamine dependence. *Neuropsychology*, **19**, 35–43.

Yamanouchi, N., Okada, S., Kodama, K. et al. (1995). White matter changes caused by chronic solvent abuse. *American Journal of Neuroradiology*, **16**, 1643–1649.

Yamanouchi, N., Okada, S., Kodama, K. et al. (1997). Effects of MRI abnormalities on WAIS-R performance in solvent abusers. *Acta Neurologica Scandinavica*, **96**, 34–39.

Yücel, M. & Lubman, D. I. (2007). Neuropsychological and neuroimaging evidence of behavioural dysregulation in human drug addiction: implications for diagnosis, treatment and prevention. *Drug and Alcohol Review*, **26**, 33–39.

Thilo Deckersbach, Cary R. Savage and Scott L. Rauch

Introduction

Neuropsychological research has emerged as a valuable tool in shaping our understanding of the pathophysiology of obsessive-compulsive disorder (OCD). Below, we review neuropsychological findings in OCD and their relationship to current neuroanatomical models of the disorder. This review extends previous ones that we have written, together with our colleagues, on the same and related topics (Anderson et al., 2004; Savage, 1998).

The cortico-striatal model of OCD

Structural and functional neuroimaging studies implicate the striatum, orbitofrontal cortex (OFC) and anterior cingulate (ACC) in the pathophysiology of OCD. Studies using positron emission tomography (PET) and single photon emission computed tomography (SPECT) in OCD have found increased regional brain activity within the OFC, ACC (Baxter et al., 1987, 1988, 1992; Machlin et al., 1991; Nordahl et al., 1989; Rubin et al., 1992; Swedo et al., 1989) and the striatum (specifically, caudate nucleus; Baxter et al., 1987, 1988). Studies employing PET (Rauch et al., 1994) and functional magnetic resonance imaging (fMRI) studies (Adler et al., 2000; Breiter et al., 1996) have revealed increased brain activity or activation within anterior/lateral OFC, ACC, as well as caudate nucleus when OCD-related obsessions were provoked using OCD-related stimuli. Response to behavioral or pharmacological treatment of OCD attenuates abnormal regional brain activity within the OFC, ACC and caudate nucleus (Baxter et al., 1992; Benkelfat et al., 1990; Hoehn-Saric et al., 1991; Perani et al., 1995; Schwartz et al., 1996). Some treatment studies suggest that lower pre-treatment activity in

OFC better predicts subsequent response to serotonergic reuptake inhibitors (Brody et al., 1998; Rauch et al., 2002; Saxena et al., 1999; Swedo et al., 1989).

These findings have been incorporated into the cortico-striatal model of OCD (see Figure 23.1) which focuses on cortico-striato-thalamo-cortical circuitry (Rauch et al., 1988, 1998). According to this model, abnormal striatal function leads to inefficient gating at the level of the thalamus, which results in hyperactivity within the OFC and ACC. Compulsions can be viewed as ritualistic behaviors that are performed to recruit the inefficient striatum to ultimately achieve thalamic gating.

In recent functional neuroimaging studies distinct patterns of brain activity/activation associated with separate OCD symptom dimensions (e.g. checking versus contamination) have begun to emerge. This includes findings of different correlations between striatal activation and the combined severity of checking compulsions and aggressive/religious/sexual obsessions compared with the severity of symmetry and ordering compulsions (Rauch et al., 1998). Saxena et al. (2004) found increased dorsal ACC glucose metabolism in non-hoarding patients with OCD compared with patients with hoarding compulsions. The provocation of checking symptoms in a study by Mataix-Cols et al. (2004) yielded predominant activations in brain regions important for motor and attentional functioning (e.g. thalamus, dorsolateral cortical regions including dorsal ACC), whereas provocation of washing symptoms was overall more associated with activation in ventromedial prefrontal regions.

Neuropsychology of OCD

Neuropsychological studies in OCD have been conducted for over two decades. While intellectual function

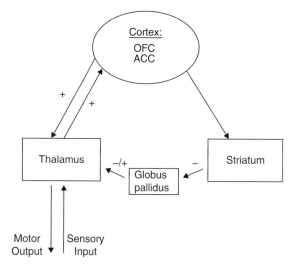

Figure 23.1. The cortico-striatal model of obsessive-compulsive disorder (adapted from Rauch *et al.*, 1998). The striatum projects via direct and indirect pathways through the globus pallidus to the thalamus which in turn projects to the neocortex. OFC = orbitofrontal cortex; ACC = anterior cingulate; excitatory connections are labeled +; inhibitory connections are labeled –.

in individuals with OCD appears to be preserved (Mataix-Cols *et al.*, 2002; Savage *et al.*, 1999, 2001), studies point to neuropsychological impairments in three cognitive domains: (1) visuospatial skills, (2) memory and (3) executive functioning.

Visuospatial skill

Visuospatial skill can be defined as the ability to perceive and manipulate objects in two- and three-dimensional space (Lezak, 1995). In OCD, impairments in this domain have been shown using a variety of tests including the Block Design subtest of the Wechsler Adult Intelligence Scale – Revised (WAIS-R; Christensen *et al.*, 1992; Head *et al.*, 1989; Hollander *et al.*, 1993), Cube Copying (Hollander *et al.*, 1990), Money's Road Map Test (Behar *et al.*, 1984), Figure Matching Test (Aronowitz *et al.*, 1994), Tactual Performance Test (Christensen *et al.*, 1992; Flor-Henry *et al.*, 1979; Insel *et al.*, 1983), Hooper Visual Organization Test (Boone *et al.*, 1991), Mental Rotations Test (Savage *et al.*, 1999), and the copy condition of the Rey–Osterrieth Complex Figure Test (RCFT; Behar *et al.*, 1984; Boone *et al.*, 1991).

Memory

Obsessive-compulsive disorder groups have been found to be impaired on both explicit and implicit

memory. Explicit memory refers to a type of memory for which contents can be declared (or brought) to mind, whereas implicit (or procedural) memory largely refers to non-conscious learning processes that take place outside an individual's awareness (Graf & Schacter, 1985). In the domain of explicit memory, impairments have been noted on a variety of tests of non-verbal memory, including the Visual Reproduction subtest of the WMS (Boone *et al.*, 1991; Christensen *et al.*, 1992), Delayed Recognition Span Test (Savage *et al.*, 1996), Benton Visual Retention Test (Aronowitz *et al.*, 1994; Cohen *et al.*, 1996), Recurring Figures Test (Zielinski *et al.*, 1991), Corsi's Block Test (Zielinski *et al.*, 1991), Memory Efficiency Battery (Dirson *et al.*, 1995), Stylus Maze Learning (Behar *et al.*, 1984), and recall conditions of the RCFT (Boone *et al.*, 1991; Deckersbach *et al.*, 2000; Savage *et al.*, 1999; 2000). More recently, there have been some findings about impaired performance in analogous tests of verbal learning and memory (Deckersbach *et al.*, 2000; Savage *et al.*, 2000) suggesting that memory impairments in OCD are not limited to non-verbal information.

For an event to be remembered it must be encoded, stored and consolidated over time, and then retrieved from storage (Kapur *et al.*, 1996). Encoding refers to the processes that convert a perceived event into an enduring cognitive representation. Retrieval is the process that reactivates a stored representation leading to the experience of explicit recollection of the past event (Kapur *et al.*, 1996). Findings suggest that OCD patients' problems affect primarily the ability to encode and retrieve new episodes, while the ability to store information over time appears to be preserved (Aronowitz *et al.*, 1994; Boone *et al.*, 1991; Cohen *et al.*, 1996; Savage *et al.*, 1999, 2000; Zielinski *et al.*, 1991). Processes of storage and retrieval can be disentangled by comparing an individual's free recall and recognition performance. Recognition tests usually require a subject to discriminate between original items and distractors. Presumably, they have fewer retrieval demands than tests of free recall. Intact recognition in the face of impaired free recall is indicative of retrieval but not retention (storage) difficulties. For example, Savage *et al.* (1996) examined recall and recognition memory and found that OCD patients were impaired on measures of non-verbal delayed recall but not on delayed recognition. Deckersbach *et al.* (2000), who used the Rey–Osterrieth Complex Figure Test, found that immediately following the initial copy trial, OCD patients had difficulties redrawing a complex geometric figure from memory. However, the comparison of recall drawings immediately following the copy trial and those obtained after a 20-minute delay indicated that patients did not have any difficulties in retaining information over the delay. Overall, these findings suggest that OCD patients have difficulties encoding and/or retrieving new memories while the ability to retain information once learned appears to be preserved.

Implicit memory in OCD has been investigated using the serial reaction time task (SRT; Nissen & Bullemer, 1987). The SRT involves the serial presentation of visual cues at one of four locations on a computer screen. Subjects respond to each cue by pressing one of four buttons on a keypad, each of which corresponds to one of the possible cue positions. While some of the sequences are random, others, unbeknownst to the subject, are presented repeatedly. Over time, subjects without explicit knowledge develop a reaction time advantage for repeated sequences, indicative of implicit memory. Neuroimaging studies have confirmed the involvement of the striatum in implicit sequence learning (Berns et al., 1997; Doyon et al., 1996; Grafton et al., 1995; Hazeltine et al., 1997; Rauch et al., 1995, 1997a, 1997b). In OCD, using the SRT and PET, consistent with the cortico-striatal model of OCD, Rauch et al. (1997b) found that OCD patients failed to activate the striatum and instead exhibited compensatory activation of medial temporal lobe structures (e.g. the hippocampal/parahippocampal region). The findings of aberrant medial temporal recruitment have been twice replicated with fMRI in independent samples (Rauch et al., 2001, 2007); the deficits in striatal recruitment have also been replicated and in a manner that suggests they may be most closely related to certain subtypes of OCD (Rauch et al., 2001, 2007). Recently, Kathmann et al. (2005) also using the SRT found impaired sequence learning in patients with OCD compared with healthy individuals. Fernandez et al. (2003) found impaired performance of OCD patients on the Tower of Hanoi task (a procedural learning task). This was associated with reduced regional cerebral blood flow in the left caudate nucleus. Interestingly, a functional neuroimaging study of the Tower task revealed deficient striatal recruitment and aberrant activation of medial temporal lobe regions in OCD (van den Heuvel et al., 2005), mirroring the results

using the SRT. This suggests that medial temporal lobe structures in procedural or implicit learning tasks are recruited to compensate for striatal dysfunction in OCD.

Executive function

The term executive function typically refers to a set of higher-order control processes that serve to control, regulate and guide lower-level processes in the service of planning and problem-solving. Investigators have long suspected that OCD is associated with executive function disturbances since so many of its central features are reminiscent of classic "frontal lobe" symptoms, such as behavioral inflexibility and stereotypy (Stuss & Benson, 1986). Impairments have been found (although inconsistently) in a variety of tests of executive functioning including the Trail Making Test, Part B (Aronowitz et al., 1994), the Category Test (Flor-Henry et al., 1979; Insel et al., 1983), visual attention tests (Dirson et al., 1995; Nelson et al., 1993), selective attention tests (Clayton et al., 1999), self-paced working-memory tests (Martin et al., 1995), Stroop (Hartston & Swerdlow, 1999), organizational measures from the RCFT (Behar et al., 1984; Deckersbach et al., 2000; Savage et al., 1999, 2000), the Wisconsin Card Sorting Test (WCST; Harvey, 1986; Head et al., 1989; Malloy, 1987 but see Abbruzzese et al., 1995b; Boone et al., 1991; Deckersbach et al., 2000; Gross-Isseroff et al., 1996; Zielinski et al., 1991 for non-significant findings) and the Object Alternation Test (OAT; Abbruzzese et al., 1995a; 1997; Gross-Isseroff et al., 1996). Overall, these measures tap into various aspects of executive functioning, such as the ability to plan, implement strategic action, and monitor and flexibly shift behavior when it is no longer appropriate.

Moderators of neuropsychological impairment

The inconsistency of results in the above-described studies suggests that other factors in addition to OCD also contribute to neuropsychological difficulties in afflicted individuals. Variables that have been discussed include OCD severity, chronicity, comorbidity, medication and OCD subtypes (or symptom dimensions). For example, Okasha et al. (2000) found that individuals with less severe OCD showed better selective attention than patients with more severe

OCD. In addition, longer duration of illness was associated with more pronounced impairment on tasks of visuospatial skill and non-verbal memory (Okasha et al., 2000). Likewise, Moritz et al. (2005) reported that impairments in tests of psychomotor speed, selected and divided attention were particularly pronounced in patients with severe OCD. Malloy (1987) noted that OCD patients who were impaired on the WCST were judged by clinicians to be "more psychotic" but Savage et al. (1999, 2000) did not find changes in the pattern of impairments when controlling for comorbidity. Abbruzzese et al. (1995b) found that medicated patients with OCD made more errors on the WCST than non-medicated OCD patients and also showed a lower level of conceptual responses, whereas in studies by Savage et al. (1999, 2000) selective serotonin reuptake inhibitor (SSRI) medicated OCD patients did not differ from non-medicated patients. Findings by Mataix-Cols et al. (2002) suggest a potentially more complex interaction between the type of medication and cognitive domain. They administered a comprehensive neuropsychological battery to assess general intelligence, attention, verbal and non-verbal working memory, declarative and procedural learning, visuoconstructive skills and executive functions. Serotonergic reuptake inhibitor (SRI) medicated OCD patients did not differ from SRI-free patients on any neuropsychological measure. However, there were significant interactions between SRIs and benzodiazepines on the perseverative errors of the WCST and on reaction times (Mataix-Cols et al., 2002). Specifically, OCD patients taking a SRI and a benzodiazepine medication made fewer perseverative errors than patients who were taking benzodiazepines alone.

With respect to OCD symptom dimensions or OCD subtypes, Rauch et al. (1998) found that the severity of checking compulsions/aggressive/religious/sexual obsessions was positively correlated with striatal activity during a continuous performance task, whereas there was a trend towards a negative correlation for symmetry and ordering compulsions (see also Rauch et al., 2007). This suggests that different symptom patterns may be associated with different types of striatal dysfunction. On the other hand, the few studies that used standardized neuropsychological tests, to our knowledge, have failed to find associations between neuropsychological impairment and OCD symptom dimensions or OCD subtypes. For example, Khanna & Vijaykumar (2000) compared

neuropsychological profiles of patients with predominantly washing or checking compulsions or pure obsessions, and failed to find differences between the groups on a battery of frontal lobe tests. Similarly, Deckersbach et al. (1999) examined the relationship between obsessive-compulsive symptom dimensions derived by Mataix-Cols et al. (1999) and performance on the California Verbal Learning Test (CVLT), and also found no significant associations between neuropsychological impairment and severity in distinct symptom dimensions. Another moderating variable that may account for the variability in findings of cognitive impairment in OCD is the use of cognitive strategies, which will be discussed in the following section.

Integrating domains of cognitive impairment

Neuropsychological tasks, especially those with higher levels of complexity, typically benefit from using cognitive strategies that enhance performance on such tasks. Recent studies in OCD suggest that some of the cognitive impairments found in the earlier described domains may be due to impairments in using cognitive strategies. For example, Veale et al. (1996) used the Tower of London Test to show that OCD subjects had delays generating alternate strategies following initially incorrect responses. They attributed this slowing to difficulty in shifting mental set. Schmidtke et al. (1998) reported that OCD subjects were impaired on measures of controlled attention (a Digit Connection Task) and strategic flexibility (Weight Sorting Task). Likewise, Purcell et al. (1998a, 1998b) found that OCD patients experienced difficulties on computerized measures of spatial working memory, especially those that required the ability to organize and execute strategies in the presence of minimal external structure. Difficulties in the ability to organize verbal and non-verbal information may also in part account for OCD patients' difficulties in tasks assessing visuospatial skills and memory. For example, our group has used the RCFT (see Figure 23.2). The RCFT is a widely used measure of visuospatial construction and non-verbal memory. In the RCFT participants are asked to copy a complex geometric figure and subsequently redraw this figure from memory. One of the critical aspects of this test is that organizing the figure into meaningful perceptual units (e.g. a large rectangle, diagonals etc.) during

(A) Rey–Osterrieth Complex Figure   (B) California Verbal Learning Test

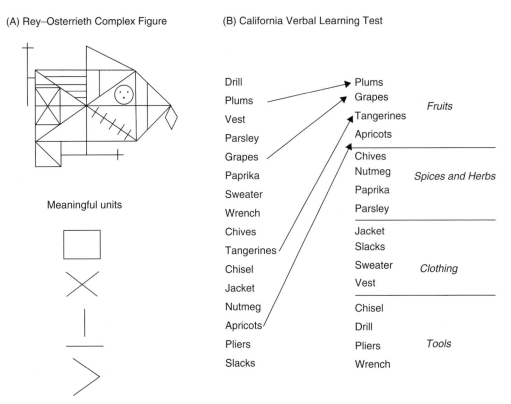

Figure 23.2. (A) The complex figure used in the Rey–Osterrieth Complex Figure Test (RCFT); meaningful organizational units are shown beneath the figure; (B) The word list used in the California Verbal Learning Test (Delis *et al.*, 1987). Words stem from four different semantic categories (fruits, spices/herbs, clothing, tools).

copy enhances its subsequent free recall from memory (see Figure 23.2). Savage *et al.* (1999) found that individuals with OCD organize the figure less well than controls during encoding (copy) associated with subsequent difficulties redrawing the figure from memory (see also Mataix-Cols *et al.*, 2003; Moritz *et al.*, 2005). Similar findings were observed in the domain of verbal memory using the CVLT. The CVLT involves learning a list of 16 words as well as long-delayed recall. Words in the list stem from four different categories (tools, spices/herbs, fruits, clothing) and are presented in a manner that a word from a given category is never followed by a word from the same category (see Figure 23.2). Grouping the words into their semantic categories during list presentation typically enhances subsequent recall from memory. This strategy is called semantic clustering. Deckersbach *et al.* (2000) and Savage *et al.* (2000) found that OCD patients use semantic strategies less than healthy individuals. This impairment may account for subsequent difficulties recalling the CVLT word list after the long delay.

Thus, it is conceivable that some of the observed impairments in visuospatial skill and memory may be secondary to impairments in executive functions, especially impairments in using cognitive strategies that typically enhance cognitive performance, particularly in complex and not well-structured tasks.

The role of cognitive strategies in OCD

Employing cognitive strategies in the service of enhancing one's performance for a task is a complex process that involves multiple steps. Different brain regions contribute to strategy initiation and implementation (Savage *et al.*, 2001). For example, neuroimaging studies investigating the use of organizational strategies during encoding have consistently demonstrated involvement of the dorsolateral prefrontal cortex (DLPFC) and inferior prefrontal cortex (IPFC) during the implementation of encoding strategies (Fletcher *et al.*, 1998; Savage *et al.*, 2001; Wagner *et al.*, 2001). Encoding studies typically explicitly instruct participants to use a particular encoding strategy. Savage *et al.* (2001) found that the degree to which healthy individuals spontaneously initiated a semantic clustering strategy during list-learning (without instruction to do so) was associated with the degree of activation in the OFC, a brain region involved in the pathophysiology of OCD (see Figure 23.1). This suggests that the OFC is involved in aspects of strategy initiation whereas other brain regions such as the DLPFC and IPFC mediate processes directly involved in strategy implementation. This view is consistent with findings from other animal and human studies. For example, the animal literature has implicated the OFC in operations underlying the motivational control of goal-directed behavior (Tremblay & Schultz, 1999), including stimulus-reward reversal and monitoring the incentive value of potential reinforcers (Dias *et al.*, 1997; Gallagher *et al.*, 1999; Tremblay & Schultz, 1999). For instance, Dias *et al.* (1997) reported that OFC lesions in monkeys impaired stimulus-reward reversals, but only during the first reversal trial. Furthermore, studies of odor discrimination learning in rats have shown that OFC neurons fire in anticipation of rewarding and aversive outcomes, early in the course of training, before reliable behavioral discriminations have developed (Lipton *et al.*, 1999; Schoenbaum *et al.*, 1998). These and other animal studies suggest a role of the OFC in early processes of tasks in the service of guiding behavior based on anticipation of future events (Schoenbaum *et al.*, 1998). Humans with lesions in the OFC often demonstrate subtle, but functionally devastating cognitive impairments (Eslinger & Damasio, 1985; Rolls, 1996; Rolls *et al.*, 1994). These difficulties have been demonstrated in the context of so-called "gambling-paradigms" (Bechara *et al.*, 1996, 1997, 1998, 1999) where patients with OFC lesions consistently fail to adopt a strategy that prevents long-term loss. This suggests that OFC lesions impair the ability to anticipate future consequences in unstructured situations. Functional imaging studies specifically targeting the OFC have found increased OFC activation associated with conditions in which subjects had to inhibit previously learned stimulus-response associations on a test of visuospatial orientation (Nobre *et al.*, 1999). This finding is consistent with other evidence in humans that the OFC mediates the ability to inhibit previously reinforced responses and shift mental set (Freedman *et al.*, 1998). The OFC has also been implicated with fMRI in "guessing" operations on a task, based on the

Bechara/Damasio gambling paradigm, in which subjects were instructed to make their best educated "guess" regarding the upcoming card suit or color (Elliott *et al.*, 1999). Specifically, OFC activation was associated with increased guessing demands, as subjects had to factor in past instances of success and failure over a number of trials to predict what the next card would be. Rogers *et al.* (1999) used a computerized "risk taking" task very similar to the Bechara/Damasio gambling paradigm. During scanning, subjects had to choose small, high-probability rewards over large, low-probability rewards. The resolution of conflicts between these competing choices was associated with activations in the right OFC and IPFC. Damasio (1996) has hypothesized that problems in OFC-lesioned patients reflect difficulty in operations that involve inhibiting immediately reinforcing responses to form a plan based on appreciation of future consequences. The "somatic marker" hypothesis proposes that OFC monitors somatic or emotional states and uses this information to allocate processing resources so that executive systems can engage effective strategies (Damasio, 1996). Anatomically, posterior OFC has reciprocal connections with limbic structures such as the amygdala, while anterior regions of OFC are predominately connected with association cortex, such as the DLPFC and anterior cingulate (Zald & Kim, 1996). The OFC is, therefore, anatomically positioned as a convergence zone for emotional (limbic) and cognitive (prefrontal) information. It is connected in such a way as to use limbic information to determine the motivational significance of stimuli and then initiate executive processes mediated in other regions of the prefrontal cortex. These abilities are most critical in novel or unstructured situations in which individuals must resolve conflicts between competing choices on the basis of ambiguous or competing information (Bechara *et al.*, 1998).

Taken together, there is evidence that OFC mediates the early inhibition of automatic behavior in favor of developing a plan for future action, especially in novel or ambiguous situations. In this context, the OFC may specifically subserve the inhibition of automatic processing, thus enabling engagement of deliberate strategic processing. Consistent with this view, a recent study by our group found that individuals with OCD were impaired in the spontaneous use of a verbal learning strategy in an unstructured verbal learning task, but did not exhibit difficulties when instructed which learning strategies to use (Deckersbach *et al.*, 2005). That is, OCD patients had difficulties spontaneously initiating a semantic clustering encoding strategy when learning a list of words, whereas there was no impairment in implementing such a strategy once instructed to do so, to the extent that their performance was indistinguishable from control participants (Deckersbach *et al.*, 2005).

Taken together, the ability to inhibit ongoing cognitive processes in favor of initiating other (strategic) cognitive processes may be a central deficit in OCD, thereby accounting for some of the variability found in studies investigating neuropsychological impairment in this disorder.

Error monitoring in OCD

Recently, there has been renewed interest in the concept of faulty action monitoring processes involved in OCD. Early studies investigating this concept had failed to demonstrate impairment in patients with OCD (Brown *et al.*, 1994; McNally & Kohlbeck, 1993). However, studies assessing event-related potentials or using fMRI have found increased activations in the dorsal ACC in patients with OCD following errors of commission in cognitive tasks (Gehring *et al.*, 2000; Johannes *et al.*, 2001; Ursu *et al.*, 2003). The dorsal ACC in multiple neuroimaging studies has been implicated in processes of error monitoring/detection (Carter *et al.*, 1998, 2000). Maltby *et al.* (2005) using a Go–No Go task and fMRI found increased dorsal ACC activation in individuals with OCD compared with healthy control participants despite correct performance. As suggested by Maltby *et al.* (2005), increased dorsal ACC activation in OCD may reflect exaggerated or false error signals (even when actions were performed correctly) that may contribute to compulsive behaviors. This interpretation is consistent with findings by Tolin *et al.* (2001) who found that in OCD confidence in memory decreases with repeated study test trials.

Conclusion and future directions

Neuropsychological studies have most consistently demonstrated cognitive impairments in OCD in the domains of visuospatial skill, memory and executive functioning, although findings vary considerably across studies. Difficulties using cognitive strategies, which would normally enhance performance on cognitive tasks, appear to be a significant impairment

that contributes to poorer performance on neuropsychological measures, and perhaps everyday functioning. Some findings suggest that individuals with OCD may be predominantly characterized by difficulties initiating cognitive strategies, whereas the ability to carry them out appears to be preserved. The notion of impaired capacity for inhibiting ongoing cognitive processes in favor of executing cognitive tasks may be one reason why considerable variability of impairments in neuropsychological studies of OCD is reported. It may even account for some of the variability found in imaging studies of OCD, which often identify abnormal OFC function. Future studies are needed to investigate how abnormal OFC functioning, memory impairments and exaggerated error signals associated with aberrant ACC activation, interact and lead to intrusive thoughts and ritualistic behaviors in OCD. In addition, the role of comorbidities, chronicity, symptom subtypes and medications and their association to neuropsychological impairment in OCD should be further explored.

References

Abbruzzese, M., Bellodi, L., Ferri, S. & Scarone, S. (1995a). Frontal lobe dysfunction in schizophrenia and obsessive-compulsive disorder: a neuropsychological study. *Brain and Cognition*, **27**, 202–212.

Abbruzzese, M., Ferri, S. & Scarone, S. (1995b). Wisconsin Card Sorting Test performance in obsessive-compulsive disorder: no evidence for involvement of dorsolateral prefrontal cortex. *Psychiatry Research*, **58**, 37–43.

Abbruzzese, M., Ferri, S. & Scarone, S. (1997). The selective breakdown of frontal functions in patients with obsessive-compulsive disorder and in patients with schizophrenia: a double dissociation experimental finding. *Neuropsychologia*, **35**, 907–912.

Adler, C. M., McDonough-Ryan, P., Sax, K. W. *et al.* (2000). fMRI of neuronal activation with symptom provocation in unmedicated patients with obsessive compulsive disorder. *Psychiatry Research*, **34**, 317–324.

Anderson, K. E. & Savage, C. R. (2004). Cognitive and neurobiological findings in obsessive-compulsive disorder. *Psychiatric Clinics of North America*, **27**, 37–47.

Aronowitz, B. R., Hollander, E., DeCaria, C. *et al.* (1994). Neuropsychology of obsessive-compulsive disorder: preliminary findings. *Neuropsychiatry, Neuropsychology and Behavioral Neurology*, **7**, 81–86.

Baxter, L. R., Phelps, M. E., Mazziotta, J. C. *et al.* (1987). Local cerebral glucose metabolic rates in obsessive compulsive disorder: a comparison with rates in unipolar depression and in normal controls. *Archives of General Psychiatry*, **44**, 211–218.

Baxter, L., Schwartz, J., Mazziotta, J. *et al.* (1988). Cerebral glucose metabolic rates in nondepressed patients with obsessive-compulsive disorder. *American Journal of Psychiatry*, **145**, 1560–1563.

Baxter, L. R. Jr., Schwartz, J. M., Bergman, K. S. *et al.* (1992). Caudate glucose metabolic rate changes with both drug and behavior therapy for obsessive-compulsive disorder. *Archives of General Psychiatry*, **49**, 681–689.

Bechara, A., Damasio, H., Damasio, A. R. & Lee, G. P. (1999). Different contributions of the human amygdala and ventromedial prefrontal cortex to decision-making. *Journal of Neuroscience*, **19**, 5473–5481.

Bechara, A., Damasio, H., Tranel, D. & Anderson, S. W. (1998). Dissociation of working memory from decision making within the human prefrontal cortex. *Journal of Neuroscience*, **18**, 428–437.

Bechara, A., Damasio, H., Tranel, D. & Damasio, A. R. (1997). Deciding advantageously before knowing the advantageous strategy. *Science*, **275**, 1293–1294.

Bechara, A., Tranel, D., Damasio, H. & Damasio, A. R. (1996). Failure to respond autonomically to anticipated future outcomes following damage to prefrontal cortex. *Cerebral Cortex*, **6**, 215–225.

Behar, D., Rapoport, J. L., Berg, C. J. *et al.* (1984). Computerized tomography and neuropsychological test measures in adolescents with obsessive-compulsive disorder. *American Journal of Psychiatry*, **141**, 363–369.

Benkelfat, C., Nordahl, T. E., Semple, W. E. *et al.* (1990). Local cerebral glucose metabolic rates in obsessive-compulsive disorder: patients treated with clomipramine. *Archives of General Psychiatry*, **47**, 840–848.

Berns, G. S., Cohen, J. D. & Mintun, M. A. (1997). Brain regions responsive to novelty in the absence of awareness. *Science*, **276**, 1272–1275.

Boone, K. B., Ananth, J., Philpott, L., Kaur, A. & Djenderedjian, A. (1991). Neuropsychological characteristics of nondepressed adults with obsessive-compulsive disorder. *Neuropsychiatry, Neuropsychology and Behavioral Neurology*, **4**, 96–109.

Breiter, H. C., Rauch, S. L., Kwong, K. K. *et al.* (1996). Functional magnetic resonance imaging of symptom provocation in obsessive compulsive disorder. *Archives of General Psychiatry*, **53**, 595–606.

Brody, A. L., Saxena, S., Schwartz, J. M. *et al.* (1998). FDG-PET predictors of response to behavioral therapy versus pharmacotherapy in obsessive-compulsive disorder. *Psychiatry Reseach Neuroimaging*, **84**, 1–6.

Brown, H. D., Kosslyn, S. M., Breiter, H. C., Baer, L. & Jenike, M. A. (1994). Can patients with obsessive-compulsive disorder discriminate between percepts and mental images? A signal detection analysis. *Journal of Abnormal Psychology*, **103**, 445–454.

Carter, C. S., Braver, T. S., Barch, D. M. *et al.* (1998). Anterior cingulate cortex, error detection, and the online monitoring of performance. *Science*, **280**, 747–749.

Carter, C. S., Macdonald, A. M., Botvinick, M. *et al.* (2000). Parsing executive processes: strategic vs. evaluative functions of the anterior cingulate cortex. *Proceedings of the National Academy of Sciences USA*, **97**, 1944–1948.

Christensen, K. J., Kim, S. W., Dysken, M. W. & Hoover, K. M. (1992). Neuropsychological performance in obsessive-compulsive disorder. *Biological Psychiatry*, **31**, 4–18.

Clayton, I. C., Richards, J. C. & Edwards, C. J. (1999). Selective attention in obsessive-compulsive disorder. *Journal of Abnormal Psychology*, **108**, 171–175.

Cohen, L. J., Hollander, E., DeCaria, C. M. *et al.* (1996). Specificity of neuropsychological impairment in obsessive-compulsive disorder: a comparison with social phobic and normal control subjects. *Journal of Neuropsychiatry and Clinical Neuroscience*, **8**, 82–85.

Damasio, A. R. (1996). The somatic marker hypothesis and the possible functions of prefrontal cortex. *Philosophical Transactions of the Royal Society of London*, **351**, 1413–1420.

Deckersbach, T., Otto, M. W., Savage, C. R., Baer, L. & Jenike, M. A. (2000). The relationship between semantic organization and memory in obsessive-compulsive disorder. *Psychotherapy and Psychosomatics*, **69**, 101–107.

Deckersbach, T., Savage, C. R., Curran, T. *et al.* (2002). A study of parallel implicit and explicit information processing in patients with obsessive-compulsive disorder. *American Journal of Psychiatry*, **159**, 1780–1782.

Deckersbach, T., Savage, C. R., Dougherty, D. D. *et al.* (2005). Spontaneous and directed application of verbal learning strategies in bipolar disorder and obsessive-compulsive disorder. *Bipolar Disorders*, **7**, 166–175.

Deckersbach, T., Savage, C. R., Mataix-Cols, D. *et al.* (1999). *Verbal memory in OCD subtypes*. Poster presented at the 33rd Annual Convention of the Association for the Advancement of Behavior Therapy, New York.

Delis, D. C., Kramer, J. H., Kaplan, E. & Ober, B. A. (1987). *The California Verbal Learning Test: Research Edition Adult Version*. San Antonio, CA: The Psychological Corporation.

Dias, R., Robbins, T. W. & Roberts, A. C. (1997). Dissociable forms of inhibitory control within prefrontal cortex with an analog of the Wisconsin Card Sort Test: restriction to novel situations and independence from "on-line" processing. *Journal of Neuroscience*, **17**, 9285–9297.

Dirson, S., Bouvard, M., Cottraux, J. & Martin, R. (1995). Visual memory impairment in patients with obsessive-compulsive disorder: a controlled study. *Psychotherapy and Psychosomatics*, **63**, 22–31.

Doyon, J., Owen, A. M., Petrides, M., Sziklas, V. & Evans, A. C. (1996). Functional anatomy of visuomotor skill learning in human subjects examined with positron emission tomography. *European Journal of Neuroscience*, **8**, 637–648.

Elliott, R., Rees, G. & Dolan, R. J. (1999). Ventromedial prefrontal cortex mediates guessing. *Neuropsychologia*, **37**, 403–411.

Eslinger, P. J. & Damasio, A. R. (1985). Severe disturbance of higher cognition after bilateral frontal lobe ablation: patient EVR. *Neurology*, **35**, 1731–1741.

Fernandez, A., Pino Alonso, M., Mataix-Cols, D. *et al.* (2003). Neuroactivation of the Tower of Hanoi in patients with obsessive-compulsive disorder and healthy volunteers. *Revista Española de Medicina Nuclear*, **22**, 376–385.

Fletcher, P. C., Shallice, T. & Dolan, R. J. (1998). The functional roles of prefrontal cortex in episodic memory. I. encoding. *Brain*, **121**, 1239–1248.

Flor-Henry, P., Yeudall, L. T., Koles, Z. J. & Howarth, B. G. (1979). Neuropsychological and power spectral EEG investigations of the obsessive-compulsive syndrome. *Biological Psychiatry*, **14**, 119–130.

Gallagher, M., McMahan, R. W. & Schoenbaum, G. (1999). Orbitofrontal cortex and representation of incentive value in associative learning. *Journal of Neuroscience*, **19**, 6610–6614.

Gehring, W. J., Himle, J. & Nisenson, L. G. (2000). Action-monitoring dysfunction in obsessive-compulsive disorder. *Psychological Science*, **11**, 1–6.

Graf, P. & Schacter, D. L. (1985). Implicit and explicit memory for new associations in normal and amnestic subjects. *Journal of Experimental Psychology, Learning Memory and Cognition*, **13**, 45–53.

Grafton, S. T., Hazeltine, E. & Ivry, R. (1995). Functional mapping of sequence learning in normal humans. *Journal of Cognitive Neuroscience*, **7**, 497–510.

Gross-Isseroff, R., Sasson, Y., Voet, H. *et al.* (1996). Alternation learning in obsessive-compulsive disorder. *Biological Psychiatry*, **39**, 733–738.

Hartston, H. J. & Swerdlow, N. R. (1999). Visuospatial priming and Stroop performance in patients with obsessive-compulsive disorder. *Neuropsychology*, **13**, 447–457.

Harvey, N. S. (1986). Impaired cognitive set-shifting in obsessive-compulsive neurosis. *IRCS Medical Science*, **14**, 936–937.

Hazeltine, E., Grafton, S. T. & Ivry, R. (1997). Attention and stimulus characteristics determine the locus of motor-sequence encoding: a PET study. *Brain*, **120**, 123–140.

Head, D., Bolton, D. & Hymas, N. (1989). Deficit in cognitive shifting ability in patients with obsessive-compulsive disorders. *Biological Psychiatry*, **25**, 929–937.

Hoehn-Saric, R., Pearlson, G. D., Harris, G. J., Machlin, S. R. & Camargo, E. E. (1991). Effects of fluoxetine on regional cerebral blood flow in obsessive-compulsive patients. *American Journal of Psychiatry*, **148**, 1243–1245.

Hollander, E., Cohen, L., Richards, M. *et al.* (1993). A pilot study of the neuropsychology of obsessive-compulsive disorder and parkinson's disease: basal ganglia disorders. *Journal of Neuropsychiatry and Clinical Neuroscience*, **5**, 104–106.

Hollander, E., Schiffman, E., Cohen, B. *et al.* (1990). Signs of central nervous system dysfunction in obsessive-compulsive disorder. *Archives of General Psychiatry*, **47**, 27–32.

Insel, T. R., Donnely, E. F., Lalakea, M. L., Alterman, I. S. & Murphy, D. L. (1983). Neurological and neuropsychological studies of patients with obsessive-compulsive disorder. *Biological Psychiatry*, **18**, 741–751.

Johannes, S., Wieringa, B. M., Nager, W. *et al.* (2001). Discrepant target detection and action monitoring in obsessive-compulsive disorder. *Psychiatry Research*, **108**, 101–110.

Kapur, S., Tulving, E., Cabeza, R. *et al.* (1996). The neural correlates of intentional learning of verbal materials: a PET study in humans. *Cognitive Brain Research*, **4**, 243–249.

Kathmann, N., Rupertseder, C., Hauke, W. & Zaudig, M. (2005). Implicit sequence learning in obsessive-compulsive disorder: further support for the fronto-striatal dysfunction model. *Biological Psychiatry*, **58**, 239–244.

Khanna, S. & Vijaykumar, D. R. (2000). Neuropsychology of obsessive compulsive disorder. *Biological Psychiatry*, **47**, 127S.

Lezak, M. D. (1995). *Neuropsychological Assessment* (3rd edn.). New York, NY: Oxford University Press.

Lipton, P. A., Alvarez, P. & Eichenbaum, H. (1999). Crossmodal associative memory representations in rodent orbitofrontal cortex. *Neuron*, **22**, 349–359.

Machlin, S. R., Harris, G. J., Pearlson, G. D. *et al.* (1991). Elevated medial-frontal cerebral blood flow in obsessive-compulsive patients: a SPECT study. *American Journal of Psychiatry*, **148**, 1240–1242.

Malloy. P. (1987). Frontal lobe dysfunction in obsessive-compulsive disorder. In E. Perecmann (Ed.), *The Frontal Lobes Revisited* (pp. 207–223). New York, NY: IRBN Press.

Maltby, N., Tolin, D. F., Worhunsky, P., O'Keefe, T. M. & Kiehl, K. A. (2005). Dysfunctional action monitoring hyperactivates frontal-striatal circuits in obsessive-compulsive disorder: an event-related fMRI study. *Neuroimage*, **24**, 495–503.

Martin, A., Wiggs, C. L., Altemus, M., Rubenstein, C. & Murphy, D. (1995). Working memory as assessed by subject-ordered tasks in patients with obsessive-compulsive disorder. *Journal of Clinical and Experimental Neuropsychology*, **17**, 786–792.

Mataix-Cols, D., Alonso, P., Hernandez, R. *et al.* (2003). Relation of neurological soft signs to nonverbal memory performance in obsessive-compulsive disorder. *Journal of Clinical and Experimental Neuropsychology*, **25**, 842–851.

Mataix-Cols, D., Alonso, P., Pifarre, J., Menchon, J. M. & Vallejo, J. (2002). Neuropsychological performance in medicated vs. unmedicated patients with obsessive-compulsive disorder. *Psychiatry Research*, **109**, 255–264.

Mataix-Cols, D., Rauch, S. L., Manzo, P. A., Jenike, M. A. & Baer, L. (1999). Use of factor-analyzed symptom dimensions to predict outcome with serotonin reuptake inhibitors and placebo in the treatment of obsessive-compulsive disorder. *American Journal of Psychiatry*, **156**, 1409–1416.

Mataix-Cols, D., Wooderson, S., Lawrence, N. *et al.* (2004). Distinct neural correlates of washing, checking, and hoarding symptom dimensions in obsessive-compulsive disorder. *Archives of General Psychiatry*, **61**, 564–576.

McNally, R. J. & Kohlbeck, P. A. (1993). Reality monitoring in obsessive-compulsive disorder. *Behaviour Research and Therapy*, **31**, 249–253.

Moritz, S., Kloss, M., Jacobsen, D. *et al.* (2005). Extent, profile and specificity of visuospatial impairment in obsessive-compulsive disorder (OCD). *Journal of Clinical and Experimental Neuropsychology*, **27**, 795–814.

Nelson, E., Early, T. S. & Haller, J. W. (1993). Visual attention in obsessive-compulsive disorder. *Psychiatry Research*, **49**, 183–196.

Nissen, M. J. & Bullemer, P. (1987). Attentional requirements of learning: evidence from performance based measures. *Cognitive Psychology*, **19**, 1–32.

Nobre, A. C., Coull, J. T., Frith, C. D. & Mesulam, M. M. (1999). Orbitofrontal cortex is activated during breaches of expectation in tasks of visual attention. *Nature Neuroscience*, **2**, 11–12.

Nordahl, T. E., Benkelfat, C., Semple, W. *et al.* (1989). Cerebral glucose metabolic rates in obsessive-compulsive disorder. *Neuropsychopharmacology*, **2**, 23–28.

Okasha, A., Rafaat, M., Mahallawy, N. *et al.* (2000). Cognitive dysfunction in obsessive-compulsive disorder. *Acta Psychiatrica Scandinavica*, **101**, 281–285.

Perani, D., Colombo, C., Bressi, S. *et al.* (1995). FDG PET study in obsessive-compulsive disorder: a clinical metabolic correlation study after treatment. *British Journal of Psychiatry*, **166**, 244–250.

Purcell, R., Maruff, P., Kyrios, M. & Pantelis, C. (1998a). Cognitive deficits in obsessive-compulsive disorder on tests of frontal-striatal function. *Biological Psychiatry*, **43**, 348–357.

Purcell, R., Maruff, P., Kyrios, M. & Pantelis, C. (1998b). Neuropsychological deficits in obsessive-compulsive disorder: a comparison with unipolar depression, panic disorder, and normal controls. *Archives of General Psychiatry*, **55**, 415–423.

Rauch, S. L., Dougherty, D. D., Shin, L. M. *et al.* (1998). Neural correlates of factor-analyzed OCD symptom dimensions: a PET study. *CNS Spectrums*, **3**, 37–43.

Rauch, S. L., Jenike, M. A., Alpert, N. M. *et al.* (1994). Regional cerebral blood flow measured during symptom provocation in obsessive-compulsive disorder using ^{15}O-labeled CO_2 and positron emission tomography. *Archives of General Psychiatry*, **51**, 62–70.

Rauch, S. L., Savage, C. R., Alpert, N. M. *et al.* (1997a). Probing striatal function in obsessive compulsive disorder: a PET study of implicit sequence learning. *Journal of Neuropsychiatry and Clinical Neurosciences*, **9**, 568–573.

Rauch, S. L., Savage, C. R., Brown, H. D. *et al.* (1995). A PET investigation of implicit and explicit sequence learning. *Human Brain Mapping*, **3**, 271–286.

Rauch, S. L., Shin, L. M., Dougherty, D. D. *et al.* (2002). Predictors of fluvoxamine response in contamination-related obsessive compulsive disorder: a PET symptom provocation study. *Neuropsychopharmacology*, **27**, 782–791.

Rauch, S. L., Wedig, M. M., Wright, C. I. *et al.* (2007). Functional magnetic resonance imaging study of regional brain activation during implicit sequence learning in obsessive-compulsive disorder. *Biological Psychiatry*, **61**, 330–336.

Rauch, S. L., Whalen, P. J., Curran, T. *et al.* (2001). Probing striato-thalamic function in obsessive-compulsive disorder and Tourette syndrome using neuroimaging methods. *Advances in Neurology*, **85**, 207–224.

Rauch, S. L., Whalen, P. J., Dougherty, D. D. & Jenike, M. A. (1988). Neurobiological models of obsessive compulsive disorders. In M. A. Jenike, L. Baer & W. E. Minichiello (Eds.), *Obsessive-Compulsive Disorders: Practical Management* (3rd edn.) (pp. 222–253). St Louis, MO: Mosby.

Rauch, S. L., Whalen, P. J., Savage, C. R. *et al.* (1997b). Striatal recruitment during an implicit sequence learning task as measured by functional magnetic resonance imaging. *Human Brain Mapping*, **5**, 124–132.

Rogers, R. D., Owen, A. M., Middleton, H. C. *et al.* (1999). Choosing between small, likely rewards and large, unlikely rewards activates inferior and orbital prefrontal cortex. *Journal of Neuroscience*, **20**, 9029–9038.

Rolls, E. T. (1996). The orbitofrontal cortex. *Philosophical Transactions of the Royal Society of London*, **351**, 1433–1444.

Rolls, E. T., Hornak, J. & McGrath, W. J. (1994). Emotion-related learning in patients with social and emotional changes associated with frontal lobe damage. *Journal of Neurology, Neurosurgery and Psychiatry*, **57**, 1518–1524.

Rubin, R. T., Villaneuva-Myer, J., Ananth, J., Trajmar, P. G. & Mena, I. (1992). Regional xenon-133 cerebral blood flow and cerebral Technetium 99m HMPAO uptake in unmedicated patients with obsessive-compulsive disorder and matched normal control subjects. *Archives of General Psychiatry*, **49**, 695–702.

Savage, C. R. (1998). Neuropsychology of obsessive-compulsive disorder: research findings and treatment implications. In M. A. Jenike, L. Baer & W. E. Minichiello (Eds.), *Obsessive-Compulsive Disorders: Practical Management* (3rd edn.), (pp. 254–275). St Louis, MO: Mosby.

Savage, C. R., Baer, L., Keuthen, N. J. *et al.* (1999). Organizational strategies mediate nonverbal memory impairment in obsessive-compulsive disorder. *Biological Psychiatry*, **45**, 905–916.

Savage, C. R., Deckersbach, T., Heckers, S. *et al.* (2001): Prefrontal regions supporting spontaneous and directed application of verbal learning strategies. Evidence from PET. *Brain*, **124**, 219–231.

Savage, C. R., Deckersbach, T., Wilhelm, S. *et al.* (2000). Strategic processing and episodic memory impairment in obsessive-compulsive disorder. *Neuropsychology*, **14**, 141–151.

Savage, C. R., Keuthen, N. J., Jenike, M. A. *et al.* (1996). Recall and recognition memory in obsessive-compulsive disorder. *Journal of Neuropsychiatry and Clinical Neuroscience*, **8**, 99–103.

Saxena, S., Brody, A. L., Maidment, K. M. *et al.* (1999). Localized orbitofrontal and subcortical metabolic changes and predictors of response to paroxetine treatment in obsessive-compulsive disorder. *Neuropsychopharmacology*, **21**, 683–693.

Saxena, S., Brody, A. L., Maidment, K. M. *et al.* (2004). Cerebral glucose metabolism in obsessive-compulsive hoarding. *American Journal of Psychiatry*, **161**, 1038–1048.

Schmidtke, K., Schorb, A., Winkelmann, G. & Hohagen, F. (1998). Cognitive frontal lobe dysfunction in obsessive-compulsive disorder. *Biological Psychiatry*, **43**, 666–673.

Schoenbaum, G., Chiba, A. A. & Gallagher, M. (1998). Orbitofrontal cortex and basolateral amygdala encode expected outcomes during learning. *Nature Neuroscience*, **1**, 155–159.

Schwartz, J. M., Stoessel, P. W., Baxter, L. R. Jr., Martin, K. M. & Phelps, M. E. (1996). Systematic changes in cerebral glucose metabolic rate after successful behavior modification. *Archives of General Psychiatry*, **53**, 109–113.

Stuss, D. T. & Benson, D. F. (1986). *The Frontal Lobes.* New York: Raven Press.

Swedo, S. E., Shapiro, M. B., Grady, C. L. *et al.* (1989). Cerebral glucose metabolism in childhood-onset obsessive-compulsive disorder. *Archives of General Psychiatry*, **46**, 518–523.

Tolin, D. F., Abramowitz, J. S., Brigidi, B. D. *et al.* (2001). Memory and memory confidence in obsessive-compulsive disorder. *Behaviour Research and Therapy*, **39**, 913–927.

Tremblay, L. & Schultz, W. (1999). Relative reward preference in primate orbitofrontal cortex. *Nature*, **398**, 704–708.

Ursu, S., Stenger, V. A., Shear, M. K., Jones, M. R. & Carter, C. S. (2003). Overactive action monitoring in obsessive-compulsive disorder: evidence from functional magnetic resonance imaging. *Psychological Science*, **14**, 347–353.

van den Heuvel, O. A., Veltman, D. J., Groenewegen, H. J. *et al.* (2005). Disorder-specific neuroanatomical correlates of attentional bias in obsessive-compulsive disorder, panic disorder, and hypochondriasis. *Archives of General Psychiatry*, **62**, 922–933.

Veale, D. M., Sahakian, B. J., Owen, A. M. & Marks, I. M. (1996). Specific cognitive deficits in tests sensitive to frontal lobe dysfunction in obsessive-compulsive disorder. *Psychological Medicine*, **26**, 1261–1269.

Wagner, A. D., Maril, A., Bjork, R. A. & Schacter, D. L. (2001). Prefrontal contributions to executive control. fMRI evidence for functional distinctions within lateral prefrontal cortex. *Neuroimage*, **14**, 1337–1347.

Zald, D. H. & Kim, S. W. (1996). Anatomy and function of the orbital frontal cortex, I: Anatomy, neurocircuitry, and obsessive-compulsive disorder. *Journal of Neuropsychiatry and Clinical Neuroscience*, **8**, 125–138.

Zielinski, C. M., Taylor, M. A. & Juzwin, K. R. (1991). Neuropsychological deficits in obsessive-compulsive disorder. *Neuropsychiatry, Neuropsychology, and Behavioral Neurology*, **4**, 110–126.

Neuropsychological investigation in mood disorders

Paul Keedwell, Simon A. Surguladze and Mary Philips

Introduction

In this chapter we will consider the various approaches to defining neuropsychological abnormalities underlying major depressive disorder and bipolar disorder. We will consider the methodological limitations, the implications for defining vulnerability markers and the priorities for further research.

Major depressive disorder

Introduction

Major depressive disorder (MDD) remains one of the most debilitating psychiatric illnesses worldwide with an estimated lifetime prevalence of 16% (Kessler *et al.*, 2003). By the year 2020 depressive disorder is predicted to become the second largest cause of disability after ischemic heart disease (World Health Organization, 1999). Major depressive disorder is associated with lost productivity, physical morbidity and suicide (Üstün & Chatterji 2001). Each depressive episode increases risk for subsequent episodes (Mueller *et al.*, 1999; Solomon *et al.*, 1997). Depression is thought to occur due to an interaction between a genetic diathesis and environmental stress (Andreasen, 1997; Caspi *et al.*, 2003; Kendler, 1998). However, there are problems with defining a valid phenotypic marker for genetic vulnerability (a "trait marker"). Such a marker should persist throughout episodes of illness and remission, co-segregate within families of affected individuals, and bear some conceptual relationship to MDD (Kraemer *et al.*, 2002). If found it could help to define the endophenotype – a neurological target for treatment.

Negative cognitions

Information processing models focus on cognitive processes that guide the selection, transformation, encoding, storage, retrieval and generation of information. These models suggest that negative cognitive biases are essential elements of depression (state phenomena), but they may also represent predisposing factors in vulnerable individuals (trait phenomena). Thus, cognitive theories of depression propose that negatively biased associative processing, especially negative self-referent information, confers cognitive vulnerability to depression (Abramson *et al.*, 1989; Beck *et al.*, 1979; Ingram *et al.*, 1998; Teasdale, 1988). Paradigms that uncover these neurocognitive vulnerability factors could be amenable to integration with neuroimaging and genetic research in order to define an endophenotype. For example, neuropsychological studies of working memory have proved successful in identifying genes involved in the abnormal functioning of the prefrontal cortex of individuals with schizophrenia (Egan *et al.*, 2001).

Emotional bias and executive control in major depression (state effects)

It has been proposed (Phillips *et al.*, 2003) that abnormalities in emotion processing in major depression are associated with structural and functional anomalies in ventral (orbitofrontal cortex, ventral anterior cingulate gyrus, ventral striatum, amygdala) and dorsal (dorsolateral prefrontal cortex, dorsal anterior cingulate gyrus, dorsomedial prefrontal cortex) neural systems. Neuropsychological assessment offers an opportunity to probe particular psychological properties related to these neural systems. Here, we discuss current findings reporting abnormal performance on tests of social cognition and emotional processing as potential predictors of depressive disorder.

Individuals with depression show poor interpersonal functioning (Gotlib & Whiffen, 1989; Libet &

Lewinson, 1973), which may in part be due to faulty appraisal of socially salient stimuli. It was found that people with depressive disorder were impaired in recognition of facial expressions of emotion, accompanied by negative reactions to others' emotions (Persad & Polivy, 1993). Other studies have revealed emotion-specific abnormalities in depressed individuals, who were demonstrating negative perceptual bias, i.e. recognizing significantly more sadness in facial expressions compared with healthy volunteers (Bouhuys et al., 1999; Gur et al., 1992; Hale et al., 1998; Matthews & Antes, 1992). There have been additional reports of depressed individuals having impaired recognition of positive facial expressions (Suslow et al., 2001), and diminished emotional responses to pleasant pictorial stimuli (Sloan et al., 1997, 2001). A previous study conducted at the Section of Neuroscience and Emotion, Institute of Psychiatry, London reported a bias away from happy faces in individuals with major depression (Surguladze et al., 2004). There have been, however, contradictory results reported by some other investigators. For example, Asthana et al. (1998) demonstrated impairments in performance of both non-emotive visuospatial tasks and emotion expression recognition in depressed individuals (identification of neutral, happy, sad, fearful and angry expressions); this was suggestive of a general visual perception deficit rather than a specific emotion recognition deficit, although a serious limitation of this study was the lack of control of medication effects. In contrast, Feinberg et al. (1986) found that whilst depressed individuals were not significantly impaired in tasks requiring matching of pictures of emotional faces, they were significantly impaired in verbal labeling of all emotional (anger, happiness, sadness, fear, disgust, surprise) and neutral faces.

When specific comparisons are made between the perception of happy and sad faces, an attentional bias toward sad faces has been demonstrated in depressed patients compared with healthy controls (Erickson et al., 2005; Murphy et al., 1999). Together with evidence of the impact of negative emotional context (perceived failure) upon executive control task performance (Elliott et al., 1996), these findings support the theory that perceptual bias is caused by a negative cognitive set. In a recent study, impaired performance of depressed patients on visuospatial and executive control tasks was modulated by the affective rather than the informational context of the task (Murphy et al., 2003); the performance of depressed individuals

on a visual discrimination and reversal task was affected by misleading negative feedback, demonstrated by an increased tendency to switch responding to the 'incorrect' stimulus following negative reinforcement, relative to that of controls.

Regarding performance on "non-emotion" processing tasks, there have been reports of impaired performance of depressed individuals on executive functions such as cognitive flexibility, problem-solving, planning and monitoring (Austin et al., 1992; Beats et al., 1996; Dalla et al., 1995; Moreaud et al., 1996; Veiel, 1997), as well as episodic and declarative memory (for meta-analysis see Zakzanis et al., 1998). These findings are consistent with evidence from neuroimaging studies of attenuated prefrontal cortical activity during task performance in depressed patients (Elliott et al., 1997; George et al., 1997).

The evidence to date supports the presence of an attentional bias towards sad stimuli and impaired executive control in depression; with the former causing further interference with the latter. The observed neurocognitive abnormalities in major depression therefore appear to reflect a complex interaction between biased emotion processing and impaired executive control. Further research is needed to study the nature of this interaction.

Information processing in remission

Studies that have examined cognitive changes in previously depressed individuals have found that reasoning styles in these individuals are largely state-dependent and appear to normalize upon recovery (Coyne & Gotlib, 1983; Segal & Dobson, 1992). Mikhailova et al. (1996) also found improvement in the ability to recognize emotions from pictures of facial expressions when depression remitted.

Similarly, neuroimaging studies suggest state-dependent abnormalities in MDD which are notable during an episode of illness, but then resolve following pharmacotherapy (Fu et al., 2004; Keedwell et al., 2008; Mayberg et al., 2000; Sheline et al., 2001). In these studies, abnormally increased activity in neural regions underlying emotion processing pre-treatment ameliorated with treatment, while activity in neural regions underlying executive control increased after treatment. Nonetheless, some studies have shown persistent abnormalities in remitted individuals with a history of MDD. There are reports that the negative-emotion attentional bias persists during remission (Hammen *et al.*, 1985; Koschack *et al.*, 2003), as do the strong associations between the self and negative adjective descriptors (Dozois & Dobson, 2001). Elliott *et al.* (1997) found an abnormal response to negative feedback in individuals remitted from the depressive episode. It is possible that neurocognitive abnormalities may become more apparent following "priming" of putative negative constructs, in otherwise apparently healthy patients with relevant memory prompts prior to testing (Chamberlain & Sahakian, 2004).

Tavares *et al.* (2003) advocate the use of "hot cognitions" to assess such phenomena, which are relevant to personal experience in the context of affective Go–No Go or probabilistic reversal learning tasks. Another useful approach is proposed by dual-process theorists (Beevers, 2005), who suggest using paradigms that elicit automatic cognitive bias by manipulating controlled (reflective) processes. Autobiographical memory prompts have been commonly employed in neuroimaging tasks which attempt to provoke sad mood (Keedwell *et al.*, 2005; Liotti *et al.*, 2002; Mayberg *et al.*, 1999). However, the neuroimaging research examining persistent abnormalities in remitted patients is sparse. In one study (Liotti *et al.*, 2002), a unique effect of sad mood provocation in the pregenual cortex (BA24) was demonstrated in remitted depressed patients, but not in depressed patients and healthy controls. It was suggested that this might be a trait marker, but the remitted group were taking antidepressants so it may represent a treatment effect. Furthermore, the abnormality should have been present in the acutely depressed group.

An important and still unresolved issue is that neurocognitive abnormalities that persist during remission may represent a post-episode "scar" rather than a trait deficit. For example, Bos *et al.* (2005) reported an increased negative-emotion attentional bias during an affective prosody task in individuals with a history of recurrent depression, but not after a single episode of depression. This was not explained by residual symptoms of depression, suggesting that such a bias may develop during the course of the illness.

Similarly, Paelecke-Habermann *et al.* (2005) argued that attentional and executive deficits (planning and monitoring) seem to develop in the course of MDD, persist in the remitted state and increase with further periods of illness. This suggests a kind of "kindling" effect of depression on neurocognitive

deficit and perceptual bias, although the effect of treatment cannot be excluded, and it is important to exclude subsyndromal symptoms that commonly persist after apparent recovery. Residual depression symptoms may correlate with putative vulnerability factors (Coyne & Whiffen, 1995).

One way to avoid these confounds in separating state versus trait is to examine "high-risk" individuals who have never experienced a depressed episode, but who are at high genetic risk due to their proximity to relatives with a history of MDD.

Trait investigations: studies of high-risk individuals

Studies examining the heritability of the negative perceptual bias in MDD suggest that the presence of recurrent thoughts of death and suicide in a proband predicts risk of depression in relatives (Kendler *et al.*, 1999). A recent study of 100 female triads found that attachment styles and personality vulnerabilities to depression (self-criticism and insecure attachment) persisted across three generations of women (Besser & Priel, 2005). The authors concluded that these characteristics could be heritable vulnerability markers for depression.

Further support for the heritability of cognitive and emotion processing abnormalities, and in particular negative-emotion attentional bias, comes from studies of familiality of personality traits. Reports have indicated that first-degree relatives may share some traits such as optimism (Schulman *et al.*, 1993), neuroticism (Hecht *et al.*, 2005; Jang *et al.*, 2002) and rigidity (Lauer *et al.*, 1997; Maier *et al.*, 1992).

The Cardiff depression study found familiality of personality traits such as sensation-seeking (Farmer *et al.*, 2001), extraversion and neuroticism (Farmer *et al.*, 2002). Importantly, the Temperament and Character Inventory (TCI; Cloninger *et al.*, 1993) scores on harm avoidance, reward dependence, novelty seeking and self-directedness dimensions were reported to represent stable traits premorbidly as well as in unaffected individuals, possibly behaving as vulnerability markers for depressive disorder (Farmer *et al.*, 2003).

Despite these findings, it is difficult to exclude common environmental factors. Furthermore, some retrospective assessments are problematic. Personality tests recorded during an episode of depression will be unreliable. For example, neuroticism scores from the Eysenck Personality Questionnaire (EPQ; Eysenck & Eysenck, 1975) have been shown to be highest amongst those relatives of depressed individuals who were themselves depressed at the time of the study (Katz & McGuffin, 1987). Scores on the TCI questionnaire have also shown a correlation with depression as measured by the Beck Depression Inventory (Peirson & Heuchert, 2001). So, it is important to ensure that large genetic studies exclude syndromal and subsyndromal depression from the analysis. Unaffected relatives must be the focus of this kind of enquiry.

Importantly, there is a suggestion that only a minority of depressed patients have had abnormal premorbid personalities (McGuffin, 1997), and that these can be clustered into a depression-spectrum disorder along with personality disorder and alcoholism. "Pure" depression may occur either sporadically or due to familial diathesis and may not be contaminated by abnormal premorbid personality (Winokur, 1974). Personality tests are possibly too crude to be specific for the testing of neurocognitive vulnerability, and underline the need for more carefully constructed neurocognitive tests – more specifically, tasks examining emotion attentional bias, executive function and the relationship between these two functional domains are required. This would help to identify potential markers of vulnerability, which can then be examined alongside neuroimaging investigations.

Conclusions on findings in MDD

It is now well established that individuals with MDD demonstrate bias in emotion recognition away from happy stimuli and towards sad stimuli. This attentional bias compounds more general difficulties with executive function through an emotional Stroop effect, and may help to maintain depression. However, it is still debated whether these effects reverse upon successful treatment, with executive function and emotion recognition becoming comparable with that of healthy volunteers. This question is vexated by the confounding factors of residual symptomatology and treatment. Hence, some studies examining remitted patients show persisting deficits and some do not. Furthermore, studies of remitted patients cannot ultimately identify trait markers without further evidence of their presence premorbidly. Trait markers can only be determined with relative certainty by examining "at risk" individuals prior to illness onset and their relatives. Once neurocognitive markers have been established, we can use neuroimaging and

linkage analysis to define the endophenotype more closely. This could lead to the important breakthroughs in targeted prevention and treatment that are so urgently needed to improve outcomes in depression.

Bipolar disorder
Introduction

Bipolar disorder has a poor prognosis in terms of admission rates, occupational functioning and disability. Residual inter-episode symptomatology is common and contributes to poor functional recovery (Altshuler et al., 2006). However, until recently it has been a comparatively neglected target for research. The neurocognitive markers of mania are discussed in Chapter 25. Here we will focus on deficits relating to euthymic bipolar patients, and the implications for defining an endophenotype. Data from imaging literature suggest that there may be stable differences in brain morphology in bipolar disorder compared with healthy comparison individuals, particularly in the basal ganglia (Baumann et al., 1999; Osuji & Cullum, 2005; Surguladze et al., 2003). It has been proposed that these differences reflect genetically driven population variation in the function of critical networks controlling cognition and emotion recognition; although much more research is required to exclude confounds and to explore any overlap with unipolar depression. We wish to uncover a stable neurodevelopmental abnormality, possibly multifactorial in origin, which could be a target for treatment and prevention. However, we must attempt at the same time to exclude three other potential causes of neurocognitive dysfunction in bipolar disorder, which may be independent or interact: (1) changes secondary to treatment, (2) reversible deficits related to acute or residual mood disturbance or (3) a progressive neurodegeneration that results from the disease process. Furthermore, there is some degree of familial clustering of both unipolar and bipolar disorder, suggesting that there may be overlapping of (genetically determined) endophenotype markers.

Neurocognitive dysfunction and relationship to clinical status

It is now well established that there are neurocognitive deficits associated with bipolar disorder. However, some authors have suggested that these deficits can be accounted for by acute or residual (subsyndromal) symptomatology. For example, depressive symptoms are more common in the so-called euthymic bipolar population than in the general population. Thompson et al. (2005) examined 63 euthymic, mostly medicated, patients with bipolar disorder and found widespread neurocognitive deficits ranging in frequency from 3% to 42%; these included difficulties with sustained attention, executive function, immediate spatial memory and verbal and visuospatial declarative memory. As expected, depressive symptom scores were higher than healthy comparisons for the group as a whole, but the cognitive findings appeared to be robust when controlling for these depressive symptoms. Bearden et al. (2006) included patients with varying mood states, from mania to euthymia to depression. They found that bipolar patients recalled and recognized fewer words than controls in a declarative memory paradigm, independent of clinical status. In contrast, a previous study with a similar design (Dixon et al., 2004) suggested that clinical status was important – executive function deficits were most evident during mania and were particularly associated with formal thought disorder. Murphy et al. (1999) found contrasting effects for different mood states, with depressed subjects having difficulty shifting their attention, and manic patients having more difficulty with sustained attention and inhibitory control. However, despite variations across different mood states, there is evidence that suggests that a number of deficits remain independent of mood change. For example, Dixon et al. (2004) found that deficits in response initiation, strategic thinking and inhibitory control were seen in the depressive, manic and euthymic phases of bipolar disorder.

Affect processing

Bipolar disorder is associated with functional and structural abnormalities in the brain circuits involved in processing emotional stimuli. It is logical to assume, therefore, that affect processing paradigms may prove to have great utility in defining an endophenotypic marker in bipolar disorder. Mood congruent memory bias has been found to be a consistent finding in both major depressive disorder and depressed bipolar patients – subjectively unpleasant material is recalled over pleasant material in both explicit and implicit (priming) experiments (Watkins

et al., 1996). Murphy et al. (1999) used a novel affective shifting task to demonstrate that depressed bipolar patients were biased towards negative stimuli, in common with findings in unipolar depression, whilst manic patients were biased towards positive stimuli. In contrast, Kerr et al. (2005) found no differences between manic, euthymic and depressed bipolar patients in their response to Emotional Stroop (Lyon et al., 1999), with all patients being worse than matched controls. However, numbers were possibly too small to detect modal differences in response to happy or sad word meanings in these clinical groups. Getz et al. (2003) investigated the performance of 25 manic bipolar patients and 25 healthy participants on tests of facial recognition and facial affect recognition and found that, whilst the groups did not differ significantly on the Benton Facial Recognition Test, the performance of the bipolar group was significantly worse than the comparison group on a novel facial affect labeling task. This result suggested that patients with bipolar disorder are able to recognize faces, but have difficulty processing facial affective cues; however, the abnormalities may disappear when bipolar patients are euthymic. Young et al. (2004) examined emotional bias to facial expressions in euthymic bipolar patients and matched controls and found no differences, although the sample size was small. In contrast, Bora et al. (2005) examined affect recognition together with social cognition in euthymic patients with bipolar disorder. They demonstrated impairments in performance on Theory of Mind tests (employing the Eyes and Hints tests), but there were also deficits in emotion recognition, which could have partially explained the results. Harmer et al. (2002) assessed the ability of 20 euthymic patients with bipolar disorder to recognize different facial expressions of emotion, compared with matched controls. In contrast to the small impairments seen in the non-emotional categorization task, patients with bipolar disorder showed a robust facilitation in the discrimination of disgusted facial expressions. The recognition of other basic negative and positive emotions was unchanged.

Affect processing and neuroimaging

Emotion recognition paradigms, covert or voluntary, can be employed in combination with neuroimaging paradigms to probe hypothesized cortical and limbic/paralimbic abnormalities. The research to date in this area is surprisingly sparse. Lennox et al. (2004) found that bipolar patients with mania had a specific, mood-congruent, negative bias in sad facial affect recognition, which was associated with an attenuation of activation in the subgenual anterior cingulate and bilateral amygdala, and increased activation in the posterior cingulate and posterior insula during functional imaging. Lawrence et al. (2004) measured neural responses to mild and intense expressions of fear, happiness and sadness in patients with MDD, bipolar disorder and healthy volunteers using an event-related covert mood recognition paradigm. Bipolar patients were free of any syndromal mood disturbance, but scored higher on measures of depression than the healthy control subjects. Compared with healthy controls, bipolar patients demonstrated increased activation within the ventral prefrontal cortex to expressions of intense sadness and increased left amygdala responses to expressions of intense fear. The latter finding is consistent with the literature on MDD suggesting an overlap in endophenotypic markers, probably not accounted for by residual symptoms given that no positive correlations were found between depression symptom severity and neural responses in the amygdala in the bipolar patients. Interestingly, bipolar patients had a greater response to mild happy expressions in the ventral prefrontal cortex, amygdala and striatum than controls, suggesting an enhanced sensitivity to happy facial expressions. However, the controls had a greater response than bipolar patients in the caudate and amygdala/uncus. Yurgelun-Todd et al. (2000) had previously found an increase in amygdalar activation in response to fearful facial affect in bipolar patients compared with healthy controls. In addition, although the bipolar patients completed the task demands, they demonstrated an impaired ability to correctly identify fearful facial affect, but not happy facial affect. These findings, together with structural MRI data, add support to the hypothesis that amygdala pathology is responsible for abnormal mood regulation in bipolar disorder.

Medication effects

Medication is an important confound to consider, given that bipolar disorder usually necessitates long-term treatment with a mood stabilizer. For example, lithium may have effects on a number of domains, including psychomotor speed and verbal memory

(Kocsis et al., 1993); although some authors do not find such an association (Engelsmann et al., 1998), and, furthermore, posit a neuroprotective function for lithium (Bauer et al., 2003). Mood stabilizers are commonly combined with antidepressants and antipsychotic medications. The effect of these combinations is hard to predict. For example Frangou et al. (2005) determined that current antipsychotic treatment predicted worse performance across all executive function tests in bipolar patients. It is probably wise to exclude any patients with a history of ECT treatment from studies of neurocognitive markers, given that the long-term effect of ECT on memory function is still a contentious issue.

Specificity

When looking for a specific trait deficit for a particular condition it is beneficial to compare patients from different diagnostic categories. Frangou et al. (2006) studied 43 patients with bipolar I disorder, 54 with schizophrenia and 46 matched healthy controls. They hypothesized that the prefrontal abnormalities found in both schizophrenia and bipolar disorder, suggested by neuropsychiatric and neuroimaging paradigms, might recruit different functional circuits. They reported that both bipolar and schizophrenia patients had deficits in performing the Stroop and Winsconsin Card Sorting tests; and while verbal fluency was only markedly impaired in the schizophrenic group, the bipolar group fared better in the congruent color-word matches in the Stroop. One conclusion that could be drawn from this study is that neurocognitive abnormalities in bipolar disorder lack specificity. Again, medication could be a factor which hides trait differences. A meta-analysis of cognitive functioning in bipolar disorder and schizophrenia concluded that patients with bipolar disorder did consistently better than schizophrenic patients, but unique patterns of deficit did not emerge for the bipolar patients (Krabbendam et al., 2005).

Disease process

Neurocognitive deficits may reflect disease process rather than disease vulnerability. The finding that patients with more severe illness and greater number of episodes have greater neurocognitive decline seems to support the former interpretation (Denicoff et al., 1999; Kessing et al., 1998; van Gorp et al., 1998). Furthermore, greater impairments are seen in patients who are older, or who had an earlier onset of the disease (Osuji & Cullum, 2005). More specifically, Frangou *et al.* (2005) found a relationship between number of years of treatment and loss of inhibitory control, but longitudinal cohort studies are needed to explore associations of this kind. It can equally be argued that those with greater neuro-cognitive deficit premorbidly may be more likely to progress to severe illness.

Pediatric bipolar studies

Sufficiently powerful longitudinal studies are, of course, difficult to conduct, but some researchers have examined young people with bipolar disorder who are at an earlier stage of the disease process. This group may represent a more "pure" sample for the purpose of uncovering vulnerability markers. They are also at an earlier stage of their treatment careers. There might well be a positive relationship between the effect of years of treatment and degree of cognitive deficit, although this has not been confirmed or refuted. Doyle *et al.* (2007) found problems with sustained attention, working memory and processing speed in 57 young people with bipolar disorder. Moderate decrements were also found in the Stroop test, abstract problem-solving and verbal declarative learning, consistent with the adult literature; but these deficits did not achieve significance. Another study (McClure *et al.*, 2005) specifically explored social cognition, motor inhibition and response flexibility in pediatric bipolar disorder. They found that bipolar patients were more impaired than controls in recognizing facial expressions, even if euthymic, consistent with the findings of Bora *et al.* (2005) in adults.

First-degree relatives

The study of first-degree relatives of bipolar disorder patients reveals subtle neurocognitive impairments, suggesting that at least some of the impairments seen in patients may represent trait susceptibility markers rather than disease processes or medication effects. Sobczak *et al.* (2003) discovered deficits in unaffected probands of bipolar patients in memory, focused attention, divided attention and psychomotor performance. The effects were more pronounced in relatives of bipolar I patients than in bipolar II patients, who in turn had greater deficits than matched healthy controls. The contrast with controls was even more pronounced following a tryptophan depletion challenge. Ferrier *et al.* (2004) have published a preliminary report on the performance of 17 unaffected first-degree relatives of bipolar patients and 17 demographically matched controls on a range of neuropsychological tests. Relatives were significantly impaired on Backward Digit Span, Spatial Span and on tasks of visuospatial declarative memory in comparison with controls. This is in keeping with their previous report of deficits in euthymic bipolar patients, suggesting they may be useful endophenotypic markers of genetic vulnerability to bipolar disorder. Clark *et al.* (2005b) examined cognitive flexibility and verbal learning in relatives of patients with bipolar disorder and in euthymic patients with recurrent major depression. They demonstrated abnormalities in attentional set shifting but no deficits in verbal learning, delayed recall and recognition using the California Verbal Learning Test, which is not inconsistent with the findings of Ferrier *et al.* (2004). However, another study by the same group demonstrated that deficits in sustained attention were found in euthymic bipolar patients but not in first-degree relatives (Clark *et al.*, 2005a) which may reflect methodological differences.

Conclusions on findings in bipolar disorder

In conclusion, there are some clinically and statistically significant neurocognitive deficits that appear to be a feature of bipolar disorder, some dependent and some independent of clinical status, and which are presumed to have a significant impact on social and occupational functioning. These include problems with set shifting and visuospatial memory, which can also be found in unaffected high-risk relatives. In addition, emotion recognition and social cognition paradigms reveal abnormalities in bipolar disorder, some of which appear to be independent of clinical status. Responses to fear and disgust seem to be important in euthymic patients and may represent underlying pathology in subcortical structures. However, more research is needed in the area of affect processing in unaffected first-degree relatives.

General conclusions

Follow-up studies are required of high-risk individuals for mood disorder. The neuropsychological approach is important, but should be combined with functional and structural imaging, neurophysiology and genotyping of candidate genes. Provocations, either through mood induction, stressful stimuli, or biological challenge, such as tryptophan depletion, can help to uncover a latent diathesis. Given the fact that both bipolar disorder and unipolar disorder cluster in the same families, it should be recognized that some overlap is likely in terms of neurobiology. Emotion recognition paradigms could be useful in combination with cognitive tests and may prove to have greater utility in terms of targeting abnormalities in mood regulation circuits. Abnormalities in prefrontal cortical function are found together with subcortical abnormalities in neuroimaging paradigms, illustrating the importance of a variety of approaches.

Our ability to find useful results when applying neuropsychological tests to mood disorders depends on our ability to take a simultaneously syndromal and dimensional approach. We are unlikely to find a single vulnerability marker for MDD or bipolar disorder that defines a target for a single treatment, but we may find several vulnerabilities, some shared and some more specific for MDD or bipolar disorder. These are unlikely to fit syndromal boundaries perfectly, but may underlie separate symptom dimensions, each modified in character by individual life experience, and interacting in synergistic or competitive ways.

References

Abramson, L. Y., Metalsky, G. I. & Alloy, L. B. (1989). Hopelessness depression: a theory-based subtype of depression. *Psychological Review*, **96**, 358–372.

Altshuler, L. L., Post, R. M., Black, D. O. *et al.* (2006). Subsyndromal depressive symptoms are associated with functional impairment in patients with bipolar disorder: results of a large, multisite study. *Journal of Clinical Psychiatry*, **67**, 1551–1560.

Andreasen, N. C. (1997). Linking mind and brain in the study of mental illness: a project for a scientific psychopathology. *Science*, **275**, 1586–1593.

Asthana, H. S., Mandal, M. K., Khurana, H. & Haque-Nizamie, S. (1998). Visuospatial and affect recognition deficit in depression. *Journal of Affective Disorders*, **48**, 57–62.

Austin, M.-P., Ross, M., Murray, C. *et al.* (1992). Cognitive functions in major depression. *Journal of Affective Disorders*, **25**, 21–30.

Bauer, M., Alda, M., Priller, J. & Young, L. T. (2003). Implications of the neuroprotective effects of lithium for the treatment of bipolar and neurodegenerative disorders. *Pharmacopsychiatry Supplement*, **36**, 250–254.

Baumann, B., Danos, P., Krell, D. *et al.* (1999). Reduced volume of limbic system-affiliated basal ganglia in mood disorders: preliminary data from a postmortem study. *Journal of Neuropsychiatry and Clinical Neurosciences*, **11**, 71–78.

Bearden, C. E., Glahn, D. C., Monkul, E. S. *et al.* (2006). Sources of declarative memory impairment in bipolar disorder: mnemonic processes and clinical features. *Journal of Psychiatric Research* **40**, 47–58.

Beats, B. C., Sahakian, B. J. & Levy, R. (1996). Cognitive performance in tests sensitive to frontal lobe dysfunction in the elderly depressed. *Psychological Medicine*, **26**, 591–603.

Beck, A. T., Rush, A. J., Shaw, B. F. & Emery, G. (1979). *Cognitive Therapy of Depression*. New York, NY: Guilford Press.

Beevers, C. G. (2005). Cognitive vulnerability to depression: a dual process model. *Clinical Psychology Review*, **25**, 975–1002.

Besser, A. & Priel, B. (2005). The apple does not fall far from the tree: attachment styles and personality vulnerabilities to depression in three generations of women. *Personality and Social Psychology Bulletin*, **31**, 1052–1073.

Bora, E., Vahip, S., Gonul, A. S. *et al.* (2005). Evidence for theory of mind deficits in euthymic patients with bipolar disorder. *Acta Psychiatrica Scandinavica*, **112**, 110–116.

Bos, E. H., Bouhuys, A. L., Geerts, E. *et al.* (2005). Cognitive, physiological, and personality correlates of recurrence of depression. *Journal of Affective Disorders*, **87**, 221–229.

Bouhuys, A. L., Geerts, E. & Gordijn, M. C. M. (1999). Depressed patients' perceptions of facial emotions in depressed and remitted states are associated with relapse: a longitudinal study. *Journal of Nervous and Mental Disease*, **187**, 595–602.

Caspi, A., Sugden, K., Moffitt, T. E. *et al.* (2003). Influence of life stress on depression: moderation by a polymorphism in the 5-HTT gene. *Science*, **301**, 386–389.

Chamberlain, S. R. & Sahakian, B. J. (2004). Cognition in mania and depression: psychological models and clinical implications. *Current Psychiatry Reports*, **6**, 451–458.

Clark, L., Kempton, M. J., Scarna, A., Grasby, P. M. & Goodwin, G. M. (2005a). Sustained attention-deficit confirmed in euthymic bipolar disorder but not in first-degree relatives of bipolar patients or euthymic unipolar depression. *Biological Psychiatry*, **57**, 183–187.

Clark, L., Sarna, A. & Goodwin, G. M. (2005b). Impairment of executive function but not memory in first-degree relatives of patients with bipolar I disorder and in euthymic patients with unipolar depression. *American Journal of Psychiatry*, **162**, 1980–1982.

Cloninger, C. R., Svrakic, D. M. & Przybeck, T. R. (1993). A psychobiological model of temperament and character. *Archives of General Psychiatry*, **50**, 975–990.

Coyne, J. C. & Gotlib, I. H. (1983). The role of cognition in depression: a critical appraisal. *Psychological Bulletin*, **94**, 472–505.

Coyne, J. C. & Whiffen, V. E. (1995). Issues in personality as diathesis for depression: the case of sociotropy-dependency and autonomy-self-criticism. *Psychological Bulletin*, **118**, 358–378.

Dalla, B. G., Parlato, V., Iavarone, A. & Boller, F. (1995). Anosognosia, intrusions and 'frontal' functions in Alzheimer's disease and depression. *Neuropsychologia*, **33**, 247–259.

Denicoff, K. D., Ali, S. O. & Mirsky, A. F. (1999). Relationship between prior course of illness and neuropsychological functioning in patients with bipolar disorder. *Journal of Affective Disorders*, **56**, 67–73.

Dixon, T., Kravariti, E., Frith, C., Murray, R. M. & McGuire, P. K. (2004). Effect of symptoms on executive function in bipolar illness. *Psychological Medicine*, **34**, 811–821.

Doyle, A. E., Wilens, T. E., Kwon, A. *et al.* (2007). Neuropsychological functioning in youth with bipolar disorder. *Biological Psychiatry*, **58**, 540–548.

Dozois, D. J. A. & Dobson, K. S. (2001). A longitudinal investigation of information processing and cognitive organization in clinical depression: stability of schematic interconnectedness. *Journal of Consulting and Clinical Psychology*, **69**, 914–925.

Egan, M. F., Goldberg, T. E., Kolachana, B. S. *et al.* (2001). Effect of COMT Val108/158 Met genotype on frontal lobe function and risk for schizophrenia. *PNAS*, **98**, 6917–6922.

Elliott, R., Baker, S. C., Rogers, R. D. *et al.* (1997). Prefrontal dysfunction in depressed patients performing a complex planning task: a study using positron emission tomography. *Psychological Medicine*, **27**, 931–942.

Elliott, R., Sahakian, B. J., Herrod, J. J., Robbins, T. W. & Paykel, E. S. (1997). Abnormal response to negative feedback in unipolar depression: evidence for a diagnosis specific impairment. *Journal of Neurology, Neurosurgery and Psychiatry*, **63**, 74–82.

Elliott, R., Sahakian, B. J., McKay, A. P. *et al.* (1996). Neuropsychological impairments in unipolar depression: the influence of perceived failure on subsequent performance. *Psychological Medicine*, **26**, 975–989.

Engelsmann, F., Katz, J., Ghadarian, A. M. *et al.* (1998). Lithium and memory: a long-term follow-up study. *Journal of Clinical Psychopharmacology*, **8**, 207–211.

Erickson, K., Drevets, W. C., Clark, L. *et al.* (2005). Mood-congruent bias in affective go/no-go performance of unmedicated patients with major depressive disorder. *American Journal of Psychiatry*, **162**, 2171–2173.

Eysenck, H. J. & Eysenck, S. B. G. (1975). *Manual of the Eysenck Personality Inventory*. London: Hodder & Stoughton.

Farmer, A., Mahmood, A., Redman, K. *et al.* (2003). A sib-pair study of the Temperament and Character Inventory scales in major depression. *Archives of General Psychiatry*, **60**, 490–496.

Farmer, A., Redman, K., Harris, T. *et al.* (2001). Sensation-seeking, life events and depression. The Cardiff Depression Study. *British Journal of Psychiatry*, **178**, 549–552.

Farmer, A., Redman, K., Harris, T. *et al.* (2002). Neuroticism, extraversion, life events and depression. The Cardiff Depression Study. *British Journal of Psychiatry*, **181**, 118–122.

Feinberg, T. E., Rifkin, A., Schaffer, C. & Walker, E. (1986). Facial discrimination and emotional recognition in schizophrenia and affective disorders. *Archives of General Psychiatry*, **43**, 276–279.

Ferrier, I. N., Chowdhury, R., Thompson, J. M., Watson, S. & Young, A. H. (2004). Neurocognitive function in unaffected first-degree relatives of patients with bipolar disorder: a preliminary report. *Bipolar Disorders*, **6**, 319–322.

Frangou, S., Dakhil, N., Landau, S. & Kumari, V. (2006). Fronto-temporal function may distinguish bipolar disorder from schizophrenia. *Bipolar Disorder*, **8**, 47–55.

Frangou, S., Donaldson, S., Hadjulis, M., Landau, S. & Goldstein, L. H. (2005). The Maudsley Bipolar Disorder Project: executive dysfunction in bipolar disorder I and its clinical correlates. *Biological Psychiatry*, **58**, 859–864.

Fu, C. H., Williams, S. C., Cleare, A. J. *et al.* (2004). Attenuation of the neural response to sad faces in major depression by antidepressant treatment: a prospective, event-related functional magnetic resonance imaging study. *Archives of General Psychiatry*, **61**, 877–889.

George, M. S., Ketter, T. A., Parekh, P. I. *et al.* (1997). Blunted left cingulate activation in mood disorder subjects during a response interference task (the Stroop). *Journal of Neuropsychiatry and Clinical Neuroscience*, **9**, 55–63.

Getz, G. E., Shear, P. K. & Strakowski, S. M. (2003). Facial affect recognition deficits in bipolar disorder. *Journal of the International Neuropsychology Society*, **9**, 623–632.

Gotlib, I. H. & Whiffen, V. E. (1989). Depression and marital functioning: an examination of specificity of gender differences. *Journal of Abnormal Psychology*, **98**, 23–30.

Gur, R. C., Erwin, R. J., Gur, R. E. *et al.* (1992). Facial emotion discrimination: II. Behavioral findings in depression. *Psychiatry Research*, **42**, 241–251.

Hale, W. W., III, Jansen, J. H., Bouhuys, A. L. & van den Hoofdakker, R. H. (1998). The judgement of facial expressions by depressed patients, their partners and controls. *Journal of Affective Disorders*, **47**, 63–70.

Hammen, C., Marks, T., Mayol, A. & deMaryo, R. (1985). Depressive self-schemas, life stress, and vulnerability to depression. *Journal of Abnormal Psychology*, **94**, 308–319.

Harmer, C. J., Clark, L., Grayson, L. & Goodwin, G. M. (2002). Sustained attention deficit in bipolar disorder is not a working memory impairment in disguise. *Neuropsychologia*, **40**, 1586–1590.

Hecht, H., Genzwurker, S., Helle, M. & van Calker, D. (2005). Social functioning and personality of subjects at familial risk for affective disorder. *Journal of Affective Disorders*, **84**, 33–42.

Ingram, R., Miranda, J. & Segal, Z. V. (1998). *Cognitive Vulnerability to Depression*. New York, NY: Guilford Press.

Jang, K. L., Livesley, W. J., Angleitner, A., Riemann, R. & Vernon, P. A. (2002). Genetic and environmental influences on the covariance of facets defining the domains of the five-factor model of personality. *Personality and Individual Differences*, **33**, 83–101.

Katz, R. & McGuffin, P. (1987). Neuroticism in familial depression. *Psychological Medicine*, **17**, 155–161.

Keedwell, P. A., Andrew, C., Williams, S. C. R., Brammer, M. J. & Phillips, M. L. (2005). A double dissociation of ventromedial prefrontal cortical responses to sad and happy stimuli in depressed and healthy individuals. *Biological Psychiatry*, **58**, 495–503.

Keedwell, P. A., Drapier, D., Surguladze, S. *et al.* (2008). Neural markers of symptomatic improvement during antidepressant therapy in severe depression: subgenual cingulate and visual cortical responses to sad, but not happy, facial stimuli are correlated with symptom score. *Journal of Psychopharmacology* (Epub ahead of print).

Kendler, K. S. (1998). Major depression and the environment: a psychiatric genetic perspective. *Pharmacopsychiatry*, **31**, 5–9.

Kendler, K. S., Gardner, C. O. & Prescott, C. A. (1999). Clinical characteristics of major depression that predict risk of depression in relatives. *Archives of General Psychiatry*, **56**, 322–327.

Kerr, N., Scott, J. & Phillips, M. L. (2005). Patterns of attentional deficits and emotional bias in bipolar and major depressive disorder. *British Journal of Clinical Psychology*, **44**, 343–356.

Kessing, L. V., Andersen, P. K. & Mortensen, P. B. (1998). Recurrence in affective disorder. I. Case register study. *British Journal of Psychiatry*, **172**, 23–28.

Kessler, R. C., Berglund, P., Demler, O. *et al.* (2003). The epidemiology of major depressive disorder: results from the National Comorbidity Survey Replication (NCS-R). *Journal of the American Medical Association*, **289**, 3095–3105.

Kocsis, J. H., Shaw, E. D., Stokes, P. E. *et al.* (1993). Neuropsychologic effects of lithium discontinuation. *Journal of Clinical Psychopharmacology*, **13**, 268–275.

Koschack, J., Hoschel, K. & Irle, E. (2003). Differential impairments of facial affect priming in subjects with acute or partially remitted major depressive episodes. *Journal of Nervous and Mental Disease*, **191**, 175–181.

Krabbendam, L., Arts, B., van Os, J. & Aleman, A. (2005). Cognitive functioning in patients with schizophrenia and bipolar disorder: a quantitative review. *Schizophrenia Research*, **80**, 137–149.

Kraemer, H. C., Schultz, S. K. & Arndt, S. (2002). Biomarkers in psychiatry: methodological issues. *American Journal of Geriatric Psychiatry*, **10**, 653–659.

Lauer, C. J., Bronisch, T., Kainz, M. *et al.* (1997). Pre-morbid psychometric profile of subjects at high familial risk for affective disorder. *Psychological Medicine*, **27**, 355–362.

Lawrence, N. S., Williams, A. M., Surguladze, S. *et al.* (2004). Subcortical and ventral prefrontal cortical neural responses to facial expressions distinguish patients with bipolar disorder and major depression. *Biological Psychiatry*, **55**, 578–587.

Lennox, B. R., Jacob, R., Calder, A. J., Lupson, V. & Bullmore, E. T. (2004). Behavioural and neurocognitive responses to sad facial affect are attenuated in patients with mania. *Psychological Medicine*, **34**, 795–802.

Libet, J. & Lewinson, P. (1973). Concept of social skills with special reference to the behavior of depressed persons. *Journal of Consulting and Clinical Psychology*, **40**, 304–313.

Liotti, M., Mayberg, H. S., McGinnis, S., Brannan, S. L. & Jerabek, P. (2002). Unmasking disease-specific cerebral blood flow abnormalities: mood challenge in patients with remitted unipolar depression.[comment] *American Journal of Psychiatry*, **159**, 1830–1840.

Lyon, H. M., Startup, M. & Bentall, R. P. (1999). Social cognition and the manic defense: attributions, selective attention, and self-schema in bipolar affective disorder. *Journal of Abnormal Psychology*, **108**, 273–282.

Maier, W., Lichtermann, D., Minges, J. & Heun, R. (1992). Personality traits in subjects at risk for unipolar major depression: a family study perspective. *Journal of Affective Disorders*, **24**, 153–163.

Matthews, G. R. & Antes, J. R. (1992). Visual attention and depression: cognitive biases in the eye fixation of the dysphoric and non-depressed. *Cognitive Therapy and Research*, **16**, 359–371.

Mayberg, H. S., Brannan, S. K., Tekell, J. L. *et al.* (2000). Regional metabolic effects of fluoxetine in major depression: serial changes and relationship to clinical response. *Biological Psychiatry*, **48**, 830–843.

Mayberg, H. S., Liotti, M., Brannan, S. K. *et al.* (1999). Reciprocal limbic-cortical function and negative mood: converging PET findings in depression and normal sadness. *American Journal of Psychiatry*, **156**, 675–682.

McClure, E. B., Treland, J. E., Snow, J. *et al.* (2005). Deficits in social cognition and response flexibility in pediatric bipolar disorder. *American Journal of Psychiatry*, **162**, 1644–1651.

McGuffin, P. (1997). Affective disorders. In R. Murray, P. Hill & P. McGuffin (Eds.), *The Essentials of Postgraduate Psychiatry* (pp. 310–351). Cambridge: Cambridge University Press.

Mikhailova, E. S., Vladimirova, T. V., Iznak, A. F., Tsusulkovskaya, E. J. & Sushko, N. V. (1996). Abnormal recognition of facial expression of emotions in depressed patients with major depression disorder and schizotypal personality disorder. *Biological Psychiatry*, **40**, 697–705.

Moreaud, O., Naegele, B., Chabannes, J. P. *et al.* (1996). Frontal lobe dysfunction and depression: relation with the endogenous nature of the depression. *Encephale*, **22**, 47–51.

Mueller, T. I., Leon, A. C., Keller, M. B. *et al.* (1999). Recurrence after recovery from major depressive disorder during 15 years of observational follow-up. *American Journal of Psychiatry*, **156**, 1000–1006.

Murphy, F. C., Sahakian, B. J., Rubinsztein, J. S. *et al.* (1999). Emotional bias and inhibitory control processes in mania and depression. *Psychological Medicine*, **29**, 1307–1321.

Murphy, F. C., Michael, A., Robbins, T. W. & Sahakian, B. J. (2003). Neuropsychological impairment in patients with major depressive disorder: the effects of feedback on task performance. *Psychological Medicine*, **33**, 455–467.

Osuji, I. J. & Cullum, C. M. (2005). Cognition in bipolar disorder. *Psychiatric Clinics of North America*, **28**, 427–441.

Paelecke-Habermann, Y., Pohl, J. & Leplow, B. (2005). Attention and executive functions in remitted major depression patients. *Journal of Affective Disorders*, **89**, 125–135.

Peirson, A. R. & Heuchert, J. W. (2001). The relationship between personality and mood: comparison of the BDI and the TCI. *Personality and Individual Differences*, **30**, 391–399.

Persad, S. & Polivy, J. (1993). Differences between depressed and nondepressed individuals in the recognition of and response to facial cues. *Journal of Abnormal Psychology*, **102**, 358–368.

Phillips, M. L., Drevets, W. C., Rauch, S. L. & Lane, R. (2003). Neurobiology of emotion perception. II: implications for major psychiatric disorders. *Biological Psychiatry*, **54**, 515–528.

Schulman, P., Keith, D. & Seligman, M. E. P. (1993). Is optimism heritable? A study of twins. *Behavioural Research and Therapy*, **31**, 569–574.

Segal, Z. V. & Dobson, K. S. (1992). Cognitive models of depression: report from a consensus development conference. *Psychological Inquiry*, **3**, 219–224.

Sheline, Y. I., Barch, D. M., Donnelly, J. M. *et al.* (2001). Increased amygdala response to masked emotional faces in depressed subjects resolves with antidepressant treatment: an fMRI study. *Biological Psychiatry*, **50**, 651–658.

Sloan, D. M., Strauss, M. E. Quirk, S. W. & Sajatovic, M. (1997). Subjective and expressive emotional responses in depression. *Journal of Affective Disorders*, **46**, 135–141.

Sloan, D. M., Strauss, M. E. & Wisner, K. L. (2001). Diminished response to pleasant stimuli by depressed women. *Journal of Abnormal Psychology*, **110**, 488–493.

Sobczak, S., Honig, A., Schmitt, J. A. & Riedel, W. J. (2003). Pronounced cognitive deficits following an intravenous L-tryptophan challenge in first-degree relatives of bipolar patients compared to healthy controls. [see comment] *Neuropsychopharmacology*, **28**, 711–719.

Solomon, D. A., Keller, M. B., Leon, A. C. *et al.* (1997). Recovery from major depression. A 10-year prospective follow-up across multiple episodes. *Archives of General Psychiatry*, **54**, 1001–1006.

Surguladze, S., Keedwell, P. A. & Phillips, M. (2003). Neural systems underlying affective disorders. *Advances in Psychiatric Treatment*, **9**, 446–455.

Surguladze, S. A., Young, A. W., Senior, C. *et al.* (2004). Recognition accuracy and response bias to happy and sad facial expressions in patients with major depression. *Neuropsychology*, **18**, 212–218.

Suslow, T., Junghanns, K. & Arolt, V. (2001). Detection of facial expressions of emotions in depression. *Perceptual and Motor Skills*, **92**, 857–868.

Tavares, J. V., Drevets, W. C. & Sahakian, B. J. (2003). Cognition in mania and depression. *Psychological Medicine*, **33**, 959–967.

Teasdale, J. D. (1988). Cognitive vulnerability to persistent depression. *Cognition and Emotion*, **2**, 247–274.

Thompson, J. M., Gallagher, P., Hughes, J. H. *et al.* (2005). Neurocognitive impairment in euthymic patients with bipolar affective disorder. *British Journal of Psychiatry*, **186**, 32–40.

Üstün, B. T. & Chatterji, S. (2001). Global burden of depressive disorders and future projections. In A. Dawson & A. Tylee. (Eds.), *Depression: Social and Economic Timebomb* (pp. 31–43). London: British Medical Journal.

van Gorp, W. G., Altshuler, L., Theberge, D., Wilkins, J. & Dixon, W. (1998). Cognitive impairment in euthymic bipolar patients with and without prior alcohol abuse: a preliminary study. *Archives of General Psychiatry*, **55**, 41–46.

Veiel, H. O. F. (1997). A preliminary profile of neuropsychological deficits associated with major depression. *Journal of Clinical and Experimental Neuropsychology*, **19**, 587–603.

Watkins, P. C., Vache, K., Verney, S. P. *et al.* (1996). Unconscious mood-congruent memory bias in depression. *Journal of Abnormal Psychology*, **105**, 34–41.

Winokur, G. (1974). The division of depressive illness into depression spectrum disease and pure depressive disease. *International Pharmacopsychiatry*, **9**, 5–13.

World Health Organization (1999). *The World Health Report 1999: Making a Difference*. Geneva: World Health Organization.

Young, A. H., Gallagher, P., Watson, S. *et al.* (2004). Improvements in neurocognitive function and mood following adjunctive treatment with mifepristone (RU-486) in bipolar disorder. *Neuropsychopharmacology*, **29**, 1538–1545.

Yurgelun-Todd, D. A., Gruber, S. A. & Kanayama, G. (2000). fMRI during affect discrimination in bipolar affective disorder. *Bipolar Disorders*, **2**, 248.

Zakzanis, K. K., Leach, L. & Kaplan, E. (1998). On the nature and pattern of neurocognitive function in major depressive disorder. *Neuropsychiatry, Neuropsychology and Behavioral Neurology*, **11**, 111–119.

Chapter 25

Manic distractibility and processing efficiency in bipolar disorder

David E. Fleck, Paula K. Shear and Stephen M. Strakowski

Bipolar disorder is a dynamic illness characterized by cycling among emotional extremes. Patients experience marked euphoria and irritability, which are the defining symptoms of mania, along with depression that either alternates or co-occurs with mania. However, the disorder can be diagnosed only in the presence of mania, according to DSM–IV (American Psychiatric Association, 1994), and the occurrence of mania predicts subsequent affective episodes in 80–90% of cases (Goodwin & Jamison, 1990). Based on the specificity of mania as a phenomenological expression of bipolar disorder, much of the neuropsychological research to date has been focused on cognitive processing during acute manic episodes.

In keeping with this focus, this chapter will examine cognitive performance in patients with DSM–IV bipolar I disorder in the manic state relative to euthymic patients, in whom mood syndromes are absent by definition, and healthy comparison subjects. Our emphasis will be on an information-processing perspective of cognitive dysfunction in bipolar disorder. Virtually by definition, during manic episodes patients experience clinically significant cognitive dysfunction (Basso et al., 2002; Bearden et al., 2001). This dysfunction may persist, albeit usually in attenuated form (Bearden et al., 2001), during periods of euthymia as well (Olley et al., 2005; Rubinsztein et al., 2000; Zubieta et al., 2001), which likely contributes to the substantial morbidity risks associated with bipolar disorder (Goldberg et al., 1995; Keck et al., 1998; Strakowski et al., 1996, 1998; Tohen et al., 1990, 2000). However, bipolar disorder is generally not considered to involve global processing deficits (Bearden et al., 2001), as is commonly described in patients with schizophrenia (Gold & Harvey, 1993). Unlike the relatively stable negative syndrome that

characterizes the end-state in schizophrenia, cognition, mood, and neurovegetative factors continually fluctuate throughout the course of bipolar disorder (Goodwin & Jamison, 1990).

With extreme fluctuations in mood and cognition, it becomes difficult to predict and model behavior with linear systems. As seen in Figure 25.1, the relationship between manic symptoms (as measured on the Young Mania Rating Scale; YMRS) and verbal recognition discriminability (the ability to discriminate between previously studied words and new distractor words) in manic and euthymic patients forms a cubic function (represented by the curved solid line and dashed lines representing the 95% confidence interval). Note that although neither a linear (represented by the horizontal solid line) nor a quadratic model (not shown) was significant for the full sample, a linear model was independently significant for the euthymic group and a quadratic model accounted for marginally significant performance variability for the manic group (data adapted from Fleck et al., 2003). Complicated findings of this type suggest that mood/performance relationships change as information processing adaptations occur in response to increasing symptoms or changing mood states.

The fact that cognitive performance changes across mood states during the normal course of bipolar disorder is in keeping with evidence that cognitive and emotional systems operate in dependent, and sometimes antagonistic, fashion in the healthy human brain (Drevets & Raichle, 1998; Yamasaki et al., 2002). Drevets & Raichle (1998) describe regional cerebral blood flow increases in brain regions implicated in either emotional processing (amygdalae, orbitofrontal cortex, ventral anterior cingulate) or cognitive processing (dorsolateral prefrontal cortex,

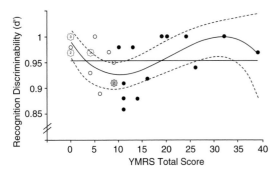

Figure 25.1. Scatter plot of recognition discriminability performance (d') as a function of Young Mania Rating Scale (YMRS) total scores for bipolar patients. Opened and filled circles represent observed data for euthymic and manic patient groups, respectively. Points of data overlap are represented by numeric information within circles, and the gray circle represents overlap in the manic and euthymic groups (data adapted from Fleck *et al.*, 2003 with permission).

dorsal anterior cingulate) during experimentally induced emotional states or demanding attention tasks, respectively. However, regional blood flow was found to be decreased in emotional processing regions during cognitive task performance, and also in cognitive processing regions during emotional task performance. The dissociation between cognitive and emotional processing has been segregated into anatomically distinct dorsal and ventral tracts that are integrated by anterior cingulate cortex (Yamasaki *et al.*, 2002). With respect to bipolar disorder, cognitive processing may deteriorate when brain regions subserving cognition are "deactivated" because attentional resources are being allocated to process heightened emotions such as mania. Although a lengthy description of functional neuroimaging work is beyond the scope of this chapter, recent imaging results are beginning to bear this out (Strakowski *et al.*, 2004). The question that remains is by what cognitive constructs we might begin to account for cognitive processing and neurophysiological abnormalities in bipolar disorder.

Manic distractibility and bipolar disorder

Distractibility (i.e. attention too easily drawn to unimportant or irrelevant external stimuli) is a primary cognitive symptom of mania (DSM–IV). Because manic patients often struggle to resist attentional distraction, it could be hypothesized that it would be more difficult for them to complete complex tasks

or otherwise control and regulate ongoing thoughts and behaviors (Aston-Jones *et al.*, 1999). Although the DSM–IV describes external sources of distraction from the environment as being prominent in bipolar disorder, internal sources may also be involved (Harnishfeger, 1995). For instance, the manifestation of mania itself (i.e. abnormally and persistently elevated, expansive, or irritable mood) may heighten distractibility, especially considering the potentially antagonistic relationship between emotional and cognitive brain circuitry previously described. During syndromal remission (i.e. euthymic periods) when mania scores are relatively low, error rates on cognitive tasks generally improve, possibly due to increased spare processing capacity or resources in the absence of distraction. However, certain other measures of effort, psychomotor processing speed and strategy use may still be affected, indicating a susceptibility to distraction.

Formal neuropsychological studies have indicated relative processing deficits in a number of specific cognitive abilities during manic episodes that may be related to, or result from, distractibility. The most common deficits reported include decrements in *sustained attention*, *verbal memory impairment* and decreased *executive functioning* (Clark *et al.*, 2001; Malhi *et al.*, 2004; Martinez-Aran *et al.*, 2004; Quraishi & Frangou, 2002; Savitz *et al.*, 2005). Below is a brief description of recent findings in these three domains. In each case, there is evidence for decreased performance during mania with at least some normalization during euthymia.

Cognitive domains implicated in bipolar mania
Sustained attention (vigilance)

Inability to sustain attention is an obvious behavioral consequence of mania (Bearden *et al.*, 2001). Decreased accuracy and increased reaction time (RT) on continuous performance tasks (CPTs) have been identified in mania (Addington & Addington, 1997; Sax *et al.*, 1995, 1999), and are among the most reliable cognitive indicators of manic episodes (Liu *et al.*, 2002; Nuechterlein *et al.*, 1991). In contrast, research shows that during euthymia, patients have attenuated error rates on CPTs compared with healthy controls (Strakowski *et al.*, 2004; Wilder-Willis *et al.*, 2001), although they may continue to exhibit RT slowing (Fleck *et al.*, 2001; Wilder-Willis *et al.*, 2001).

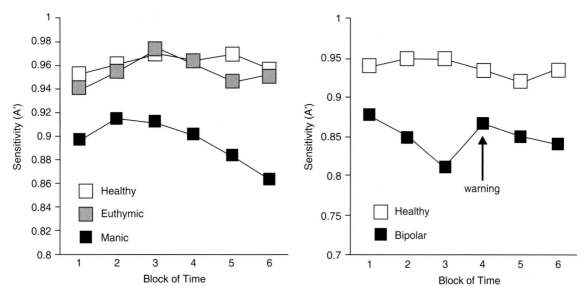

Figure 25.2. Group comparison of continuous performance task (CPT) sensitivity (A') without performance feedback (left) (unpublished data). Group comparison of CPT sensitivity (A') with performance feedback (right) (data adapted from Sax et al., 1995).

Figure 25.2 (left) depicts a sustained attention deficit specific to manic patients, as indicated by a monotonically decreasing sensitivity function relative to an independent sample of euthymic patients and healthy subjects. Note that sustained attention was assessed over an 8-minute vigil (80-s blocks) rather than reported as an average value to visualize the performance decrement. These data are consistent with previous reports suggesting that sustained attention deficits are *episode indicators* of bipolar disorder (Neuchterlein *et al.*, 1991). Episode indicators are most evident during acute mood states, but then normalize during euthymia. However, longitudinal studies will be needed to verify this contention, which is primarily based on cross-sectional findings.

As depicted in Figure 25.2 (right panel), a similar performance decrement was statistically ameliorated, although still inferable, when patients were provided with warnings to redirect attention, encouragement or other forms of feedback per standard CPT instructions (data adapted from Sax *et al.*, 1995). Although "warnings" are intended to facilitate task-appropriate behavior, they undermine construct validity by focusing attention, artificially limiting distractibility and inflating performance. Externally generated, periodic auditory warnings likely influence performance by imposing top-down monitoring of current goals (Burgess & Robertson, 2002). It is precisely this top-down monitoring mechanism (e.g. the Supervisory Attentional System; Norman & Shallice, 1986) that is likely compromised by mania.

Verbal memory

There is also a wealth of evidence suggesting that bipolar mania is characterized by prominent deficits in verbal declarative memory (Altshuler *et al.*, 2004; Basso *et al.*, 2002; Clark *et al.*, 2001; Deckersbach *et al.*, 2004; Krabbendam *et al.*, 2000; Martinez-Aran *et al.*, 2004; van Gorp *et al.*, 1998, 1999). Not all aspects of verbal memory are affected equally, however. Recall is often impaired in manic and euthymic patients relative to healthy subjects, although recognition deficits are generally restricted to mania (Altshuler *et al.*, 2004; Basso *et al.*, 2002; Clark *et al.*, 2001; Deckersbach *et al.*, 2004; Krabbendam *et al.*, 2000; Martinez-Aran *et al.*, 2004; van Gorp *et al.*, 1999). These findings suggest that, like sustained attention, poor recognition performance may be an episode indicator influenced by mood, while poor recall represents a stable vulnerability indicator of bipolar disorder that persists to the same degree in the absence of abnormal mood episodes. Similar to the attentional findings, RT slowing has been shown to account for certain verbal memory deficits. Kieseppä *et al.* (2005) reported that information processing speed had a significant effect on memory and verbal learning differences found between

367

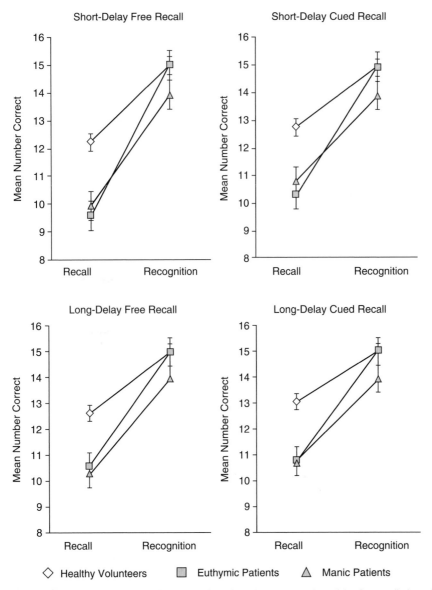

Figure 25.3. Group comparison of mean number of words correct on short-delay free recall, short-delay cued recall, long-delay free recall and long-delay cued recall relative to recognition hits on the California Verbal learning Test (CVLT) (data adapted from Fleck *et al.*, 2003 with permission).

euthymic bipolar twins and non-bipolar co-twins. After adjusting test performance for RT, group differences between bipolar twins and controls were ameliorated for working-memory span, memory encoding and learning efficiency, but remained significant on recall measures (Kieseppä *et al.*, 2005).

Figure 25.3 displays group means for manic, euthymic and healthy volunteers on a variety of long-term memory measures from the California Verbal Learning Test (CVLT) relative to recognition

performance (note that the recognition data are the same in each dataset; data adapted from Fleck *et al.*, 2003). In each comparison, the manic and euthymic groups performed significantly worse than the healthy group on the recall measure, but only the manic group performed significantly worse than the healthy group on recognition (Fleck *et al.*, 2003). These interactions suggest that highly retrieval-dependent verbal recall deficits may be stable vulnerability indicators, while more encoding-dependent verbal recognition deficits may be episode indicators in bipolar disorder. Retrieval failure on recall may be consistent with chronic subcortical abnormalities identified in structural and functional neuroimaging studies of bipolar disorder (Strakowski *et al.*, 2005).

Executive functioning

A number of investigators have reported impaired executive abilities during the manic state of bipolar disorder (Clark *et al.*, 2001; McGrath *et al.*, 1997). However, there is still debate about whether or not these abilities improve in the euthymic state (McGrath *et al.*, 1997; Rossi *et al.*, 2000) or remain impaired (Altshuler *et al.*, 2004; Tam *et al.*, 1998; Zubieta *et al.*, 2001). There is recent evidence to suggest that during euthymia, accuracy measures on executive tests normalize, while response latencies remain increased (similar to findings for sustained attention and verbal memory; Dixon *et al.*, 2004; Rubinsztein *et al.*, 2000). Olley *et al.* (2005) reported no significant differences between euthymic patients and healthy controls on a variety of primary accuracy measures of executive functioning, but on secondary measures of speed the patients were slower to complete the first trial of the Stroop task and slower to initiate certain responses, indicating a possible speed/accuracy tradeoff.

Figure 25.4 presents data on executive functioning in bipolar disorder using the Wisconsin Card Sort Task (WCST). As can be seen in Figure 25.4 (top), on average the manic group completed fewer WCST categories relative to the healthy group. In Figure 25.4 (bottom) the manic group also made significantly more perseverative errors relative to the healthy group. After corrections for multiple comparisons, differences between the manic and euthymic groups were marginally significant. These data are consistent with the idea that executive dysfunctions are episode indicators of bipolar disorder. They further attest to the influence of mood state on cognitive performance and highlight the importance of developing testable theories to account for interrelationships among emotional and cognitive variables in bipolar disorder.

The above findings suggest that the three primary domains of cognitive dysfunction in acute mania are not necessarily clinically compromised during euthymia (with the possible exception of verbal recall), at least during the early disease course, but are frequently accompanied by psychomotor slowing. Unfortunately many standard neuropsychological tests, including the CVLT and WCST, do not assess performance speed,

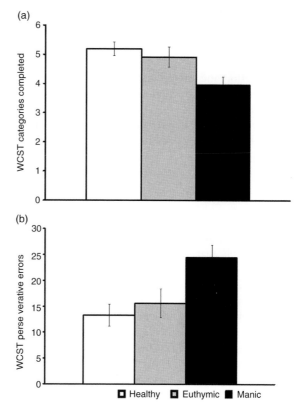

Figure 25.4. Group comparisons of Wisconsin Card Sort Test (WCST) mean categories completed (top) and mean perseverative errors (bottom) as a function of study group (unpublished data).

and even when RT measures are available, such as for CPTs, they are rarely considered as primary outcome measures. In order to better explain cognitive efficiency across mood states, speed/accuracy performance relationships should be outcome considerations in new theories of emotion and cognition in bipolar disorder.

A processing efficiency account of bipolar disorder

Processing efficiency theory (Eysenck & Calvo, 1992) was developed to account for the influence of state anxiety on cognitive performance. According to the theory, worrisome thoughts compete with the active processing and transient storage of task-relevant information. This interference is thought to impair performance on tasks with high attentional demands because the effects of anxiety on performance are mediated by the attentional system (see Eysenck, 1992 for a review). However, a Supervisory Attentional

System (SAS), thought to be mediated by frontal cortex (Norman & Shallice, 1986), may allocate additional processing resources to increase attentional processing capacity and improve performance through increased on-task effort and strategy use.

There is a distinction in processing efficiency theory between *processing efficiency* and *performance effectiveness*. Impaired processing efficiency is characterized by a tendency to increase effort or strategy use, which in turn slows RT. Examples of decreased processing efficiency include slowing response rates to enhance performance accuracy on a self-paced task, adopting a more conservative response bias by responding to fewer targets but making fewer false alarms on a signal-detection type task, or developing a more complicated strategy of memory cuing during encoding on a memory task. Impaired performance effectiveness, on the other hand, is simply characterized by increased error rates. Performance effectiveness is limited by attentional resources. However, in the context of heightened anxiety, competition for limited resources available to process attention and anxiety concurrently is expected to influence processing efficiency more than performance effectiveness (Eysenck & Calvo, 1992). That is, an individual may be able to achieve adequate performance, but at the expense of processing efficiency.

Because anxiety has traditionally been divided into two components: worry and *emotionality* (see Morris et al., 1981 for a review), processing efficiency theory may be extended to account for cognitive processing deficits in patients with anxiety and mood disorders, in that both worry and emotionality create *susceptibility to distraction* (Eysenck & Byrne, 1992). However, an adaptation of processing efficiency theory to bipolar disorder would need to account for distractibility in clinical samples because the theory was developed with subclinical samples of anxious subjects (i.e. healthy subjects with varying degrees of test anxiety). With clinically significant mania, the SAS might be expected to allocate additional processing resources as an active response to reduce susceptibility to distraction and improve attentional performance. However, in acutely manic patients, one might predict that levels of distractibility can be so high that the capacity of the SAS to exert additional attentional control is overwhelmed, and that only patients with modest symptom levels (i.e. hypomania or euthymia) would be expected to demonstrate performance benefits based on processing efficiency changes. In acute

mania the emotional demands on attention would be expected to be so great that even relatively simple tasks might be performed inaccurately.

Information processing approaches to assess processing efficiency

Processing efficiency theory relies on the information processing perspective of cognitive psychology. Information-processing studies almost invariably assess processing speed in some form, generally reaction time (RT) in milliseconds. The theoretical definition of RT is the absolute minimum time in which an individual can respond with 100% accuracy (Pachella, 1974). However, because patients with bipolar mania are not able to perform cognitive tasks in a completely accurate manner (Addington & Addington, 1997; Bearden et al., 2001; Liu et al., 2002; Nuechterlein et al., 1991; Sax et al., 1995, 1999; Strakowski et al., 2004; Wilder-Willis et al., 2001), RT necessarily covaries with response probabilities. Unfortunately, most prior studies of cognition in bipolar disorder have tended not to report RT, making it impossible to examine the influence of processing speed. In those that have, psychomotor slowing has been related to deficits in sustained attention (Fleck et al., 2001, 2005a, 2005b; Wilder-Willis et al., 2001), verbal memory (Kieseppä et al., 2005) and executive functioning (Malhi et al., 2005; Olley et al., 2005).

Therefore, it is important to formally examine speed/accuracy relationships in cognitive studies of bipolar disorder. Salthouse & Hedden (2002) suggest a number of possible approaches to do so. First, analysis of covariance (ANCOVA) can be used to hold RT constant while examining the influence of accuracy independently. Second, the ratio of accuracy over time can be used to reflect *processing efficiency* as a level of accuracy per unit time. Third, group accuracy averages can be compared across successive percentiles of a subject's RT distribution (e.g. the 25th, 50th, 75th percentile). They suggest that this type of comparison is appropriate when susceptibility to distraction is high, such as in bipolar disorder, and one would predict large differences among each subject's slowest RTs (those trials where attention lapsed).

Salthouse & Hedden (2002) also suggest that if complete speed/accuracy operating functions are available, then speed/accuracy tradeoffs can be eliminated by making comparisons of accuracy at fixed time levels or vice versa. One method to obtain more complete data is to use instructions or payoffs emphasizing varying speed and accuracy levels across different blocks of trials. A second method is to obtain different speed and accuracy combinations by using RT deadlines or response windows. By manipulating these types of variables, responses can be accurate and slow in some trials, inaccurate and fast in some trials, and intermediate in both accuracy and speed in some trials (Salthouse & Hedden, 2002). Such test manipulations might prove useful in functional neuroimaging studies as well.

Preliminary examples of a processing efficiency approach

In an initial attempt to demonstrate how processing efficiency theory can be applied to cognition in bipolar disorder, we will provide two examples of how statistical control was used to account for the influence of RT (a primary index of processing efficiency) on performance effectiveness. In this way, processing efficiency adaptations across mood state were equated, at least in a statistical sense. These examples involved the use of ANCOVA in two studies that employed either a degraded stimulus continuous performance task (DS-CPT) or a computerized, verbal recognition memory test. Based on the primary prediction of processing efficiency theory (i.e. that anxiety, or emotionality in the case of bipolar disorder, impairs processing efficiency more than performance effectiveness), we expected that when accuracy was examined independent of the influence of processing speed/efficiency, deficits in the performance effectiveness of attention and memory would be reduced.

Example 1: The degraded stimulus continuous performance task (DS-CPT)

The first example comes from a study of DS-CPT performance in manic and euthymic patients with bipolar disorder relative to healthy controls (Fleck et al., 2005a). As demonstrated in Figure 25.5 (top), healthy subjects outperformed both manic and euthymic patients at the beginning of a vigil, but by the end healthy subjects only outperformed manic patients, who demonstrated a sustained attention decrement (i.e. higher error rates as attentional demands increased over time; Corkum & Siegel, 1993; Nuechterlein, 1991). As seen in Figure 25.5 (bottom), when

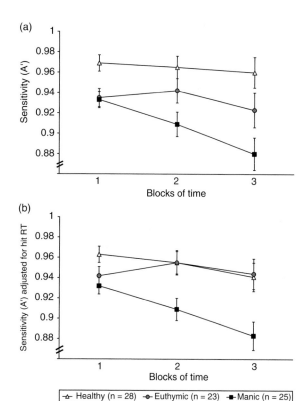

Figure 25.5. Group comparison of mean degraded stimulus continuous performance task (DS-CPT) perceptual sensitivity (A') across three successive blocks of time in ANOVA (top) and ANCOVA with Hit reaction time (RT) at block 1, 2 and 3 as the covariates (bottom) (data from Fleck et al., 2005a, with permission).

RT was removed from the model by ANCOVA, the sensitivity function for euthymic patients became indistinguishable from that of healthy subjects, suggesting that during euthymia patients may sustain attention by increasing accuracy at the expense of speed, either as an unconscious compensatory process or conscious control strategy. In fact, the euthymic group, but not the manic group, was significantly slower than the healthy group overall (559 ms, 521 ms and 499 ms, respectively), confirming a speed/accuracy tradeoff (Fleck et al., 2005a).

A discriminant function analysis based on these data yielded a model of sustained attention and symptomatology that distinguished healthy, euthymic and manic subjects on two dimensions. As can be seen in Figure 25.6, the first dimension was related to manic symptoms, and separated manic individuals from euthymic and healthy individuals. The second dimension was interpreted as a spectrum of effort and strategy use to maintain attention. Both hit RT and

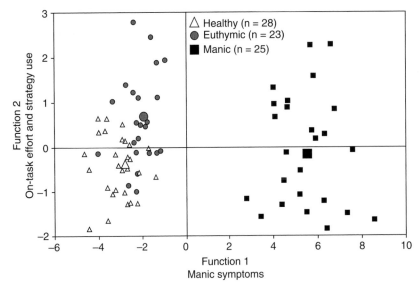

Figure 25.6. Scatter plot demonstrating the covariance between psychiatric symptoms and performance. Displayed are the group centroids on two discriminant functions derived from three performance variables (A′, β″, and hit reaction time (RT)) and three symptom rating scale variables (Young Mania Rating Scale, Hamilton Rating Scale for Depression and Scale for the Assessment of Positive Symptoms total scores) (data from Fleck et al., 2005a, with permission).

perceptual sensitivity (A′) predicted the cognitive effort and strategy use required to sustain attention. Healthy subjects required little effort to sustain perceptual sensitivity relative to both patient groups, but considerably less than euthymic patients. Euthymic patients required more effort, and responded more slowly to maintain relatively high sensitivity. Finally, manic patients responded variably across the entire spectrum of cognitive resource utilization, consistent with the performance of acutely ill patients in many cognitive domains (Fleck et al., 2005a).

Example 2: A verbal recognition memory test

A second example testing processing efficiency theory comes from a study examining verbal memory among bipolar manic, bipolar euthymic and healthy control subjects using a directed forgetting in recognition paradigm (Fleck et al., 2005b). Directed forgetting is used to explore the ability to comply with instructions to forget irrelevant information. In the item method of directed forgetting, individual words are presented one at a time and followed by a cue either to remember or forget that word. This type of stimulus presentation ensures that both "remember" and "forget" cued words are encoded prior to memory testing. A directed forgetting effect is demonstrated by poorer recognition memory for forget-cued words relative to remember-cued words on a memory test for both

word types (Basden et al., 1993; Fleck et al., 2001; MacLeod, 1989, 1999).

As seen in Figure 25.7 (top), an analysis of directed forgetting performance indicated that both recognition effectiveness (overall R- and F-cued word sensitivity combined) and directed-forgetting effectiveness (R-cued word superiority over F-cued words) were impaired in acutely manic patients. As demonstrated in Figure 25.7 (bottom), when RT was held constant using ANCOVA to examine performance effectiveness in the absence of processing efficiency differences, manic patients recognized previously presented words as accurately as euthymic and healthy subjects overall, and showed intact selective encoding indicated by a significant directed forgetting effect (Fleck et al., 2005b).

Taken together, these examples in domains of attention and memory are consistent with the notion that euthymic patients perform as accurately as healthy participants if processing efficiency is equated. Moreover, although the sustained attention deficit in manic patients remained unchanged, recognition and selective encoding deficits were ameliorated after controlling for processing efficiency differences. Bipolar patients may be less able to perform sustained attention and recognition, consistent with mood-state related changes in information-processing capacity, rather than having stable deficits in these abilities per se. Instead, sustained attention and verbal memory impairment may be secondary

(a)

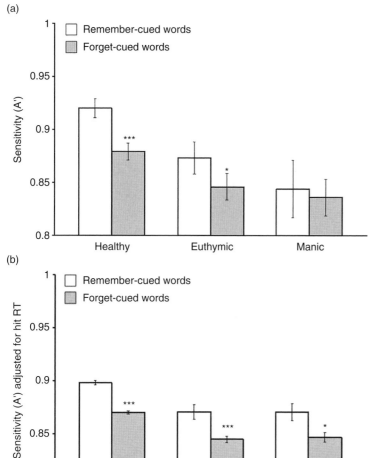

(b)

Figure 25.7. Group comparison of mean recognition sensitivity (A') to remember- and forget-cued words in ANOVA (top). Group comparison of mean recognition sensitivity (A') to remember- and forget-cued words with remember- and forget-cued hit reaction time (ms) as covariates in ANCOVA (bottom). * = within group directed-forgetting effect, $P < 0.05$. *** = within group directed-forgetting effect, $P < 0.001$ (data from Fleck et al., 2005b, with permission).

to a mediating vulnerability to distractibility by manic symptoms of bipolar disorder (Fleck et al., 2005a, 2005b). These results were not likely due to medication effects, as there were no statistically significant differences between medicated and unmedicated patients on any of the attentional variables (Fleck et al., 2005a), and medication factors were not related to memory performance (Fleck et al., 2005b).

Conclusions

The above findings suggest that there may be fewer stable vulnerability indicators of impaired cognition in bipolar disorder than currently thought. When RT was statistically controlled in the discussed examples,

cognitive differences between bipolar patients and healthy subjects were reduced or ameliorated. This may suggest that generalized psychomotor slowing is a primary means by which bipolar patients compensate for abnormalities in cognitive networks. Bipolar patients may be able to perform cognitive tasks through greater effortful control at the expense of processing efficiency, if manic symptoms do not overwhelm processing capacity, and if other factors do not intervene (e.g. comorbidities such as alcohol abuse or progressive alterations in brain structure or function resulting from a chronic course).

Increasing symptoms may act as a trigger for the cognitive system to recruit additional resources from functional cortical regions to compensate for decreased attentional capacity, especially during euthymia. In this scenario, attentional capacity is influenced not only by dynamic energy factors (e.g. effort, motivation) and physical factors (e.g. neurophysiology), but also by emotional factors such as manic distractibility. The degree of symptom-related distractibility may mediate cognitive performance across mood states, but might only be revealed during euthymia by psychomotor slowing.

Most deficits identified in euthymic samples (so-called core or trait deficits) are less severe than those seen during mania. If euthymic performance is considered in greater detail, it often becomes apparent that certain functions are spared (e.g. sustained attention as a decrement over time), even if overall performance effectiveness remains below normal. The most severe euthymic deficits are typically associated with a chronic course of illness, as indexed by an increased number of mood episodes and hospitalizations or longer mood episodes (Denicoff *et al.*, 1999; van Gorp *et al.*, 1998; Zubieta *et al.*, 2001), which may be suggestive of a neurodegenerative process. Stable vulnerability indicators, particularly in younger, less chronically ill patients, may be overestimated when speed–accuracy trade offs, cognitive strategies and motivation and effort are not considered.

The characteristics of a stable vulnerability indicator in relation to bipolar disorder need to be better defined. For instance, should they be entirely consistent across mood state? Are they always present in high-risk subjects? How many standard deviations below normal should they be? It should be noted that, although a processing efficiency theory of bipolar disorder would predict fewer true stable vulnerability indicators (that is stable in the sense of cognitive impairment with frank brain lesions), certain deficits, such as retrieval deficits (e.g. verbal recall), may be relatively more stable characteristics of bipolar disorder. If an identified cognitive deficit persists after accounting for processing efficiency differences through either statistical, or more appropriately methodological control, then the case for considering it a biomarker of bipolar disorder would be strengthened considerably. The ability to identify subtle deficits that are consistent across mood states will become more likely as our understanding of the influence of clinical factors (e.g. symptom severity, substance use, medications) and energy/effort/motivational factors (e.g. processing efficiency) continues to develop.

Psychomotor slowing may be a more accurate mediating vulnerability indicator of bipolar disorder than are deficits in specific cognitive abilities of attention, memory and executive control, because it provides an index of available processing capacity. Reaction time can not only be used in relation to error-based measures to assess processing efficiency, but may also be an important outcome measure in its own right. Therefore, increased RT should not be interpreted as a medication effect by default, but this possibility should always be tested. If medication effects can be ruled out or at least minimized, then RT slowing might be thought to reflect attentional distractibility brought on by physical, effortful or emotional means. For instance, psychomotor slowing may indicate a reduction in the efficiency of white matter networks that subserve attention in bipolar disorder. Diffusion tensor imaging studies are beginning to reveal that tracts within the frontal lobes are disarrayed in bipolar disorder (Adler *et al.*, 2004). Functional MRI studies further demonstrate a high degree of potentially effortful compensatory processing, which may serve to counteract attentional abnormalities, during euthymia (Strakowski *et al.*, 2004). Another interpretation of slow RT could be that disruption of attentional networks alters awareness or alertness (Posner & Rueda, 2002). This might suggest that cognitive dysfunction in bipolar disorder can be conceived of as a disorder of consciousness as described in Section 4.

The present exposition is only a starting point for reconsidering cognitive dysfunction in bipolar disorder. In the future, neuropsychological investigations might benefit by providing more complete speed/accuracy operating functions, examining cognitive performance across an extended range of symptom scores, and using longitudinal assessments across mood states when possible. Additionally, cognitive studies of bipolar disorder might place more emphasis on assessing global process deficits that cut across domains in addition to assessing specific cognitive abilities (e.g. attention, memory, executive function). Global processing deficits in bipolar disorder might involve an inability to resist distraction in numerous domains, as described here, or globally increased impulsivity, which has received recent research attention and holds promise as a cross-cutting deficit (Swann *et al.*, 2003, 2005). Adopting such techniques, in the context of a processing efficiency perspective, may help to clarify the nature of non-linear mood/performance relationships in bipolar disorder that make it such a difficult illness to characterize in neuropsychological terms.

References

Addington, J. & Addington, D. (1997). Attentional vulnerability indicators in schizophrenia and bipolar disorder. *Schizophrenia Research*, **23**, 197–204.

Adler, C. M., Holland, S. K., Schmithorst, V. *et al.* (2004). Abnormal frontal white matter tracts in bipolar disorder: a diffusion tensor imaging study. *Bipolar Disorders*, **6**, 197–203.

Altshuler, L. L., Ventura, J., van Gorp, W. G. *et al.* (2004). Neurocognitive function in clinically stable men with bipolar I disorder or schizophrenia and normal control subjects. *Biological Psychiatry*, **56**, 560–569.

American Psychiatric Association (1994). *Diagnostic and Statistical Manual of Mental Disorders* (4th edn.) (DSM–IV). Washington, DC: APA.

Aston-Jones, G. S., Desimone, R., Driver, J., Luck, S. J. & Posner, M. I. (1999). Attention. In M. J. Zigmond, F. E. Bloom, S. C. Landis, J. L. Roberts & L. R. Squire (Eds.), *Fundamental Neuroscience* (pp. 1385–1409). San Diego, CA: Academic Press.

Basso, M. R., Lowry, N., Neel, J., Purdie, R. & Bornstein, R. A. (2002). Neuropsychological impairment among manic, depressed, and mixed-episode inpatients with bipolar disorder. *Neuropsychology*, **16**, 84–91.

Bearden, C. E., Hoffman, K. M. & Cannon, T. D. (2001). The neuropsychology and neuroanatomy of bipolar affective disorder: a critical review. *Bipolar Disorders*, **3**, 106–150.

Burgess, P. W. & Robertson, I. H. (2002). Principles of the rehabilitation of frontal lobe function. In D. T. Stuss & R. T. Knight (Eds.), *Principles of Frontal Lobe Function* (pp. 557–572). New York, NY: Oxford University Press.

Clark, L., Iversen, S. D. & Goodwin, G. M. (2001). A neuropsychological investigation of prefrontal cortex involvement in acute mania. *American Journal of Psychiatry*, **158**, 1605–1611.

Corkum, P. V. & Siegel, L. S. (1993). Is the continuous performance task a valuable research tool for use with children with attention-deficit-hyperactivity disorder? *Journal of Child Psychology and Psychiatry and Allied Disciplines*, **34**, 1217–1239.

Deckersbach, T., Savage, C. R., Reilly-Harrington, N. *et al.* (2004). Episodic memory impairment in bipolar disorder and obsessive-compulsive disorder: the role of memory strategies. *Bipolar Disorders*, **6**, 233–244.

Denicoff, K. D., Ali, S. O., Mirsky, A. F. *et al.* (1999). Relationship between prior course of illness and neuropsychological functioning in patients with bipolar disorder. *Journal of Affective Disorders*, **56**, 67–73.

Dixon, T., Kravariti, E., Frith, C., Murray, R. M. & McGuire, P. K. (2004). Effects of symptoms on executive function in bipolar illness. *Psychological Medicine*, **34**, 811–821.

Drevets, W. C. & Raichle, M. E. (1998). Reciprocal suppression of regional cerebral blood flow during emotional versus higher cognitive processes: implications for interactions between emotion and cognition. *Cognition and Emotion*, **12**, 353–385.

Eysenck, M. W. (1992). *Anxiety: The Cognitive Perspective*. Hove, UK: Lawrence Erlbaum Associates.

Eysenck, M. W. & Byrne, A. (1992). Anxiety and susceptibility to distraction. *Personality and Individual Differences*, **13**, 793–798.

Eysenck, M. W. & Calvo, M. G. (1992). Anxiety and performance: the processing efficiency theory. *Cognition and Emotion*, **6**, 409–434.

Fleck, D. E., Sax, K. W. & Strakowski, S. M. (2001). Reaction time measures of sustained attention differentiate bipolar disorder from schizophrenia. *Schizophrenia Research*, **52**, 251–259.

Fleck, D. F., Shear, P. K. & Strakowski, S. M. (2005a). Processing efficiency and sustained attention in bipolar disorder. *Journal of the International Neuropsychological Society*, **11**, 49–57.

Fleck, D. E., Shear, P. K. & Strakowski, S. M. (2005b). Processing efficiency and directed forgetting in bipolar disorder. *Journal of the International Neuropsychological Society*, **11**, 871–880.

Fleck, D. E., Shear, P. K., Zimmerman, M. E. *et al.* (2003). Verbal memory in mania: effects of clinical state and task requirements. *Bipolar Disorders*, **5**, 375–380.

Gold, J. M. & Harvey, P. D. (1993). Cognitive deficits in schizophrenia. *Psychiatric Clinics of North America*, **16**, 295–312.

Goldberg, J. F., Harrow, M. & Grossman, L. S. (1995). Course and outcome in bipolar affective disorder: a longitudinal follow-up study. *American Journal of Psychiatry*, **152**, 379–384.

Goodwin, F. K. & Jamison, K. R. (1990). *Manic-Depressive Illness*. New York, NY: Oxford University Press.

Harnishfeger, K. K. (1995). The development of cognitive inhibition: theories, definitions, and research evidence. In F. N. Dempster & C. J. Brainerd (Eds.), *Interference and Inhibition in Cognition* (pp. 175–204). San Diego, CA: Academic Press.

Keck, P. E. Jr., McElroy, S. L., Strakowski, S. M. *et al.* (1998). 12-month outcome of patients with bipolar disorder following hospitalization for a manic or mixed episode. *American Journal of Psychiatry*, **155**, 646–652.

Kieseppä, T., Tuulio-Henriksson, A., Haukka, J. *et al.* (2005). Memory and verbal learning functions in twins with bipolar-I disorder, and the role of information-processing speed. *Psychological Medicine*, **35**, 205–215.

Krabbendam, L., Honig, A., Wiersma, J. *et al.* (2000). Cognitive dysfunction and white matter lesions in patients with bipolar disorder in remission. *Acta Psychiatrica Scandinavica*, **101**, 274–280.

Liu, S. K., Chiu, C-H., Chang, C-J. *et al.* (2002). Deficits in sustained attention in schizophrenia and affective disorders: stable versus state-dependent markers. *American Journal of Psychiatry*, **159**, 975–982.

MacLeod, C. M. (1989). Directed forgetting affects both direct and indirect tests of memory. *Journal of Experimental Psychology: Learning, Memory, and Cognition*, **15**, 13–21.

MacLeod, C. M. (1999). The item and list methods of directed forgetting: test differences and the role of demand characteristics. *Psychonomic Bulletin and Review*, **6**, 123–129.

Malhi, G. S., Ivanovski, B., Szekeres, V. & Olley, A. (2004). Bipolar disorder: it's all in your mind? The neuropsychological profile of a biological disorder. *Canadian Journal of Psychiatry*, **49**, 813–819.

Malhi, G. S., Lagopoulos, J., Sachdev, P. S., Ivanovski, B. & Shnier, R. (2005). An emotional Stroop functional MRI study of euthymic bipolar disorder. *Bipolar Disorders*, **7**, 58–69.

Martinez-Aran, A., Vieta, E., Reinares, M. *et al.* (2004). Cognitive function across manic or hypomanic, depressed, and euthymic states in bipolar disorder. *American Journal of Psychiatry*, **161**, 262–270.

Morris, L. W., Davis, M. A. & Hutchings, C. H. (1981). Cognitive and emotional components of anxiety: literature review and a revised worry-emotionality scale. *Journal of Education Psychology*, **73**, 541–555.

Norman, D. A. & Shallice, T. (1986). Attention to action: willed and automatic control of behavior. In R. J. Davidson, G. E. Schwartz & D. Shapiro (Eds.), *Consciousness and Self-Regulation* (Vol. 4, pp. 1–18). New York, NY: Plenum Press.

Nuechterlein, K. H. (1991). Vigilance in schizophrenia and related disorders. In S. R. Steinhauer, J. H. Gruzelier & J. Zubin (Eds.), *Handbook of Schizophrenia. Neuropsychology, Psychophysiology, and Information Processing* (Vol. 5, pp. 397–433). Amsterdam: Elsevier Science.

Nuechterlein, K. H., Dawson, M. E., Ventura, J., Miklowitz, D. & Konishi, G. (1991). Information

processing anomalies in the early course of schizophrenia and bipolar disorder. *Schizophrenia Research*, **5**, 195–196.

Olley, A. L., Malhi, G. S., Bachelor, J. *et al.* (2005). Executive functioning and theory of mind in euthymic bipolar disorder. *Bipolar Disorders*, **7**, 43–52.

Quraishi, S. & Frangou, S. (2002). Neuropsychology of bipolar disorder: a review. *Journal of Affective Disorders*, **72**, 209–226.

Pachella, R. G. (1974). The interpretation of reaction time in information processing research. In B. Kantowitz (Ed.), *Human Information Processing: Tutorials in Performance and Cognition*. New York: Lawrence Erlbaum.

Posner, M. I. & Rueda, M. R. (2002). Mental chronometry in the study of individual and group differences. *Journal of Clinical and Experimental Neuropsychology*, **24**, 968–976.

Rubinsztein, J. S., Michael, A., Paykel, E. S. & Sahakian, B. J. (2000). Cognitive impairment in remission in bipolar affective disorder. *Psychological Medicine*, **30**, 1025–1036.

Salthouse, T. A. & Hedden, T. (2002). Interpreting reaction time measures in between-group comparisons. *Journal of Clinical and Experimental Neuropsychology*, **24**, 858–872.

Savitz, J., Solms, M. & Ramesar, R. (2005). Neuropsychological dysfunction in bipolar affective disorder: a critical opinion. *Bipolar Disorders*, **7**, 216–235.

Sax, K. W., Strakowski, S. M., McElroy, S. L., Keck, P. E. Jr., & West, S. A. (1995). Attention and formal thought disorder in mixed and pure mania. *Biological Psychiatry*, **37**, 420–423.

Sax, K. W., Strakowski, S. M., Zimmerman, M. E. *et al.* (1999). Frontosubcortical neuroanatomy and the continuous performance test in mania. *American Journal of Psychiatry*, **156**, 139–141.

Strakowski, S. M., Adler, C. M., Holland, S. K., Mills, N. & DelBello, M. P. (2004). A preliminary FMRI study of sustained attention in euthymic, unmedicated bipolar disorder. *Neuropsychopharmacology*, **29**, 1734–1740.

Strakowski, S. M., DelBello, M. P. & Adler, C. M. (2005). The functional neuroanatomy of bipolar disorder: a review of neuroimaging findings. *Molecular Psychiatry*, **10**, 105–116.

Strakowski, S. M., Keck, P. E. Jr., McElroy, S. L. *et al.* (1998). Twelve-month outcome after a first hospitalization for affective psychosis. *Archives of General Psychiatry*, **55**, 49–55.

Strakowski, S. M., McElroy, S. L., Keck, P. E. Jr. & West, S. A. (1996). Suicidality among patients with mixed and manic bipolar disorder. *American Journal of Psychiatry*, **153**, 674–676.

Swann, A. C., Dougherty, D. M., Pazzaglia, P. J. *et al.* (2005). Increased impulsivity associated with severity of suicide attempt history in patients with bipolar disorder. *American Journal of Psychiatry*, **162**, 1680–1687.

Swann, A. C., Pazzaglia, P., Nicholls, A., Dougherty, D. M. & Moeller, F. G. (2003). Impulsivity and phase of illness in bipolar disorder. *Journal of Affective Disorders*, **73**, 105–111.

Sweeney, J. A., Kmiec, J. A. & Kupfer, D. J. (2000). Neuropsychological impairment in bipolar and unipolar mood disorders on the CANTAB neurocognitive battery. *Biological Psychiatry*, **48**, 674–685.

Tohen, M., Hennen, J., Zarate, C. M. Jr. *et al.* (2000). Two-year syndromal and functional recovery in 219 cases of first-episode major affective disorder with psychotic features. *American Journal of Psychiatry*, **157**, 220–228.

Tohen, M., Waternaux, C. M. & Tsuang, M. T. (1990). Outcome in mania: a 4-year prospective follow-up of 75 patients utilizing survival analysis. *Archives of General Psychiatry*, **47**, 1106–1111.

van Gorp, W. G., Altshuler, L., Theberge, D. C. & Mintz, J. (1999). Declarative and procedural memory in bipolar disorder. *Biological Psychiatry*, **46**, 525–531.

van Gorp, W. G., Altshuler, L., Theberge, D. C., Wilkins, J. & Dixin, W. (1998). Cognitive impairment in euthymic bipolar patients with and without prior alcohol dependence. *Archives of General Psychiatry*, **55**, 41–46.

Wilder-Willis, K. E., Sax, K. W., Rosenberg, H. L. *et al.* (2001). Persistent attentional dysfunction in remitted bipolar disorder. *Bipolar Disorders*, **3**, 58–62.

Yamasaki, H., LaBar, K. S. & McCarthy, G. (2002). Dissociable prefrontal brain systems for attention and emotion. *PNAS*, **99**, 11447–11451.

Zubieta, J-K., Huguelet, P., O'Neil, R. L. & Giordani, B. J. (2001). Cognitive functioning in euthymic bipolar I disorder. *Psychiatry Research*, **102**, 9–20.

Renée Testa, Stephen J. Wood and Christos Pantelis

Introduction

A review of the other chapters within this book provides a detailed description of the neurocognitive profile of schizophrenia. As a result the current chapter will focus upon the course or progression of neuropsychological impairment in the disorder. Using findings derived from both cross-sectional and longitudinal studies, this chapter will first present a brief overview of the neuropsychological deficits that are associated with schizophrenia, both in established illness and at first presentation (including studies of at-risk populations). To reconcile the cognitive differences that have been identified in these groups, a framework will then be considered, which describes how different cognitive profiles may be accounted for at different stages of the illness. The importance of examining schizophrenia within a longitudinal and developmental framework will be discussed. Finally, future directions will be presented, which hope to progress our understanding of the timing and emergence of cognitive deficits, and various factors that may contribute to the onset of psychosis.

Schizophrenia is a serious psychiatric disorder that is characterized clinically by abnormal experiences and beliefs, disturbances of emotion and affect, as well as behavioral disturbances and impaired social functioning (Jablensky, 1995). The prevailing view is that schizophrenia is a neurodevelopmental disorder in which structural brain changes, caused by an early antenatal or perinatal insult, predispose to the development of schizophrenia, but are not progressive beyond the onset of symptoms. According to the neurodevelopmental model the lesion produced by an early insult interacts with normal post-pubertal brain maturation to produce the clinical symptoms of schizophrenia, which remain stable following the

onset of illness. Others consider that a neurodegenerative course is also apparent, and may result from vulnerability consequent on a neurodevelopmental lesion (Moller & von Zerssen, 1995; Pantelis & Barnes, 1996).

Studies examining neurocognition, specifically examining the presence and/or progression of cognitive deficits throughout the course of the schizophrenic disorder, have been particularly informative with regard to our understanding of disease-related mechanisms occurring pre- and post-presentation of psychotic disorder. Past findings have confirmed that neuropsychological deficits are prominent and can be identified at all stages of the illness, from first episode (and even before) through to established illness, and have been identified in a wide range of cognitive domains including attention, working memory, executive functioning and memory (Heinrichs & Zakzanis, 1998; Pantelis *et al.*, 2001; Wood *et al.*, 2002, 2003, 2006, 2007). The differentiation of the cognitive profile of individuals at different stages of the illness has proved useful to document the timing and progression of cognitive deficits. These findings have begun to challenge developmental notions regarding the emergence or progression of cognitive dysfunction in schizophrenia, with evidence suggestive of both neurodevelopmental and neurodegenerative processes.

Cross-sectional studies in high-risk, first-episode and established schizophrenia

Schizophrenia is associated with impairment in four principal domains of cognition: attention, working memory, verbal learning and executive functioning. Cross-sectional studies have traditionally dominated the neuropsychological literature and have provided useful information regarding the cognitive profile of individuals placed at different stages of the illness – high-risk, first-episode and chronic schizophrenia. As is demonstrated by the review below, differences are evident across the three clinical groups in the different domains of cognition, which may suggest either that cognitive functioning is associated with long-term outcome and/or that dynamic processes occur from the inception to the chronic stages of the illness.

In regards to the later, more chronic stages of schizophrenia, two relatively recent meta-analyses have been conducted. Fioravanti et al. (2005) identified significant and consistent impairments in intelligence, memory, language, attention and executive functions in chronically unwell patients in their large meta-analysis. However, significant variability between studies was also reported, suggestive of the multifaceted nature of cognitive deficits within the schizophrenia population. Rajji & Mulsant (2008) examined schizophrenia in later life and found marked impairments in executive functions, visuospatial ability and verbal fluency, with relatively less impairment found in memory, attention and working memory. Interestingly, these are the domains that are most markedly dysfunctional early in the course of the disease, which may suggest that early deficits are not progressive in nature, whilst those that appear later are more progressive and continue to deteriorate over time.

Deficits in working memory have been identified as a prominent feature of schizophrenia. Patients with schizophrenia are impaired on visuospatial working memory tasks, such as delayed response (DR) tasks (Badcock et al., 2005; Brewer et al., 1996; Fleming et al., 1997; Keefe et al., 1995, 1997; Park & Holzman, 1992; Partiot et al., 1992; Raine et al., 1992), the "self-ordered" spatial working-memory task (Hutton et al., 1998; Pantelis et al., 1997; Vance et al., 2006; Sacchetti et al., 2008) and the 'N-back' task (Bertolino et al., 2000; Krieger et al., 2005; Brahmbhatt et al., 2006). Impairments in verbal working memory have also been described in schizophrenia using Brown–Peterson paradigms, in which verbal stimuli are followed by a distraction task before subjects are asked to recall the original stimuli (Fleming et al., 1995; Randolph et al., 1992). Twamley et al. (2006) examined verbal short-term memory (Digits Forward (DF)) and working-memory capacity (Digits Backwards (DB) and Letter Number Sequencing (LNS)) in a large schizophrenia cohort and reported that patients showed impairment for all tasks, with worse negative symptoms associated with poorer performance. However, some degree of dissociation was identified, with DB being predictive of LNS performance and not DF. Kim et al. (2004) examined components of working memory using visuospatial and verbal delayed-response tasks, with findings suggesting that maintenance and central executive aspects of working memory were impaired. However, results suggested that the central executive may be affected to a greater degree. This was also supported by Silver et al. (2003) who investigated verbal and spatial working-memory deficits and their effect on other cognitive, executive measures. Findings suggested that working-memory deficits were a principal feature of cognitive dysfunction in schizophrenia and, as such, this deficit was restricting or limiting other cognitive skills to function optimally.

In their study of spatial working memory, Pantelis et al. (1997) directly compared patients with chronic schizophrenia with other neurological groups. Patients with schizophrenia were similar to parkinsonian patients in showing impaired visual short-term memory capacity, and were similar to both parkinsonian patients and patients with frontal lesions in showing deficits in spatial working memory and impaired ability to generate a systematic strategy. In contrast, patients with temporal lobe lesions were unimpaired on this task (Owen et al., 1996). The results were consistent with Petrides' (1994) notion that different regions of the dorsal prefrontal cortex are involved in schizophrenia, providing support for the notion that both ventrolateral and dorsolateral frontal circuits (as well as their interaction) are compromised (for discussion see Pantelis et al., 1997). Liederman & Strejilevich (2004) also identified deficits in single and dual spatial and object working-memory tasks in schizophrenic patients. The authors proposed that these findings were indicative of deficits in visuospatial working memory systems and the central executive (rather than a short-term memory maintenance deficit) given that dual-task performance was significantly worse than the single-task paradigm. More recently, in an adolescent-onset schizophrenia cohort, Vance et al. (2006) also reported visuospatial working memory deficits, but not on measures of spatial short-term memory span and strategy. The authors suggested that these data supported a model of frontal-striatal-parietal dysfunction, which is a proposal that has been examined by a number of other studies using imaging techniques. For example, using diffusion tensor imaging (DTI),

Karlsgodt *et al.* (2008) examined frontal-parietal connections in a recent-onset schizophrenia cohort. They reported structural abnormalities in the superior longitudinal fasciculus, with deficits more pronounced on the left side. Furthermore, the integrity of the white matter fibers was found to predict performance on a verbal working-memory task in patients. Barch & Csernansky (2007) conducted an fMRI study to investigate whether prefrontal and parietal regions in chronic patients demonstrated abnormal activity in verbal and non-verbal working memory tasks (2-back). They further investigated whether any dysfunction identified was specific to the nature of the information being used, or whether domain-general processes were involved. Results were suggestive of deficits in prefrontal and parietal brain activation, areas associated with the central executive components of working memory, rather than domain-specific storage systems (see also Schlösser *et al.*, 2008).

The numerous studies of memory in schizophrenia have generally concluded that memory function is impaired both in chronically unwell patients (Saykin *et al.*, 1991) and in those in their first episode of a psychotic illness, as earlier described (Riley *et al.*, 2000; Saykin *et al.*, 1994). Generally, verbal memory deficits appear to be more robust than visuospatial ones, and verbal memory shows little improvement over the first few years of illness (Hoff *et al.*, 1999). Nonetheless, a meta-analysis of 70 studies of memory in schizophrenia provided strong support for a deficit in recall and recognition for both verbal and visual material, as well as short-term memory and working memory (forward and backward digit span; Aleman *et al.*, 1999). Surprisingly, negative symptoms were associated with memory deficits, which are usually thought to be related to impairments of prefrontal function, especially involving DLPFC (Liddle *et al.*, 1992; Pantelis *et al.*, 2001). However, the analysis did not investigate whether the impairment of memory was over and above the recognized impairments of global cognitive function (as measured by IQ), attention or working memory. This is significant given that previous studies have found that lowered performance on specific cognitive measures has been attributable to a general decline in intelligence or poor working-memory capacity, for example. This need to account for other domains of cognition, and even developmental trajectories, has more recently come to the foreground in the literature. This is particularly in light of studies such as Woodberry *et al.* (2008), who conducted a meta-analysis examining intelligence in schizophrenia and reported that patients consistently demonstrated a significant impairment in premorbid IQ that was evident well before the onset of psychotic symptoms (one half of a standard deviation). Further, the onset of psychosis was found to be associated with an even greater deterioration in the intellectual level of patients.

Despite this finding, studies that have accounted for lower intelligence to permit a more accurate interpretation of results have found that specific deficits endure. Investigations such as those by Weickert *et al.* (2000) and Pantelis *et al.* (1999) both identified deficits in the WCST and IDED (CANTAB) tasks respectively in chronically unwell patients, that could not be explained by IQ differences. Further, Badcock *et al.*'s (2005) investigation which examined subgroups of schizophrenic patients with preserved, compromised or deteriorated intellectual skills demonstrated that even those with an average estimated IQ displayed deficits in executive functions that were significantly more impaired than normal controls; however, performance was still significantly better than either the compromised or deteriorated groups. Reaction time was found to be equally impaired across all three clinical groups.

More recently the need to account for developmental trajectories to understand cognitive dysfunction throughout the progression and in different subgroups of the disorder has been reported. White *et al.* (2006) examined the effect of age of onset of illness (AOI) on the cognitive status of patients in an adolescent onset group (AOI = 16.5 years) and an adult onset group (AOI = 24.4 years). Two normal control groups matched for age were also included. Results found that the adolescent-onset group performed worse that the adult group on measures of working memory, language and motor functioning. Furthermore, the normal adolescent group was also found to perform worse than adult controls on measures of working memory and language (although better on measures of motor function). When these normal developmental differences were taken into consideration for the two patient groups, differences between the adolescent and adult onset groups for working memory and language were no longer found. This study highlights the need to account for trajectories of cognition, which is especially pertinent given that investigation of cognitive dysfunction in schizophrenia is now targeted at prodromal groups that are yet to reach complete brain maturation.

It is evident from the above evidence that chronic illness in schizophrenia is associated with marked and significant impairments. However, understanding the underlying nature and possible progression of these cognitive deficits is limited when investigation is undertaken within only chronically unwell patients. Greater insight has only more recently been obtained by examining individuals earlier in the course of the illness, including first-episode and even prodromal, high-risk cohorts, which permit more opportunities to examine when cognitive deficits occur throughout the course of the illness and whether when present, further deterioration of these deficits in specific cognitive domains is evident.

Studies examining the pattern of cognitive deficits in first-episode groups have generally reported that deficits are not as severe as in chronic groups, but are more marked and occur in a greater number of cognitive domains than high-risk cohorts (Brewer et al., 2005; Eastvold et al., 2007; Fusar-Poli et al., 2007; Joyce et al., 2005; Simon et al., 2007). Gonzalez-Blanch et al. (2007) reported significantly poorer performance in eight different cognitive domains in patients at the very early stages of the illness. These included verbal learning/memory, verbal comprehension, motor speed and impulsivity, with the most marked deficits in speed of processing, executive functions, motor dexterity and sustained attention. Significant verbal-learning deficits early in the disorder have been reported previously (Riley et al., 2000), although such deficits have been significantly associated with a poorer ability to use organizational strategies to permit more efficient learning. Reported marked deficits in select executive functions in first-episode cohorts have included planning, the capacity to initiate strategies, inhibition, sustained and shifting attention, cognitive switching, attention allocation, working memory and verbal fluency (Chan et al., 2006; Hutton et al., 1998, 2002; Joyce et al., 2005).

There is some suggestion that the early phase of the illness might be accompanied by cognitive decline. Lappin et al. (2007) examined duration of untreated psychosis (DUP) in a first-episode cohort and its relationship to efficient encoding and recall. They found that longer DUP was associated with poorer performance in verbal intelligence tasks, verbal learning and verbal working memory; visual learning and speed of processing was not affected. Joyce et al. (2005) also reported that longer DUP was correlated with poorer attentional set-shifting abilities.

Research examining whether deficits exhibited by first-episode patients are more marked than or as severe as chronic schizophrenia patients has been inconsistent. The issue of whether cognitive deterioration occurs throughout the course of the illness is debated, with studies including Moritz et al. (2002) demonstrating that first-episode and chronic patients differed significantly in neurocognitive tasks from controls, but not from each other, suggesting that deficits do not worsen over the course of the illness. Studies of attentional set shifting, however, have been suggestive of deterioration, with chronic patients demonstrating worse deficits than first-episode cohorts (Hutton et al., 1998; Pantelis et al., 2009a). Indeed, attentional set-shifting ability has received much interest in the schizophrenia literature. A number of studies have confirmed that patients with chronic schizophrenia perform poorly on these tasks, which require subjects to shift attention between different stimulus dimensions on the basis of reinforcing feedback. Using such a task Elliott & Sahakian (1995) found that patients with moderately severe schizophrenia fail due to a tendency to perseverate, akin to frontal lesion patients. In their study, Pantelis et al. (1999) directly compared a more chronic group of patients with schizophrenia with a cohort of patients with frontal lobe lesions, and found more severe deficits in schizophrenia.

Studies examining neurocognition in high-risk and first-episode patients generally report normal or near-normal intelligence (Hawkins et al., 2004). However, even in the high-risk, prodromal stage of the illness, this has been found to occur within the context of significant cognitive deficits in several domains. These include lower performances in verbal paired associative learning, spatial recognition memory, visual processing and spatial working memory (Bartok et al., 2005). Whyte et al. (2006) reported deficits in immediate and delayed verbal memory (story recall) in a high-risk group, while there was a suggestion that those converting to illness showed poorer baseline verbal learning performance. Significant cognitive deficits were also reported by Pflueger et al. (2007) who found that high-risk individuals performed most poorly and were subsequently best discriminated from healthy controls on measures assessing verbal intelligence, executive functions and most specifically working memory. These results were also supported by Eastvold et al. (2007) who found comparable findings in a neurocognitive study examining high-risk, first-episode patients and controls. Deficits in spatial working memory and verbal anel visual memory have also been consistently identified in the Melbourne UHR studies. Wood *et al.* (2003) reported deficits in spatial working memory and visual memory in a UHR group. Those who later became psychotic performed more poorly than those who did not. Brewer *et al.* (2005) examined global memory processes in a UHR cohort and similarly found significantly poorer scores for those that later developed psychosis. Significant working memory and executive dysfunction in a high-risk cohort has also been captured via questionnaires such as the Behavioural Rating Inventory of Executive Functioning (BRIEF), which measures real life, everyday dysexecutive behavior (Niendam *et al.*, 2007).

In a comparative study of high-risk patients with previously reported neuropsychological data from first-episode and chronic patients from other studies, Hawkins *et al.* (2004) found that high-risk patients were more cognitively intact than either a first-episode or chronic group, but still performed below normal expectations. Differential levels of deficit severity were also noted. The high-risk group performed similarly to the chronic group on a test of verbal fluency and visual memory (immediate recall), but better on tests of visual memory (delayed recall), processing speed, and verbal memory than either the chronic or first-episode groups. Although such comparisons across studies are useful as a wider sample can be utilized, it is limited by many issues such as sampling and methodological differences.

Further differentiation of the progression of cognitive deficits can be achieved by comparing individuals at high risk with those at ultra-high risk. Simon *et al.* (2007) identified marked deficits again in working memory (verbal), verbal fluency and declarative verbal memory (word list) in high-risk (showing basic predictive symptoms) and ultra-high-risk groups, that were not as marked as deficits found in a first-episode group, but poorer than normal performance. Interestingly, differences in performance were found between the high-risk and ultra-high-risk, where the ultra-high-risk group exhibited fewer deficits than the first-episode cohort, but performed more poorly than the high-risk group. Similarly, Myles-Worsley *et al.* (2007) attempted to better understand the prodrome by comparing normal controls to individuals that were either clinically high risk or genetically high or low risk (with a proportion

of each group exhibiting some symptomatology). Findings demonstrated that whilst the genetically high-risk group exhibited deficits in verbal memory, verbal working memory, sustained attention and fine motor skills, those that exhibited psychosis additionally performed more poorly on measures of spatial working memory and visual-organizational skills (perceptual organization scale on the Wechsler Adult Intelligence Scale (WISC–III)). Further, increased symptomatology was not associated with more severe neurocognitive deficits, with no significant interaction between genetic risk and clinical status and cognition. This study suggests that cognitive impairments were more broadly mediated by genetic status rather than clinical symptomatology; however, impending psychosis was associated with emerging deficits in visuospatial processing skills.

In sum, individuals with an at-risk mental state for psychosis already show impairment of neuropsychological functions prior to the onset of the first psychotic episode, particularly in the domains of executive function and working memory. Given the relative sparing of deficits in high-risk or ultra-high-risk groups, it suggests that interventions targeted at slowing or delaying the onset of psychosis would be warranted. However, further longitudinal investigations (as discussed later in the chapter) would be required to better understand the trajectory and/or progression of deficits and help to determine whether and at what point interventions would need to be targeted to delay the onset or progression of deficits.

Limitation of adopting a cross-sectional approach

The adoption of a cross-sectional design when investigating a disorder that is likely to be both neurodevelopmental and neuroprogressive in nature (for discussion see Pantelis *et al.*, 2005) presents several obstacles. As described earlier, neurocognitive studies have delineated different cognitive profiles in individuals at different stages of schizophrenia (high-risk, first-episode and chronic), suggesting that changing and unpredictable processes are occurring throughout the disorder. Therefore, the trajectory of the illness, including the effects that the disease-related processes have had on specific individuals is difficult to determine.

Because of this, participant-related differences across studies can hinder accurate comparisons of research findings. It is impossible to ensure that patient variables, including the severity of the illness, genetic loading of schizophrenia, duration of untreated psychosis, illness chronicity, number of psychotic episodes and medications, are equitable, and therefore represent major confounding variables. This issue is difficult to overcome when comparing patients across different studies or even different sample populations within one investigation, and also creates innumerable difficulties when selecting comparative groups. This questions many cross-sectional studies that have evaluated or contrasted individuals at different stages of illness (e.g. high-risk individuals, those prodromal for psychosis, within first-episode and chronic cohorts). It cannot be assumed that the outcome of a chronic group would necessarily be the foreseeable outcome for the first-episode group.

Further, the varied and diverse range of deficits identified at different stages throughout the illness (i.e. high-risk, first-episode, chronic), but also within each of these stages makes it difficult to accurately document cognitive changes in different cohorts. It can be difficult to ascertain when to assess patients to obtain the most accurate picture of deficits that are occurring in the sample of patients, where factors such as medication can confound results. Gonzalez-Blanch et al. (2007), for example, compared a first-episode cohort with controls in an initial assessment and then three months post antipsychotic treatment. Whilst initial assessment demonstrated significant impairments in executive functions, verbal memory, working memory, sustained attention and visuomotor processing speed, marked improvements were identified in several domains including executive functions, immediate verbal memory and visuomotor processing following administration of medication. The time at which the assessment is undertaken can therefore significantly affect the identification of deficits within sample groups.

Methodological factors can also play a significant role, with the type and number of measurements used also creating difficulties and making direct comparisons difficult. Even seemingly minor differences in cognitive requirements in neuropsychological tests can produce different results, especially when other inter-related cognitive abilities are not accounted for.

The best means to overcome the abovementioned difficulties is to conduct longitudinal studies that can accurately document the progression of the illness in the same individuals at each stage of the illness.

Only longitudinal studies can reliably document the course of the illness and the relationship between different cognitive and neurological facets of the illness, and thus determine whether schizophrenia is a progressive disorder. The adoption of a longitudinal, as opposed to cross-sectional approach also provides greater insight into developmental patterns of cortical change. Longitudinal studies are required to examine growth trajectories so that the fluid nature of the relationships between cognitive and cortical measures can be examined. They also permit greater understanding of the neurobiological processes at illness inception, with studies from before illness onset and over the initial stages of psychosis required to determine the nature of progressive changes over time, and to determine which indices may be predictive markers of the illness or its course. Such studies also provide evidence about which biological indices may represent "state" versus "trait" ("endophenotypic") illness markers, and can provide further evidence as to whether abnormalities present in those with established illness reflect neurobiological processes at earlier illness or pre-illness stages (Pantelis et al., 2009b). Thus, while it has been suggested that these structural and cognitive abnormalities have their basis in early brain development (Murray & Lewis, 1987; Weinberger, 1987), it is now apparent as we understand this disorder better that elucidating the nature, timing and course of underlying neurobiological changes from cross-sectional studies can only provide a somewhat limited and incomplete picture.

Longitudinal investigations in high-risk, first-episode and established schizophrenia

The differences in the degree of neuropsychological impairment found across the stages of schizophrenia noted above could be regarded as suggesting progressive decline with continued illness. However, there does not appear to be much support for such a notion. Although there were early reports of progressive cognitive deficits in schizophrenia (Bilder et al., 1991; Goldberg et al., 1987), a review of the field in 1998 largely confirmed the idea of static impairments (Rund, 1998). A further ten years' work has not changed the essential picture of cognition as manifesting stable deficits in established schizophrenia. A recent meta-analysis of 2476 chronic patients in 53 studies examined longitudinal change over an average of 12 months, and found significant improvement in almost every cognitive test studied (Szöke et al., 2008). Indeed, only one test (Boston Naming) showed even a non-significant decline, suggesting that far from progressive impairments, schizophrenia patients could show meaningful recovery in function. However, a comparison with the changes over time seen in controls indicated similar improvement implying that practice was a more likely explanation. A comparable finding was also reported by Goldberg et al. (2007) who noted in their study of first-episode and control patients that improvements in cognition following administration of two commonly prescribed antipsychotic medications (olanzapine and risperidone) were primarily due to practice effects, given that the degree of improvement was comparable to that observed in healthy control patients.

A similar pattern exists in studies of first-episode psychosis – largely stable cognitive deficits over the first 12–24 months of illness, with any improvements attributable to practice effects (Addington et al., 2005; Gold et al., 1999; Hill et al., 2004; Hoff et al., 1999). This stability is somewhat surprising given the findings of progressive decline in structural brain measures across a similar timeframe (for review see DeLisi, 2008; Pantelis et al., 2005), but to date there is only a weak relationship between structural and cognitive change (Ho et al., 2003; Zipparo et al., 2008), if any (Hoff et al., 1999).

Instead, progressive impairments may be revealed over a much longer interval. When the follow-up interval is around ten years, patients with first-episode psychosis show less or a lack of improvement compared with controls (Hoff et al., 2005; Stirling et al., 2003) in a number of cognitive domains, but particularly memory. This is supported by our own recently completed longitudinal study in early psychosis. We assessed 27 patients and 13 controls on two occasions, an average of six years apart. Although most cognitive abilities remained stable over this period we found significant decline in two tests – visuospatial paired associate learning (Wood et al., 2006) and attentional set-shifting (Pantelis et al., 2006).

As well as these changes that may be occurring over the first decade after the onset of psychosis, there is evidence for cognitive changes as the illness develops. In one of the earliest studies by Caspi et al. (2003), 44 first-episode patients were enrolled who had had a cognitive assessment four or five years

earlier at recruitment to the Israeli military service. Compared with 44 healthy controls, patients showed deterioration on measures of abstract reasoning and concentration between the two time points – although the patients were already significantly impaired at baseline. More recently, we have examined progressive changes in cognitive function over the transition to psychosis as part of the Melbourne ultra-high risk studies (Wood et al., 2007). Sixteen ultra-high risk patients (seven of whom developed psychosis) were assessed neuropsychologically at baseline and after transition to psychosis (or after 12 months). While performance on most tests was stable or improved, visuospatial memory, verbal fluency and attentional switching showed significant decline over the transition to psychosis. These progressive impairments were not seen in the non-psychotic ultra-high-risk group. These data would seem consistent with progressive brain structural changes over transition to psychosis (for review see Wood et al., 2008), and suggest that potential endophenotypes may not be stable over the transition to illness (Pantelis et al., 2009b).

These data in an ultra-high-risk cohort do not support findings from the Edinburgh High Risk Study, who were selected only on genetic risk criteria. In that study, the cognitive performance of 13 people who became ill was compared with that of 105 who did not, at two time points at least 1000 days apart. Deficits were clearly apparent for story recall in the high-risk sample as a whole compared with controls and these deficits were stable over time. However, there were no specific deficits or progressive changes in those who developed schizophrenia (Whyte et al., 2006).

Discussion and future directions

Although there do seem to be differences in cognitive impairments by stage of illness (as assessed by cross-sectional studies), the findings from longitudinal studies are equivocal at best. The more parsimonious explanation is that cognitive impairments are present from the start of the illness and do not progress appreciably. Some decline may occur across the transition to frank disorder, however. Nonetheless, continued study is indicated, especially in the few years either side of onset.

We argue that a better understanding may be achieved by exploring growth curves and the developmental trajectories of cognitive abilities, and in particular those of the executive function system (see Testa & Pantelis, Chapter 9). Whilst growth curves can inform us about the cognitive dysfunctions experienced by individuals who develop schizophrenia and neurodevelopmental disorders, we also argue that they may prove to be particularly informative in regards to understanding the timing of illness onset. Arguably, earlier age of onset would be associated with more profound deficits, though there is limited evidence to support this as yet, and this may depend upon whether the neural substrate has already been damaged at earlier developmental stages, such that patients "grow into deficit" (Lipska et al., 1993; Lipska & Weinberger, 2000; Weinberger, 1987). Further to this, earlier age of onset may be associated with greater genetic loading and environmental risk for the illness, such that the "threshold" for the development of psychosis is reached earlier given the relative weighting of the factors earlier discussed. But how this comes about is still undetermined. We argue that examination of the normal and aberrant growth curves in schizophrenia may be the key to understanding this.

Using the framework of growth curves and documenting the developmental trajectory of normal cognitive (particularly executive) skills, it would be possible to compare this trajectory with that of an individual at high risk that goes on to develop psychosis. Such a "cognitive map" would aptly illustrate how cognition is affected over a longitudinal time period and offer more insight than cross-sectional studies by permitting comparisons of the developmental trajectories of specific executive abilities that are known to be essential to intact neurocognition.

References

Addington, J., Saeedi, H. & Addington, D. (2005). The course of cognitive functioning in first episode psychosis: changes over time and impact on outcome. *Schizophrenia Research*, **78**, 35–43.

Aleman, A., Hijman, R., de Haan, E. H. F. et al. (1999). Memory impairment in schizophrenia: A meta-analysis. *American Journal of Psychiatry*, **156**, 1358–1366.

Badcock, J. C., Dragovic, M., Waters, F. A. et al. (2005). Dimensions of intelligence in schizophrenia: evidence from patients with preserved, deteriorated and compromised intellect. *Journal of Psychiatric Research*, **39**, 11–19.

Barch, D. M. & Csernansky, J. G. (2007). Abnormal parietal cortex activation during working memory in schizophrenia: verbal phonological coding disturbances versus domain-general executive dysfunction. *American Journal of Psychiatry*, **164**, 1090–1098.

Bartok, E., Berecz, R., Glaub, T. et al. (2005). Cognitive functions in prepsychotic patients. *Progress in Neuropsychopharmacology and Biological Psychiatry*, **29**, 621–625.

Bertolino, A., Esposito, G., Callicott, J. H. et al. (2000). Specific relationship between prefrontal neuronal N-acetylaspartate and activation of the working memory cortical network in schizophrenia. *American Journal of Psychiatry*, **157**, 26–33.

Bilder, R. M., Lipschutz-Broch, L., Reiter, G. et al. (1991). Neuropsychological deficits in the early course of first episode schizophrenia. *Schizophrenia Research*, **5**, 198–199.

Brahmbhatt, S. B., Haut, K., Csernansky, J. & Barch, D. (2006). Neural correlates of verbal and nonverbal working memory deficits in individuals with schizophrenia and their high-risk siblings. *Schizophrenia Research*, **87**, 191–204.

Brewer, W. J., Edwards, J., Anderson, V. et al. (1996). Neuropsychological, olfactory, and hygiene deficits in men with negative symptom schizophrenia. *Biological Psychiatry*, **40**, 1021–1031.

Brewer, W. J., Francey, S. M., Wood, S. J. et al. (2005). Memory impairments identified in people at ultra-high risk for psychosis who later develop first-episode psychosis. *American Journal of Psychiatry*, **162**, 71–78.

Caspi, A., Reichenberg, A., Weiser, M. et al. (2003). Cognitive performance in schizophrenia patients assessed before and following the first psychotic episode. *Schizophrenia Research*, **65**, 87–94.

Chan, R. C., Chen, E. Y. & Law, C. W. (2006). Specific executive dysfunction in patients with first-episode medication-naive schizophrenia. *Schizophrenia Research*, **82**, 51–64.

DeLisi, L. E. (2008). The concept of progressive brain change in schizophrenia: implications for understanding schizophrenia. *Schizophrenia Bulletin*, **34**, 312–321.

Eastvold, A. D., Heaton, R. K. & Cadenhead, K. S. (2007). Neurocognitive deficits in the (putative) prodrome and first episode of psychosis. *Schizophrenia Research*, **93**, 266–277.

Elliott, R. & Sahakian, B. J. (1995). The neuropsychology of schizophrenia: relations with clinical and neurobiological dimensions. *Psychological Medicine*, **25**, 581–594.

Fioravanti, M., Carlone, O., Vitale, B. et al. (2005). A meta-analysis of cognitive deficits in adults with a diagnosis of schizophrenia. *Neuropsychology Review*, **15**, 73–95.

Fleming, K., Goldberg, T. E., Gold, J. M. *et al.* (1995). Verbal working memory dysfunction in schizophrenia: use of a Brown–Peterson paradigm. *Psychiatry Research*, **56**, 155–161.

Fleming, K., Goldberg, T. E., Binks, S. *et al.* (1997). Visuospatial working memory in patients with schizophrenia. *Biological Psychiatry*, **41**, 43–49.

Fusar-Poli, P., Perez, J., Broome, M. *et al.* (2007). Neurofunctional correlates of vulnerability to psychosis: a systematic review and meta-analysis. *Neuroscience and Biobehavior Review*, **31**, 465–484.

Gold, S., Arndt, S., Nopoulos, P. *et al.* (1999). Longitudinal study of cognitive function in first-episode and recent-onset schizophrenia. *American Journal of Psychiatry*, **156**, 1342–1348.

Goldberg, T. E., Weinberger, D. R., Berman, K. F. *et al.* (1987). Further evidence for dementia of the prefrontal type in schizophrenia? A controlled study of teaching the Wisconsin Card Sorting Test. *Archives of General Psychiatry*, **44**, 1008–1014.

Goldberg, T. E., Goldman, R. S., Burdick, K. E. *et al.* (2007). Cognitive improvement after treatment with second-generation antipsychotic medications in first-episode schizophrenia: is it a practice effect? *Archive of General Psychiatry*, **64**, 1115–1122.

Gonzalez-Blanch, C., Crespo-Facorro, B., Alvarez-Jimenez, M. *et al.* (2007). Cognitive dimensions in first-episode schizophrenia spectrum disorders. *Journal of Psychiatric Research*, **41**, 968–977.

Hawkins, K. A., Addington, J., Keefe, R. S. *et al.* (2004). Neuropsychological status of subjects at high risk for a first episode of psychosis. *Schizophrenia Research*, **67**, 115–122.

Heinrichs, R. W. & Zakzanis, K. K. (1998). Neurocognitive deficit in schizophrenia: a quantitative review of the evidence. *Neuropsychology*, **12**, 426–445.

Hill, S. K., Schuepbach, D., Herbener, E. S. *et al.* (2004). Pretreatment and longitudinal studies of neuropsychological deficits in antipsychotic-naive patients with schizophrenia. *Schizophrenia Research*, **68**, 49–63.

Ho, B.-C., Andreasen, N. C., Nopoulos, P. *et al.* (2003). Progressive structural brain abnormalities and their relationship to clinical outcome: a longitudinal magnetic resonance imaing study early in schizophrenia. *Archives of General Psychiatry*, **60**, 585–594.

Hoff, A. L., Sakuma, M., Wieneke, M. *et al.* (1999). Longitudinal neuropsychological follow-up study of patients with first-episode schizophrenia. *American Journal of Psychiatry*, **156**, 1336–1341.

Hoff, A. L., Svetina, C., Shields, G. *et al.* (2005). Ten year longitudinal study of neuropsychological functioning subsequent to a first episode of schizophrenia. *Schizophrenia Research*, **78**, 27–34.

Hutton, S. B., Puri, B. K., Duncan, L.-J. *et al.* (1998). Executive function in first-episode schizophrenia. *Psychological Medicine*, **28**, 463–473.

Hutton, S. B., Murphy, F. C., Joyce, E. M. *et al.* (2002). Decision making deficits in patients with first-episode and chronic schizophrenia. *Schizophrenia Research*, **55**, 249–257.

Jablensky, A. (1995). Schizophrenia: the epidemiological horizon. In S.W. Hirsch (Ed.), *Schizophrenia* (pp. 206–252). Oxford: Blackwell Science.

Joyce, E. M., Hutton, S. B., Mutsatsa, S. H. *et al.* (2005). Cognitive heterogeneity in first-episode schizophrenia. *British Journal of Psychiatry*, **187**, 516–522.

Karlsgodt, K. H., van Erp, T. G., Poldrack, R. A. *et al.* (2008). Diffusion tensor imaging of the superior longitudinal fasciculus and working memory in recent-onset schizophrenia. *Biological Psychiatry*, **63**, 512–518.

Keefe, R. S., Lees-Roitman, S. E. & Dupre, R. L. (1997). Performance of patients with schizophrenia on a pen and paper visuospatial working memory task with short delay. *Schizophrenia Research*, **26**, 9–14.

Keefe, R. S., Roitman, S. E., Harvey, P. D. *et al.* (1995). A pen-and-paper human analogue of a monkey prefrontal cortex activation task: spatial working memory in patients with schizophrenia. *Schizophrenia Research*, **17**, 25–33.

Kim, M. S., Ha, T. H. & Kwon, J. S. (2004). Neurological abnormalities in schizophrenia and obsessive-compulsive disorder. *Current Opinion in Psychiatry*, **17**, 215–220.

Krieger, S., Lis, S., Cetin, T., Gallhofer, B. & Myer-Linderberg, A. (2005). Executive function and cognitive subprocesses in first-episode, drug-naive schizophrenia: an analysis of N-back performance. *American Journal of Psychiatry*, **162**, 1206–1208.

Lappin, J. M., Morgan, K. D., Morgan, C. *et al.* (2007). Duration of untreated psychosis and neuropsychological function in first episode psychosis. *Schizophrenia Research*, **95**, 103–110.

Leiderman, E. A. & Strejilevich, S. A. (2004). Visuospatial deficits in schizophrenia: central executive and memory subsystems impairments. *Schizophrenia Research*, **68**, 217–223.

Liddle, P. F., Friston, K. J., Frith, C. D. *et al.* (1992). Cerebral blood flow and mental processes in schizophrenia. *Journal of the Royal Society of Medicine*, **85**, 224–227.

Lipska, B. K. & Weinberger, D. R. (2000). To model a psychiatric disorder in animals: schizophrenia as a reality test. *Neuropsychopharmacology*, **23**, 223–239.

Lipska, B. K., Jaskiw, G. E. & Weinberger, D. R. (1993). Postpubertal emergence of hyperresponsiveness to stress and to amphetamine after neonatal excitotoxic hippocampal damage: a potential animal model of schizophrenia. *Neuropsychopharmacology*, **9**, 67–75.

Moller, H. J. & von Zerssen, D. (1995). Course and outcome of schizophrenia. In S.W. Hirsch (Ed.), *Schizophrenia* (pp. 106–127). Oxford, UK, Blackwell Science.

Moritz, S., Andresen, B., Perro, C. et al. (2002). Neurocognitive performance in first-episode and chronic schizophrenic patients. *European Archive of Psychiatry and Clinical Neuroscience*, **252**, 33–37.

Murray, R. M. & Lewis, S. W. (1987). Is schizophrenia a neurodevelopmental disorder? [editorial]. *British Medical Journal*, **295**, 681–682.

Myles-Worsley, M., Ord, L. M., Ngiralmau, H. et al. (2007). The Palau Early Psychosis Study: neurocognitive functioning in high-risk adolescents. *Schizophrenia Research*, **89**, 299–307.

Niendam, T. A., Horwitz, J., Bearden, C. E. et al. (2007). Ecological assessment of executive dysfunction in the psychosis prodrome: a pilot study. *Schizophrenia Research*, **93**, 350–354.

Owen, A. M., Morris, R. G., Sahakian, B. J. et al. (1996). Double dissociations of memory and executive functions in working memory tasks following frontal lobe excisions, temporal lobe excisions or amygdalo-hippocampectomy in man. *Brain*, **119**(5), 1597–1615.

Pantelis, C. & Barnes, T. R. (1996). Drug strategies and treatment-resistant schizophrenia. *Australia and New Zealand Journal of Psychiatry*, **30**, 20–37.

Pantelis, C., Barber, F., Barnes, T. R. E. et al. (1999). Comparison of set-shifting ability in patients with chronic schizophrenia and frontal lobe damage. *Schizophrenia Research*, **37**, 251–270.

Pantelis, C., Barnes, T. R. E., Nelson, H. E. et al. (1997). Frontal-striatal cognitive deficits in patients with chronic schizophrenia. *Brain*, **120**, 1823–1843.

Pantelis, C., Proffitt, T., Wood, S. J. et al. (2006). Spatial working memory and attentional set-shifting after the onset of psychosis: data from the EPPIC medium-term follow-up study. *Schizophrenia Research*, **81** (Suppl. 1), 128.

Pantelis, C., Stuart, G. W., Nelson, H. E. et al. (2001). Spatial working memory deficits in schizophrenia: relationship with tardive dyskinesia and negative symptoms. *American Journal of Psychiatry*, **158**, 1276–1285.

Pantelis, C., Wood, S. J., Proffitt, T. M. et al. (2009a). Attentional set-shifting ability in first-episode and established schizophrenia: Relationship to working memory. *Schizophrenia Research*, **112**, 104–113.

Pantelis, C., Yücel, M., Wood, S. J. et al. (2005). Structural brain imaging evidence for multiple pathological processes at different stages of brain development in schizophrenia. *Schizophrenia Bulletin*, **31**, 672–696.

Pantelis, C., Yücel, M., Wood, S. J. et al. (2009b). Neurobiological endophenotypes of psychosis and schizophrenia: are there biological markers of illness onset? In P. D. McGorry & H. J. Jackson (Eds.), *Recognition and Management of Early Psychosis: A Preventive Approach*. Cambridge: Cambridge University Press.

Park, S. & Holzman, P. S. (1992). Schizophrenics show spatial working memory deficits. *Archives of General Psychiatry*, **49**, 975–982.

Partiot, A., Pierson, A., Dodin, V. et al. (1992). Information process in depressives. *Biological Psychiatry*, **31**, 1175–1177.

Petrides, M. (1994). Frontal lobes and working memory: evidence from investigations of the effects of cortical excisions in nonhuman primates. In F. G. J. Boller (Ed.), *Handbook of Neuropsychology*, (pp. 59–82). Amsterdam: Elsevier.

Pflueger, M. O., Gschwandtner, U., Stieglitz, R. D. et al. (2007). Neuropsychological deficits in individuals with an at risk mental state for psychosis – working memory as a potential trait marker. *Schizophrenia Research*, **97**, 14–24.

Raine, A., Lencz, T., Reynolds, G. P. et al. (1992). An evaluation of structural and functional prefrontal deficits in schizophrenia: MRI and neuropsychological measures. *Psychiatry Research*, **45**, 123–137.

Rajji, T. K. & Mulsant B. H. (2008). Nature and course of cognitive function in late-life schizophrenia: a systematic review. *Schizophrenia Research*, **102** (1–3), 122–140.

Randolph, C., Gold, J. M., Carpenter, C. J. et al. (1992). Release from proactive interference: determinants of performance and neuropsychological correlates. *Journal of Clinical and Experimental Neuropsychology*, **14**, 785–800.

Riley, E. M., McGovern, D., Mockler, D. et al. (2000). Neuropsychological functioning in first-episode psychosis – evidence of specific deficits. *Schizophrenia Research*, **43**, 47–55.

Rund, B. R. (1998). A review of longitudinal studies of cognitive functions in schizophrenia patients. *Schizophrenia Bulletin*, **24**, 425–435.

Sacchetti, E., Galluzzo, A., Panariella, A., Parrinello, G. & Cappa, S. F. (2008). Self-ordered pointing and visual conditional associative learning tasks in drug-free schizophrenia spectrum disorder patients. *BMC Psychiatry*, **8**, 6.

Saykin, A. J., Gur, R. C., Gur, R. E. et al. (1991). Neuropsychological function in schizophrenia. Selective impairment of memory and learning. *Archives of General Psychiatry*, **48**, 618–624.

Saykin, A. J., Shtasel, D. L., Gur, R. E. et al. (1994). Neuropsychological deficits in neuroleptic naïve patients with first-episode schizophrenia. *Archives of General Psychiatry*, 51, 124–131.

Schlosser, R. G., Koch, K., Wagner, G. *et al.* (2008). Inefficient executive cognitive control in schizophrenia is preceded by altered functional activation during information encoding: an fMRI study. *Neuropsychologia*, 46, 336–347.

Simon, A. E., Cattapan-Ludewig, K., Zmilacher, S. *et al.* (2007). Cognitive functioning in the schizophrenia prodrome. *Schizophrenia Bulletin*, 33, 761–771.

Silver, H., Feldman, P., Nilker, W. & Gur, R. (2003). Working memory deficit as a core neuropsychological dysfunction in schizophrenia. *American Journal of Psychiatry*, 160, 1809–1816.

Stirling, J., White, C., Lewis, S. W. *et al.* (2003). Neurocognitive function and outcome in first-episode schizophrenia: a 10-year follow-up of an epidemiological cohort. *Schizophrenia Research*, 65, 75–86.

Szöke, A., Trandafir, A., Dupont, M.-E. *et al.* (2008). Longitudinal studies of cognition in schizophrenia: meta-analysis. *British Journal of Psychiatry*, 192, 248–257.

Twamley, E. W., Palmer, B. W., Jeste, D., Taylor, M. & Heaton, R. K. (2006). Transient and executive function working memory in schizophrenia. *Schizophrenia Research*, 87, 185–190.

Vance, A., Hall, N., Bellgrive, M. *et al.* (2006). Visuospatial working memory deficits in adolescent onset schizophrenia. *Schizophrenia Research*, 87, 223–227.

Weickert, T. W., Goldberg, T. E., Gold, J. M. *et al.* (2000). Cognitive impairments in patients with schizophrenia displaying preserved and compromised intellect. *Archives of General Psychiatry*, 57, 907–913.

Weinberger, D. R. (1987). Implications of normal brain development for the pathogenesis of schizophrenia. *Archives of General Psychiatry*, 44, 660–669.

White, T., Ho, B. C., Ward, J. *et al.* (2006). Neuropsychological performance in first-episode adolescents with schizophrenia: a comparison with first-episode adults and adolescent control subjects. *Biological Psychiatry*, 60, 463–471.

Whyte, M.-C., Brett, C., Harrison, L. K. *et al.* (2006). Neuropsychological performance over time in people at high risk of developing schizophrenia and controls. *Biological Psychiatry*, 59, 730–739.

Wood, S. J., Brewer, W. J., Koutsouradis, P. *et al.* (2007). Cognitive decline following psychosis onset: data from the PACE clinic. *British Journal of Psychiatry*, 191, s52–s57.

Wood, S. J., Pantelis, C., Proffitt, T. *et al.* (2003). Spatial working memory ability is a marker of risk-for-psychosis. *Psychological Medicine*, 33, 1239–1247.

Wood, S. J., Pantelis, C., Velakoulis, D. *et al.* (2008). Progressive changes in the development toward schizophrenia: studies in subjects at increased symptomatic risk. *Schizophrenia Bulletin*, 34, 322–329.

Wood, S. J., Proffitt, T., Mahony, K. *et al.* (2002). Visuospatial memory and learning in first-episode schizophreniform psychosis and established schizophrenia: a functional correlate of hippocampal pathology? *Psychological Medicine*, 32, 429–438.

Wood, S. J., Proffitt, T., O'Brien, C. *et al.* (2006). Cognitive change after a first psychotic episode – data from the EPPIC medium-term follow-up study. *Biological Psychiatry*, 59, 213S.

Woodberry, K. A., Giuliano, A. J., Seidman, L. J. (2008). Premorbid IQ in schizophrenia: a meta-analytic review. *American Journal of Psychiatry*, 165, 579–587.

Zipparo, L., Whitford, T. J., Hodge, M. A. R. *et al.* (2008). Investigating the neuropsychological and neuroanatomical changes that occur over the first 2–3 years of illness in patients with first-episode schizophrenia. *Progress in Neuro-Psychopharmacology and Biological Psychiatry*, 32, 531–538.

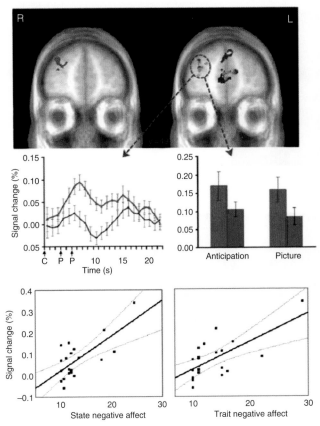

Plate 5.3. It illustrates greater activation for aversive than neutral trials across anticipation and picture periods in right dorsolateral prefrontal cortex (DLPFC) (Nitschke et al., 2006). The brain image in the top left panel displays the results of a conjunction analysis, which identifies areas that activate more for aversive than neutral trials during both the anticipation period and the picture period when analyzed separately. For the top right brain image, colored areas showed a Valence main effect for the voxel-wise Period × Valence ANOVA ($P < 0.05$, corrected). Blue areas also showed greater activation for aversive than neutral trials during the antici- pation period but not the picture period (aversive–neutral con- trasts as indicated by corresponding voxel-wise t tests, $P < 0.05$, corrected). In contrast, purple areas also showed greater activation for aversive than neutral trials during the picture period but not the anticipation period (aversive–neutral contrasts, as noted above). Yellow areas showed greater activation for aversive than neutral trials for the Valence effect and for the aversive–neutral contrast for each period, whereas green areas for the Valence main effect did not meet the $P < 0.05$ (corrected) threshold for either contrast. The middle left panel shows time series plots of the circled clusters illustrating average percentage signal change across all time points of the aversive (red) and neutral (blue) trials. The onset of the 1-s picture presentation (P) occurred 3 s after warning cue (W) onset on half of the trials and 5 s after cue onset on the other half. In the middle right panel, bar graphs of the circled clusters illustrate average percentage signal change for the anticipation period and picture period separately. Error bars for time series plots and bar graphs are for confidence intervals (Cumming & Finch, 2005) around the mean after adjusting for between-subject variance (Loftus & Masson, 1994). The bottom panel shows scatter plots illustrating the positive relationship between negative affect and right DLPFC activation during the anticipation of aversive pictures.

Plots illustrate the relationship of greater activation for aversive than neutral trials during the anticipation period in the right dorsolateral prefrontal area depicted in the top panel to increases in state negative affect (left bottom panel; $r = 0.71, P < 0.001$) and trait negative affect (right bottom panel; $r = 0.67, P < 0.001$), as measured by the Positive and Negative Affect Schedule (PANAS; Watson et al., 1988). R = right. L = left.

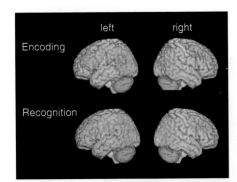

Plate 7.2. Brain regions involved in associative memory processes (unpublished functional magnetic resonance neuroimaging data from the authors). Note the important role of coordinated anterior-posterior activity associated with both encoding and retrieval processes. Data acquired from n = 17 healthy control subjects completing verbal encoding and retrieval tasks.

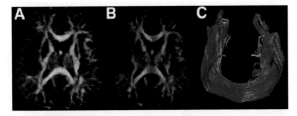

Plate 16.6. Representations of diffusion tensor imaging datasets. (A) A fractional anisotropy (FA) axial slice from a single subject. (B) FA slice, colored to represent directions: red, left-right; green, anterior-posterior; blue, superior-inferior. (C) Tractography performed on the genu of the same subject (From Kanaan et al., 2005 with permission. Copyright © 2005 Society of Biological Psychiatry).

De-activation during talking

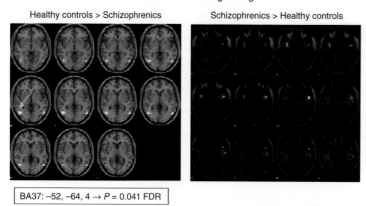

Healthy controls > Schizophrenics   Schizophrenics > Healthy controls

BA37: −52, −64, 4 → $P = 0.041$ FDR

Plate 15.1. Group contrast for Rest–Talk, showing activations exceeding $P < 0.05$, uncorrected levels with middle temporal gyrus mask. On the left are shown voxels where healthy controls have greater de-activation than patients during talking, and on the right, where patients have greater de-activation than controls. Voxels exceeding the $P < 0.05$ FDR are indicated by arrows, and the location is given as a Brodmann area and an x, y, z coordinate.

STG-masked correlation maps
Broca's-masked correlation maps

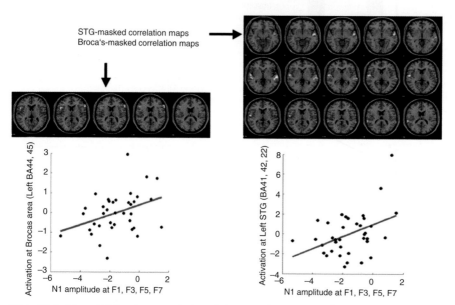

Plate 15.4. (Upper left) Broca's area-masked correlation maps showing areas of Broca's area where activation is associated with N1 suppression during talking recorded from F1, 3, 5, 7 ($P < 0.05$, uncorrected). This relationship is plotted in the lower left for left Broca's area. Subjects with more N1 suppression had greater Broca's activation during talking. (Upper right) Superior temporal gyrus (STG)-masked correlation maps showing areas of STG where activation is associated with N1 suppression ($P < 0.05$, uncorrected). This relationship is plotted in the lower right for left STG.

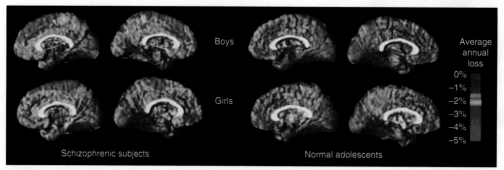

Plate 16.1. Dynamic changes of gray matter loss in boys and girls in both groups of schizophrenic subjects and normal adolescents. These maps show similar patterns of deficits for both sexes in both groups of subjects (from Vidal *et al.*, 2006, with permission).

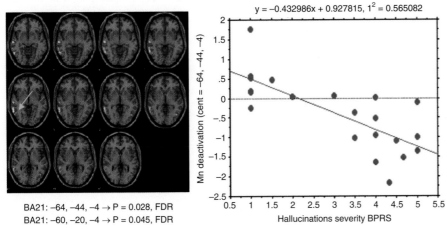

$$y = -0.432986x + 0.927815, \, r^2 = 0.565082$$

BA21: −64, −44, −4 → P = 0.028, FDR
BA21: −60, −20, −4 → P = 0.045, FDR

Plate 15.2. De-activation of middle temporal gyrus (MTG) versus hallucinations severity. MTG masked correlation maps showing areas of MTG where de-activation is associated with more severe hallucinations, $P < 0.05$, uncorrected. The voxels surviving the $P < 0.05$ correction for FDR are shown with an arrow and their location is given as a Brodmann area and as x, y, z coordinates. The correlation between hallucination severity and Talk–Rest mean activation height for left BA21 is $R = 0.74$, $P < 0.0001$. This relationship is plotted on the right. Patients with less left MTG de-activation during talking had significantly more severe auditory hallucinations.

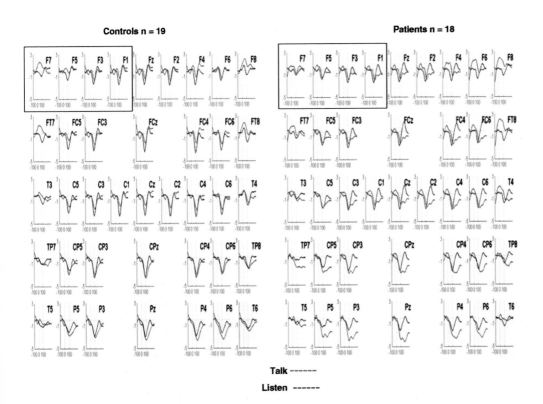

Plate 15.3. Event-related potentials to speech onset are shown for controls (left) and patients (right) during Talking (red) and Listening (blue). Single trials were corrected for eye movements and blinks. Negativity is plotted down. Even numbered electrode sites are over right hemisphere, odd numbered sites are over left hemisphere; F = frontal, T = temporal, C = central, P = parietal, Z = midline. Sites are positioned on figure as they appear on the head.

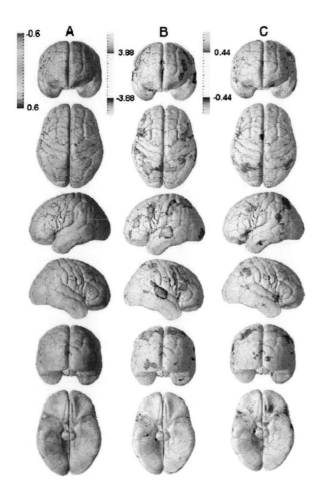

Plate 16.7. Combined structural and functional magnetic resonance imaging data of first-episode schizophrenia patients and matched healthy control subjects. Views from top to bottom: frontal, superior, left lateral, right lateral, posterior and inferior. Brodmann areas are warped into the probabilistic model of the brain surface. (A) Unthresholded correlation maps of cortical gray matter thickness by group. Positive values indicate increased gray matter while negative values indicate reduced gray matter in patients, particularly in the right anterior temporal lobe, prefrontal, frontal and parietal cortex and hippocampus. (B) Combined group BOLD response as a function of task difficulty when performing the Tower of London task showing increasing activation in the prefrontal and parietal cortex and a negative BOLD response predominantly in the superior and middle temporal gyrus. (C) Correlation maps of cortical gray matter thickness by BOLD response suggest reduced BOLD response with decreased cortical gray matter thickness in the left prefrontal, right orbitofrontal, right superior temporal and bilateral parietal cortices across groups (From Rasser *et al.*, 2005 with permission. Copyright © 2005 Published by Elsevier Inc.)

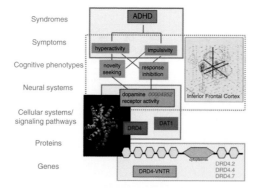

Plate 18.4. An atlas is an integrated collection of "maps" (indexed information sources). In the Neuropsychiatric Phenomics Atlas (NPA) maps must span multiple levels and scales, and support zooming to see finer granularity of concepts and/or data within levels. ADHD = attention-deficit hyperactivity disorder.

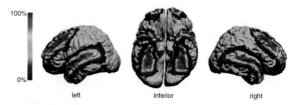

Plate 18.6. Probability maps for three cortical structures. Probabilistic data from the LPBA40 atlas was mapped back to the space of one of the atlas subjects. The surface model has been colored according to the probability values for middle frontal gyrus, superior temporal gyrus and fusiform gyrus to indicate the likelihood of one of those structures at a given surface point. From Shattuck *et al.*, 2008, with permission.

Integration and synthesis: are mental illnesses disorders of consciousness? A trialogue between neuroscientific, philosophical and psychiatric perspectives

This volume closes with a fascinating "trialogue" on the issue of whether mental illnesses can be considered disorders of consciousness. We felt that this was an appropriate section with which to end the volume for a number of reasons. First, as is evident from the preceding chapters, many of the primary symptoms of mental illnesses (e.g. delusions, hallucinations, depressed mood, fear), and the basic neuropsychological processes associated with them (e.g. attention, emotion, working memory, executive cognition), are phenomena that distinctively impact on consciousness. Second, although consciousness has at times been considered outside the domain of science, recent developments in philosophy and neuroscience are suggesting that we are increasingly able to develop a scientific understanding of consciousness (Zalazo, *et al.* 2007), including the "hard problem" of why we have conscious experience (Chalmers, 1995). Finally, the examination of the role of consciousness in mental illness provides an integrative view of the range of neuropsychological processes and specific disorders that have been covered in this volume. As such, it may point to more fundamental and innovative research questions that need to be addressed by future studies.

We have assembled an eminent panel that consists of a pair of philosophers of mind and psychopathology (G. Lynn Stephens and George Graham), a neuroscientist (Jaak Panksepp) and a psychiatrist (Kai Vogeley) writing with a philosopher colleague (Albert Newen). Each of these groups was asked to address the question of whether mental illnesses are disorders of consciousness, to comment on each others' views, and finally to respond to the others' commentaries. The result is an intriguing and lively exchange that points out the overlaps and differences in the view that those with philosophical, scientific and medical training take of the issue, and points the way towards an integrative neuropsychological understanding of the role of consciousness in mental illness.

References

Chalmers, D. (1995). Facing up to the problem of consciousness. *Journal of Consciousness Studies*, **2**(3), 200–219.

Zalazo, P. D., Moscovitch, M. & Thompson, E. (2007). *The Cambridge Handbook of Consciousness.* Cambridge: Cambridge University Press.

Chapter 27

Mental illness and the consciousness thesis

G. Lynn Stephens and George Graham

Introduction

Writing more than seventy years ago the editors of a Carnegie Corporation funded study of mental disorders wrote as follows:

> The nature of mental disorder has clearly called for special concepts, distinctive methods, and a unique training.... [But] the logic of the case has not been clarified by a tenacious tradition of two distinct but related series of events, [viz. the] bodily and mental.
>
> (Bentley & Cowdry, 1934)

If, however, mental events are not distinct, in some ultimate sense, from bodily or neural events, then what happens to the category of mental illness? There arises a definitional problem for the category of mental illness that goes something like this: to explain how mentality has a constitutive or definitional role to play in an illness or disorder (viz. mental illness or disorder), without presupposing that the domain of mental is distinct from the domain of the physical and neurobiological.

In this chapter we briefly outline and defend a solution to the definitional problem. The heart of our solution is something we call the *consciousness thesis* (or 'CT' for short). This is the thesis that mental illness is an illness in and of consciousness.[1] We also explain how CT is compatible with assuming that the brain is the base of mental illness and thus that neuroscience plays a critical, if not exclusive, role in understanding and treating mental illness.

The definitional problem

The *Diagnostic and Statistical Manual of Mental Disorders* (DSM–IV) has eliminated the term "organic mental disorders," under which previous editions had grouped delirium, dementias and other amnestic and cognitive disorders. The authors explain their reasons for this deletion as follows:

> In DSM–III–R these disorders were placed in a section titled "Organic Mental Syndromes and Disorders." The term "organic mental disorder" is no longer used in DSM–IV because it incorrectly implies that "nonorganic" mental disorders do not have a biological basis."
>
> (American Psychiatric Association, 1994, p. 123)

We doubt whether the authors or informed readers of DSM–III–R understood the terminological distinction between "organic" and "nonorganic" to have any such implication. Nevertheless, the rationale for the revision is clear enough. All mental disorders have a biological basis. Therefore, the terms "organic mental disorder" and "nonorganic mental disorder," taken literally, fail to mark any real distinction between types of disorder. No mental disorders have their basis in some "nonorganic" or immaterial substance.

What, however, should happen to the term "mental disorder" itself? Supposing that all medical disorders have a biological basis, what is the point, then, of distinguishing between mental illness and other maladies to which our flesh is heir? Might not an unwary reader read "non-biological" when he sees the word "mental," and think "non-mental" when he sees the word "biological"? What real distinction among disorders do the terms "mental disorder" and "non-mental disorder" pick out?

Here is one hypothesis. Call it the *somatic basis hypothesis*. It goes like this: "Mental disorder" marks off illnesses that have their biological or organic basis in the patient's brain from disorders based in other bodily or somatic organs, such as the heart, liver or digestive system. Note, however, that if the intent is

The Neuropsychology of Mental Illness, ed. Stephen J. Wood, Nicholas B. Allen and Christos Pantelis. Published by Cambridge University Press. © Cambridge University Press 2009.

to formulate a somatic or neural base hypothesis for mental illness, might it make more sense to replace the terms "mental" with "neurological" and "mental illness" with "brain disease"? This is precisely the semantic revision of mental illness talk recommended by some students of psychopathology.

In his opening editorial in *Archives for Psychology and Nervous Disease*, the journal's founder Wilhelm Griesinger wrote:

> Psychiatry has undergone a transformation in its relation to the rest of medicine. This transformation rests principally on the realization that patients with so-called 'mental illness' are really individuals with illnesses of the nerves and brain.
>
> (Bentall, 2003, p. 150)

Writing more than a century later, Michael Allen Taylor reaffirms this revisionist program in his textbook on clinical neurology.

> Psychiatry and neurology [is] one field. [M]ental illness is not 'mental' at all, but the behavioral disturbance associated with brain dysfunction and disease.
>
> (Taylor, 1999, p. viii)

As advocates of CT we wish to argue against the sort of revisionism endorsed by Griesinger and Taylor. Although we share their conviction that mental disorders have a neurological basis, we believe that such authors unduly restrict the descriptive and explanatory implications of this conviction. The slogan "Mental disorders have a neurological basis," properly understood, fails to entail either that so-called mental disorders are not mental at all, or that mental illness is just a brain disease. There are at least two theoretical possibilities for interpreting the slogan: (1) One (apparently assumed by Griesinger and Taylor) has the effect of making the idea of mental illness a simple verbal contradiction. There is only the base (the brain); it is not open to speak of minds. The category of mental illness is eliminated.[2] (2) The other (the interpretation assumed by us) leaves open the question whether there is a distinctive subset of neurologically based disorders usefully categorized as "mental disorders."

In what follows and in the spirit of (2) above, we try to elucidate the distinction between mental and non-mental medical disorders, as well as to more accurately work out some of the implications of acknowledging that mental disorder has a neurological basis.[3]

Consciousness

We believe that mental disorders form a distinctive subclass of medical disorders or human health maladies. What distinguishes them is that conscious activity or experience plays a distinctive and multidimensional role in mental disorder. This complex role will be described in CT. Consciousness does not perform such a role in other medical disorders.

But, first, before we describe CT, what is consciousness? "Consciousness" has no precise, univocal or generally recognized meaning. We use the term to pick out a range of phenomena.

Let us start with the expression "conscious experiences." What are conscious experiences? These are particular, occurrent episodes in a person's life, such as seeing the setting sun on some specific occasion; realizing that the sun is setting now; being alarmed, or saddened, or elated at the thought that the sun is setting; inferring that it must be 6 pm local time; recalling that one promised earlier to meet Gloria for dinner at 6; deciding to remain on the beach until dark; imagining Gloria's reaction to being stood-up; and so on.

Conscious experiences prototypically involve consciousness in two ways. First, they involve being conscious of something: you somehow apprehend, attend to or represent to yourself some actual or possible situation. This feature of consciousness is what philosophers call its *Intentionality* or *Representationality*. Second, conscious experiences can themselves be objects of consciousness. When you see the sun set, typically, you know that you see it. If this causes you a pang of regret, you are aware that you feel regretful. This is to say not just that you may be aware that *you* feel regretful (though of course you may),[4] but that it's regret that you *feel*.[5] That is also not to say that one is always aware of one's conscious experiences. However, conscious experiences are the sorts of things of which one will normally be aware if one reflects on one's current state, and to which we, as persons, refer when we describe or try to explain ourselves to ourselves or others. That is to say, references to conscious experience form a significant part of the resources we deploy in common sense or "folk" psychological explanation.

The term "consciousness" also designates extended episodes that involve sequences of conscious experiences. These may include such experiences as reciting *The Wasteland* silently to yourself or worrying all night about your financial difficulties or practicing the opening movement of the *Hammerkla-vier* sonata. Likewise, it covers dispositional states that typically are manifest in conscious experience. So, for example, a person with a reptile phobia needs to be having no particular sort of conscious experience at any given time, but would have a conscious experience of terror on finding a snake in his path. Similarly for beliefs, desires, intentions, and so on, which are dispositional states normally manifest in consciousness. Finally, we include in "consciousness" faculties or capabilities whose exercise involves conscious experience, such as visual perception, autobiographical memory, volition and emotion.

The contrast class for consciousness viz. nonconscious states includes two sorts of states of special interest in the current context. First, those that include "unconscious" states, typically postulated by Freudian or other psychodynamic accounts of disorders, which are mental in origin. Such states are assumed to exhibit Intentionality: I unconsciously fear that my father wants to kill me or desires to have sex with another man. However, such states are nonconscious or unconscious; not simply in the sense that we may fail to attend to or self-consciously notice them, but in the sense that they are inaccessible to unaided introspection and reflection. Indeed, according to Freud's theory, they must be inaccessible if they are to do their causal work. Second are "sub-personal" processes that figure, for instance, in the brain's construction of a visual scene from specific sensory inputs; they translate conscious speech intentions into fluent phonological output, or orchestrate the specific sequence of bodily movements by which we execute intended actions, such as hitting a baseball or climbing stairs. Even 20 years of psychotherapy would not allow you to understand your sub-personal dynamics, given that we are primarily aware of such processes by studying EEG read-outs and single neuron recordings, not by introspection. Nevertheless, it has proved fruitful in cognitive science to think of sub-personal activities in terms of information processing, and perhaps they also involve some sort of Intentionality and thereby qualify as mental.

Although it is evident why we don't regard the above phenomena as conscious, it is still uncertain as to why they should not be included in a discussion of the mental in mental illness? Is it not possible that disorders in or of the unconscious, in the Freudian way, of beliefs and desires, or even sub-personal information processing, should also be regarded as

mental disorders? Why consider (as we do) only disorders of consciousness in our effort to vindicate a distinction between mental and non-mental disorders?

The short answer is that we're skeptical about the reality of a Freudian Unconscious (i.e. of unconscious activity according to the Freudian model). We're not persuaded that things that are unconscious in this sense play any role in human mental disorders. While we do not doubt the reality of sub-personal information processing, or that such activity plays a role in mental disorders, we are reluctant to admit that a disorder in which the relevant dysfunction or deficit occurs only in sub-personal and consciously inaccessible activity should count as a *mental* disorder.[6] Impersonal entities such as thermostats and servo-control mechanisms operate or can also be fruitfully described in information processing terms. So also can activities of the digestive system (Gershon, 1998), the immune system, and the thermo-regulatory system. Certainly breakdowns of such systems do not count as mental disorders. In any case, we do not want our defense of the reality or categorical distinctiveness of mental disorders to rest on the assumption that such disorders are best understood in information-processing terms. In our opinion, this is not what the controversy concerning the definitional problem of mental illness is about.

The consciousness thesis

Nearly every instance of disease or illness affects the patient's consciousness, sooner or later, and becomes part of a patient's consciousness. Illness tends to bring with it unpleasant sensations – pains, chills, dizziness – anxious thoughts, distressing emotions, desires for relief, and so on. So ubiquitous are such effects that they cannot provide a useful distinction between mental and non-mental illness.

Some diseases, however, would still count as disorders and as threats to the patient's well-being, even if they had no effect on the patient's consciousness. For example, patients suffering from polycythemia vera – a bone marrow disease involving overproduction of blood cells – typically become highly irritable: they are restless, demanding, easily moved to anger. Although such conscious experiences contribute to the patient's distress, they do not constitute the real problem. In polycythemia vera, the threat to the patient's health lies in the increased risk of forming clots and the resultant increase in risk of heart attack and stroke. A course of benzodiazepine therapy that relieved the patient's irritability would not cure the polycythemia vera. The conscious effects of the condition are not what make it a disorder. It is a disorder that, while it expresses itself in consciousness, is in itself not a mental disorder.

In suffering from unipolar depression, on the other hand, the patient's conscious state *is* the problem. The threat this condition presents to the patient's well-being lies precisely within the manner that the patient thinks and feels, and which is associated with depression. The persistent global sadness and pessimism are deviations from norms of psychological health and lead directly to failure to meet social responsibilities and neglect of self-care.

Depression may also lead to changes in the patient's bodyweight. Such changes may adversely affect the patient's health. However, a treatment that restored the patient's premorbid weight without altering conscious experience would not be an effective treatment for depression.

To put the point in general terms: a characteristic feature of mental illness is that the nature of the patient's disorder cannot be described without making reference to the patient's consciousness. Even if the conscious effects of an illness are significant so that a differential diagnosis could be made, they do not represent the distinctive threat posed to the patient by polycythemia vera, for example, and one could suffer from that disease even if conscious effects were absent. Not so for depression.

A second mark of mental illness lies in the functions played by conscious experience in the etiology of and treatment for a disorder. Consider etiology briefly first.

Alzheimer's disease involves a breakdown of the patient's conscious faculties, and its effects on conscious activity are central to what makes it a disorder. However, according to the literature, the patient's conscious "history," i.e. his premorbid conscious experience over the course of his life, has nothing to do with whether the patient develops Alzheimer's disease. It also likely has little effect on the specific time of onset, or the progress or course of the disease. On the other hand, there is considerable evidence that a person's conscious history figures significantly in the etiology of depression, panic disorder and obsessive-compulsive disorder.[7]

On the matter of treatment: in the case of some disorders it is therapeutically beneficial to encourage the patient to reflect on his own condition and to undertake deliberate efforts to change how he thinks or feels, for example, by use of cognitive-behavioral therapy to teach the patient to control panic attacks. The conscious constituents of mental disorders can be altered regardless of the patient's deliberate efforts, for example, by use of antidepressant drugs to alleviate dysphoric mood or electroconvulsive therapy to eliminate disturbing memories. But, we take it as a mark of distinctively mental disorders that effective therapy must engage the patient's mind, i.e. his understanding of his illness, recognition of situational vulnerabilities, history of conscious experience, and so on.[8]

We are now in a position to describe what we mean by the very idea of a mental illness or disorder. The description takes the form of CT.

Consciousness thesis (CT)

A disorder is a mental disorder when: (1) essential reference is made to consciousness in characterizing the nature of the disorder or the threat that the disorder poses to the patient's well-being, (2) consciousness plays a significant role in the etiology of the disorder and (3) changes in the conscious experience of the patient, achieved via conscious concourse with the patient, provide significant therapeutic benefits.

Within our framework, disorders that fully satisfy the above description qualify as mental. Disorders that fail to satisfy CT in any of its parts are non-mental. Disorders that satisfy some parts of CT but not others are "hard cases" for the application of the concept of mental illness. Such disorders may be best classified as mental in part. We also propose, although the following point cannot be pursued here, that contextual parameters often figure in the application of the concept of mental disorder, and in the identification of the conscious experiences proper to a mental disorder. To illustrate, in Culture X a certain set of conscious experiences may be accepted parts of depression, whereas in Culture Y similar experiences may merely mean that a person is properly grieving, in a socially reinforced manner (e.g. the loss of a tribal chief). Finally, it is logically possible that no illness satisfies CT and thus no illness, in our way of thinking, qualifies as mental. To mention one hypothetical example, suppose it is discovered that schizophrenics remain disabled in their social functioning, even after their cognitive and emotional status returns to normal. This would indicate a need to revise our understanding of the nature of the disorder. Schizophrenia might no longer qualify as a mental illness. Call this feature of CT the *empirical conditionalization* of CT. Whether any particular disorder satisfies CT is an empirical question. It is conditional upon empirical discovery and the analysis of the disorder.

Now we turn to the definitional challenge of whether CT can be used, not just to draw a distinction between mental and non-mental disorders, but can be deployed in a manner that is compatible with assuming that mental disorder possesses a neurological or physical base.

Mental illness and brain disease

"Let us return to the contention that mental illness... is not 'mental' at all, but that the behavioral disturbance is associated with brain dysfunction and disease" (Taylor's claim), or that patients with so-called "mental illness are really individuals with illnesses of the nerves and brain" (Griesinger's claim). As noted by our mention of the empirical conditionalization of CT, we do not claim that "some people suffer from mental illness" expresses a synthetic a priori truth, immune to revision in the light of scientific inquiry. Should it prove to be the case that there are no disorders wherein consciousness plays the role outlined in CT, we would readily concede that there are no such illnesses as mental illnesses. However, we doubt that Griesinger's or Taylor's rejection of "mental illness" rests on a case-by-case review of the clinical evidence or upon detailed examination of the role of consciousness in illness. We suspect, rather, that it arises from the conviction that the notion of mental illness presupposes a mind-body dualism rendered untenable by the progress of medical science. Substantial immaterial minds are not a theoretical option for informed medical science, which is supported by basic physicalistic commitments. In Griesinger's and Taylor's view, the proposition that so-called "mental" disorders have their somatic basis in the anatomy, physiology and neurobiology of the brain also entails that "mental" illnesses really are diseases of the brain: that they are biological, not "mental" disorders.

Once again, we do not dispute that all mental disorders have their biological basis in the brain. We do dispute that this entails either that there are no mental illnesses as such or that all mental disorders

just are disorders of the brain. To explain why we reject this implication, we need, first, to say how we understand the idea that mental disorders have a biological or neurological basis.

We assume that mental disorders have their basis in physical reality. We believe that this holds for all things mental and, indeed, for all particular things generally. Elementary particle physics provides the best, most credible, account of the ultimate constituents of physical phenomena. Mental phenomena – biological phenomena, sociological phenomena, economic phenomena, etc. – exist insofar as they are realized in or embodied in systems of physical particles and forces. The account of reality provided by elementary physics constrains the accounts of reality provided by the so-called "special sciences." What biology talks about, viz. cells, hormones, digestion, natural selection, and so on, must be realizable in particles and forces. There can be cells only if cellular structures and functions are realized in a system of elementary physical particles. However, biological concepts like that of the cell abstract away from ground-level physical details, and biological explanations that advert to patterns of physical events must be salient to the special concerns of biology. Typically, it is theoretically cumbersome and, often practically speaking, epistemically impossible to capture the concepts and generalizations of biology in the "lower-level" language of elementary particle physics. The same proposition holds true for the dependence of psychology or psychiatry on biology. Conscious activities, ordered and disordered, perception and hallucination, cognition and delusional thinking, and so on, have their base in neurobiological structure and function, so that the things studied in psychopathology must be realizable in neurology. But, psychiatry and psychology often do and must abstract away from neurological details in search of descriptions and explanations that are salient for understanding certain types or features of human distress and disorder. These, in our opinion, are the disorders identified in the language of CT viz. distresses that are not just expressed in consciousness but *of* consciousness. Such are the distresses distinctive of mental illnesses.

So understood, the proposition that mental disorders have their basis in biological reality does not entail that there are no mental disorders, any more than the proposition that biological activities that have their basis on the activity of physical particles and forces, entails that there are no biological phenomena. Recognizing (what philosophers call) the ontological dependence or supervenience of the mental on the biological in no way discredits the reality of mental disorder. Nor, perhaps surprisingly, does the acknowledgment that the basal location of mental illness in the brain entails that any and all mental disorders are disorders or diseases of the brain. Griesinger and Taylor assert that "mental" illness is, or is associated with, "brain dysfunction and disease." But mental dysfunction need not involve brain dysfunction. It is possible to have a sick mind (i.e. an illness in consciousness) but a healthy brain.

Consider the drug addict. He fails to exercise prudent control over his consumption of some substance, alcohol, perhaps. He drinks more than is good for him: sacrificing more important interests (occupational and family responsibilities, etc.) to maintain his consumption of alcohol. A significant part of his problem is that when he refrains from or limits his drinking he feels bad: anxious, uncomfortable or depressed. That is to say, he goes through "withdrawal." This motivates him to continue drinking despite its otherwise negative consequences. To make matters worse, he finds that he must continually increase his consumption in order to avoid going through withdrawal. He therein develops an increasing "tolerance" for alcohol. With increase in consumption also comes increased cost; financial and personal. The addict becomes trapped in a cycle of compulsive, escalating consumption much to the detriment of his own well-being and that of others for whom or to whom he is responsible.

Through science we now understand a good deal about the neurobiological and neurochemical basis of addiction, in particular, about tolerance and withdrawal. The neurological roots of these phenomena lie in the brain's mesolimbic dopamine system: a system of neurons projecting from the ventral tegmental area to the nucleus accumbens that use dopamine as their neurotransmitter. Addictive drugs increase the availability of dopamine in the nucleus accumbens, either by inhibiting re-uptake or by binding to neurons that would otherwise inhibit dopamine production in the ventral tegmental area. Increased dopamine availability reinforces those activities that produce it. Hence, the mesolimbic dopamine system is sometimes called the "brain reward" or "dopamine reward" system. However, as repeated drug consumption increases concentrations of dopamine in the nucleus accumbens, it also stimulates the production

of dynorphin, which in turn reduces dopamine availability by inhibiting dopamine production in the ventral tegmental area. The operation of this feedback loop sets up a situation in which dopamine reward delivered by a given dose of the drug continually decreases in response to repeated doses at the same levels; hence, there arises increased tolerance for the drug. Increasing the dose will temporarily restore the original level of dopamine reward, but it will also stimulate increased dynorphin production thus reducing the dopamine payoff produced by the dosage increase and so on. On the other hand, should the user reduce or eliminate the dosage, dopamine production/sensitivity in the brain reward system will remain inhibited for some time (a matter of days) before returning to normal. Until the system returns to normal, it will not provide the level of dopamine reward that the patient has come to "expect" in response to day-to-day activities: hence, withdrawal.[9]

We take drug addiction to be a mental disorder. But we also assume that the mental disorder of drug addiction has its basis in the operation of the brain's dopamine reward system. Should we conclude, then, that drug addiction represents a disease or disorder in the brain reward system? That would be a very hasty inference. The same brain reward system subserves a whole variety of psychological and biological functions: notably learning and response to injury or other sorts of stress. In decreasing the dopamine reward for repeated instances of the same stimulus, the brain may be functioning just as Mother Nature (natural selection) designed it to function. That there are specific neurological mechanisms that underlie the addictiveness of drug consumption and contribute to substance abuse is consistent with those mechanisms functioning adequately, neurologically speaking, insofar as they underlie the adaptive activities of learning and response to injury. "Fixing" the brain reward system so that it delivered the same reward with each exposure to a given stimulus (drug) might well disable the person by interfering with learning and exploratory behavior. Facilitating prudent consumption of a recreational drug simply is not what the system was designed to do. So, from a neurobiological point of view, the brain might be functioning well, even if in doing so, the brain reward system underwrites an addict's mental disorder.

Is there a general lesson about mental illness here? Yes, there is, and it goes like this. One should not assume that the neurological basis of a mental disorder is itself a neurological disorder. Some disorders qualify as mental even though their neurological base is not unhealthy.

Of course, in response, one might insist that any pattern of neural activity that subserves or serves as the supervenience base for mental disorder counts, for this reason alone, as a brain disorder. However, such a concept of brain disorder would be conceptually or semantically parasitic on the concept of mental disorder, and on the normative standards for proper psychological functioning. They would be disorders, not in virtue of some primary, neurologically specifiable breakdown in the brain, as revisionists seem to presuppose, but simply because relevant neurological activities contribute to some condition that is psychologically undesirable. It would be pointless to offer "brain disorder," so understood, as a substitute or replacement for "mental disorder." Such a notion of brain disorder presupposes and is defined by prior reference to the notion of mental disorder.

One might concede that not every mental disorder is associated with a neurological disorder, but insist that the slogan "Mental disorders are brain disorders" nevertheless expresses an important truth. The brain is where the causal-explanatory action is regarding mental disorders. Explanation by reference to consciousness or conscious activity, for example, in the case of alcoholism can be explained by reference to the brain's reward system. So, if every mental disorder is realized in the brain, will not questions regarding the etiology (and treatment) of a disorder be answered by reference to brain events? We argue that this is not the case. Rather, explanation of how a person comes to be mentally ill must include an explanation of how the patient's brain came to be in a certain condition. Causal connections that are specified at the level of conscious experience, say, between certain patterns of thinking or desiring and a given mental disorder must be realizable at the level of neurophysiology. But this does not mean that *all* the factors relevant to explaining (and treating) mental illness must be describable in neuroscientific terms.

Again, consider the drug addict, in particular someone addicted to heavy drinking. Suppose that an alcoholic with a craving for a drink is able to resist his impulse to drink now, while his boss is present or if there is a raging fire in his house. He consciously judges that he has good reason to refrain, viz. fear of job loss or of being consumed in a blaze, and he acts accordingly, prudently. Shouldn't we say that

reference to conscious activity is necessary to explain such features of his drinking behavior? It seems to us that we should. Or suppose such a person cannot refrain from drink when he perceives that the reward of alcohol is more proximate than other rewards and unthreatened otherwise? Again, it seems that we need to answer questions about why he drinks in such circumstances, not just by reference to the brain's reward system, but also by referring to his perception of alcohol's proximity. Surely, we know that the consciously perceived proximity of reward links up with addiction even if we can't say exactly how such perception links up with neural mechanisms.[10] As one clinician sensitive to the role of conscious experiences in addiction observes: "Notice the bargaining that goes on in [an alcoholic's conscious] mind, and [the] profound ambivalence about giving up alcohol."[11] Bargaining has its source in a person's conscious ambivalence about the desirability and long-term implications of self-control.

Perhaps alcoholics cannot consciously and emotionally bridge the gap between seeing themselves as heavy drinkers and seeing themselves as nondrinkers. Alcoholism and other addictions, Andrew Garner and Valerie Hardcastle point out, "might be such life-defining habits, [that] addicts can't stop because they can't genuinely imagine their lives – their particular lives – without addiction. To stop means to become someone else, someone unknown. And for most of us, that is a scary thought" (Garner & Hardcastle, 2004, p. 376). The fact that such conscious activities of imagination and others play such causal-explanatory roles in addictive behavior means that even though drug addiction is neurally based, it qualifies as a mental disorder: as a disorder in and of consciousness.

So in our proposal, we posit that in certain contexts and with respect to certain disorders, knowledge of what goes on in conscious experience may offer us more useful guidance in the explanation (and treatment) of a patient's problems than knowledge of his neurological condition alone, and also that this argument is completely compatible with the basal dependence of mental disorder on the brain. It is in terms of such knowledge that psychiatry might manage to preserve a category of mental illness or disorder.

The crucial question behind the category of mental illness, then, is one that neuroscientists should readily pursue with philosophers of psychiatry. It is not whether mental disorders have careers in the brain (of course they do), but whether reference to conscious events together with reference to neural mechanisms is likely to result in a better or more complete understanding of certain illnesses than neuroscience can craft on its own or in its exclusive terms. Our understanding and treatment of mental illness requires a complementary partnership between the languages of neuroscience and that of conscious experience. To understand human mental illness and disorder, one has to respect conscious activity. This is not because human consciousness is not brain based, but because mental illness is illness in and of the conscious mind.

Acknowledgments

We wish to thank Professors Heidi Maibom, Eddy Nahmias and Jennifer Radden for helpful comments on an earlier draft of this paper.

Endnotes

1. We first presented this thesis (though not by the name of CT) in Graham & Stephens (2006).

2. The notion of mental illness also has critics who reject the proposition that the human problems so designated represent illnesses, biological or otherwise, rather than problems of living. Such critics wish to preserve reference to the mental, but decline to describe any mental condition as an illness. In the current paper we ask our readers to indulge our disinclination to deal with this line of criticism of the concept of mental illness. See Graham & Stephens (2006) for discussion.

3. As will be evident in due course, for us to say that mental illness has a neurobiological basis does not, of itself, entail that mental illness is a brain illness or disease. The brain may serve as the basis of mental illness without the brain being ill.

4. See G. Lynn Stephens and George Graham, "Philosophical Psychopathology and Self-Consciousness" in S. Schneider and M. Velmans (eds.), *A Companion to Consciousness* (Medford, MA: Blackwell 2006) for discussion of the self-attribution or self-awareness of conscious states and processes that occurs in certain specific sorts of mental illness.

5. Philosophically complex issues about privileged first-personal access to the character or identity of one's conscious states lurk within this sentence. We must avoid discussion of those issues here.

6. One reason that at least one of us is disinclined to categorize deficits in sub-personal information processing as mental illness is because, arguably, mere information processing lacks genuine intentionality and therein fails to qualify as mental. See Graham *et al.* (2006), for discussion.

7. It is worth noting, and see Graham and Stephens ('Psychopathology', 2006, op cit) for discussion, that cultural, environmental, and situational influences in the etiology of psychiatric disorders usually work through the patient's conscious representation of himself and his world. Exposure to radiation or asbestos dust causes disease just as readily in those who do not know they have been exposed as in those who do know. By contrast, spiders trigger phobic reactions in vulnerable people only if they are aware of the spider. For a review of the evidence regarding the role of consciousness specifically in depression, see Bentall (2003, pp. 233–269).

8. We briefly explore some of the issues connected with the treatment of mental illness in Graham & Stephens (2006). The issues are complex. It is not our view that conscious concourse with a victim of mental illness, roughly, psychotherapy, is or should be sufficient for the treatment and amelioration of each and every sort of mental illness. Given the neural base of mental disorder, and the many possible variations in that base that are present within different persons or the same person at different times, drugs (and other neurochemical treatments) and psychotherapy likely often work better in tandem than either form of treatment alone. For one outspoken plea for the integration and mutual adjustment of psychotherapy and drugs in the treatment of mental illness, see Hobson & Leonard (2002).

9. The above account of drug addiction and of its neurological basis is drawn from Nestler & Malenka (2004). See also Montague & Dayan (1998).

10. See for an examination of the causal-explanatory role of perceived proximity in cases of addiction, Ainslie (2001).

11. See Mitchell (2001). Words in brackets added.

References

Ainslie, G. (2001). *Breakdown of Will*. Cambridge: Cambridge University Press.

American Psychiatric Association (1994). *Diagnostic and Statistical Manual of Mental Disorders* (4th edn) (DSM–IV) (pp. 339–367). Washington, DC: APA.

Bentall, R. P. (2003). *Madness Explained* (p. 150). London: Penguin Press.

Bentley, M. & Cowdry, E. V. (Eds.) (1934). *The Problem of Mental Disorder* (pp. 1–2). New York, NY: McGraw-Hill.

Garner, A. & Hardcastle, V. G. (2004). Neurobiological models: an unnecessary divide – neural models in psychiatry. In J. Radden (Ed.), *The Philosophy of Psychiatry: A Companion* (p. 376). Oxford: Oxford University Press.

Gershon, M. D. (1998). *The Second Brain: A Groundbreaking New Understanding of Nervous Disorders of the Stomach and Intestine*. New York, NY: Harper and Collins.

Graham, G., Horgan, T. & Tienson, J. (2006). Consciousness and intentionality. In S. Schneider & M. Velmans (Eds.), *A Companion to Consciousness*. Medford, MA: Blackwell.

Graham, G. & Stephens, G. L. (2006). Psychopathology: minding mental illness. In P. Thagard (Ed.), *Philosophy of Psychology and Cognitive Science: A Volume of the Handbook of the Philosophy of Science* (Vol. 12, pp. 339–367). Amsterdam: North Holland.

Hobson, J. A. & Leonard, J. (2002). *Out of Its Mind: Psychiatry in Crisis – A Call for Reform*. Cambridge, MA: Perseus.

Mitchell, J. E. (2001). *Points of View: Stories of Psychopathology*. Philadelphia, PA: Brunner-Routledge.

Montague, P. R. & Dayan, P. (1998). Neurobiological modeling. In W. Bechtel & G. Graham (Eds.),

A Companion to Cognitive Science (pp. 526–541). Medford, MA: Blackwell.

Nestler, E. J. & Malenka, R. C. (2004). The addicted brain. *Scientific American*, **290**, 78–85.

Stephens, G. L. & Graham, G. (2006). Philosophical psychopathology and self-consciousness. In S. Schneider & M. Velmans (Eds.), *A Companion to Consciousness*. Medford, MA: Blackwell.

Taylor, A. T. (1999). *The Fundamentals of Clinical Neuropsychiatry (Contemporary Neurology)* (p. viii). New York, NY: Oxford University Press.

Chapter 28

A non-reductive physicalist account of affective consciousness

Jaak Panksepp

No matter what metaphysical position you take there remains an impenetrable mystery in the fact that subjective experience exists in a physio-chemical world.
(*Robert Holt*, Freud Reappraised)

Because of advances in our understanding of the brain, some aspects of subjective experience are finally penetrable with the tools of neuroscience. Substantive scientific progress is finally being made on the nature of basic emotional feelings, and this has important implications for the development of psychiatry as a scientific discipline. I will restrict my discussion to *emotional* affects (there are others such as sensory and homeostatic ones) since changes in valenced feelings (varieties of positive and negative affects) seem to lie at the very heart of psychiatrically significant distress. There exist core emotional processes possessed by each organism as gifts of nature, as psychological endophenotypes whose underlying principles can be deciphered with animal brain research. These core emotional processes contribute substantially to psychiatrically significant emotional distress, and they are a shared heritage of all humans. In addition, epigenetic cognitive processes imbue human affective experience with a host of associated cognitive meanings, and an emotional self-awareness that can vary enormously among individuals. Neuroscience (especially the animal brain research variety) is not yet well positioned to study such individual variability in the cognitive layering of experience, but it is ready to decipher the core affective nature of primary-process emotional arousals. Accordingly, I believe we must distinguish between emotional awareness, especially self-awareness, and raw (i.e. basic) emotional experience, since only the latter is open to dramatic cross-species neural clarification.

The neurophilosophical underpinnings of affective neuroscience

Without dramatic changes in felt experiences, categories of emotional/psychiatric illness would make little sense. Thus, one key to understanding all psychiatric disorders must be unraveling the nature of raw affective experience within the brain. Because of its subjective nature, this has been an enormous scientific dilemma, at least until the recent brain-imaging revolution. Most neuroscientists have long agreed that affective experience is not a workable scientific problem; those working on animal models of emotions experienced even more epistemological despair. Practically all assumed that our inability to have scientific access to the experiences of other animals was a foregone conclusion, leading almost all investigators to shun talk about affective experiences in the animals they studied. Further, due to the stifling weight of intellectual history in experimental psychology (Panksepp, 1990), most still do. A few epistemological diehards like myself, interested in the fundamental nature of psychiatrically significant emotional distress, have argued that the nature of affective consciousness has long been a tractable neuroscientific problem in animals albeit not humans, where detailed neuroscientific work cannot be ethically pursued. That kind of understanding must come through the judicious use of animal models where ancient brain emotional circuits, probably shared by all mammals, can be clarified (Panksepp, 1998a, 2005a). My assumption is that there exists a deep ancestry to our basic emotional feelings, and that with a few reasonable evolutionary assumptions about neural homologies, and hypothetico-deductive approaches that rely on the *weight of evidence*

The Neuropsychology of Mental Illness, ed. Stephen J. Wood, Nicholas B. Allen and Christos Pantelis. Published by Cambridge University Press. © Cambridge University Press 2009.

rather than scientifically untenable notions of *proof*, this "World Knot" could be untangled using a cross-species psychobiological strategy (Panksepp, 2005a, 2005b). This project now offers a vision of affective consciousness that has realistic scientific and therapeutic implications for biological psychiatry (Panksepp, 2004, 2006) and evolutionary psychology (Panksepp, 2007; Panksepp & Panksepp, 2000).

Affective neuroscience is a view that concurrently respects the role of psychological determinism in the genesis of psychiatric disorder, along with a more subtle view of psychoneural materialism about basic emotional experiences than is currently widely accepted in neuroscience. It is based on the premise that for most psychological matters, the "neuron doctrine" has too fine a resolution to be as useful as a "network doctrine," which recognizes the likelihood that basic genetically provided psychological processes, such as an array of basic affective feelings, arise from endogenous neuronal ensemble activities that contain the keys to intentionality (i.e. they generate "intentions in action" that are inherent in instinctual emotional action patterns). The most workable emotional target of inquiry are those brain states that have been evolutionarily prepared to become responsive to the world in certain behaviorally clear and significant ways – in ways that have traditionally been considered to be *instinctual*. By working out the neuroanatomies, neurochemistries, neurodynamics and developmental epigenetics of such higher-order instinctual brain processes, we can shed substantial light on the neural nature of basic emotional feelings – especially the big-ticket items that commonly accompany major psychiatric disorders.

This strategy offers a novel, deeply natural way to envision the emotional symptoms of psychiatric syndromes. It also provides an alternative to the currently popular neuroscience view that the automatic "information" processing at subcortical levels is always implicit and unconscious. That common claim has always been an enormous assumption rather than a demonstrated fact. Likewise, the assumption that consciousness intrinsically implies conscious *awareness* of one's experiences avoids dealing with primary-process phenomenal consciousness. From my perspective and other related views (e.g. Parvizi & Damasio, 2001, 2003), we must increasingly consider the possibility that subcortical brain functions, especially those mediating emotional and motivational values, can elaborate raw phenomenal experiences that deserve the label primary-process consciousness. In fact, humans born with practically no neocortical tissues show clear outward evidence of internal emotional feelings that can value and devalue their primary-process perceptual experiences (Shewmon et al., 1999). Similar brain-mind capacity seems evident in experimental animals surgically deprived of neocortical functions (Kolb & Tees, 1990; Panksepp et al., 1994). Still, at present most thinkers believe that consciousness requires awareness of one's own experiential states (i.e. the self-reflexive/self-awareness), and that consciousness intrinsically implies propositional attitudes and intentions *to* act in certain ways. Such common beliefs may be deeply flawed because they do not recognize that primary-process intentionality – intentions *in* action – are an evolved aspect of all basic emotional systems (Panksepp, 2003). I believe raw affective experience should be deemed a foundational form of consciousness that is essential for any higher-order awareness and intentionality.

My vision of affective brain organization also attacks the Achilles heel of radically ruthless neural-reductionism that seeks to eliminate mentality from neural dynamics. According to the standard fine-grained "neuron doctrine" view of brain function, mentality is simply a temporary semantic heuristic that we use before we fully understand how the brain-machine operates. In my own materialistic view, endogenous core mentalities do exist as complex emergent network properties of rather ancient "instinctual" regions of the brain. My non-reductive materialistic approach is premised on the likelihood that we can begin to access these properties scientifically by studying the neural underpinnings of instinctive emotional processes, shared homologously by all mammals. Perhaps one of the more dramatic demonstrations of this is the fact that human male orgasm is closely related to the instinctual sexual behavior circuits of deep subneocortical regions of the brain (Holstege et al., 2003).

In short, by understanding the instinctual emotional behavior circuits that all mammals share, we can begin to study the full biology of emotional circuits, and thereby decipher the neural sources of affective feelings, without claiming that a knowledge of the parts explains the whole (Bennett & Hacker, 2003), nor that a study of the circuitry eliminates the need to also conceptualize and study the psychobehavioral functionality of these systems. By capitalizing on well-selected animal models – for instance those that evaluate separation-distress, nurturance, playfulness, aggressive angriness, and the varieties of desire and anxiety – we can clarify the affective infrastructure of the mind-brain (Panksepp, 2005a, 2005b). This view leads to a host of falsifiable predictions from the animal to the human level, especially with regard to neurochemical vectors that control the types and intensities of affective feelings (Panksepp & Harro, 2004). For instance, our work on the opioid control of social motivation and attachment in various animal models predicted which neurochemicals control human sadness (Panksepp, 1981); predictions that have only recently been empirically confirmed (Zubieta et al., 2003). Thus, it is well within the mainstream of science, at least variants that subscribe to standard hypothetico-deductive methods, and this provides a counterpoint to views suggesting that all that "really" exists in the brain are action potentials and the other details of neural machinery in action. These brain circuits intrinsically create experienced and causally efficacious mentalities that are thoroughly neurobiological.

This *dual-aspect monism* view asserts that since affective mentality emerges from complex network properties of the brain, psychological analysis has as important a role to play in understanding what neural machinery actually does. Likewise, a conjoint mental and neuroscientific analysis is essential for understanding the various emotional disturbances that accompany psychiatric disorders. To privilege one or the other as the only path to substantive knowledge amounts to excessive scientific hubris, bordering on ruthlessly materialistic madness. To pursue neural functions, without considering mental functions in waking intact animals can lead to errors and distortions that do not accept the psychological nature of certain brain functions. Ruthless reductionism seeks to ignore one of the main aspects of complex brain networks – the generation of psychological processes – to the detriment of a full understanding of what the brain really does. Thus, to take psychology and consciousness out of the mammalian brain-behavior equation is comparable to trying to discard the experience of sweetness from certain types of tongue stimulation – a maneuver that is still common in animal research, because sweetness cannot be seen clearly with the tools of science. Still, substantial progress has been made in decoding the nature of various pleasures, including a laughter-type joy in animals using this strategy (Burgdorf & Panksepp, 2006; Panksepp & Burgdorf, 2003).

The dual-aspect monism viewpoint in affective neuroscience (an epistemologically workable variant of non-eliminative materialism, that seeks cross-species triangulations between brain, mind and behavior) can address the question of how something as insubstantial as mentality can have causal efficacy in the world. The answer is that mentality is deeply neurobiological. However, those most willing to accept such a view might also argue that mentality is so tightly linked to environmental stimulation, with considerable variability in developmental trajectories, that to assume there is some kind of intrinsic mentality within the brain puzzle, above and beyond perceptual processes strongly linked to environmental events, may not be warranted. However, if we take a neuro-evolutionary view to mentality, we must leave open the possibility that even environmentally untutored brains may have some potential for experiential capacities, an assumption that is obviously fraught with enormous epistemological difficulties. How could such core capacities for subjective experience ever be scientifically objectified? Affective feelings, such as the pleasure of sweetness to a hungry organism, are difficult to measure objectively, even though it is now well known that the newborn brain is prepared to respond to sweetness with apparent delight (Steiner et al., 2001). In my view, the raw affective processes of the brain are initially objectless, and through life experience perceptions can become associated to a variety of affects via learning-conditioning principles. If so, it is essential to conceptualize the nature of the neuroevolutionarily provided, affective tools of mind; a task that cannot be ethically accomplished without animal behavioral neuroscience.

The long-sustained standard view is to assume that animal mentality is inaccessible to the tools of science. Perhaps we can scientifically accept what humans say about their experiences, leading to some kind of superficial descriptive-normative science, but we have no access to experiences in animals without spoken language, whose brains can be "ethically" pursued within a neuroscientific framework. And so goes the mantra: to assume that other animals have comparable emotional experiences is simply not scientifically justified – "it's impossible to know what they feel" (see quote by LeDoux, in Starr, 2006). If we accept that anti-evolutionary view, it leaves us with no practical way to reveal the neural principles by which affects are engendered within the human brain. Animal brain research is the only way we can obtain detailed knowledge about the causal mechanisms of affective consciousness, and therein exists the enormous catch-22 within the current cultural climate of behavioral neuroscience. There is little consensus, at least among those well positioned to do the hard science, about whether we should cultivate the powers of predictive and face validity when confronted by such dilemmas. of course, the key pragmatic question should be: will the new neuroscientific knowledge about the apparent behaviorally indexed affective states of other animals provide credible new predictions about the biological causes of internally experienced affective changes in humans? I think they will (Panksepp, 1998b, 2005a; Panksepp & Harro, 2004; for one success, see Zubieta et al., 2003).

Thus the study of affective consciousness remains a poorly developed area of inquiry; there is little work unraveling how core affective experience emerges from either human or animal brains. In line with time-honored Cartesian dualism, most working within animal behavioral neuroscience choose to ignore the possibility that animal actions may speak as loudly about the underlying nature of their mind realities as human words do about ours.

The brain and raw subjective experience – multiple forms of consciousness

Although the capacity for consciousness is an evolved capacity of the brain, a gift of nature so to speak, most would agree that without environmental inputs, as processed by the neocortex, consciousness would be extremely impoverished. Obviously our capacity to experience the world is largely perceptual, but our raw capacity for consciousness – to have felt experience – probably is not. The raw capacity for non-propositional affective experience seems to be an ancient property of sub-neocortical regions of the brain, while our capacity for any resolved cognitive experience is strongly linked to neocortical processing. Surely our ability to reflect on our experiences – to have self-consciousness – requires higher brain-power than our raw capacity to experience ourselves as beings in the world. However, we may never understand the richness of the former without understanding the nature of the latter.

At present there are very few testable ideas about how raw experiential states emerge from brain

dynamics. The dilemma of perceptual-qualia remains the hardest question in modern consciousness studies. The nature of affective evolutionary-qualia may be much more workable if feelings are part of the instinctual emotional apparatus that can be objectively studied. Still, considering that variety is a hallmark of nature, what we can be sure about is that there will be great variety in what animals can perceive and feel. But it remains possible that there may exist core substrates of raw affective feelings – emotional, motivational and sensory. These are remarkably similar in all mammals, possibly being part of the earliest shorthand value-codes for indexing life decisions at an indeterminate era of brain evolution, in which ancient psychological abilities provided competitive advantage for survival. Further, considering the fact that all useful psychiatric drugs act on ancient neuronal networks we share with the other animals (Panksepp, 2004), it seems likely that it is within such shared neural infrastructures of neuro-evolutionary-qualia that a considerable amount of psychiatric disequilibrium may lie.

Still, the majority of investigators currently seem to believe that consciousness emerges from relatively recently evolved higher brain processes, perhaps functions that are critically dependent on neocortical expansions that are unique to certain great apes. However, based on impressive evidence that species with higher forms of consciousness would fade into vegetative states without brainstem reticular functions, a smaller group of radicals keep suggesting that the essential core of consciousness is contained within those ancient parts of the brain that are almost impossible to study, in any detail, in the human species. I believe that a substantial part of understanding in this subtle realm will require us to recognize that those sub-neocortical foundations mediate a variety of "energetic" affective states, which encode immediate survival concerns – energy needs (hunger), water balance (thirst) and thermal stability (feelings of coldness and warmth), and even more subtle variants such as raw emotional feelings – primal anger, fear, painful distress, seeking, lusty desire, comfort and joy.

I suspect an accurate evolutionary view should encourage us to consider that there are ancient forms of affective consciousness upon which the more sensorially resolved cognitive varieties depend... indeed, an ancient level of mentation from which perceptual consciousness evolutionarily emerged. Certainly the evolutionary layers of brain organization encourage such views. Presumably the older variants of consciousness are more affective and homologous across mammalian species (reflecting large-scale "energetic" states of the body and brain), while the more recent cognitive varieties that parse exteroceptive information may be evolutionary outgrowths fertilized by affective dictates. Although it may be impossible for us to know what type of cognitive tactile world images are created by the brain of a star-nosed mole or the electrosensitive bill of a platypus, perhaps we can more easily grasp what it is like for them *to energetically seek* the resources they need to survive, to *feel enraged* when thwarted and to *get fearful* when threatened, etc. The cognitive varieties of consciousness are critically dependent species-specific sensory capacities, while the ancient affective varieties may be considerably more conserved across species. Perhaps through some kind of neurodynamic resonances, the cognitive varieties of perceptual consciousness are outgrowths of the more ancient affective varieties. However, that theoretical possibility awaits more critical evidence than is available from the well-established observation that massive damage of the subneocortical emotional circuits can massively impair cognitive awareness in all mammals. Also, since a great deal of cognitive activity is energized by emotional arousals, I suspect that a scientific penetration of the widely broadcast ancient emotional varieties of feelings will yield critically important evidence for why psychiatric disorders influence the way we perceive our world, especially in our social environments.

With regard to the bottom-up controls of consciousness, the neuroscientific evidence has long affirmed that subneocortical reaches of the brain, traditionally known as the reticular activating system, are critically important for all forms of consciousness. It is becoming increasingly clear that even more ancient core systems of the brain such as the mesencephalic periaqueductal gray (PAG) are essential for normal emotional life (Watt & Pincus, 2004). Although it could be argued that such primitive brain functions as merely "permissive" for consciousness, almost as if they were nothing more than a big light switch, I suspect that arousals of those circuits *are* isomorphic and isodynamic with our deepest emotional feelings. Not only do such paramedian reticular substrates for visceral self-representation allow cortical information processing to transpire, they seem to be capable of neurosymbolically representing core

biological values as raw affective experiences. The fact that the rest of the cortico-cognitive apparatus collapses without that kind of sustenance from below, suggests that we may never untangle the Gordian knot of higher cognitive forms of consciousness without first penetrating the affective glimmers of experience that emerged earlier in brain evolution (Panksepp & Panksepp, 2000).

The mechanisms of affective consciousness

As already noted, it is now clear that animals deprived of their higher neocortical functions soon after birth are quite capable of exhibiting behavioral coherence and emotional flexibility, suggesting they can still experience the core values of existence (Panksepp, 2005a). Likewise, infants of our own species born with only fragmentary remnants of neocortex do mature into admittedly "simple-minded" emotional beings, as long as they are reared in caring, supportive environments (Shewmon et al., 1999). The emotional capacities of such neurologically impaired creatures are a remarkable challenge to anyone who still wishes to place the entire realm of experience within the cognitive-generating tissues of the neocortex. In sum, neocortical functions are obviously essential for many qualities of mental life, but the imbalanced affects that accompany all major forms of mental illness are dependent more on sub-neocortical circuits than neocortical ones. This makes understanding the nature of affective experience, through the study of both animal and human models, of paramount importance for psychiatry.

Other compelling lines of evidence for a sub-neocortical locus of control for affective experience are that all drugs of abuse, which surely sustain their motivational strength through the modulation of affective states, do so through circuits including those concentrated in basal forebrain regions (nucleus accumbens, olfactory tubercle and ventral pallidum), medial diencephalic structures of both thalamus and hypothalamus, converging on medial mesencephalic structures such as ventral tegmental area (VTA) and PAG. One especially striking example of the mountain of relevant evidence (Panksepp, 1998b, 2005a) is the demonstration of conditioned place preferences when reward-producing opiates are administered locally into brain regions such as the VTA and PAG, but not into a large number of higher brain regions

(Olmstead & Franklin, 1997). It could be argued that such localized brain stimulation derives its affective power from being "read-out" by higher neocortical systems for conscious awareness, but that is an unparsimonious assumption and a promissory note that is not supported by either classical or modern studies of neocortical activation, as can currently be achieved, non-invasively, with transcranial magnetic stimulation (Schutter *et al.*, 2004). This does not mean the cortex does not participate in emotional experiences. Obviously, it helps resolve raw feelings into emotional awareness, as well as the diverse affective object-relations that are constructed through individual learning.

The critical point for the present thesis is that a host of basic emotional systems – ones that mediate coherent emotional behaviors in response to localized electrical stimulation – are concentrated in essentially the same subcortical brain regions in all animals that have been tested. These evoked emotional actions are accompanied by positive and negative affects, as measured by a variety of behavioral choices that may reflect valuative states of the brain. Animals choose to go to places where they have received positive affective experiences, and they avoid those where they have experienced negative ones. Indeed, these are the brain regions from which one can rapidly and readily evoke emotional feeling changes in humans (Heath, 1996; Panksepp, 1985). All the basic emotional systems converge on some kind of a global integrator within the PAG. Since the visceral organs are well represented along this whole massive paramedian corridor of the midbrain and diencephalic brain stem, we have a ready explanation for why we feel so many emotions intensely within our guts, and why all emotional states are accompanied by various kinds of visceral arousal. These parts of the brain contain intrinsic visceral representations – an extended viscerosomatic homunculus. There are few compelling data that emotional feeling states arise largely from sensory readout of peripheral visceral commotions. There are abundant data that our emotional feelings arise from the dynamics of brain circuits that intrinsically elaborate visceration.

The adaptive role of such centrally generated mind states is that they immediately inform the creature of where they stand in the struggle for survival. Positive affective states, of which there are several distinct varieties, highlight that one is probably partaking of survival-enhancing activities (with a few exceptions, such as the consumption of addictive drugs, that can hijack positive affect systems by mimicking natural reward processes). Various negative affects highlight psychobehavioral conditions indicative of diminished survival probability. Consider the utility of pain. The core affects are ancestral memories that intrinsically help guide survival-promoting actions, and they probably contribute substantially to those still-mysterious "reinforcement" *processes* that help guide individual learning through the auspices of higher brain mechanisms, which represent the ever-fluctuating flow of world events. Humans as well as other animals choose to maximize affective comfort zones and to diminish discomforts. The affective dimensions of these zones are deeply sub-neocortical; the cognitive sides are highly cortical.

In sum, how primal affective experience emerges in the brain remains a momentous scientific problem for psychiatry as well as consciousness studies. The weight of evidence supports a dual-aspect monism approach that envisions affective consciousness as arising from a series of basic emotional systems interacting with ancient neural representations of "core-SELF" (Panksepp, 1998b); this is primarily visceral and somatic (as indicated by distinct instinctual types of behavioral activation accompanied by distinct kinds of autonomic arousal). A diffuse visceral homunculus (i.e. comprised of organ representations) of some description is likely distributed throughout the paramedian core of the upper brain stem, as first highlighted by the work of Walter Hess (1957). Every brain site that generates coherent emotional behavior – whether of fear, anger or desire – also generates a host of peripheral visceral and hormonal effects that help the body cope with those emotional arousals. This is not a reflective SELF, but a raw experiential one. However, these systems are not without somatic consequences, for these same brain regions are critically important for orchestrating whole-body dynamics, which are easily recognizable as instinctual emotional behaviors. In other words, the instinctual emotional action apparatus of the brain may be the fundamental source of basic emotional affects and behaviors. Thus, it is to be expected that imbalances in such a brain system could lead to both psychiatric as well as psychosomatic disorders. To properly understand such global brain functions, where ancient mind and body functions work harmoniously together, we may need to restore "energetic" dynamic network concepts back into the lexicon of psychology and psychiatric thought (Ciompi & Panksepp, 2004).

The core-SELF is re-represented and further elaborated in the paramedian limbic structures, such as cingulate and medial frontal cortices, that Northoff *et al.* (2006) have argued constitute the fundamental substrates of self-referential information processing in higher regions of the brain. An abundance of modern functional brain-imaging data in humans highlights how powerfully these medial regions of the brain, originally conceptualized as the limbic lobe (MacLean, 1990), participate in perceptual analysis of world events in self-referential, as opposed to more affectively neutral, cognitive ways (Northoff *et al.*, 2006). In contrast, the more dorsolateral frontal cortical regions become more aroused when one is simply processing exteroceptive inputs in a neutral information-processing manner. The amount of information accumulated since MacLean advanced the limbic-emotional brain concept half a century ago remains rather overwhelming; although for various historical reasons those lines of evidence gradually became under-acknowledged in the era of cognitive neuroscience, which continues to envision all mind-brain functions merely in "information-processing" terms (Panksepp, 2003). In any event, the weight of evidence indicates that medial aspects of the brain, from brainstem to telencephalon, constitute an emotional brain that is essential for all basic emotional feeling, from raw to refined. These systems are essential for affective consciousness, and from an overall perspective the amygdala is no more important in the generation of *affects* than many other regions of the limbic brain.

Of course, the exteroceptive processors of higher neocortical brain regions, which by themselves know little about affective values, do need to connect up with affective processors for the full spectrum of cognitive consciousness, which is heavily imbued with affective coloring (Ochsner, *et al.*, 2002). Indeed, the ways in which cognitive potentials are interwoven with affective ones may require us to resurrect old Freudian concepts such as cathexes, projections, repetition compulsions and repressions. New neuroscientific light can finally be shed on those old problematic concepts, but there are now some resistances to be overcome, such as the incompleteness of the "information-processing" metaphor of the mind, and most especially our continuing failure to recognize that all mammals, not just the great apes, are sentient creatures (Panksepp, 2005a).

Finale: toward a neuroscience of affects

Our understanding of the lower brain's substrates of emotion has come largely from animal brain research, much of it conducted before the cognitive revolution matured into a cognitive neuroscience perspective; and there continues to be an inadequate incorporation of the animal work into our conceptions of human nature and consciousness. In addition, the wonderful technologies that brought us modern brain imaging have some intrinsic biases and weaknesses that often reinforce a faulty view of the human mind. Positron emission tomography (PET) imaging has provided images of human affects that are more concordant with the animal data than functional magnetic resonance imaging (fMRI) (Damasio *et al.*, 2000; Zubieta *et al.*, 2003). The most commonly used form of modern brain imaging, fMRI, is better suited for highlighting rapid firing networks of higher brain regions that process exteroceptive information than the slowly firing ones that control internal states. Functional MRI approaches tend to miss the more slowly firing "energetic systems" where the power of molecules (e.g. neuropeptides) are more influential in generating affective mentality than the rates of action potentials. The small islands of arousal often depicted in brain-imaging studies do not reflect well how widespread brain networks truly operate, and we should continue to question and examine whether such spots reflect concentrations of excitatory or inhibition-producing action potentials.

Such highly biased technologies, impressive as they are, continue to reinforce some of the core myths of the cognitive revolution; that consciousness is strictly linked to the information-processing functions of higher regions of the brain. It may be wiser to cultivate the more balanced view that the information-processing functions are strongly linked to and guided by the more ancient energetic-emotional-affective brain functions – brain processes for which many of the tools of cognitive science are not well suited. Once we begin to blend these two sources of knowledge, one coming largely from research on the brain's emotional processes of other animals and the other from the remarkable cognitive capacities of the human brain, we will begin to have a coherent neuropsychology of mental illness, and we may even need new neuro-psychoanalytic perspectives, where naturalistic psycho-ethological studies of the mental apparatus will be pursued empirically (Panksepp, 1999; Solms & Turnbull, 2002).

To sum up, the neocortex, the wellspring of our detailed perceptual awareness, does not intrinsically care about much until it is captivated by the self-referential emotional energies that emerge from below. For individuals that have been reared in the lap of luxury, with few emotional challenges, perhaps the higher mental apparatus can more easily devolve toward a solipsistic aloofness and aloneness, which deserve to be stimulated by new types of emotional education. Conversely, in many stress-related mental illnesses, perhaps higher cognitive activities have been captivated excessively by negative emotional dynamics. For mental health, cognitive activities need to be integrated with a balance of many positive and a few negative emotional energies. There are many interface areas of the brain where such interactions are concentrated. The amygdala is a critically important one for fear and anger learning, sexuality too, but other comparable structures (e.g. bed nucleus of the stria terminalis, and related orbitofrontal and other basal forebrain areas) are critically important for the many self-conscious emotions that most animals may be incapable of; these range from various antisocial to prosocial feelings, including, for example, from disdain to empathy.

There are many limbic brain regions that normally bring cognitions and affects together into a seemingly psychologically seamless whole. Whenever these interface regions become deficient, disconnection syndromes may emerge where emotional feelings and cognitive perceptions no longer inter-digitate harmoniously, as is the case in schizophrenia. Emotion-cognition disconnections and excessive amplifications may be a general characteristic of many psychiatric syndromes. When the power of positive affective states is compromised, then all cognitive life suffers, leading to primary-process mental strife of psychiatric significance.

To make better sense of consciousness, in ways that can promote psychiatric understanding, we may need to develop a better appreciation of where the first glimmers of affective experience were created in brain evolution; and then step by step, try to understand how they interact with other cognitive structures to permit realistic thinking about affective circumstances in the world.

It will be a scientific challenge to understand how our uniquely human linguistically based mind functions – allowing us to think about our own and others' thoughts, and to be aware of our feelings. It will require a great deal of research to understand how our basic affective "energies" allow our cultural imagination to flourish, and for socially constructed mindscapes to emerge. Animal brain research will play no part in answering these momentous questions, and there will be little progress on those questions until we understand the neural nature of our affective consciousness. Since changes in affective experience seem to lie at the very heart of psychiatrically significant distress, it would seem that a study of the evolved nature of affective consciousness should be a key target of neuropsychological inquiry, without denying that epigenetic processes help affective consciousness to create a host of idiosyncratic cognitive meanings that neuroscience is not yet well positioned to study. Fortunately, this will forever leave abundant room for psychoanalytic descriptions and humanistic illuminations of the human comedy...and great novelists are far ahead of scientists in describing the vast idiosyncratic landscapes of affective-cognitive interactions that pervade human consciousness. It is unlikely that neurobiological science will ever clarify much of that, for those issues may largely remain inaccessible through human brain research.

References

Bennett, M. R. & Hacker, P. M. S. (2003). *Philosophical Foundations of Neuroscience*. Malden, MA: Blackwell.

Burgdorf, J. & Panksepp, J (2006). The neurobiology of positive emotions. *Neuroscience and Biobehavioral Reviews*, **30**, 173–187.

Ciompi, L. & Panksepp, J. (2004). Energetic effects of emotions on cognitions – complementary psychobiological and psychosocial finding. In R. Ellis & N. Newton (Eds.), *Consciousness and Emotions* (Vol. 1, pp. 23–55). Amsterdam: John Benjamins.

Damasio, A. R., Grabowski, T. J., Bechara, A. *et al.* (2000). Subcortical and cortical brain activity during the feeling of self-generated emotions, *Nature Neuroscience*, **3**, 1049–1056.

Heath, R. G. (1996). *Exploring the Mind-Body Relationship*. Baton Rouge, FL: Moran Printing.

Hess, W. R. (1957). *The Functional Organization of the Diencephalon*. New York, NY: Grune & Stratton.

Holstege G., Georgiadis, J. R., Paans, A. M. *et al.* (2003). Brain activation during human male ejaculation. *Journal of Neuroscience*, **23**, 9185–9193.

Kolb, B. & Tees, C. (Eds.) (1990). *The Cerebral Cortex of The Rat*. Cambridge, MA: MIT Press.

MacLean, P. D. (1990). *The Triune Brain in Evolution*. New York, NY: Plenum.

Ochsner, K. N., Bunge, S. A., Gross, J. J. & Gabrieli, J. D. E. (2002). Rethinking feelings: an fMRI study of the cognitive regulation of emotions. *Journal of Cognitive Neuroscience*, **14**, 1215–1229.

Northoff, G., Heinzel, A., de Greck, M., Bermpohl, F. & Panksepp, J. (2006). Our brain and its self – the central role of cortical midline structures, *Neuroimage*, **31**, 440–457.

Olmstead, M. C. & Franklin, K. B. J. (1997). The development of a conditioned place preference to morphine: effects of microinjections into various CNS sites. *Behavioral Neuroscience*, **111**, 1324–1334.

Panksepp, J. (1981). Brain opioids: a neurochemical substrate for narcotic and social dependence. In S. Cooper (Ed.), *Progress in Theory in Psychopharmacology* (pp. 149–175). London: Academic Press.

Panksepp, J. (1985). Mood changes. In *Handbook of Clinical Neurology. Clinical Neuropsychology*. (Vol. 1, pp. 271–285). Amsterdam: Elsevier Science.

Panksepp, J. (1990). Can "mind" and behavior be understood without understanding the brain? *New Ideas in Psychology*, **8**, 139–149.

Panksepp, J. (1998a). *Affective Neuroscience. The Foundations of Human and Animal Emotions*. New York, NY: Oxford University Press.

Panksepp, J. (1998b). The periconscious substrates of consciousness: affective states and the evolutionary origins of the SELF. *Journal of Consciousness Studies*, **5**, 566–582.

Panksepp, J. (1999). Emotions as viewed by psychoanalysis and neuroscience: an exercise in consilience, and accompanying commentaries. *NeuroPsychoanalysis*, **1**, 15–89.

Panksepp, J. (2003). At the interface of affective, behavioral and cognitive neurosciences: decoding the emotional feelings of the brain. *Brain and Cognition*, **52**, 4–14.

Panksepp, J. (Ed.) (2004). *Textbook of Biological Psychiatry*. New York, NY: Wiley.

Panksepp, J. (2005a). Affective consciousness: core emotional feelings in animals and humans. *Consciousness and Cognition*, **14**, 19–69.

Panksepp, J. (2005b). On the embodied neural nature of core emotional affects. *Journal of Consciousness Studies*, **12**, 161–187.

Panksepp, J. (2006). Emotional endophenotypes in evolutionary psychiatry. *Progress in Neuro-Psychopharmacology and Biological Psychiatry*, **30**, 774–784.

Panksepp, J. (2007). The neuroevolutionary and neuroaffective psychobiology of the pro-social brain. In R. I. M. Dunbar & L. Barrett (Eds.), *The Oxford Handbook of Evolutionary Psychology* (pp. 145–162). Oxford: Oxford University Press.

Panksepp, J. & Burgdorf, J. (2003). "Laughing" rats and the evolutionary antecedents of human joy? *Physiology and Behavior*, **79**, 533–547.

Panksepp, J. & Harro, J. (2004). Future prospects in psychopharmacology. In J. Panksepp (Ed.), *Textbook of Biological Psychiatry* (pp. 627–660). Hoboken, NJ: Wiley.

Panksepp, J. & Panksepp, J. B (2000). The seven sins of evolutionary psychology. *Evolution and Cognition*, **6**, 108–131.

Panksepp, J., Normansell, L. A., Cox, J. F. & Siviy, S. (1994). Effects of neonatal decortication on the social play of juvenile rats. *Physiology and Behavior*, **56**, 429–443.

Parvizi, J. & Damasio, A. (2001). Consciousness and the brainstem. *Cognition*, **79**, 135–160.

Parvizi, J. & Damasio, A. (2003). Neuroanatomical correlates of brainstem coma. *Brain*, **126**, 1524–1536.

Schutter, D. J. L. G., Van Honk, J. & Panksepp, J. (2004). Introducing repetitive transcranial magnetic stimulation (rTMS) and its property of causal inference in investigating the brain-function relationship. *Synthese*, **141**, 155–173.

Shewmon, D. A., Holmes, D. A. & Byrne, P. A. (1999). Consciousness in congenitally decorticate children: developmental vegetative state as self-fulfilling prophecy. *Developmental Medicine and Child Neurology*, **41**, 364–374.

Solms, M. & Turnbull, O. (2002). *The Brain and the Inner World: An Introduction to the Neuroscience of Subjective Experience*. New York, NY: Karnac.

Starr, D. (2006). Animal passions. *Psychology Today*, Mar/April 2006, 94–99.

Steiner, J. E., Glaser, D., Hawilo, M. E. & Berridge, K. C. (2001). Comparative expression of hedonic impact: affective reactions to taste by human infants and other primates. *Neuroscience and Biobehavioral Reviews*, **25**, 53–74.

Watt, D. F. & Pincus, D. I. (2004). Neural substrates of consciousness: implications for clinical psychiatry. In J. Panksepp (Ed.), *Textbook of Biological Psychiatry* (pp. 75–110). Hoboken, NJ: Wiley.

Zubieta, J. K., Ketter, T. A., Bueller, J. A. *et al.* (2003). Regulation of human affective responses by anterior cingulate and limbic mu-opioid neurotransmission. *Archives of General Psychiatry*, **60**, 1145–1153.

Chapter 29

Consciousness of oneself and others in relation to mental disorders

Kai Vogeley and Albert Newen

Consciousness and mental disorders

Consciousness is a unique phenomenon that can be characterized by the subjective experience, the so-called phenomenal quality involved in one's own mental states such as perceptions, judgments, thoughts, intentions to act, feelings or desires.

We have to refer to this subjective experiential space when we try to define mental disorders. In essence, mental disorders are norm-deviant disturbances of subjective experiences that are related to any of the following domains: changes in interactive and communicative behavior, inadequate emotional experiences or changes in sharing emotional experiences with others (emotional "resonance"), inconsistency of subjective experiences, or incongruency with experiences of others leading to a loss of a "sense of reality" that can be shared by the majority of other persons with the same cultural and traditional background. This definition of mental disorders underlines three important aspects: first, mental disorders are crucially linked to subjective experience; second, mental disorders often refer to a "change" of a certain experience that had been experienced by the same person differently before; and third, mental disorders are defined on the basis of norms that are generated or constituted by groups of people, populations or social systems. With respect to the relation of neuropsychology or neural correlates of consciousness and mental disorders, we will focus in the following on the third aforementioned aspect and on the research related to "social consciousness".

Complementary to this first-person-account of subjective experience, consciousness can be defined from a third-person-account as the integrated internal representation of the outer world and one's own organism based on situational and stored information providing reflected responses to the needs of our environment (Vogeley et al., 1999). These two accounts correspond to the distinction of a subjective space-time-system and an objective space-time-system (Kuhlenbeck, 1982). The processes required for a representation of the outer world and one's own organism within a cognitive system are based on many different cognitive processes that are a central focus of cognitive (neuro)science. A widely used definition of the term cognition summarizes it as the complex of perceptual and epistemic capacities, that are experience-based and that are relevant for the orientation in the world and the survival of the organism (Roth, 1994). Cognitive neuroscience usually focuses on research topics like perception, attention, memory, language and action planning. Methodologically, this research program crucially depends on the availability of different methodologies that provide access to the study of both structure and function of the living human brain.

Following a naturalistic account in contemporary philosophy of mind, consciousness appears to be closely linked to cognition, thus bridging the first- and third-person-accounts. Consciousness can be considered "the subjective experience of cognitive function" (Fuster, 2003, p. 249): "conscious experience can emerge from the operation of any cognitive function" (Fuster, 2003, p. 249) serving our orientation and survival in the world. Cognitive neuroscience is based on the strong intuition that "conscious experience results from the operation and interaction of several functions in complex assemblies of cortical networks" (Fuster, 2003, p. 249). However, exploring the neural correlates of consciousness is a non-trivial and complex endeavor. Consciousness is "a concomitant phenomenon of cognition" that is always "consciousness-of-something" (Fuster, 2003, p. 249); this

The Neuropsychology of Mental Illness, ed. Stephen J. Wood, Nicholas B. Allen and Christos Pantelis. Published by Cambridge University Press. © Cambridge University Press 2009.

also includes conscious states, like being tired, which only informs us about a state of our body. Furthermore, it must be considered that as a function of the nervous system that is distributed, and that recruits different brain regions and processes from one instantiation of a conscious experience to another, "Any portion of neocortex can generate conscious phenomena as a participant in cognitive function. Thus, the neocortical contribution to consciousness varies from one time to another and from one area to another. The conscious experience can change accordingly in a wide variety of ways as neural activity migrates within and between the many potential cortical networks" (Fuster, 2003, p. 256).

A special class of cognitive processes – and thus potentially also of conscious or subjective experiences – are related to self-referential and social cognitive capacities that are usually summarized under the heading of social cognition. Social cognition is essentially constituted by two different components, first, the capacity to differentiate between one's own and others' mental states (self–other differentiation) and, second, the capacity to adequately ascribe mental states to others in order to explain or predict their behavior or to communicate and interact with others successfully; the latter of which has been referred to as "theory of mind," "mentalizing" or "mindreading" (Baron-Cohen, 1995; Frith & Frith, 2003; Premack & Woodruff, 1978). These processes play a key role in the constitution of mental disorders. Neurobiologically, social cognition has recently become a key topic in cognitive neuroscience implementing a new research domain called social (cognitive) neuroscience. Neurobiologically, numerous studies have shown that the anterior medial prefrontal cortex (MPFC) and the temporoparietal cortex (TPC) are recruited during social cognitive processes. Notably, these regions are demonstrated to be active during resting states or baseline conditions that are characterized by the absence of any external instruction. This specific pattern of distribution of baseline activation has been called the "default mode of brain function" (Gusnard et al., 2001; Raichle et al., 2001). This convergence supports the hypothesis that we have a disposition for social cognition that is neurobiologically instantiated and potentially disturbed during disturbances of social cognition.

Consciousness of oneself and others

Survival in a social world clearly requires the ability to distinguish between oneself and others, and the ability

to adequately ascribe mental states to oneself or someone else as the "owner" of mental states or the "agent" of mental activities. The ability to distinguish *one's* own mental states from those of others is central to self-consciousness, which can be defined as the implicit or explicit awareness of one's own mental or bodily states as one's own, i.e. self-consciousness includes an immediate self-representation of a cognitive system, but this need not be transparent in the subjective experience. The ability to explicitly meta-represent one's mental or bodily states as one's own is thus evaluated to be a special case of self-consciousness (Newen & Vogeley, 2003). According to Gallagher (2000), a first-person perspective represents a "minimal self," which does not necessarily involve a reflective act of consciousness (in contrast to a "narrative self"). This distinction is developed into a more fine-grained view: on the basis of different forms of representation, and inferred from evidence from developmental psychology, five different levels of self-consciousness can be differentiated (Newen & Vogeley, 2003). Self-consciousness seems to emerge through the infant's interaction with others by comparing and distinguishing states of the self with those of others (Decety & Chaminade, 2003).

From an empirical view-point, it is important to define empirical indicators of self-consciousness. Essential features comprise: (1) the unity of our experiences; (2) the feeling of ownership and of agency; and (3) the perspectivity of our experiences. The unity refers to a long-term coherent whole of beliefs and attitudes (Vogeley et al., 1999). Autobiographical memory can serve as an empirical indicator of this construct of a long-term coherent whole of beliefs and attitudes (Fink et al., 1996; Piefke et al., 2003). The experience of ownership (with respect to perceptions, judgments etc.) has to be distinguished from the experience of agency (with respect to actions, thoughts etc.) (Fink et al., 1999; Jeannerod, 1994, 2001; Synofzik et al., 2008a,b; Vosgerau et al., 2008). In the case of involuntary action, both can be different: "I may acknowledge ownership of a movement – that is, I have a sense that I am the one who is moving or is being moved – (...), but I may not have a sense of causing or controlling the movement." (Gallagher, 2000, p. 16). Taking a first-person-perspective might be closely related to the multimodal experiential space around one's own body axis, thus literally creating a spatial model of one's own body upon which the experiential space is centered (Berlucchi & Aglioti, 1997; Vogeley & Fink, 2003).

Summarizing the evidence for neural correlates of self-referential cognition, there is growing evidence that a well-defined network comprising cortical midline structures, MPFC in particular, and superior temporal and temporoparietal regions might represent neural correlates of self-consciousness as suggested by several neuroimaging studies that utilized self-referential stimuli (Kelley *et al.*, 2002; Macrae *et al.*, 2004; Northoff & Bermpohl, 2004; Schilbach *et al.*, 2006; Vogeley *et al.*, 2001, 2004), including awareness of agency (David *et al.*, 2006; Frith, 2002).

Impairments in this ability of self-referential cognition or "self-monitoring" (Frith, 1992) are associated with mental disorders and can be plausibly linked to psychopathological phenomena. According to the predictive feed-forward model of motor control, an essential constituent that runs in parallel with the generation of movements is the formation of a so-called "efference-copy," as the prediction of sensory consequences of movements. Efference copy signals and the anticipated sensory consequences of the motor act are then compared with each other, thus determining the source of sensory events. Whereas self-generated actions are usually correctly predictable, just as anticipated sensory consequences and efference copy signals are congruent, externally generated actions are not associated with such efference copy signals and therefore cannot be compared and adequately detected as "self-generated" actions. This suggests that the feed-forward model explains how we are able to reliably distinguish between one's own and others' intentions to act as a specific class of mental states, thus contributing to a sense of agency (a detailed investigation shows that this model does not give us the whole story; Synofzik *et al.*, 2008a). Interestingly, this comparator function appears to be a cerebellar function, as has been shown in agency tasks (Blakemore *et al.*, 2001). Disorders of agency have been associated with mental disorders (Franck *et al.*, 2001) that might be related to an inability to compensate for the sensory consequences of actions (Lindner *et al.*, 2005), misattribution of external speech (Allen *et al.*, 2004), disturbances of verbal self-monitoring and auditory hallucinations (Johns *et al.*, 2001), and to the concept of self-monitoring disturbance in general (Carter *et al.*, 2001; Fourneret *et al.*, 2001). Additionally, disturbances of perspective-taking and agency are assumed to contribute to key symptoms in schizophrenia such as delusions of control, thought insertion and social deficits (Frith & Frith, 1999; Spence *et al.*, 1997).

With respect to perspective taking, Langdon & Coltheart found evidence of disturbed visuospatial perspective-taking in normal adults who score higher on the personality variable of schizotypy and who are known to be relatively poor mentalizers (Langdon & Coltheart, 2001). They concluded that poor mentalizing in normal adults can be understood as an impairment of visual and cognitive perspective taking. The ability of perspective taking seems to be trivial, but in fact is an essential capacity of our cognitive system that might become disturbed, for instance, in so-called out-of-body experiences (Blanke *et al.*, 2005). Although rare in psychiatric disturbances, it illustrates that particular brain regions, especially the temporoparietal junction in the case of neural implementation of one's own body schema, are of crucial importance for self-referential cognition.

Closely related to the ability to assign and maintain a self-perspective is the capacity to attribute beliefs, desires or other attitudes to others, often referred to as "theory of mind" (ToM) (Premack & Woodruff, 1978) or "mindreading" (Baron-Cohen, 1995). This is an essential social skill that can be assessed in paradigms in which mental states of another person are to be modeled. A number of functional imaging studies using PET and fMRI have previously and successfully delineated brain regions involved in "reading other minds" (Fletcher *et al.*, 1995; Gallagher *et al.*, 2000; Vogeley *et al.*, 2001). These studies have repeatedly demonstrated increased neural activity associated with ToM conditions in the anterior MPFC.

Recently, Frith & Frith (2003) drew a distinction between implicit and explicit mentalizing corresponding to ToM "online" and "offline." It is an important issue to what extent human social understanding of others – particularly in everyday-life situations – relies on actual "online" involvements in a given situation or on inferential, "offline" modes of representing the mental states of others. Neuroimaging studies have only recently begun to target aspects of "online" interactions that require personal involvement in social communication (Gallagher *et al.*, 2002; McCabe *et al.*, 2001; Sanfey *et al.*, 2003). Thus far, however, the differential effects of self-involvement on the cerebral representation of mentalizing have not been investigated. This is emphasized by Ochsner (2004), who points out that no within-study comparison of self- and other-related activations (often found in MPFC) has been carried out.

From a clinical point of view, psychiatric disorders like autism and schizophrenia present with deficits in the mentalizing ability called "mindblindness" (Baron-Cohen, 1995). Poor performance in ToM tasks has been shown in a variety of studies with patients suffering from schizophrenia (Doody *et al.*, 1998; Frith & Corcoran, 1996; Pickup & Frith, 2001).

Phenomenology and neurobiology of consciousness and its disorders

Defining consciousness as the subjective experience of one's own cognitive processes, and defining mental disorders as disturbances of subjective experiences that are deviant from the experiences of the social group, leads to a view that allows us to conceptually bridge the gap between first- and third-person accounts, and supports a naturalistic research program that tries to elucidate the cognitive and neurobiological foundations of disturbances of consciousness. Mental disorders do not appear to be linked to disturbances of our conscious awareness, but to the content of consciousness (consciousness and content should be clearly distinguished: Vosgerau *et al.*, 2008), especially to the consciousness of oneself and others or "social consciousness."

Speculating on the question of how the individual ontogenetic development might be related to the social origin of self-consciousness, we hypothesize that social consciousness comprising self-consciousness and mentalizing is the function of a dynamic interplay of social interactions in which the contents of consciousness (of oneself or another) are experienced via automatic attunement processes to others and are gradually integrated into a developing self-model (Gergely & Watson, 1996; Trevarthen, 2001). This may then establish a basic form of intentionality that predisposes for social interaction with others and – later in the development – for the acquisition of detached mental representations of social interactions. In the same line Gallagher distinguishes primary and secondary intersubjectivity as two forms of social cognition (Gallagher, 2005). Social consciousness is thus the fundamental basis of establishing and specifying social relations.

Empirical evidence for the recruitment of medial cortical activation sites during experiences related to social consciousness is provided by the concept of a so-called "default mode of the brain" put forward by Gusnard *et al.* (2001) and Raichle *et al.* (2001). According to this hypothesis, resting states reflect stimulus-independent thoughts, which are experienced as a "state of self." They also correlate with a "default mode of brain function" characterized by certain cortical activation patterns, predominantly in the anterior and posterior cingulate and medial parietal cortex. If a cognitive activity requires a higher demand, neural activation is "shifted" towards the target neuronal network to be recruited; medial frontal and parietal regions in turn tend to decrease their activity (Raichle *et al.*, 2001). According to Gusnard *et al.* (2001) this is not only a noisy signal, but might reflect a "continuous simulation of behavior" or "an inner rehearsal as well as an optimization of cognitive and behavioral serial programs for the individual's future." In short, a state of the "multifaceted self" (p. 4263). What appears as "state of self" on the phenomenal level appears as "default brain state" on the neuronal level.

Future studies in the field of social cognition have to focus on a number of research questions that should comprise at least the following: do spatial (e.g. navigational) and language-based (e.g. narrative) tasks refer to the same abstract body representation? How can we further elucidate both the subjective experience and the specific neural mechanisms underlying the "default mode of brain function?" To what extent is the body representation involved in the "default mode of brain function" as found in resting states? These research questions are of course applicable both under conditions of mental health and disorders.

However, data on neural correlates of cognitive functions in different disease states have to be interpreted carefully. It appears essential that the behavioral data of different diagnostic groups are comparable. If patients have performed significantly worse on a behavioral task, it can no longer be assumed that they recruited the relevant cognitive and neural processes to realize this task. Moreover, it must be considered that they are recruiting different brain systems that are possibly not at all responsible for the particular task to be performed. Furthermore, one has to take into consideration that regional specializations and functional specifications of given brain structures or processes might change under pathological conditions. Future studies should address the intriguing question about the connectivity between brain regions engaged in self–other representations or their potential disconnectivity that may underlie disturbances of self-consciousness, as for example occurring in schizophrenia.

In our view, there is no alternative to the dialogue of cognitive neuroscience and theoretical philosophy

411

as an inter- and transdisciplinary endeavor that serves the understanding of mental disorders. We are convinced that the integration of phenomenological and neuroscientific approaches can stimulate the development of enriched pathophysiological concepts of mental disorders.

References

Allen, P. P., Johns, L. C., Fu, C. H. *et al.* (2004). Misattribution of external speech in patients with hallucinations and delusions. *Schizophrenia Research*, **69**, 277–287.

Baron-Cohen, S. (1995). *Mindblindness*. Cambridge, MA: MIT Press. 1995.

Berlucchi, G. & Aglioti, S. (1997). The body in the brain: neural bases of corporeal awareness. *Trends in Neuroscience*, **20**, 560–564.

Blakemore, S. J., Frith, C. D. & Wolpert, D. M. (2001). The cerebellum is involved in predicting the sensory consequences of action. *Neuroreport*, **12**, 1879–1884.

Blanke, O., Mohr, C., Michel, C. M. *et al.* (2005). Linking out-of-body experience and self processing to mental own-body imagery at the temporoparietal junction. *Journal of Neuroscience*, **25**, 550–557.

Carter, C. S., MacDonald, A. W., Ross, L. L. & Stenger, V. A. (2001). Anterior cingulate cortex activity and impaired self-monitoring of performance in patients with schizophrenia: an event-related fMRI study. *American Journal of Psychiatry*, **158**, 1423–1428.

David, N., Bewernick, B., Newen, A. *et al.* (2006). The self-other distinction in social cognition – perspective-taking and agency in a virtual ball-tossing game. *Journal of Cognitive Neuroscience*, **18**, 898–910.

Decety, J. & Chaminade, T. (2003). When the self represents the other: a new cognitive neuroscience view on psychological identification. *Consciousness and Cognition*, **12**, 577–596.

Doody, G. A., Gotz, M., Johnstone, E. C., Frith, C. D. & Owens, D. G. (1998). Theory of mind and psychoses. *Psychological Medicine*, **28**, 397–405.

Fink, G. R., Markowitsch, H. J., Reinkemeier, M. *et al.* (1996). Cerebral presentation of one's own past: neural networks involved in autobiographical memory. *Journal of Neuroscience*, **16**, 4275–4282.

Fink, G. R., Marshall, J. C., Halligan, P. W. *et al.* (1999). The neural consequences of conflict between intention and the senses. *Brain*, **122**, 497–512.

Fletcher, P., Happé, F., Frith, U. *et al.* (1995). Other minds in the brain: a functional imaging study of "theory of mind" in story comprehension. *Cognition*, **57**, 109–128.

Fourneret, P., Franck, N., Slachevsky, A. & Jeannerod, M. (2001). Self-monitoring in schizophrenia revisited. *Neuroreport*, **12**, 1203–1208.

Franck, N., Farrer, C., Georgieff, N. *et al.* (2001). Defective recognition of one's own actions in patients with schizophrenia. *American Journal of Psychiatry*, **158**, 454–459.

Frith, C. D. (1992). *The Cognitive Neuropsychology of Schizophrenia*. Hillsdale, NJ: Lawrence Erlbaum Associates Ltd.

Frith, C. D. (2002). Attention to action and awareness of other minds. *Consciousness and Cognition*, **11**, 481–487.

Frith, C. D. & Corcoran, R. (1996). Exploring 'theory of mind' in people with schizophrenia. *Psychological Medicine*, **26**, 521–30.

Frith, C. D. & Frith, U. (1999). Interacting minds – a biological basis. *Science*, **286**, 1692–1695.

Frith, U. & Frith, C. D. (2003). Development and neurophysiology of mentalizing. *Philosophical Transactions of the Royal Society of London, Series B: Biological Sciences*, **358**, 459–473.

Fuster, J. M. (2003). *Cortex and Mind – Unifying Cognition*. Oxford: Oxford University Press.

Gallagher, H. L., Jack, A. I., Roepstorff, A. & Frith, C. D. (2002). Imaging the intentional stance in a competitive game. *Neuroimage*, **16**, 814–821.

Gallagher, H. L., Happe, F., Brunswick, N. *et al.* (2000). Reading the mind in cartoons and stories: An fmri study of 'theory of mind' in verbal and nonverbal tasks. *Neuropsychologia*, **38**, 11–21.

Gallagher, S. (2000). Philosophical conceptions of the self: implications for cognitive science. *Trends in Cognitive Science*, **4**, 14–21.

Gallagher, S. (2005). *How the Body Shapes the Mind*. Oxford: Oxford University Press.

Gergely, G. & Watson, J. S. (1996). The social biofeedback theory of parental affect-mirroring: the development of emotional self-awareness and self-control in infancy. *International Journal of Psycho-Analysis*, **77**, 1181–1212.

Gusnard, D. A., Akbudak, E., Shulman, G. L. & Raichle, M. E. (2001). Medial prefrontal cortex and self-referential mental activity: relation to a default mode of brain function. *Proceedings of the National Academy of Sciences USA*, **98**, 4259–4264.

Jeannerod, M. (1994). The representing brain: neural correlates of motor intention and imagery. *Behavior and Brain Sciences*, **17**, 187–245.

Jeannerod, M. (2001). Neural simulation of action: a unifying mechanism for motor cognition. *Neuroimage*, **14**, S103–S109.

Johns, L. C., Rossell, S., Frith, C. *et al.* (2001). Verbal self-monitoring and auditory verbal hallucinations in patients with schizophrenia. *Psychological Medicine*, **31**, 705–715.

Kelley, W. M., Macrae, C. N., Wyland, C. L., *et al.* (2002). Finding the Self? An event-related fMRI study. *Journal of Cognitive Neuroscience*, **14**, 785–794.

Kuhlenbeck, H. (1982). *The Human Brain and its Universe*. Basel, Switzerland: Karger Verlag.

Langdon, R. & Coltheart, M. (2001). Visual perspective-taking and schizotypy: evidence for a simulation-based account of mentalizing in normal adults. *Cognition*, **82**, 1–26.

Lindner, A., Thier, P., Kircher, T. T., Haarmeier, T. & Leube, D. T. (2005). Disorders of agency in schizophrenia correlate with an inability to compensate for the sensory consequences of actions. *Current Biology*, **15**, 1119–1124.

Macrae, C. N., Moran, J. M., Heatherton, T. F., Banfield, J. F. & Kelley, W. M. (2004). Medial prefrontal activity predicts memory for self. *Cerebral Cortex*, **14**, 647–654.

McCabe, K., Houser, D., Ryan, L., Smith, V. & Trouard, T. (2001). A functional imaging study of cooperation in two-person reciprocal exchange. *Proceedings of the National Academy of Sciences*, **98**, 11832–11835.

Newen, A. & Vogeley, K. (2003). Self-representation: searching for a neural signature of self-consciousness. *Consciousness and Cognition*, **12**, 529–543.

Northoff, G. & Bermpohl, F. (2004). Cortical midline structures and the self. *Trends in Cognitive Science*, **8**, 102–107.

Ochsner, K. N. (2004). Current directions in social cognitive neuroscience. *Current Opinion in Neurobiology*, **14**, 254–258.

Pickup, G. J. & Frith, C. D. (2001). Theory of mind impairments in schizophrenia: symptomatology, severity and specificity. *Psychological Medicine*, **31**, 207–220.

Piefke, M., Weiss, P. H., Zilles, K., Markowitsch, H. J. & Fink, G. R. (2003). Differential remoteness and emotional tone modulate the neural correlates of autobiographical memory. *Brain*, **126**, 650–668.

Premack, D. & Woodruff, D. (1978). Does the chimpanzee have a "theory of mind"? *Behavior and Brain Sciences*, **4**, 515–526.

Raichle, M. E., MacLeod, A. M., Snyder, A. Z. *et al.* (2001). A default mode of brain function. *Proceedings of the National Academy of Sciences USA*, **98**, 676–682.

Roth, G. (1994). *Das Gehirn und seine Wirklichkeit*. Frankfurt: Suhrkamp.

Sanfey, A. G., Rilling, J. K., Aronson, J. A., Nystrom, L. E. & Cohen, J. D. (2003). The Neural basis of economic decision-making in the Ultimatum Game. *Science*, **3000**, 1755–1758.

Schilbach, L., Ritzl, A., Kraemer, N. C. *et al.* (2006). On being with others: neural correlates of social interaction. *Neuropsychologia*, **44**, 718–730.

Spence, S. A., Brooks, D. J., Hirsch, S. R. *et al.* (1997). A PET study of voluntary movement in schizophrenic patients experiencing passivity phenomena (delusions of alien control). *Brain*, **120**, 1997–2011.

Synofzik, M., Vosgerau, G. & Newen, A. (2008a). Beyond the comparator model: a multifactorial two-step account of agency. *Consciousness and Cognition*, **17**, 219–239.

Synofzik, M., Vosgerau, G. & Newen, A. (2008b). I move, therefore I am: a new theoretical framework to investigate agency and ownership. *Consciousness and Cognition*, **17**, 411–424.

Trevarthen, C. (2001). The neurobiology of early communication: intersubjective regulations in human brain development. In A. F. Kalverboer & A. Gramsbergen (Eds.), *Handbook on Brain and Behavior in Human Development*. Dordrecht: Kluwer.

Vogeley, K. & Fink, G. (2003). Neural correlates of first-person-perspective. *Trends in Cognitive Science*, **7**, 38–42.

Vogeley, K., Bussfeld, P., Newen, A. *et al.* (2001). Mind reading: neural mechanisms of theory of mind and self-perspective. *Neuroimage*, **14**, 170–181.

Vogeley, K., Kurthen, M., Falkai, P. & Maier, W. (1999). The prefrontal cortex generates the basic constituents of the self. *Consciousness and Cognition*, **8**, 343–363.

Vogeley, K., May, M., Ritzl, A. *et al.* (2004). Neural correlates of first-person perspective as one constituent of human self-consciousness. *Journal of Cognitive Neuroscience*, **16**, 817–827.

Vosgerau, G., Schlicht, T. & Newen, A. (2008). Orthogonality of phenomenality and content. *American Philosophical Quarterly*, **45**, 329–348.

Chapter 30

Trialogue: commentaries on "Are mental illnesses disorders of consciousness?"

Comments on Panksepp and on Vogeley & Newen

G. Lynn Stephens and George Graham

In a contribution to an earlier collection on the neurobiology of mental illness, George Heninger (1999, p. 89) remarks as follows: "At an idealistic theoretical level it would greatly simplify matters if all mental disorders were as straightforward as phenylketonuria." Why does Heninger say that? Because, he writes, "here there is a specific biochemical pathogenesis" (p. 89). However, we hasten to note that phenylketonuria, assuming that our Consciousness Thesis is correct, really is not a mental illness. Although phenylketonuria is a syndrome with a mental deficiency, it is not a disorder in and of conscious experience. So, it fails to qualify as a mental illness. Heninger seems to admit as much, noting that its best descriptions are in neurology and not psychiatry texts (p. 91).

We are encouraged that each of our distinguished co-contributors to this section of the current volume seems to agree with us on that specific score. Mental illnesses occur in and of conscious experience. What makes them mental as opposed to non-mental is not their non-physicality (no room for mind-body dualism here), but the experiential influences that course through them.

Perhaps Panksepp is correct that one type of conscious experience in particular – namely, a loss of certain positive and basic emotional experiences of sorts shared by human beings with some species of non-human animals – leads to "mental strife of

psychiatric significance". Certainly, this hypothesis seems a promising partial explanation of what happens, for example, in various anxiety disorders. Human beings, just as certain species of non-human animals, possess an evolved tendency to respond fearfully to some situations (the presence of snakes, for example), but not to others (the presence of trees, for example). Call these tendencies, as they are sometimes called in the literature, lurking fears. Our emotional equilibrium is disrupted by lurking fears and some individuals (perhaps those prone to anxiety attacks) may be oversensitive to the perceived presence of relevantly fearful stimuli in their environment.

We are dubious (is Panksepp also?) whether neuroanatomically locating which "brain states...have been evolutionarily prepared to be responsive" to the world in fearful ways will help us to decide between competing accounts of the origins of anxiety disorders. We doubt whether a mere anatomical hypothesis will identify which of two causal neurobiological routes is responsible for an anxiety attack; a "leftover" evolutionary one in terms of the continued salience of ancient stimuli or one in terms of classically conditioned stimuli. Competition between two such hypotheses must consider behavioral data as well as the learning histories of individual organisms (see Coltheart, 2006 for related discussion). Even if we locate the neural base of lurking fears in particular areas or systems of the brain, location alone will tell us little if anything about how those areas represent, encode and instantiate the processes responsible for anxiety attacks. Does an area help to produce attacks by encoding ancient response patterns, or by implementing mechanisms of classical conditioning that have the power to transform any current stimulus into one that elicits oversensitive fear?

The Neuropsychology of Mental Illness, ed. Stephen J. Wood, Nicholas B. Allen and Christos Pantelis. Published by Cambridge University Press. © Cambridge University Press 2009.

Kai Vogeley and Albert Newen (hereafter "V&N") claim that "the ability to distinguish one's own mental states from those of others" is central to self-consciousness, i.e. to "awareness of one's mental states as one's own" and to "the capacity to adequately ascribe mental states to others in order to explain and predict their behavior." Clearly, understanding how we acquire and exercise this ability represents an important part of our understanding of normal cognitive development. It may also contribute to our understanding of mental disorders. V&N draw attention particularly to autism and to certain phenomena associated with schizophrenia, such as thought insertion, experiences of alien control and verbal hallucinations.

We agree with V&N that both autism and delusions such as thought-insertion involve a failure to "differentiate between one's own and other's mental states." We want to point out, however, that a patient's problems with "self–other differentiation" are quite different in the two sorts of cases. These differences indicate the scope and complexity of problems that must be faced in trying to understand how people distinguish their own mental states from those of others, or may fail to do so in cases of mental disorder. We have written extensively about such problems elsewhere (see, for examples, Graham, 2004; Stephens & Graham, 2000). Here we wish to further elucidate their relevance to V&N's helpful discussion.

First, consider autism. According to a now widely (though not universally) accepted account, autistic subjects (and normal 3-year-olds) perform as they do on false belief tests because they lack a "theory of mind." In the case of autistic subjects, the lack is due to impairment and not expressive of a normal stage of conceptual development. Autistic children suffer from a deficient understanding of mentality. (Of course, "autism" is an extremely complicated and varied diagnosis, and no such generalization covers all cases. However, we assume that the just-mentioned attribution of impairment is sound for present illustrative purposes.) Uta Frith (1989), for example, explains that children suffering from autism do not "appreciate the difference between their own beliefs and someone else's beliefs, and that there can be different beliefs about a single event" (p. 159). They fail, she says, "to realize fully what it means to have a mind and to think, know, believe, and feel differently from other people" (p. 173).

Now contrast with thought insertion. Thought insertion also represents a striking breakdown in a subject's ability to differentiate his own thoughts from the purported thoughts of others. However, thought insertion represents a very different sort of problem of self–other differentiation from the one found in autism.

Normally, introspection enables persons not just to identify both the content of their thoughts or attitudes and their attitude type, but also their own self as the thinker or believer. I believe that *the car looks red*. I *believe* that the car looks red. *I* believe that the car looks red. In thought insertion, however, the subject finds specific episodes of thinking or believing occurring in his stream of consciousness which, judging from his introspective reports, he somehow fails to recognize as his own. Indeed, he takes them to be somebody else's thoughts.

Unlike young victims of autism on Uta Frith's (1989) account, persons suffering from delusions of thought insertion are not cognitively "blind" to the existence of minds *qua* minds: either their own or those of other persons. They recognize and employ the distinction between their own thoughts and those of others, even if, with regard to certain thoughts, they draw the distinction differently. Nor are they oblivious to the possibility that their own thoughts and those of others may differ in content. They have learned the general distinction between my thoughts and other peoples' thoughts, although in certain and often striking instances, they apparently mistake their own thoughts for someone else's thoughts. These thoughts appear to them to be alien.

It is not obvious just what precise mistake in attribution the subject makes in thought insertion. The subject locates the alien thoughts in his own mind or stream of consciousness, as opposed to believing, for example, that he is directly aware of or eavesdropping upon someone else's stream. However, since the thoughts he claims to occur in him (in his mind) he also claims to be someone else's, he seems to be reporting something that is self-contradictory. How can one and the same mental episode be both mine (in me) and not mine (someone else's)? Is there a coherent interpretation of the subject's delusion?

V&N offer a distinction that helps with this interpretative problem. V&N speak of two different ways of ascribing mental states to oneself, one of which involves an experience of agency and the other of ownership. In our own work we draw a similar distinction between what we describe as an experience of agency and an experience of subjectivity. (We prefer to speak of subjectivity rather than of ownership because, in part, the language of ownership may connote a form of personal appropriation, of "owning up" to or taking responsibility for an episode. No such acceptance of responsibility occurs on the subjectivity side of the experiential ledger in thought insertion.) These distinctions help to remove the apparent contradiction in a person's claim that someone else's thoughts occur in his mind. They also suggest, as we have argued elsewhere, that there is a psychological link or similarity between thought insertion and various specific symptoms of schizophrenia, including delusions of control and of voices or verbal auditory hallucinations (see Stephens & Graham, 2000).

The main idea goes something like this: I may acknowledge (in the case of my body) that a fist clenching counts as my activity, in the sense that it happens to my body rather than someone else's body, but then deny that I myself clenched the fist (i.e. that I did it deliberately or voluntarily). Just so, I may say that the thought "Kill God" occurs in my mind (I am the subject), but deny that I am the author of or agent behind the thought. "Kill God" is not something that I, as a mental agent, *think*.

V&N mention a hypothesis of Christopher Frith which states that persons who experience their own activities, mental or bodily, as those of another agent or as due to an alien agency do so because they suffer from a breakdown in subpersonal cognitive systems that monitor connections between intentions and resulting activities. However, in our view, something other or more than monitoring failure is involved in the disorder. Although inserted thoughts seem to the person to be disconnected from his mental economy, they do not have the random character normally associated with transient, non-voluntary thoughts running through one's head. They seem purposive or characteristic of a mind, but not just one's own mind, and it is because of this appearance of being purposive that they are attributed to or experienced as those of another agent.

Ours may not be the right or remotely complete explanation of the experience of alienation (i.e. the experience of one's own thoughts as those of another), but clearly some explanation is needed. Just as clearly confusion about one's own mind and how it differs from another's lies at the heart of the conscious experience of a number of different mental disorders.

References

Coltheart, M. (2006). What has functional neuroimaging told us about the mind (so far)? *Cortex*, **42**, 323–331.

Heninger, G. (1999). Special challenges in the investigation of the neurobiology of mental illness. In D. Charley *et al.* (Eds.), *Neurobiology of Mental Illness* (pp. 89–99). Oxford: Oxford University Press.

Frith, U. (1989). *Autism: Explaining the Enigma*. Oxford: Blackwell.

Graham, G. (2004). Self-ascription: thought insertion. In J. Radden (Ed.), *The Philosophy of Psychiatry* (pp. 89–105). Oxford: Oxford University Press.

Stephens, G. L. & Graham, G. (2000). *When Self-Consciousness Breaks: Alien Voices and Inserted Thoughts*. Cambridge, MA: MIT Press.

Affective consciousness and the psychiatric comfort zones of experienced life

Jaak Panksepp

Consciousness is such a multidimensional topic that many overlapping perspectives need to be considered for scientific illumination of this core problem of modern neuroscience. I found the contributions by Stephens & Graham (S&G) and Vogeley & Newen (V&N) to be synergistic with my own perspectives. The vigorous advocacy of S&G for a full acceptance of the phenomenology of conscious experience within psychiatric practice and our research endeavors is essential for dealing with human troubles in humane ways, and such visions can pave the road for the discovery of new, more subtle mind medicines through neuroscientific investigations. V&N provide a highly resolved cognitive view of consciousness with which I agree, but I encourage them to incorporate affective experience more explicitly into their analysis. I suspect that most cognitive abilities ultimately arose, in mammalian brain evolution, to service affective needs. Affect may be the most ancient form of consciousness, since it seems directly related to essential biological needs. Along with a few others (e.g. Denton, 2006), I have argued that the decoding of the affective strata of mind is an essential gateway for progress on the cognitive processes that may have evolved to optimize organismic search for the affective "comfort zones" that support life. Of course, in humans cognitive activity has achieved a seeming self-sufficiency not evident in other species.

My own goal has been to understand the evolutionary underbelly of cognitive consciousness that is surely deeply affective – so deep, that some are prone to envision it as part of the dynamic unconscious. In line with Freud's perspectives, I think affects are fully experienced, but rarely talked about. V&N advocated conceptualizing consciousness in more cognitive terms than would I, even though the critically important aspect of cognitive views is the recognition of how deeply enmeshed our emotional processes are with our thoughts, as well as environmental events (i.e. situated cognitions). Of course, the critical scientific question is how we craft epistemological strategies for unraveling how experience is actually created within the brain, especially in a way that can positively impact psychiatric therapeutics. I suspect it will be rather easier to generate a clinically productive neuroscience of affect than of cognition. Much of what we have to say at the cognitive level will already have been said at one time or another, but the *detailed* neural analysis of higher cognitive functions is incredibly more difficult than that of lower affective functions, because the animal models are less robust. Although many who do not pursue detailed functional neuroscience have little motivation to distinguish between cognitive and affective processes of the mind–brain, since they are completely interpenetrant in intact organisms, the aim of science is to dissect the complexity of nature. There are many credible ways to distinguish affects and cognitions (Ciompi & Panksepp, 2004). Such distinctions provide potentially critically important considerations for clinically productive neuroscientific analysis (Panksepp, 2003, 2006).

For instance, I think the lack of ownership of experience that is often seen in schizophrenia, highlights how cognitive and affective processes become dissociated in this disconnection syndrome. In schizophrenia, higher and lower brain functions no longer operate as a coherent whole. Thus, the functional dissection of affect from cognition may be an essential scientific stepping stone for any evolutionarily coherent and psychiatrically relevant science of consciousness. Evidence abundantly indicates that psychiatrically relevant imbalances in consciousness reside heavily at affective levels, even though it is amplified and modulated by all sorts of ruminative activities. Affective imbalance may most commonly

be the first-order symptoms of schizophrenia and other psychiatric disorders, while cognitive changes are second-order symptoms. Thus, I was a bit concerned that my esteemed colleagues focused such modest attention on affective consciousness.

My commentary arises largely from one pragmatic consideration: what can we scientifically achieve that is truly lasting and important, at the present time? I do feel abundant neuroscientific payoffs would emerge if we focused much more effort on primary-process forms of emotional-affective consciousness, the main *forces* for mental disequilibrium, than on the more visible cognitive (information-processing) dimensions of mind. Without affective turmoil, cognitions alone would rarely fall into the kinds of disequilibrium that lie at the core of psychiatrically significant problems in living, and the faulty object-relations they foster. However, I would qualify this claim: the sensory and homeostatic affects (e.g. as explicated by Denton, 2006), are surely of tertiary importance as compared with imbalances in raw emotional feelings – i.e. less important than cognitive factors.

Still, from the emotional vantage, the analysis of both V&N and S&G, although well within the mainstream of modern consciousness studies, may need to become immersed in the emotional forces that drive cognitive disequilibrium. Parenthetically I would add that for me a disciplined definition of "cognitive" is the permutation of information harvested by the external senses. Affects are largely intrinsic, within-brain evaluative processes, where information-processing metaphors no longer do much work. For instance, I would not define "consciousness as the subjective experience of one's own cognitive processes" as do V&N. There needs to be a clear distinction between raw primary-process experience and one's cognitive reflections on those experiences. I think we must begin to think in terms of evolutionary layering of consciousness, raising the possibility that more fundamental forms of consciousness may often become inhibited by the emergence of higher forms, and that extreme primary-process variants begin to re-emerge in sustained psychiatric distress.

Although cognitive reflections and affective feelings are highly interactive in many clinically pregnant ways, perhaps various primary emotional processes can serve as *endophenotypes* that can promote breakthrough thinking in psychiatric thinking and practice (Panksepp, 2006). Each meaningful psychiatric syndrome surely has a distinct set of critically important emotional state processes that have become imbalanced, and it will be interesting to study how cognitions become enmeshed in those poorly regulated emotional *energies*. Indeed, if we readjust the imbalanced affective states, often it will be much easier to deal with cognitive disequilibrium. As noted by Kraemer (1993), psychiatric difficulties often resolve simply from pharmacological re-establishment of affective homeostasis with little need for cognitive intervention.

Of course, there is a downside to the powerful biological interventions that are now available. The discovery of hundreds of molecules to modify affect has now helped create a biological psychiatry without any clear vision of the mental apparatus. This is not good, even though it served as a corrective to the first half of the 20th century, where we had complex psychoanalytic ideas about mental processes, with no equally sophisticated neuroscience to bolster those ideas. It can be hoped that the goal of 21st century psychiatry will be to restore a balanced program, where the mind is brought fully back into neuroscientific views. Clear conceptions of how the brain generates core affective processes and the resulting cognitive entanglements must be a substantial part of that agenda.

Still, I abundantly agree with S&G's and V&N's emphasis of the importance of social-consciousness and cognitive-dynamics in psychiatric practice. The interface between human beings is both deeply affective and profoundly cognitive. Thus, the power of intersubjectivity has been one of the essential tools of all forms of psychotherapy, where the qualities of the therapist are commonly more important than the formal (manualized) qualities of the treatment. Presumably, at the foundation of all intersubjectivity there is a fairly small set of raw affective feelings that are critical for the quality of interaction, ranging from whether one is feeling lonely, insecure and feeling the pain of isolation or whether one is immersed in feelings of security, warm acceptance and trust. I would suggest such feelings are critically dependent on the degree of activity in the separation-distress (PANIC) networks of the brain, systems that are especially vigorously controlled by endogenous opioid, oxytocin and prolactin circuits. When such systems are satisfied (in homeostatic balance), then one can work more effectively with sexual feeling, nurturant tendencies, and certainly the degree of playfulness that can fill the intersubjective field.

Consider the PLAY circuits of the brain, barely recognized in psychiatric practice, that provide endless opportunities for enjoyable interactions that can be soul-healing (assuming, of course, that the "soul" is completely biological). I would go so far as to say that a child therapist who is not able to actually engage in rough-and-tumble playfulness with a young child, as opposed to simply partaking in toy- and game-facilitated interactions, is not using the full power of play therapy. Child psychiatrists who learn to put their toys to the side, and engage in real physical play, will open a very wide therapeutic door to all other interventions. The use of abundant rough-and-tumble play, each and every day, is much underutilized in developing children where we would like to abort the emergence of ADHD type symptoms (Panksepp *et al.*, 2003). Indeed, a case can be made that much of the symptomatic (but not sustained) therapeutic effect of psychostimulants in ADHD children is due to the robust anti-playful effects of such agents (Panksepp *et al.*, 2002a).

Also, most adult therapeutic environments would improve if a certain degree of the ineffable lightness of being, which can emerge from playful attitudes would more abundantly permeate the therapeutic interactions. There is a great deal of evidence suggesting that affective consciousness tends to be reciprocally related to higher cognitive activities – namely that lower limbic affectivity may not get fully aroused during abundant neocortical activity (Liotti & Panksepp, 2004). Obviously, thinking can sustain emotions as one dwells specifically on their troubles, but equally importantly, cognitive activity can also inhibit emotionality. Words can often get in the way. Thus, the uncovering and full acceptance of emotional feelings is as useful as any other aspect of consciousness within productive psychiatric interactions. We can anticipate that in the future there will be new medications that can work at the level of individual emotions, and some, perhaps oxytocinergics, may even help therapists to stay more effectively in the living moment.

In this context it is critically important to recognize the medial frontal cortical participation in feelings such as social cohesiveness, highlighted in V&N's important focus on the resting "self" work in brain imaging. Equally important to emphasize is that these brain regions participate in self-referential processing of all kinds of external perceptions (Northoff *et al.*, 2006), allowing lower and higher brain functions to be blended. However, it is puzzling that a great deal of modern thinking, based on meager evidence, continues to assume that affect emerges fairly high in the neuroaxis even up to neocortical levels. Damasio's advocacy of a somatic-marker hypothesis is perhaps the most prominent of many examples of trying to place affect within the "read-out" processes of higher regions of the brain. Those regions, especially anterior medial and insular cortices, surely contribute much to how we experience life, but they may be incapable of affectivity without the lower sub-neocortical substrates we share with the other animals.

S&G also emphasize the role of experienced life in psychiatric disorders and changes in mental life that accompany addictions. I agree with their analysis. It allows us to better see how much of drug addiction is an attempt to self-medicate so as to improve affective homeostasis, and it is worth considering exactly what kinds of feelings certain addictive drugs promote. For instance, it is pretty clear that opioids can alleviate loneliness and replace the need for social relations (Panksepp, 1981). On the other hand, psychostimulants amplify euphoric engagement with the world, and promote states of social dominance (Panksepp et al., 2002b).

Overall, I think all of us agree that neurophilosophically informed views of mental life, where lived subjective experience is never marginalized, provide better opportunities for major advances in psychiatric knowledge and practice than any form of ruthless "never-mind" reductionism that denies causal efficacy to the felt qualities of brain activities. A sophisticated and well-targeted consciousness view, where the positive social feelings of mutually experienced intersubjectivity is recognized as part of the healing equation, will allow us to use much lower doses of mind-modulating drugs. Indeed, we may then begin to look for new and more precise and gentle mind medicines, such as neuropeptide modulators, that may control very specific affective states (Panksepp & Harro, 2004). It is possible that such medicines, as well as the older ones that operate on more generalized brain-state regulatory mechanisms (e.g. the biogenic amine whole-brain "spritzers" that revolutionized psychiatry half a century ago), can be used at much lower doses in optimal psychotherapeutic environments. After all, psychotherapy can change brain dynamics and chemistries in richer, more symphonic ways than will ever be achieved with drugs.

It does seem that I am enamored by a more primitive (i.e. evolutionarily ancient) level of neuro-phenomenological analysis than either S&G or V&N. This comes from my own understanding of how the brain is organized in evolutionary layers, with the lower layers providing fundamental homeostatic-affective substrates for the experienced life, while the higher levels provide ever-increasing cognitive resolution to the opportunities and dangers of the world. Both levels of analysis are essential for any comprehensive picture, but perhaps the lower levels are currently much more susceptible to a rigorous neuroscientific analysis, if for no other reason than we have robust animal models where underlying causal issues can be studied in some detail. Information-processing approaches to mind tend to neglect that underbelly of mental life. Overall, affective neuroscience may advance psychiatric practice and understanding more than cognition-based views of consciousness.

References

Ciompi, L. & Panksepp, J. (2004). Energetic effects of emotions on cognitions – complementary psychobiological and psychosocial finding. In R. Ellis & N. Newton (Eds.), *Consciousness and Emotions* (Vol. 1, pp. 23–55). Amsterdam: John Benjamins.

Denton, D. (2006). *The Primordial Emotions: The Dawning of Consciousness*. New York, NY: Oxford University Press.

Kraemer, P. D. (1993). *Listening to Prozac*. New York, NY: Viking.

Liotti, M. & Panksepp, J. (2004). On the neural nature of human emotions and implications for biological psychiatry. In J. Panksepp (Ed.), *Textbook of Biological Psychiatry* (pp. 33–74). New York, NY: Wiley.

Northoff, G., Henzel, A., de Greck, M. et al. (2006). Self-referential processing in our brain – a meta-analysis of imaging studies of the self. *Neuroimage*, 31, 440–445.

Panksepp, J. (1981). Brain opioids: a neurochemical substrate for narcotic and social dependence. In S. Cooper (Ed.), *Progress in Theory in Psychopharmacology* (pp. 149–175). London: Academic Press.

Panksepp, J. (2003). At the interface between the affective, behavioral and cognitive neurosciences: decoding the emotional feelings of the brain. *Brain and Cognition*, 52, 4–14.

Panksepp, J. (2006). Emotional endophenotypes in evolutionary psychiatry. *Progress in Neuro-Psychopharmacology and Biological Psychiatry*, 30, 774–784.

Panksepp, J. & Harro, J. (2004). The future of neuropeptides in biological psychiatry and emotional psychopharmacology: goals and strategies. In J. Panksepp (Ed.), *Textbook of Biological Psychiatry* (pp. 627–660). New York, NY: Wiley.

Panksepp, J., Burgdorf, J., Gordon, N. & Turner, C. (2002a). Treatment of ADHD with methylphenidate may sensitize brain substrates of desire. *Consciousness and Emotion*, 3, 7–19.

Panksepp, J., Burgdorf, J., Gordon, N. & Turner, C. (2003). Modeling ADHD-type arousal with unilateral frontal cortex damage in rats and beneficial effects of play therapy. *Brain and Cognition*, 52, 97–105.

Panksepp, J., Knutson, B. & Burgdorf, J. (2002b). The role of emotional brain systems in addictions: a neuro-evolutionary perspective. *Addiction*, 97, 459–469.

The definition and the constitution of mental disorders and the role of neural dysfunctions

Kai Vogeley and Albert Newen

Comments

The two contributions by Panksepp and Stephens & Graham (S&G) provide important insights into the nature of mental diseases and its relation to consciousness. They focus on the role of emotional affects and pre-reflective processes for the constitution of mental diseases (Panksepp) and the relation between consciousness, mental diseases and their neural implementation (S&G).

Panksepp focuses on the significant scientific progress that has been made with respect to the nature of emotional affects and its neural implementation. As neuroscience is not yet able to read out any conscious experience individually, such as emotional awareness and self-awareness, Panksepp recommends that we should focus instead on raw emotional experiences that are assumed to be common to all human beings and probably even across mammalian species. His central claim with respect to mental disorders is that a major cause of mental disorders, at least with respect to affective disorders, can be traced back to a disturbance of raw emotional experience.

He proposes in a cross-species approach that psychological processes comprising basic or raw affective feelings arise from endogenous activity of neuronal assemblies. These have been evolutionarily prepared to become responsive to the world in certain behaviorally basic and significant, "instinctual" ways that evolved within a certain environment. Panksepp emphasizes the role of the non-conceptual dimension of consciousness for mental disorders that constitutes "primary-process consciousness." These raw feelings mediate emotional and motivational values and are essential for any higher-order awareness and intentionality. They are assumed to be a property of sub-neocortical brain processes that are considered a trans-species universal in the representation of raw feelings and which constitute a representation of a viscerosomatic homunculus or "the core self." Its localization in the paramedian area of the midbrain and diencephalon might well be correlated with the visceral and proprioceptive or interoceptive phenomena that are associated with emotions. As a pragmatic argument, Panksepp puts forward that psychopharmacological drugs such as antidepressants influence systems that are related to early and evolutionarily old processes. An ancient level of mentation might have thus been the foundation of higher-order consciousness that evolutionarily evolved or emerged from those simple and primitive forms of mental states. Subsequently, raw feelings can be transposed into emotional awareness of the reflexive type after being read out by the neocortex.

Panksepp emphasizes, as we do, that there is a basic type of consciousness that is a non-conceptual (or pre-reflexive) form of consciousness, and may include primitive "intentions in action" independent from any propositional attitudes. In greater detail we argue in favor of a distinction of five levels of self-consciousness including the non-conceptual self-acquaintance (Newen & Vogeley, 2003). Essentially, he argues against the widespread view that consciousness has to include self-consciousness (self-reflexive states), and that it has to be connected with propositional attitudes and intentions to act. We want to comment that mental disorders should not only be analyzed with respect to raw or affective feelings, instead we want to stress that in addition to these raw feelings, high-level cognitive emotions also considerably contribute to mental disorders (for the difference between "basic emotions" and "cognitive emotions" see Zinck & Newen, 2008). Often emotional experiences do not only involve basic phenomenal experiences, but are also essentially shaped by cognitive attitudes such as beliefs and expectations about social relations (e.g. partnership).

Related to the cross-species approach is of course the question as to how the interspecies relation can be bridged concerning mental phenomena. With respect to this "problem of other minds," the traditional view is that we are able to "read" other persons' mental states because of a principal similarity of another person's mental experiences and my own. The most important issue in this respect appears to be the finding that children already understand other subjects long before they acquire a full-blown "theory of mind." To account for that fact, we follow the proposal of Gallagher (2005) who distinguishes between primary intersubjectivity comprising non-conceptual forms of social understanding and secondary subjectivity. This account is in concordance with Panksepp's claim that focuses on non-conceptual (pre-reflexive) consciousness to systematically investigate the neural processes of primary intersubjectivity.

This is related to a basic question that is addressed by all three contributions, which is the question of whether these processes are subpersonal or personal in nature. In contrast to S&G, Panksepp and we argue that one cannot exclude subpersonal or "unconscious" processes in the explanation of mental disorders. As pointed out by Panksepp, information-processing functions are presumably guided by ancient energetic-emotional-affective brain functions. It is plausible to assume that we can only reach a complete understanding of mental diseases after incorporating affective components and cognitive components into a common framework. In accordance to Panksepp, we prefer to develop an informational-processing account to characterize the complex interaction of conscious and unconscious emotions and cognitions. It is, however, by no means clear whether this should be a Neo-Freudian neuropsychoanalytic account.

A more fundamental issue covered in all three contributions is the relation of mental and neural phenomena and subsequently the relation between psycho- and neuropathology. In concordance with our position, Panksepp follows a non-reductionistic monistic view or a dual-aspect theory proposing that neither the first-person-experiential nor the third-person-scientific perspective provide a complete explanation of mental phenomena. We argue for an account that is explanatorily non-reductive, but

ontologically reductive, i.e. psychological and neuro-biological explanations are non-reductive, but they refer to one and the same monistic world of physical phenomena. A complete description of the functional role of a mental state does not only include neural processes but also inner experiences of the cognitive system and the relation to the external situation. This relation between mental or physical processes can be either spelled out in terms of an identity or a functionalist theory (Newen & Cuplinskas, 2002; Vogeley, 1995). We ourselves prefer the latter because it can account for multiple realizations of the same class of mental phenomena that might be instantiated in different ways in different individuals. However, for one individual or a group of individuals with similar brain organizations, we may be able to characterize mental phenomena in terms of a type-to-type variant of the identity theory. So our functionalist view is compatible with a domain-restricted identity theory.

Although S&G appear to share with us the general position claiming an epistemological non-reductionism with the core idea that a complete description and explanation of mental disorders is dependent on a description in psychological terms, they underestimate the potential contributions of the neurosciences for understanding and explaining mental diseases. With respect to mental illnesses, S&G focus on the so-called "consciousness thesis" that proposes that mental illness can only be properly understood as a disorder of consciousness and that mental disorders cannot be explained without reference to consciousness and psychological terminology. Subsequently, therapy can only be successful on the grounds of conscious concourse. Consciousness is characterized by four distinct features: first, the occurrence of conscious experiences involves the experience of being conscious-of-something, also referred to as "intentionality," second, conscious experiences can themselves be objects of consciousness, third, consciousness may involve extended episodes of sequences of conscious experiences, and fourth, the talk about consciousness refers to the characterization of dispositions, but relevant here are only those abilities whose exercise involves conscious experience.

Their core intuition is that diseases either have a clear bodily or somatic nature (e.g. polycythemia vera) or a mental nature (e.g. schizophrenia), thus implicitly introducing an ontological dualism: if a disorder is of a mental nature we won't be able to identify an organic course of this disease. Such an identification of a somatic cause of a mental disorder would in fact be a misclassification, thus leading to an exclusive view on mental and somatic disorders, which would subsequently imply that it is not a mental disorder we propose. Even if we had a medical treatment such that schizophrenia as diagnosed today would lead to a complete recovery, this would still not make the psychological description of the disorder superfluous. The description of the behavior of patients suffering from schizophrenia remains essentially dependent on psychological terms even if we would discover a complete "bodily" cause. This is the critical question that makes the difference between our view and their position. This has strong consequences for the conceptual differentiation of "organic" and "non-organic mental disorder" in operationalized classification systems such as the DSM–IV. Conceptually, we do not agree, as S&G do, with this distinction because mental disorders in our view always have an "organic" substrate and a "non-organic" facet of subjective experience that describes how it is to be in a particular conscious state at a given time. Our view thus corresponds to the revisionist position of classical psychiatry that the authors cite as the "somatic basis hypothesis." However, the terms "mental" and "mental illness" cannot be replaced by "neurological" or "brain disease" because the latter terminology does not adequately reflect the world of subjective experiences. Nevertheless, the two terminologies correspond to each other because they both refer, philosophically speaking, to the same extension; that is, the brain with all its neural processes in a given environment.

Following this we clearly disagree with the statement that a sick mind might be related to a healthy brain. In contrast, we propose that mental dysfunctions must correspond to some sort of brain dysfunction. For instance, there is nothing wrong with a proposition such as "Drug addiction represents a disorder in the brain reward system." The comments S&G make at this point are related to problems of granularity of description of neural phenomena. Of course, these brain systems are "unspecific" in that they subserve a variety of psychological functions: the reward system is involved in the complex phenomenon of drug addiction but is, of course, also involved in other non-pathological conscious experiences such as a desire. However, the phenomenon of a desire is also similarly "unspecific" because it can occur under pathological conditions (drug addiction disturbance),

as well as under healthy circumstances. This corresponds to a mereological fallacy: we cannot ascribe a particular psychopathological syndrome that is adequately described only on a personal level to a particular brain system that is isolated from the context of other neural processes of the suffering person. Instead, we have to consider brain systems always as a part of a complex set of systems that constitute a nervous system of a human being. Pathology presumably does not involve only one particular brain system, but might be related to an imbalance of different brain systems. This is presumably a matter of degrees of disturbances and balances between different interacting subsystems of the brain, which are not yet fully understood. However, from the fact that we still do not have neuroscientific data, it cannot be inferred that neuropathology can never explain mental disorders.

It is thus non-adequate to infer that mental disorders do not qualify as neurological disorders. In fact, it is the only plausible position that they correlate with dysfunctions of the nervous system. The authors reject this view as "parasitic" because neurobiology would be forced to refer to normative standards for proper psychological functioning that are to be correlated with neural processes, whereby implying an implicit, strong and implausible dualistic account with a certain hierarchy between the mental and the neural. We rather argue that the mental world from which we can be taught about normative values can be of great heuristic value for neurosciences. Moral decisions and cultural differences must also be realized in the brain. That we do not understand much at the moment about culture-dependent differences in cognitive neuroscience does not argue against a monistic view in principle. All mental phenomena have a neural correlate. If this is so, we have to incorporate cultural contexts, individual dispositions and so forth into a complete picture of the neural instantiation of mental phenomena in a given environment. This is exactly the interesting point, but this proposal of course increases the interest for brain functions instead of eliminating them.

According to S&G mental disorders are defined by the fact that consciousness is essentially involved in the cause, the etiology and also in the treatment of the disease. Of course, we accept that cause, development and treatment are important dimensions for the definition of a nosological concept, but the key factor concerning mental disorders is the degree of deviation from standard psychological competences: *A disorder of a person is a mental disorder if the person has psychological states, processes or abilities which deviate essentially from the standard psychological states, processes and abilities, such that this results in an important change of the conscious experience or the personality traits.* This definition has the advantage that it takes into account that (1) a standard mental disease (e.g. schizophrenia) still remains to be a mental disorder even if we would be able to discover a complete physical cause and an adequate medical treatment, and (2) that mental disorders are essentially culture-dependent. To define mental disorders along deviations from standards that are determined by the society or a culture by no means contradicts that this has an organic correlate of the disorder.

Using descriptions from two different terminologies that reflect a subjective view on the conscious experiences and an objective view on the cognitive and neural processes underlying consciousness does neither imply a methodological nor an ontological dualism. There is still room for integrating the two different perspectives. We agree with the explanatory non-reductionism, but not with the ontological claim. In our opinion, the challenge here is not to weaken the explanatory value of neuroscience. Rather, it is to strengthen the view that mental disorders can only be further explored with the deep understanding that these diseases are involving different levels of description, which have to be integrated in an approach of multi-level explanations that are not competitive but cooperative in nature. In summary, we defend a monistic account including epistemically non-reductive explanations. But these different explanations could be essentially connected and integrated with each other. Conceptually, it is most important and fruitful to transfer mental illness to brain disorder because this is a major strategy to understand the pathophysiology, including its genetic basis, of diseases and to provide new strategies for therapies.

References

Gallagher, S. (2005). *How the Body Shapes the Mind*. Oxford: Oxford University Press.

Newen, A. & Cuplinskas, R. (2002). Mental causation: a real phenomenon in a physicalistic world without epiphenomenalism or overdetermination. *Grazer Philosophische Studien*, **65**, 141–169.

Newen, A. & Vogeley, K. (2003). Self-representation: the neural signature of self-consciousness. *Consciousness and Cognition*, **12**, 529–543.

Vogeley, K. (1995). *Repräsentation und Identität*. Duncker und Humblot.

Zinck, A. & Newen, A. (2008). Classifying emotions: a developmental account. *Synthese*, **161**, 1–25 .

Response to commentaries

G. Lynn Stephens and George Graham

Are we dualists? Kai Vogeley and Albert Newen believe that we are. This is because we talk in our target chapter of the roles of conscious experience in mental illness as if (to them) we intend to refer to something non-neurobiological. Also, they ask: when we say that a disordered mind may be embodied in a healthy or normally functioning brain, aren't we denying that mental illness is physical? And, finally: Are we more or less neglectful – as Jaak Panksepp worries – of the roles of emotion, mood and affect in mental disorder? Do we wish to downplay those roles?

These are three significant, if not the only questions posed to us by our section colleagues in their commentaries. Below we address them in order. (1) Suppose that each and every mental state is somehow nothing but a type of brain state. Call this a version of The Base Thesis. This is the thesis (mentioned in our target chapter) that mind and mental illness has a neurophysical base. There are other versions of the base thesis, but this particular version presupposes that the metaphysical thesis of physical monism is true. Other versions do not. What follows from this monist inspired version of the base thesis – call it the Basal Identity Thesis (BIT) – about how mental illness is best understood and explained?

Not much, we claim. Metaphysical monism does not entail explanatory monism.

We claim (in CT, our consciousness thesis) that mental illness is illness in and of conscious experience or activity, broadly understood. By this we mean that it has to be understood and explained in robust part in terms of the language of conscious experience. The language of neuroscience by itself is insufficient to understand and account for mental illness even if BIT is true.

Consider the following analogy. A physicist from the Martian Institute of Technology (MIT) lands on planet earth and observes a baseball game at Yankee Stadium. He knows a lot about physics, but nothing about the rules of baseball. Each and every move of each and every player in the game is physical. Can physics fully explain why the players act as they do? No, of course not, for while each player is in motion (and physics addresses that fact), not everybody *merely* is in motion. The players are following the rules of the game and their actions cannot be understood without reference to those rules and to each player's knowledge of them.

Now suppose that someone suffers from a mental disorder, say, alcohol addiction. (Assume, for the sake of illustration, that alcohol addiction is a mental disorder in the manner identified by CT.) Can the Martian understand why this person consumes alcohol as imprudently as they do? Not, on our view, unless the Martian also identifies various relevant conscious events and experiences of the victim as well as the explanatory roles that such events play in the disorder. Our saying such things about mental illness, our privileging consciousness, does not make us metaphysical dualists or anti-monists. It makes us realists about mental illness. If mental illness is real honest-to-goodness illness and is distinct from brute somatic disorder ('brute', meaning that consciousness plays no critical role), it has to be understood, in part, in phenomenological terms. A neurophysicist from MIT observing an alcoholic in action needs to know the 'rules' or conscious experiences and tendencies responsible, at least in part, for the disorder. (2) Suppose, again, that BIT is true. Does this mean that each and every mental illness is a brain disease or neurological disorder? No, it does not. We believe that some mental disorders are not disorders of the brain even if BIT is true. Consider the following analogy.

An inexperienced baker is baking bread in an oven. He wonders what the temperature of the loaf is. So, he foolishly takes an oral thermometer from his medicine cabinet and sticks it into the piping hot loaf. The thermometer's mercury rises immediately and bursts the device. Does this mean that the thermometer is functioning improperly? No, the answer is, not at all. Not every burst of an oral thermometer is of a thermometer that fails to function as it should. The baker used his thermometer improperly. It's meant to be placed under the tongue and not in a hot loaf.

Alcoholics behave improperly. Mother Nature designed the brain to regulate consumption, learning, memory and much else besides. The brain may also help to produce addiction, just as a thermometer may be deployed to determine the temperature of a hot loaf. However, when a person is addicted, this does not mean that the brain is failing to behave as it should, any more than an oral thermometer is at fault in a hot loaf. The person is not behaving as *he* should. He is suffering from a mental disorder that is not also a brain disorder, even if the disorder is a physical state of the brain. It can be a physical state without also being a disordered physical state. Again: Not every mental disorder is a disorder of the brain, even if every mental disorder is physical. (3) We regret that we do not have space here to discuss our views about the role of emotion in mental disorder. In our commentary to Jaak Panksepp's target chapter, we did not wish to convey the impression that we regard that role as relatively less important or weaker than that of the cognitive aspects of mental illness. For one, we believe that the conscious experience of stress may tilt (to use a metaphor of J. Allan Hobson) the brain's chemistry towards "emotional problems acting as triggers for a wide range of mental problems" (Hobson & Leonard, 2001, p. 239). Elsewhere we have written (though not in detail) about the role of emotional stress and other aspects of emotion in mental disorder (see Graham & Stephens, 2007). Interested readers may wish to consult that paper. That paper also contains complementary discussion of the points we make in (1) and (2) above.

One final point with which to close: nothing is "monolingual" about understanding mental disorder. From a medical-scientific point of view, it is eminently desirable that all sorts of information from neuroscience contribute to our understanding of mental illness, even though that information, given the truth of CT, is ultimately incomplete. So, for example, if certain stress-related memories (to use the language of consciousness), stored in the amygdala (to use a term from neuroanatomy), but normally inactive, can in certain settings become active and set off fight or flee responses (to use the language of behavioral neuroscience that applies as well to non-human animals), then such a complex fact may help to explain the onset of debilitating anxiety or phobia. At their individual bests, such multiple languages or schemes cohere like close brothers and sisters. Each helps with certain explanatory responsibilities that their siblings cannot discharge on their own.

References

Graham, G. & Stephens, G. L. (2007). Psychopathology: minding mental illness. In P. Thagard (Ed.), *Philosophy of Psychology and Cognitive Science* (pp. 339–367). Amsterdam: Elsevier.

Hobson, J. A. & Leonard, J. (2001). *Out of Its Mind: Psychiatry in Crisis: A Call for Reform.* Cambridge, MA: Perseus.

Understanding affects: toward a neurobiology of primary process mentalities

Jaak Panksepp

One of the most infamous statements in biological psychiatry is that "Behind every crooked thought there lies... a crooked molecule" (see Pincus (2000) and Slater (1999) for the context of this famous quote by Ray Fuller, one of Prozac's co-inventors at Eli Lilly). This kind of thinking neglects the importance of lived lives in managing psychiatric distress. This resembles the concern raised by Stephens & Graham about my advocacy for a neuroscientific approach to affective consciousness, which reflects both my main scientific and psychiatric concerns. They wisely question whether anything about the anatomy (and presumably other detailed features) of brain emotional systems "will help us to decide between competing accounts of the origins of, say, anxiety disorders?" My answer to this is "yes" and "no." Brain facts will certainly not help us fathom the individual life trajectories that have led an individual down the path of disabling anxiety. However, they may help us generate a better *evidence-based* psychiatry (with all the equivocations we must have about such laudable goals – see Little, 2003).

For instance Don Klein (1964) provided an early example of how two anxiety syndromes, panic attacks and generalized anxiety disorders, could be distinguished on the basis of one responding much better to tricyclic antidepressants while the other was quelled selectively by the early benzodiazepines. Although this rule of thumb has been muddied by the utility of more potent benzodiazepines (i.e. alprazolam is effective in panic), it highlights the multiple neurobiological paths to anxiety, an active field of animal investigations (Vianna & Brandão, 2003). There are probably life history and phenomenological differences among anxieties that correspond to brain differences. For instance, different anxieties emerge from FEAR and separation-distress/PANIC systems of the brain (Panksepp *et al.*, 2009). Also, as these systems *sensitize* from traumatic vicissitudes of life, the changing morphologies, gene-expression patterns, and neurochemical titres – the substrates of primary-process mentality – should be of considerable importance for psychiatric understanding and effective management of emotional distress. The biological views and life trajectory views surely need to work better together.

I thank Newen & Vogley for their insightful synopsis of my views on cross-species "subpersonal" aspects of emotional life. I affirm their call for scientific approaches to psychiatrically relevant consciousness studies that face up to the enormous empirical challenges posed by primary-process brain mechanisms. I find their preference for a "functionalist" over my so-called "identity" account of affective processing to be an appropriate move for the higher cortico-cognitive aspects of emotional processing, but perhaps not as useful for understanding evolutionarily provided emotional tools found at the subpersonal, subcortical level. Those modes of processing may blend within convergent-integrative higher limbic zones.

Can we agree that a most critical scientific issue for all of psychiatry is clarification of the biophysical nature of primary-process affective experience? There are hardly any neuro-mechanistic proposals in the area (but see Panksepp, 1998). Existing evidence suggests that the most psychiatrically useful biological knowledge may emerge from understanding the evolved subpersonal, subcortical realms (the depth neuro-psycho-biologies of our animalian "souls"), rather than by describing the diverse life experiences of individuals. It certainly appears that our minds are grounded on a very complex and presently unfathomed subcortical core-SELF structure, homologous in all mammals, laid out in viscero-somatic action coordinates. Here is where a great deal of psychiatrically significant distress is probably felt, and where the general principles must be sought for a scientific understanding of affective experience. It may well be that all forms of consciousness are still grounded to the basic values of primary affective states. If so, cognitions, defined as information-processing states, may derive their psychiatrically significant power from affects and less the other way around.

The evidence-based "identity view," derived from abundant evolutionary-functional homologies within subcortical limbic circuits, encourage us to consider that animal models are the most robust scientific ways to understand the foundations of human affective consciousness. When we accept that we are "just" mammals, the epistemology in this murky area becomes straightforward: as one studies the neural substrates for genetically ingrained instinctual responses, one is harvesting critical knowledge about those subpersonal emotional feelings, deeply experienced by those in psychiatrically significant distress. Within the massive random-access associative spaces of neocortex, a functionalist view has many more degrees of freedom for individualized mental navigation. To the extent that psychiatric disorders reside more in those neuromental spaces, we have less hope (certainly fewer strategies) for deriving therapeutically useful general principles from any fine-scaled neuroscientific analysis, and hence clinical wisdom will prevail.

We must elucidate details of evolutionarily provided subpersonal emotional systems for major progress in psychiatric medicinal development and for understanding the shared substrates of emotional imbalances in psychiatric disorders. This does not contradict the critical importance of individual lives in psychiatry; N&V correctly encourage us to also focus on "the importance of other high-level cognitive emotions for mental disorders" – I did not only because of space limitations and the inability of animal models to access cognitive issues as effectively as basic affective ones. Still, perhaps the best basic science investments in this area will be in decoding the cross-species subcortical affective substrates in animal models, which may offer sufficiently detailed general principles of neural action that can advance biological psychiatric therapeutics. Comparable investments on cognitive issues are less likely to provide robust general principles, if for no other reason than massive cross-species and individual differences at that level of analysis. Might "functionalist" variability in higher brain mechanisms generating comparable psychological effects be a barrier to robust scientific progress?

Many foundational neuropeptides and other neuro-chemistries remain to be functionally characterized and harnessed for development of more precise psychiatric therapeutics (Panksepp & Harro, 2004). A neuroscientific confrontation with those mysteries should percolate naturally into practical clinical concerns: when we understand the neurochemistries of RAGE circuitry, we may have anti-anger medicines, quite useful for regulating that endophenotype in many psychiatric syndromes. Consider that separation-anxiety is quelled better by opiates than benzodiazepines: since social loss is a major vector in depression, might we wish to consider non-addictive mixed opiate receptor agonists/antagonists such as buprenorphine in the treatment of depression (Watt & Panksepp, 2009)? Preliminary evidence affirms the remarkable efficacy of such approaches (Bodkin et al., 1995).

The issue of *emergence* will continue to haunt us as long as our knowledge remains incomplete. However, if emotion and affect in brain–mind evolution served as the primary-process for all subsequent developments in consciousness, solid scientific progress at higher levels may remain linked to our understanding of brain–mind substrates. I believe that evolutionarily, consciousness likely emerged from the coding of biological survival values (unless we believe in a *panexperientialist* quantum "mind dust" permeating the physical universe). A compelling but vastly ignored idea is that our remarkable cognitive abilities are grounded in core survival themes (primary affects), allowing cognitions to rapidly weigh alternative courses of action that may facilitate or hinder survival. That, I believe, is the ultimate function of affective consciousness, and why affects, as Freud surmised, are never unconscious, while many cognitive activities work effectively when out of mind. Despite the success of cognitive-behavioral therapies, emotional homeostasis will be most rapidly adjusted through a better understanding and use of affective issues, both biological and psychological. Concurrently, clients' cognitive concerns should never be minimized.

How to facilitate emotional awareness, in both clinical as well as scientific practice, remains a momentous challenge for both biological psychiatry and cognitive neuroscience. We have barely initiated systematic inquiries into the "heart of darkness" that affective experience poses for our scientific understanding of lived lives.

I appreciate this most interesting opportunity to discuss topics of momentous importance for psychiatric thought. I hope the scientific community will pursue, more courageously, illumination of the neurobiological underpinning of affective consciousness. It is finally a do-able task, because emotional feelings are closely linked to instinctual action networks of the brain. By contrast, obtaining *causal* understanding of individual human cognitive experiences remains, regrettably, next to impossible. Perhaps that makes the topic less workable for development of *new* evidence-based medical practices. Psychoanalysis, especially when it comes to be based on modern neuroscience, will remain the most comprehensive way to understand individual mental landscapes.

References

Bodkin, J. L., Zornberg, G. L., Lucas, S. E. & Cole, J. O. (1995). Buprenorphine treatment of refractory depression. *Journal of Clinical Psychopharmacology*, **16**, 49–57.

Klein, D. (1964). Delineation of two drug-responsive anxiety syndromes. *Psychopharmacology*, **5**, 397–408.

Little, M. (2003). 'Better than numbers...' A gentle critique of evidence-based medicine. *Australia and New Zealand Journal of Surgery*. **73**, 177–182.

Panksepp, J. (1998). The periconscious substrates of consciousness: affective states and the evolutionary origins of the SELF. *Journal of Consciousness Studies*, **5**, 566–582.

Panksepp, J. & Harro, J. (2004). The future of neuropeptides in biological psychiatry and emotional psychopharmacology: goals and strategies. In J. Panksepp (Ed.), *Textbook of Biological Psychiatry* (pp. 627–660). New York, NY: Wiley.

Panksepp, J., Fuchs, T. & Iacobucci, P. (2009). The basic neuroscience of emotional experiences: the case of FEAR and implications for clinical anxiety in animals and humans. *Applied Animal Behaviour Science*, in press.

Pincus, D. (2000). Mind and brain sciences in the 21st century. *Psychoanalytic Psychology*, **17**, 600–607.

Slater, L. (1999). *Prozac Diary*. London: Hamish Hamilton.

Vianna, D. M. L. & Brandão, M. L. (2003). Anatomical connections of the periaqueductal gray: specific neural substrates of different kinds of fear. *Brazilian Journal of Medical and Biological Research*, **36**, 557–566.

Watt, D. F. & Panksepp, J. (2009). Depression: an evolutionarily conserved mechanism to terminate separation-distress? A review of aminergic, peptidergic, and neural network perspectives. *Neuropsychoanalysis*, **11**, in press.

Replies to comments by Jaak Panksepp and by G. Lynn Stephens & George Graham

Kai Vogeley and Albert Newen

Comments

Again, we are grateful for the considerations of our colleagues on our contributions that consider both basic aspects of consciousness as well as clinical issues. Summarizing our view on consciousness, a solid concept of consciousness has to cover both conceptual and non-conceptual properties and cannot be confined to a reflexive, "cognitive" domain, but should also include intuitive, pre-reflexive experiences. Panksepp refers to the latter with the term of "raw primary-process experience." What the evolutionary relevance of this "layering" of consciousness might be is an interesting question and cannot be fully answered on empirical grounds yet. In our view, a theory of cognition has definitely high relevance for the understanding of consciousness. In addition, we generally agree with Panksepp that affective experiences need to be incorporated into a full account and understanding of consciousness and its role for mental disorders. Such a pre-reflexive self is not only constituted by affective states, but there are at least the additionally important dimensions of (1) motor activities while acting in an environment, (2) perception-based representations of consciously experienced objects and (3) social interactions with other people.

Let us consider the particular aspect of social interaction in greater detail. In addition to affective feelings, a core factor of the development of mental disorders is social interaction. Panksepp accepts that general claim, but holds that social interaction is essentially determined by fundamental affective feelings. Of course, the interaction with a person is usually presupposing a positive affective feeling towards a person. Nevertheless, the social interaction is only essentially constrained by the affective feeling if those are either extremely positive or aversive. If there are only "standard" affective feelings involved – as it is presumably the case in most of our interactions with others – then the actual interaction is more important and may be the main factor leading to an affective evaluation of the person. It may happen that the low-level negative affective evaluation at the first glance is changed by the everyday interaction into a strong positive affective stance. The actual interaction includes not only language-based, but also non-verbal communication including gesture, gaze, posture and other essentially embodied means of communications.

We agree with Panksepp that the influence of emotions has to be taken into account to understand mental disorders, but there is of course again the danger of reducing mental disorders to affective disorders. In his comments Panksepp is making a quite strong claim, namely, that affective forces drive cognitive processes. We are suspicious whether emotional experiences have always been the root for cognitive processes. On the one hand, there exist alternative theoretical accounts that try to reconstruct emotions as cognitive processes (as proposed for instance by Antonio Damasio). In our own work, we also argue that we have to distinguish basic emotions that are essentially independent from complex emotions that involve high-level cognitive processes. The latter are classified as primary and secondary cognitive emotions (Zinck & Newen, 2008). On the other hand, there are concepts under debate that try to reconstruct the core deficit of psychiatric disturbances on the basis of fundamental information processing, for instance organization of behavior in the temporal domain (Vogeley & Kupke, 2007). We are in favor of a multifactorial concept of mental disorders that investigates the interrelations between the important factors of emotion, perception, action and abstract thinking. We are of the opinion that neither the cognitive abilities nor the social interaction can be reduced to fundamental affective states. To fully account for mental diseases we have to investigate the complex interaction between affective, cognitive and social competences as they are realized by neural processes. To reach this aim we should develop a close connection between neuropsychiatry of adults and the developmental psychology and cognitive neuroscience investigating the ontogenesis of children and the genesis of mental diseases.

With respect to the clinical domain, Stephens and Graham (S&G) point out that "a patient's problems with 'self-other differentiation' are quite different" within different diagnostic groups. They further propose that these "differences indicate the scope and complexity of problems that must be faced in trying to understand how people distinguish their own mental states from those of others or may fail to do so in cases of mental disorder."

We are grateful for the fine-grained considerations that are pointed out by S&G with respect to a necessary distinction with respect to self-other differentiation and self-other exchange. Let us first consider disturbances of self-other exchange that cover the phenomena of delusion and social cognitive disturbance of autism according to our concept. Chris Frith has recently put forward a very fruitful distinction separating "hypermentalizing" and "hypomentalizing" (Frith, 2004). The best example for the hypermentalizing disturbance is the phenomenon of delusion as a first-rank Schneiderian symptom for schizophrenia, during which more than necessary information is read out from random datasets which are usually not considered informative during non-disturbed ("ortho"-)mentalizing processes. A specific phenomenon might gain extraordinary importance during the delusional experience such as a black shirt of another person that might indicate sudden death. According to our view, delusional experiences are disturbances of the ability of self-other-exchange or perspective taking. The person suffering from delusional experience is no longer able to share his or her experiences with others; this experience has become highly private and rigid and can no longer be corrected by others.

In contrast, hypomentalizing is true for the diagnostic group of autism in which mentalizing is weak or impossible. The disturbance or inability to take the perspective of others ("standing in someone else's shoes") is the most prominent symptom of autism that occurs along the entire spectrum of the disorder (low- and high-functioning autism). Autistic persons have difficulties in imagining what other persons think or feel, in understanding implicit messages (including irony, metaphors etc.), and non-verbal communication. This disturbance or inability has severe consequences for their social life.

The phenomenon of thought insertion is clearly different. Thought insertion as another Schneiderian first-rank symptom besides delusions belongs to the group of phenomena covered by the term ego-psychopathology ("Ich-Stoerungen"). In our view, this is a typical example for a disturbance of the ability of self-other differentiation that usually allows us to ascribe a mental phenomenon to oneself or to other persons. This ascription is obviously no longer adequate if a mental phenomenon such as a thought is ascribed to someone else. To fully account for this phenomenon we need to distinguish affective and cognitive levels in a two-step account that distinguishes a disturbance of the feeling of ownership from the cognitive judgment of ownership (Vosgerau & Newen, 2007). Meanwhile the analogous distinction of feeling of agency and judgment of agency is relevant to account for delusions of control (Synofzik *et al.*, 2008).

The interplay of self-other differentiation and exchange is definitely an intricate complex of different cognitive and affective processes that need to be balanced in a subtle and fine-tuned way, in order to allow everyday interaction and communication with others. Functional imaging studies focusing on self-referential and social cognitive processes suggest that both processes recruit similar brain regions including the anterior medial prefrontal cortex and the temporoparietal junction. The fact that these regions are also part of a so-called "default mode of brain function" (Raichle *et al.*, 2001) that correlates with resting activity might be an indication of the fact that our brain has a natural disposition for these self-referential and social cognitive processes. This, however, is yet only a speculative hypothesis and sets up another research agenda that must be followed up in more detail in future research programs.

References

Frith, C. D. (2004). Schizophrenia and theory of mind. *Psychological Medicine*, **34**, 385–389.

Raichle, M. E., MacLeod, A. M., Snyder, A. Z. *et al.* (2001). A default mode of brain function. *Proceedings of the National Academy of Sciences USA*, **98**, 676–682.

Synofzik, M., Vosgerau, G. & Newen, A. (2008). Beyond the comparator model: a multifactorial two-step account of agency. *Consciousness and Cognition*, **17**, 411–424.

Vogeley, K. & Kupke, C. (2007). Disturbances of time consciousness from a phenomenological and a neuroscientific perspective time. *Schizophrenia Bulletin*, **33**, 157–165.

Vosgerau, G. & Newen, A. (2007). Thoughts, motor actions and the self. *Mind and Language*, **22** (1), 22–43.

Zinck, A. & Newen, A. (2008). Classifying emotions. *Synthese*, **161**, 1–25.

Index

acrotomophilia 17

action
attention to 106–107
link with perception 26, 27
semantics 27

adaptive testing 275

addictive behavior 326–336
as brain dysfunction 395
decision-making deficits 138,
146–148
as disorder of consciousness 396, 421
pathways leading to 335, 336
premorbid vulnerability 331–333
specific drugs 326–331
vulnerability of adolescents 333–335
see also metamphetamine (MA)
dependence, substance abuse

ADHD *see* attention-deficit
hyperactivity disorder

adolescents
affective disorder risk factors 9–10
assessment 6
brain development 124–127, 320
collaborative brain function 320
eating disorders *see* eating disorders
maturation of executive functions
125–126
neurodevelopmental vulnerability
to addiction 333–335
neuromotor dysfunction 29
psychiatric illness risk factors 7–10
schizophrenia risk factors 8–9
social information processing
network (SIPN) 320–321
spatial working memory (SWM)
123
substance use risk factors 331–333

affective consciousness 399–406,
418–421
animals 399–400, 400–401,
401–402, 416
brain and 402–403
mechanisms 403–405
neuroscientific concept 405–406,
416, 422, 427–429

affective disorders *see* mood disorders

affective neuroscience 399–402

affective processing
bipolar disorder 357
neuroimaging studies 357–358
eating disorders 320–321

affective stimulus 37–38

affective word lists 209–210

affiliation (social closeness) 302
genetic influences 306
neurobehavioral systems 302–306

affiliative reward
multidimensional model of
personality disturbance 310
neurobiology 304–306

affordances 26–27

age differences
ease of ADHD diagnosis 287–288
neuropsychological test results 199

agency 409, 410, 417–418
disorders of 410
social behavior 302

aggression: fear 310

agreeableness 302
neurobehavioral systems 302–306
personality disorder categories
and 300–301

alcohol abuse
adolescent brain development
and 334
as brain disorder 395
decision-making deficits 146–148
as disorder of consciousness 396
neuropsychological sequelae
326–327

alien hand 27

alienation, experience of 418

Alzheimer's disease 69, 393

ambiguity
decision-making under 139
lexical 77–78

amphetamine
effects of chronic use 329–330

neurochemistry 261, 305
see also metamphetamine (MA)
dependence

amputation, desire for 17

amputees
attraction to other 17
phantom sensations 16

amygdala 42
anxiety processing 306–307
attentional biases and 111
decision-making 141, 144
emotion perception 38, 160, 167
emotion production and
experience 39
executive functions 118
face perception 159
fear processing 308
mood regulation in bipolar
disorder 358
schizophrenia 99–100
social cognition 161, 165
theory of mind 160–161

anarchic hand phenomenon 26–27

anger 50

angular gyrus, neuromotor
dysfunction 32–33

animals
emotional systems 404, 416
studies of emotions 399–400,
400–401, 401–402

anomia 69

anorexia nervosa (AN)
binge-eating/purging type (BPAN)
316
limitations of literature 316–317
neurodevelopmental model
319–321
neuropsychological functioning
317–319
restricting type (RAN) 316
treatment approaches 321

anosognosia 18

anterior cingulate cortex (ACC)
attentional control 107, 108